# Impotence: Diagnosis and Management of Male Erectile Dysfunction

# Impotence: Diagnosis and Management of Male Erectile Dysfunction

**R. S. Kirby** MA, MD, FRCS
Consultant Urologist, Department of Urology, St Bartholomew's Hospital, London, UK

**Culley C. Carson** MD
Professor of Surgery, Division of Urology, Duke University Medical Center, Durham, North Carolina, USA

**G. D. Webster** MB, FRCS
Department of Surgery, Division of Urology, Duke University Medical Center, Durham, North Carolina, USA

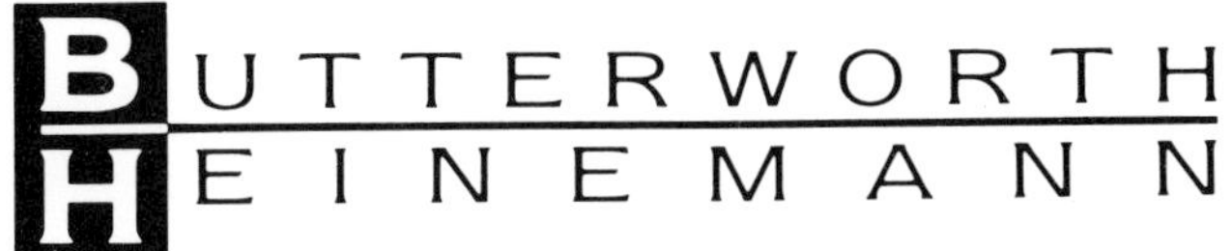

Butterworth-Heinemann Ltd
Linacre House, Jordan Hill, Oxford OX2 8DP

 PART OF REED INTERNATIONAL BOOKS

OXFORD LONDON BOSTON
MUNICH NEW DELHI SINGAPORE SYDNEY
TOKYO TORONTO WELLINGTON



First published 1991



**British Library Cataloguing in Publication Data**
Kirby, R. S.
Impotence: Diagnosis and Management of Male Erectile Dysfunction.
I. Title II. Webster, G. D.
III. Carson, Culley C.
616.6

ISBN 0 7506 1362 9

**Library of Congress Cataloguing in Publication Data**
Impotence: Diagnosis and Management of Male Erectile Dysfunction/[edited by]
R. S. Kirby, Culley C. Carson, G. D. Webster.
p. cm.
Includes bibliographical references and index.
ISBN 0 7506 1362 9
1. Impotence. I. Kirby, R. S. (Roger S.) II. Carson, Culley C.
III. Webster, George D., 1943–
[DNLM: 1. Impotence—diagnosis. 2. Impotence—therapy. WJ 709
D535]
RC889.D52 1991
616.6′92—dc20
DNLM/DLC
for Library of Congress 91-13783
CIP

Composition by Genesis Typesetting, Laser Quay, Rochester, Kent
Printed and bound in Great Britain by Bath Press Ltd, Bath, Avon

# Foreword

Male erectile dysfunction – the phrase attacks the very essence of a man's stature. The implications surpass the simple concept of the inability to obtain a satisfactory erection for intercourse: male erectile dysfunction adversely affects the wellbeing of the man in a broader sense, often implying that he is inadequate, unsuccessful, worthless, emasculate and impotent.

Male erectile dysfunction is common, affecting an estimated one in ten men, with prevalence much higher in certain subgroups. Inumerable tactics have been utilized through the centuries to strengthen or reestablish erectile function, including superstitious ceremonial experiences, herbal medicines, mechanical supports, hormonal manipulations and transplantations, as well as various ablative and reconstructive surgical measures.

Demand motivates wisdom. Over the last decade there has been phenomenal progress – gone forever is the Freudian attribution of erectile dysfunction exclusively to psychogenic factors. In its place, a more liberal perception has emerged. When consistent, male erectile dysfunction is more likely than not to be the consequence of primary organic pathophysiology, in conjunction with secondary psychological factors. This modern concept has been associated with advances in the field, in the areas of basic research, diagnostic evaluation and therapeutic options.

The fundamental principles of the phenomenon of erection have been known since the pioneering work of Eckhardt and Langley. New discoveries, however, have elucidated several of the neurotransmitters involved in the mechanism of penile erection, and future research will continue to explore and unravel the intricacies of the process. Such knowledge will continue to fuel expected diagnostic and therapeutic advances.

The evaluation of the male with erectile dysfunction has enabled the rational compartmentalization of the syndrome into various aetiological categories: psychogenic, hormonal, neurogenic, arteriogenic and venogenic. In particular, advances have been made in neurological testing, where for the first time, direct assessment of the integrity of corporal autonomic innervation is achievable. Progress in vascular testing over the last decade has been remarkable. Dynamic state testing has provided for the examination of venous outflow resistance during erection, especially in the presence of complete corporal smooth muscle relaxation. Future clinical evaluations in the dynamic state will enhance the appreciation of venous outflow resistance by assessing the ability of the corporal bodies to store pressure energy over time.

Therapeutic advances have paralleled progress in diagnosis and basic science. Non-prosthetic treatment alternatives, such as vacuum constrictive devices and intracavernosal administration of vasoactive agents, have enabled tens of thousands to resume erectile potency without surgical intervention. It should be expected that in the future, newer, more potent pharmacological agents will be developed for oral, topical and intracavernosal administration. Vascular reconstructive surgery, the only treatment option able to restore natural erections without mechanical or pharmacological assistance, has advanced dramatically – success in restoring erectile potency has been achieved in almost three-quarters of patients with localized arterial occlusion, typically induced by blunt perineal or pelvic injury. Lastly, penile prosthetic devices have improved significantly; a wide variety is available, with a high success rate proved.

This book attempts to cover these new developments, linking together basic research, diagnostic approaches and therapeutic options. Internationally renowned authorities have provided their insight into the latest developments and balanced this with up-to-date information on previously well established techniques. The book will not only be of use to practising urologists, but also to those who wish to achieve an overview of the current and evolving concepts of penile erection, impotence diagnosis and management.

Irwin Goldstein MD
Boston University School
of Medicine, Boston, USA

# Preface

It has been estimated that the sum total of scientific knowledge doubles every 5 years. In the field of erectile impotence this is probably an underestimate, for our level of understanding before the 1980s was scarcely more than rudimentary. The stimulus for the past decade's intense activity came from the discovery that both the smooth-muscle relaxant papaverine and the alpha-blocker phentolamine could produce a pharmacological erection when injected intracorporeally. This opened the way for the burgeoning use of these agents in both diagnosis and therapy of the impotent male. The fact that erectile impotence affects one in 10 of the male population in the developed world (i.e. 10 million men in the USA alone) and that the population over the age of 60 is predicted to double over the next 25 years, has provided further impetus for clinical research, and specialized impotence clinics have been set up to cater for seemingly limitless patient demand.

In this book we have set out to condense within a single volume the received wisdom from the world's leading experts in the field, in a readable and understandable form. Starting with the basic science of the mechanisms of erection and the ways in which these may be distributed by disease, we move on to a practical guide to diagnosis and management. We have tried to cover both the well-accepted treatment approaches such as pharmacotherapy and prosthetic implantation, as well as the more controversial areas including venous ligation surgery and arterial revascularization. In the final sections of the book we discuss some of the specific problem areas of management in erectile dysfunction.

We hope that we have created a book that is useful for the increasing numbers of physicians, surgeons, and psychotherapists, both in practice and in training, who deal with this condition which is a source of embarassment and distress to so many millions of men, but which can now be effectively treated in the majority of cases.

Roger Kirby
Cully Carson
George Webster

# List of Contributors

**Karl-Erik Andersson** MD, PhD
*Professor and Head, Department of Clinical Pharmacology, University Hospital of Lund, S-22185 Lund, Sweden*

**Pat Barnes** MEd (Counselling), BA(Econ)
*Relate Sex Therapist*

**William J. Barwick** MD
*Assistant Professor, Division of Plastic and Reconstructive Surgery, Duke University Medical Center, Durham, NC, USA*

**A. K. Batra** MD
*Department of Urology, Temple University Medical School, Philadelphia, Pennsylvania, USA*

**Pierre-Marc Bouloux** BSc(Hons), MD, MRCP
*Senior Lecturer in Endocrinology, Academic Department of Medicine, Royal Free Hospital, London, UK*

**G. S. Brindley** MD, FRCP, HonFRCS, FRS
*Professor of Physiology, Institute of Psychiatry, de Crespigny Park, London, UK*

**G. Burnstock** DSc, FAA, FRCP(Hon), FRS
*Professor, Department of Anatomy and Developmental Biology, University College, London, UK*

**Culley C. Carson** MD
*Division of Urologic Surgery, Duke University Medical Center, Durham, NC, USA*

**Rahima Crowe** BSc, PhD
*Associate Senior Research Fellow, Department of Anatomy and Developmental Biology, University College, London, UK*

**K. M. Desai** ChM, FRCS
*Senior Registrar, Department of Urology, Southmead Hospital, Bristol, UK*

**Ian Eardey** MA, MChir
*Clinical Lecturer and Senior Registrar in Urology, Addenbrookes Hospital, Cambridge, UK*

**Christine Evans MD, FRCS**
*Glan Clwyd Hospital, Bodelwydden, Rhyl, Wales*

**C. J. Fowler**

**E. Gale**

**H. G. Gilbert**

**H. W. Gilbert** FRCS
*Research Fellow, Department of Urology, Southmead Hospital, Bristol, UK*

**J. G. Gingell** FRCS
*Consultant Urological Surgeon, Southmead Hospital, Bristol, UK*

**P. Grech** MB, ChB, MRCP, FRCR
*Senior Registrar in Radiology, St Mary's Hospital, London, UK*

**F. Hedlund**

**Max Hirschkowitz** PhD, ACP
*Co-director, Veterans' Affairs Sleep Research Center; Associate Clinical Director, Baylor College of Medicine Sleep Disorders Center, Baylor College of Medicine, Houston, Texas, USA*

**F. Holmquist**

**Ismet Karacan** MD, DSc(Med)
*VAMC-Research, Houston, Texas, USA*

**Roger S. Kirby** MA, MD, FRCS
*Consultant Urologist, St Bartholomew's Hospital, London, UK*

**J. Lincoln** BSc, PhD
*Research Fellow, Department of Anatomy and Developmental Biology, University College, London, UK*

**Joseph LoPiccolo** PhD
*Professor, Department of Psychology, University of Missouri-Columbia; Director of Psychological Services, Sexual Medicine Center of Mid-Missouri, Missouri, USA*

**Tom F. Lue** MD
*Associate Professor of Urology, University of California School of Medicine, San Francisco, California, USA*

**John S. P. Lumley** MS, FRCS
*Professor of Vascular Surgery, University of London; Consultant Surgeon, St Bartholomew's Hospital, London, UK*

**Inge Nockler** FRCR
*Department of Radiology, St Bartholomew's Hospital, London, UK*

**J. A. H. Wass**
*Professor of Endocrinology, St Bartholomew's Hospital, London, UK*

**E. Wespes** MD, PhD
*Service d'Urologie, Hopital Erasme, Cliniques Universitaires de Bruxelles, Brussels, Belgium*

**Gordon Williams** MS, FRCS
*Consultant Urologist, Hammersmith Hospital; Hon. Senior Lecturer, Royal Postgraduate Medical School, London, UK*

**Roy Witherington** MD
*Professor of Surgery and Chief of Urology, The Medical College of Georgia, Augusta, Georgia, USA*

**R. O'N. Witherow** MS, FRCS
*Consultant Urologist, St Mary' sHospital, London, UK*

**C. R. J. Woodhouse** MB, FRCS
*Senior Lecturer in Urology, The Institute of Urology; Consultant Urologist, St George's Hospital and the Royal Marsden Hospital; Honorary Consultant Urologist, St Peter's Hospitals and Hospital for Sick Children, Great Ormond Street, London, UK*

**Adrian W. Zorgniotti** MD
*Professor of Clinical Urology, New York University School of Medicine, New York, USA*

# Contents

# Section One

# Mechanisms of erection and causes of impotence

1

# Neuropeptides and impotence

J. Lincoln, R. Crowe and G. Burnstock

## Introduction

Penile erection is a haemodynamic event under autonomic nervous control. There has been considerable progress in our understanding of the nervous control of the vasculature in recent years, such that it can no longer be regarded solely in terms of the release of noradrenaline (NA) from perivascular sympathetic nerves with variable antagonistic action of acetylcholine (ACh) released from parasympathetic nerves. In addition to NA and ACh, adenosine 5′-triphosphate (ATP), serotonin (5-hydroxytryptamine, 5-HT), and many neuropeptides including vasoactive intestinal polypeptide (VIP), calcitonin gene-related peptide (CGRP), neuropeptide Y (NPY) and substance P (SP) have been localized in perivascular nerves and considered as neurotransmitter candidates. The concepts of the co-localization of more than one transmitter in the same neurone, co-transmission and neuromodulation have become accepted mechanisms in autonomic nervous control (Burnstock, 1987, 1988a, b, 1990). In addition, since the discovery by Furchgott and Zawadzki in 1980 that vasodilatation by ACh requires the presence of an intact endothelium, the role of the endothelium in the control of vascular tone must also be considered (Burnstock, 1988b).

In order to elucidate the role of neuropeptides in erection and thus their contribution to impotence, they have to be considered in terms of (1) the sequence of vascular events that take place during erection and detumescence; (2) the nervous supply of the penis; (3) the actions and interactions of transmitters in penile vessels and erectile tissues; and (4) the role of the endothelium in the erectile process.

## Vascular events during erection

Blood reaches the penis via terminal branches of the right and left pudendal arteries. Vessels carry blood to the erectile tissues, which consist of two corpora cavernosa lying side by side on the dorsal aspect of the penis, and the corpus spongiosum surrounding the urethra. When the penis is flaccid, there appears to be a blockade of the vascular supply to the corpora cavernosa and the trabecular smooth muscle is maintained in a contractile state (Aoki *et al.*, 1986; Lue and Tanagho, 1987). During the change from the flaccid to the erect state, there is increased blood flow, raised intracorporeal pressure and the blood becomes diverted to the erectile tissue, filling the vascular spaces which results in tumescence. Newman and Northup (1981) have reviewed a number of theories to account for this transformation.

It is generally accepted that vasodilatation of the penile arteries rapidly followed by relaxation of the cavernous smooth muscle are primarily responsible for the initiation of erection (Newman and Northup, 1981; Aboseif and Lue, 1988). However, the process by which blood becomes diverted to the cavernous spaces has not been clearly defined. It has been postulated that relaxation of 'polsters' would allow increased blood flow into the cavernous spaces (see Newman and Northup (1981) for review). However, such structures have been suggested to develop as a response to ageing, stress, atherosclerosis or as an adaptive change to turbulent blood flow (Ruzbarsky and Michal, 1977; Benson *et al.*, 1980; Wespes, Depierreux and Schulman, 1987). It has recently been proposed that vasoconstriction of 'shunt' arteries may be a crucial mechanism in producing and maintaining erection, rather than relaxation of 'polsters' (Wagner *et al.*, 1982). Thus, constriction of 'shunt' arteries has been claimed to divert blood, which normally passes directly to the corpus spongiosum, into the helicine arteries which fill the cavernous spaces resulting in tumescence.

The role of venous outflow restriction in erection is also controversial. It has been stated that a venoconstrictor mechanism is not required for cavernous filling (Andersson, Bloom and Mellander, 1984) and that, during tumescence, venous outflow increases in parallel with arterial inflow and it is only once erection has been attained that venous constriction appears (Aoki *et al.*, 1986). However, it

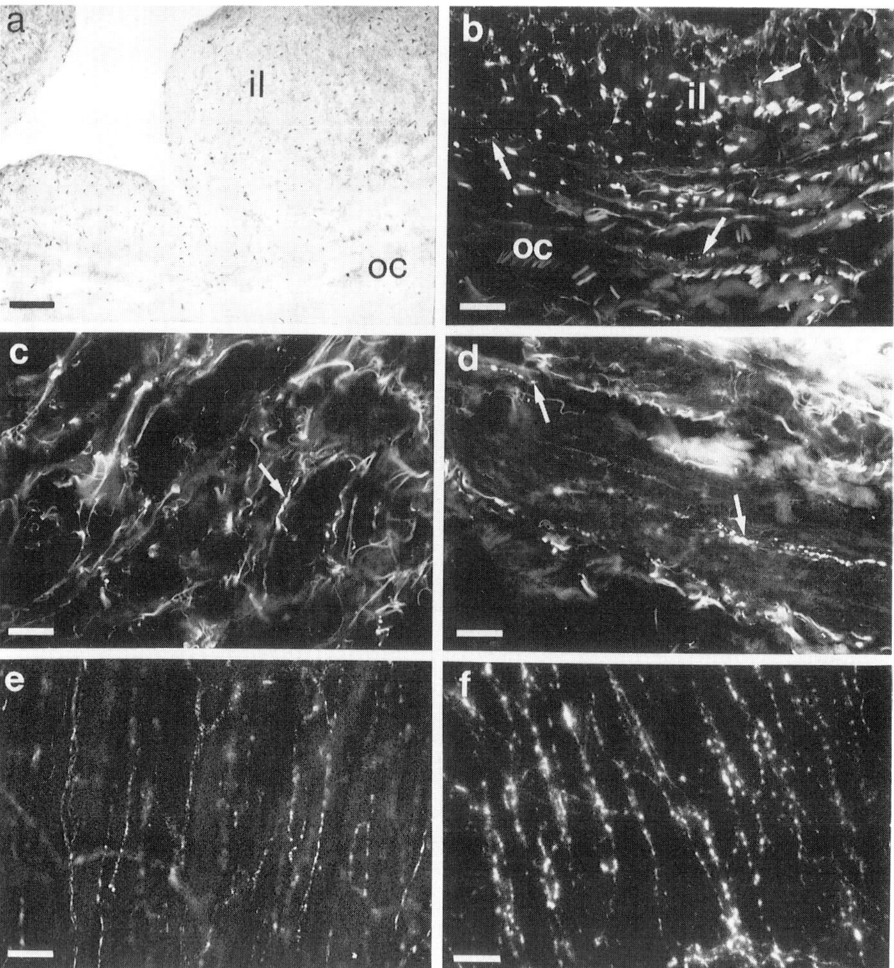


**Figure 1.1** The deep dorsal vein of human and rat penis: histological staining and immunohistochemical and histochemical localization of NPY-, VIP- and catecholamine-containing nerves: (a) van Giesen-stained transverse section of human deep dorsal vein showing the lumen and the inner longitudinal (il) and outer circular (oc) arrangement of the smooth muscle layers of the media. Calibration bar = 125 μm; (b) NPY-immunoreactive nerve fibres in a transverse section of the human deep dorsal vein. White arrows indicate fluorescent NPY-containing nerve fibres within the inner longitudinal (il) and outer circular (oc) smooth muscle layers of the media. Note the presence of autofluorescence in the preparation. Calibration bar = 80 μm; (c) a higher magnification of NYP-immunoreactivity in a transverse section of the inner longitudinal muscle of the human deep dorsal vein. White arrow indicates NPY-containing nerve fibres within the inner longitudinal smooth muscle layer of the media. Calibration bar = 30 μm; (d) a higher magnification of NPY-immunoreactivity in a transverse section of the outer circular smooth muscle of the human deep dorsal vein. White arrows indicate NPY-containing nerve fibres running along the longitudinal axis of the outer circular smooth muscle layer of the media. Note the connective tissue (top right hand corner) is autofluorescent. Calibration bar = 30 μm; (e) VIP-immunoreactivity in a stretch preparation of the rat deep dorsal vein. VIP-containing nerves form a dense plexus at the adventitial–medial border of the vessel. Note that some of the nerves are out of the plane of focus. Calibration bar = 30 μm; (f) glyoxylic acid fluorescence staining of catecholamine-containing nerve fibres in a stretch preparation of the rat deep dorsal vein. Catecholamine-containing nerve fibres form a dense plexus at the adventitial–medial border of the vessel. Calibration bar = 30 μm

has also been proposed that venous outflow restriction takes place during erection and is necessary not only to maintain erection but also to induce it (Juenemann, Lue and Tanagho, 1986). It is recognized that venous leakage can cause impotence (Wespes *et al.*, 1984). Where obstruction of venous drainage has been demonstrated in erection, it has not been ascertained whether this occurs by an active or passive mechanism (Dorr and Brody, 1967). There is evidence to suggest that contraction of the deep dorsal vein may be actively controlled in erection (Casey and Woods, 1982; Wespes *et al.*, 1988); the vein has a rich supply of autonomic nerves (Figure 1.1). However, obstruction of the venous network of the erectile tissue is believed to occur by a passive mechanism, secondary to arterial vasodilatation and filling of the vascular spaces which results in compression by the relatively indistensible tunica albuginea (Juenemann *et al.*, 1986; Lue and Tanagho, 1987).

All of these vascular events must be considered when attempting to define the autonomic mechanisms involved in controlling erection. *In vitro* studies of cavernous smooth muscle have to take into account the fact that, under physiological conditions, the muscle would normally be contracted. Agents, with little or no effect at basal tone, may be able to cause relaxation of preparations under raised tone. Most studies have concentrated on vasodilator mechanisms but it is apparent that vasoconstriction of the appropriate vasculature may also be involved. Finally, it cannot be assumed that the same agent will have the same effect in all the components of the penile vascular bed.

## Nervous supply of the penis

Initially erection was thought to be entirely mediated by a sacral spinal reflex involving sensory input via the pudendal nerve and parasympathetic output via the pelvic nerves to the penis producing 'reflexogenic' erections. The major role of the sympathetic nervous system was assigned to detumescence and seminal emission. While these pathways are undoubtedly of primary importance, studies of patients with spinal cord injury revealed that some patients with complete sacral lesions were still able to have erections but only after psychogenic stimuli and not after reflexogenic stimuli. 'Psychogenic' erections have been proposed to occur via sympathetic pathways originating in the thoracolumbar region of the spinal cord which are in communication with higher centres in the brain. In normal man psychogenic and reflexogenic stimuli can often act synergistically to produce erections. However, it is also recognized that certain psychogenic stimuli can inhibit the erection reflex (see Weiss (1972) for review). Thus both the parasympathetic and the sympathetic divisions of the autonomic nervous system have to be considered in erection.

Preganglionic parasympathetic axons arise from neurones in the sacral region of the spinal cord and form the pelvic nerve which provides excitatory input to parasympathetic ganglion cells in the pelvic plexus. Postganglionic parasympathetic axons travel via the penile and cavernous nerves to supply the blood vessels and erectile tissue of the penis.

The sympathetic supply to the penis is more complex and appears to follow more than one route. Preganglionic sympathetic nerves leave the spinal cord from the lower thoracic and upper lumbar anterior roots and pass to the sympathetic chain ganglia. Some preganglionic sympathetic axons travel together with postganglionic axons in the hypogastric nerve and meet the parasympathetic supply in the pelvic plexus (Lue *et al.*, 1984; Dail *et al.*, 1986; de Groat and Steers, 1988). In the rat it has been reported that the cavernous tissue, but not the blood vessels, of the penis is supplied by short adrenergic nerves rather than the classic long postganglionic adrenergic nerves arising from the paravertebral and prevertebral sympathetic ganglia. Such short sympathetic nerves originate from local ganglion cells in the pelvis situated close to the target organ (Dail and Evan, 1974). Other sympathetic nerves travel down the sympathetic chain and reach the male sexual organs via the pelvic and pudendal nerves arising from the sacral regions of the spinal cord (de Groat and Steers, 1988). The sympathetic supply to the penis has been divided into two portions: sympathetic erectile and sympathetic anti-erectile, although the nature of this division is still controversial and the particular pathways involved are not established (Brindley, 1988). In the rabbit the two groups appear to be anatomically separate, the erectile fibres running in the hypogastric plexus and the anti-erectile fibres in the sympathetic chains (Sjöstrand and Klinge, 1979). Stimulation of the hypogastric nerve elicits penile erection in the rabbit, cat and man (Sjöstrand and Klinge, 1979; Brindley, 1986a; Andersson *et al.*, 1987), no response in the rat (Dail, Walton and Olmsted, 1989) and a mixed response in the baboon (Brindley, 1986a).

It is now recognized that transmission in sensory nerves can occur in peripheral terminals as well as in the spinal cord, i.e. 'axon reflexes' following antidromic stimulation of collateral branches (Burnstock, 1987, 1988a, 1990; Maggi and Meli, 1988). In addition to the transmission of sensory signals to the central nervous system, dorsal root ganglia communicating with the pelvic organs are likely to have multiple functions, including modulation of local blood flow and autonomic ganglionic and neuromuscular transmission (see de Groat (1987) for review). Sensory input to the sacral region of the spinal cord from the penis occurs via the pudendal nerve.

Somatomotor nerves supplying the striated muscle surrounding the proximal shaft (ischiocavernous muscle) are also derived from the pudendal nerve. Although it has been stated that the ischiocavernous muscles do not play an essential role in erection (Weiss, 1972), it has recently been proposed that pudendal nerve stimulation of these muscles is of importance in producing penile rigidity (Juenemann *et al.*, 1989).

Clearly there is considerable opportunity for interaction between the sympathetic, parasympathetic and sensory nerve supplies of the penis. This is particularly evident when one considers the complexity of the pelvic plexus where the sympathetic and parasympathetic components become difficult to separate (Newman and Northup, 1983). In the rat, the main penile nerve has been shown to contain postganglionic sympathetic and parasympathetic axons as well as sensory fibres. Further, there are numerous autonomic ganglion cells in the penile nerve which receive input from both the hypogastric and the pelvic nerves and may share a common role in producing erection (Dail *et al.*, 1986, 1989; Dail and Hamill, 1989; Dail, Walton and Olmsted, 1989). A recent study has also shown that the nervous control of erection can change following injury. Following interruption of the pelvic nerve, hypogastric nerve stimulation results in increased penile pressure in the rat, a response which is not seen in controls. This has been postulated to occur by sprouting of hypogastric axons to innervate decentralized parasympathetic ganglion cells in the pelvic plexus (Dail, Walton and Olmsted, 1989) as has been shown in the bladder (de Groat and Kawatani, 1989).

## The role of neuropeptides in erection

It has been known for some time that the autonomic nervous control of penile erection does not conform to the classic concepts of adrenergic and cholinergic mechanisms (Benson, 1983). It is generally accepted that constriction of the penile arteries and cavernous smooth muscle is mediated by NA released from sympathetic nerves acting on α-adrenoceptors (Luduena and Grigas, 1966; Hedlund and Andersson, 1985a). Adrenergic nerves have been localized in blood vessels and erectile tissue (McConnell, Benson and Wood, 1979; Gu *et al.*, 1983) and are thought to maintain the flaccid state and be involved in detumescence (Carati *et al.*, 1985; Brindley, 1988). There is considerable evidence that the vasodilatation response resulting in tumescence and penile erection cannot be accounted for by a simple mechanism involving release of ACh acting on muscarinic receptors in the vasculature. Acetylcholinesterase (AChE)-containing nerves have been demonstrated in the penis together with choline uptake, ACh synthesis and ACh release following electrical stimulation of nerves in the cavernous smooth muscle (McConnell and Benson, 1982; Blanco *et al.*, 1988; Dail and Hamill, 1989; Stief *et al.*, 1989). However, *in vitro* studies of cavernous smooth muscle have found either no response to cholinergic agonists or relaxation (McConnell, Benson and Wood, 1979; Benson *et al.*, 1980; Hedlund and Andersson, 1985a; de Tejada, Goldstein and Krane, 1988). Responses to ACh *in vivo* are variable: no response, partial erectile response and full erection have all been reported (Dorr and Brody, 1967; Domer *et al.*, 1978; de Tejada, Goldstein and Krane, 1988; Stief *et al.*, 1989). Although this may in part be explained by species differences, there is general agreement that atropine can, at most, only partially block the erectile response to ACh or to nerve stimulation, both *in vitro* and *in vivo*, and in a variety of species (Luduena and Grigas, 1966; Dorr and Brody, 1967; Bowman and Gillespie, 1983; Andersson, Bloom and Mellander, 1984; Brindley, 1986b; de Tejada, Goldstein and Krane, 1988; Stief *et al.*, 1989). Ganglionic blockade reduces the response to pelvic nerve stimulation and to ACh *in vivo*, indicating that local ganglion cells are probably involved in erection (Dorr and Brody, 1967; Stief *et al.*, 1989). While sympathetically activated vasodilatation has been observed, there is little evidence for a major physiological role for β-adrenoceptor mechanisms in erection (Domer *et al.*, 1978; Adaikan, Kottegoda and Ratnam, 1986; Brindley, 1986b; 1988; de Tejada, Goldstein and Krane, 1988). Much of the current research has now focused on the roles of neuropeptides as non-adrenergic, non-cholinergic (NANC) transmitters in the penis, particularly with regard to inhibitory responses in vascular smooth muscle.

### Vasoactive intestinal polypeptide (VIP)

The most convincing evidence for the identity of the NANC inhibitory transmitter in erection exists for VIP. Numerous immunohistochemical studies have demonstrated VIP in autonomic nerves in penile arteries, corpus cavernosum and corpus spongiosum from a variety of species including man. We have localized VIP in varicose nerve fibres in the corpus cavernosum and in nerve bundles in the tunica albuginea of humans (Figure 1.2a and b), in the dorsal penile artery of the rat (Crowe *et al.*, 1983; Lincoln *et al.*, 1987) and in the deep dorsal vein of the rat (Figure 1.1e). In a study of several different peptides, VIP-containing nerves exhibited the greatest density of innervation and exceeded the density of adrenergic nerves (Gu *et al.*, 1983). The highest number of VIP-containing nerves is in the trabecular smooth muscle of the corpus cavernosa and in arteries where the nerves are largely confined

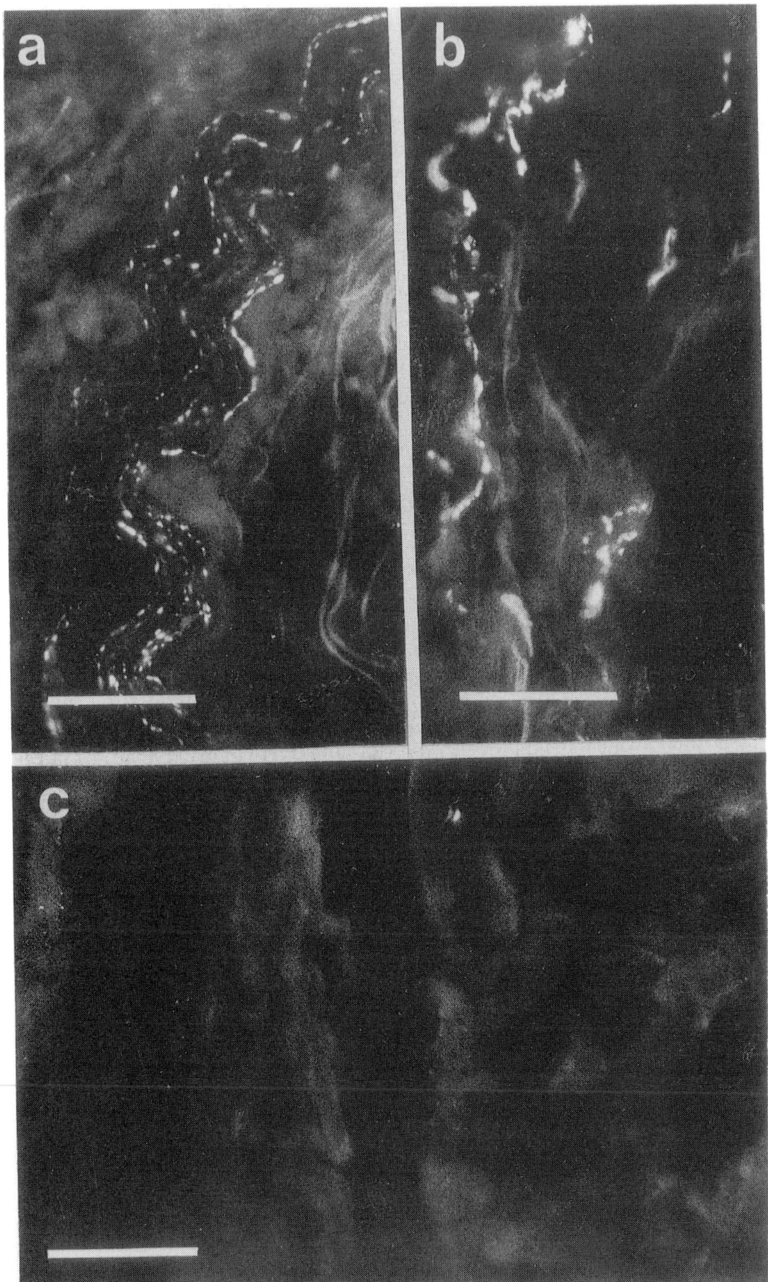


**Figure 1.2** VIP immunoreactivity in transverse sections of human corpus cavernosum and tunica albuginea from diabetic and non-diabetic impotent patients: (a) arrow indicates fluorescent VIP-containing nerve fibres within a nerve bundle in the tunica albuginea from a non-diabetic impotent patient; (b) arrows indicate fluorescent VIP-containing nerve fibres within the corpus cavernosum from a non-diabetic impotent patient; (c) VIP-immunoreactivity in the corpus cavernosum from a diabetic impotent patient. Note the marked reduction in VIP-containing nerve fibres. Calibration bars = 80 μm. (From Lincoln *et al.* (1987) with permission of the publisher)

to the adventitial–medial border, although occasionally they penetrate the adventitia of the pudendal arteries (Polak *et al.*, 1981; Willis *et al.*, 1981, 1983; Andersson *et al.*, 1983). VIP has been demonstrated in varicosities containing large dense-cored vesicles either alone or in combination with small agranular vesicles (Gu *et al.*, 1983; Steers, McConnell and Benson, 1984; de Groat and Steers, 1988). However, until specific markers such as colloidal gold particles (Merighi *et al.*, 1988) are used to identify the localization of neurotransmitters at the ultrastructural level, no clear correlation of vesicle type and transmitter content is possible. The distribution of VIP-containing nerves resembles that of AChE-positive nerves, although not invariably, since some large nerve bundles in the trabeculae of the corpus cavernosum are positive for AChE but not for VIP (Gu *et al.*, 1983). VIP has also been localized in neuronal cell bodies scattered throughout the base of the corpus cavernosum (Gu *et al.*, 1983; Polak and Bloom, 1984). In the bladder, it has been shown that pelvic denervation does not decrease VIP levels. If a similar situation exists in the penis, then this would support the view that local ganglia are the main origin of VIP-containing nerves in the urogenital tract (Polak and Bloom, 1984). Sinuses and veins of unspecified location within the penis have been reported to be devoid of VIP-containing nerves (Gu *et al.*, 1983). However, we have observed VIP-containing nerves at the adventitial–medial border of deep dorsal vein and its associated vasa vasorum (unpublished observations) and in the rat (Figure 1.1e). It should be noted that VIP has also been localized in cell bodies in lumbosacral dorsal root ganglia receiving input from the urinary tract and sex organs, indicating that VIP could also be involved as a transmitter in afferent pathways to the sacral spinal cord (see de Groat (1987) for review).

*In vitro* studies of strips of erectile tissue have revealed that VIP causes a concentration-dependent relaxation of raised tone preparations but has little effect at basal tone (Sjöstrand, Klinge and Himberg, 1981; Andersson *et al.*, 1983; Steers, McConnell and Benson, 1984; Carati *et al.*, 1985). The relaxatory response to VIP is not affected by sympathetic and parasympathetic antagonists, ganglionic blockade or by tetrodotoxin indicating that VIP is acting directly on the smooth muscle (Willis *et al.*, 1983; Adaikan, Kottegoda and Ratnam, 1986). In one study, both VIP and carbachol caused relaxation of precontracted erectile tissue whereas in the cavernous artery only VIP produced this effect (Hedlund and Andersson, 1985b). VIP has also been shown to inhibit the contractile response to electrical stimulation of nerves, and this effect appears to be particularly prominent in erectile tissue (Hedlund and Andersson, 1985c; Adaikan, Kottegoda and Ratnam, 1986). The deep dorsal vein of the penis also responds to VIP in a dose-dependent manner by relaxation (Adaikan, Kottegoda and Ratnam, 1986; Kimoto and Ito, 1987).

Studies of VIP *in vivo* have produced less consistent results. Intracorporeal injection of VIP has been reported to have no effect on the monkey penis and even caused detumescence of erection induced by cavernous nerve stimulation (Steers, McConnell and Benson, 1984). Conversely, in dogs, VIP has been shown to cause penile erection and antiserum to VIP to block the maintenance of neurostimulation-induced penile erection (Juenemann *et al.*, 1987). Other studies in dogs and man have reported that VIP can cause tumescence but not induce full erection (Andersson, Bloom and Mellander, 1984; Adaikan, Kottegoda and Ratnam, 1986; Wagner and Gerstenberg, 1987). VIP has been shown to be released following pelvic nerve stimulation, increased levels being measured in penile blood effluent. The time course of release paralleled the vasodilatation response. It was noted that the response to VIP infusion closely resembled the curtailed erectile response produced by pelvic nerve stimulation in the presence of atropine (Andersson, Bloom and Mellander, 1984). Further it has been demonstrated that when intracavernous injection of VIP is combined with visual sexual stimulation and vibration then full erection can be achieved (Wagner and Gerstenberg, 1987).

It has to be emphasized that it is probable that no single putative transmitter, when administered into the penis, can possibly mimic all the events that take place during erection. Nerve stimulation *in vivo*, rather than causing the release of a single transmitter, is likely to activate several different nerve types which by their combined action induce erection (see p. 5). Further, local release from nerves under physiological conditions confines the effect of a particular transmitter to the appropriate vasculature. Exogenous administration of VIP or other transmitters may result in an inappropriate response in vasculature which physiologically would not be exposed to that transmitter during erection. This is particularly relevant when one considers that 'shunt' arteries have been described in the penis which may need to constrict for erection to take place (see p. 3). Despite the fact that the precise mechanisms involved have not been elucidated, current evidence favours that VIP does play a significant role in the erectile process.

## Substance P (SP) and calcitonin gene-related peptide (CGRP)

SP and CGRP are neuropeptides which have frequently been found to be co-localized in sensory nerves. Both SP and CGRP have been localized in sacral dorsal root ganglion cells and, on occasions,

SP has been shown to be co-localized with VIP (de Groat, 1987).

SP has been localized immunohistochemically in nerves in the penis with a markedly different distribution from that described for VIP. Innervation of the erectile tissue and blood vessels by SP-containing nerves was sparse. SP immunoreactivity was largely concentrated in corpuscular receptors in the glans penis, probably indicating its presence in sensory nerves. No SP-containing cell bodies were observed (Gu *et al.*, 1983). We have observed sparse innervation of the deep dorsal vein by SP-containing nerves which were confined to nerve bundles (unpublished observations).

*In vitro* studies of the response to SP have revealed that at basal tone SP causes vasoconstriction of the corpus cavernosum and corpus spongiosum but has little effect on the cavernous artery. When preparations were pre-contracted with NA, SP caused moderate relaxation in corpus cavernosum and corpus spongiosum which, in the corpus spongiosum, was often followed by contraction. The response of the cavernous artery to SP was variable (Andersson *et al.*, 1983; Hedlund and Andersson, 1985c). In an *in vivo* study of the dog, SP infusion produced a clearcut though submaximal erectile response, the pattern of which was similar to the effect of pelvic nerve stimulation in the presence of atropine. SP levels in the venous effluent after pelvic nerve stimulation were variable. In five out of eight experiments SP levels increased, sometimes dramatically; however, in others the levels dropped. In no case were the increased SP levels maintained throughout the period of vasodilatation (Andersson, Bloom and Mellander, 1984).

CGRP has only recently been investigated with respect to penile erection. Varicose CGRP-containing nerve fibres have been localized in the walls of the cavernous arteries and within the trabecular smooth muscle of the corpus cavernosum of dogs. Intracavernous injection of CGRP increased cavernous arterial inflow and induced cavernous smooth muscle relaxation which subsequently resulted in venous outflow occlusion (Stief *et al.*, 1990). CGRP has also been localized in nerves of the bovine penile artery, where it causes relaxation by direct action on the smooth muscle and not by an endothelium-dependent mechanism (Alaranta, Hautamäki and Klinge, 1990). A high concentration of CGRP binding sites has been reported in extracts of rat penile tissue (Wimalawansa, Enson and MacIntyre, 1987).

At present, it is considered unlikely that SP plays a primary role in the haemodynamic events of erection, although CGRP has been implicated (Stief *et al.*, 1990). However, both SP and CGRP are involved in the transmission of sensory signals to the sacral region of the spinal cord which is involved in the reflex activation of the erectile process. It is possible that local release of these neuropeptides from sensory collaterals within the penis may assist in vasodilatation of the penile arteries and/or erectile tissue during reflexogenic erection as has been shown in axon reflex vasodilatation in the skin (Burnstock, 1987, 1988b, 1990). Such a mechanism may be of particular importance in the glans, where the sensory nerves are concentrated. While cavernous nerve stimulation in the rat induces erection of the penile body, it has been reported to be ineffective in producing erection of the glans (Quinlan *et al.*, 1989). Thus the nerves controlling the erectile tissue of the glans appear to differ from those of the corpus cavernosum.

## Neuropeptide Y (NPY)

NPY is frequently co-localized with NA in sympathetic perivascular nerves. Unlike VIP, CGRP and SP, which have direct actions on specific postjunctional receptors in the vasculature, NPY has little or no effect on vascular tone when administered exogenously to most peripheral arteries. In the penis, NPY has been shown to have no effect on the cavernous artery, corpus cavernosum or corpus spongiosum either at resting tension or when pre-contracted (Hedlund and Andersson, 1985c). It has been proposed that NPY does not act as a cotransmitter in most perivascular sympathetic nerves, but rather is a neuromodulator of the actions of the transmitters with which it is co-localized. In many vessels NPY acts postjunctionally by enhancing the contractile response to NA (Burnstock, 1987, 1990). In the smooth muscle of the corpus cavernosum and corpus spongiosum, however, NPY has no effect on the contractile response to nerve stimulation (Hedlund and Andersson, 1985c).

Immunohistochemical studies in humans have demonstrated dense innervation by NPY-containing nerve fibres in the corpus cavernosum and in the tunica of arteries. No NPY-containing cell bodies were observed and the NPY content of the glans was low (Adrian *et al.*, 1984; Wespes *et al.*, 1988). In most of the blood vessels, innervation was confined to the adventitial–medial border. However, heavy innervation by NPY was also observed in the subendothelial cushions of the helicine arteries. The smooth muscle cells forming these cushions may be functionally involved in regulating access to the sinuses (Schmalbruch and Wagner, 1989). In addition, in the deep dorsal vein which consists of an external circular muscle layer with inner longitudinal muscle, NPY has been localized in nerves penetrating the muscle layers (Wespes *et al.*, 1988). We have also observed this unusual pattern of NPY innervation (Figure 1.1a–d). VIP- and catecholamine-containing nerves were confined to the adventitial–medial border of this vessel, a dense plexus being readily demonstrated in stretch preparations from the rat (Figure 1.1e, f). Thus, NPY could be present in a population of nerves in the deep dorsal vein which do not contain either NA or VIP.

Observations on the co-localization of NPY with other transmitters in the blood vessels and erectile tissue of the corpus cavernosum have been made. A similarity has been noted in the distribution of NPY-containing and adrenergic nerves in the corpus cavernosum of rat and man, although double staining was not carried out. This would conform to the usual pattern of NPY and NA being co-localized in sympathetic nerves (Adrian *et al.*, 1984; Carrillo *et al.*, 1989). In monkeys, double-labelling techniques have been used and these revealed that NPY and VIP appear to be localized in the same nerves (Schmalbruch and Wagner, 1989). Further studies are required to examine the effects of NPY on vascular flow in the penis. In particular, it is necessary to investigate whether NPY has a specific role to play in the constriction of the deep dorsal vein and the 'shunt' arteries.

## Other neuropeptides

Several other neuropeptides have been investigated in relation to erection. Using immunohistochemistry, no met-enkephalin, leu-enkephalin, neurotensin, bombesin or cholecystokinin could be localized in the blood vessels and erectile tissue of the human corpus cavernosum (Gu *et al.*, 1983). We were also unable to localize enkephalin in the human deep dorsal vein (unpublished observations). Neurotensin and enkephalin had no effect on the penile arteries and cavernous smooth muscle *in vitro* from a variety of species except in the rabbit when enkephalin caused contraction of the erectile tissue (Sjöstrand, Klinge and Himberg, 1981). Sparse innervation by somatostatin-containing nerves has been observed in the penis (Gu *et al.*, 1983). However, somatostatin has little effect *in vitro* except at high concentrations when it causes contraction of the corpus caverosum, corpus spongiosum and cavernous artery (Sjöstrand, Klinge and Himberg, 1981; Hedlund and Andersson, 1985c). Thus there is little evidence that these neuropeptides contribute to the erectile process. Vasopressin (VP) has powerful vasoconstrictor effects on the corpus cavernosum, corpus spongiosum and cavernous artery at resting tone, but no effect on preparations precontracted with NA. A source for the VP in the penis has not been established (Hedlund and Andersson, 1985c).

## Interactions of transmitters

Recent advances in our understanding of autonomic neuroeffector mechanisms have established that there are interactions between neurotransmitters or neuromodulators at the neuromuscular junction (see Burnstock, 1987, 1990). These involve the prejunctional modulation of the release and/or postjunctional modulation of the effect of a transmitter. This can be achieved by a transmitter or neuromodulator localized in the same nerve or in different nerve types in the vicinity. Clearly, such interactions are likely to have a profound effect on the autonomic control of erection but to date they have received little direct investigation.

Two groups of workers have studied adrenergic/cholinergic interactions in the corpus cavernosum and corpus spongiosum *in vitro*. Both have shown that activation of prejunctional $\alpha_2$-adrenoceptors inhibits the release of NA during nerve stimulation while $\alpha_2$-antagonists increase release. Muscarinic agonists reduced the release of NA from nerves and attenuated the contractile response to nerve stimulation; these effects were reversed by atropine (Hedlund, Andersson and Mattiasson, 1984; de Tejada, Goldstein and Krane, 1988; de Tejada *et al.*, 1989b). In the presence of prazosin ($\alpha_1$-blockade), nerve stimulation of cavernous smooth muscle resulted in relaxation. The relaxation response was enhanced by physostygmine (an AChE inhibitor) and partially blocked by atropine. The effect of physostygmine was not prevented by bretylium (an inhibitor of adrenergic transmission) (de Tejada *et al.*, 1988). The overall interpretation of these results is that cholinergic mechanisms do not act directly to cause relaxation, but rather, cause prejunctional and postjunctional inhibition of adrenergic excitatory mechanisms (Hedlund, Andersson and Mattiasson, 1984; de Tejada *et al.*, 1988, 1989b). In addition, it is possible that ACh also acts as a neuromodulator in the penis to enhance the release and/or postjunctional effect of a NANC transmitter, suggested to be VIP (de Tejada *et al.*, 1988). Synergistic interaction between ACh and VIP co-localized in the same nerves has been demonstrated in the salivary gland (Lundberg, 1981). VIP inhibited adrenergically-mediated contractions in the corpus cavernosum but had no effect on the release of NA induced by electrical stimulation of nerves. Thus, if VIP does modulate the action of adrenergic nerves it is likely to be by a postjunctional rather than a prejunctional mechanism (Hedlund and Andersson, 1985c; de Tejada *et al.*, 1989b).

Apart from a report that NPY has no direct effect on erectile tissue or on the contractile response to nerve stimulation (Hedlund and Andersson, 1985c), little is known of the actions of NPY in the penis or its interactions with other transmitters localized in the same tissue. Similarly SP and CGRP do not appear to have been investigated in this respect. Since NPY, in separate studies, has been suggested to be co-localized with NA or with VIP in erectile tissue, it is not unreasonable to speculate that such interactions may exist.

## The role of the endothelium

Since it was first reported that the vasodilatation response to ACh requires the presence of an intact endothelium, the role of the endothelium in the regulation of vascular tone has attracted considerable interest. Numerous substances have been shown to produce endothelium-dependent responses, including ACh, SP, ATP, 5-HT, VP, angiotensin II (AgII), histamine and bradykinin (see Lincoln and Burnstock (1990) for review). Action of such substances on endothelial receptors stimulates the production of prostaglandins, endothelium-derived relaxing factors (EDRF) or constricting factors (EDCF) which subsequently modify vascular tone. EDRF has been identified as nitric oxide while endothelin (ET) is considered to be one of the constricting factors (Ignarro, Byrns and Wood, 1986; Palmer, Ferrige and Moncada, 1987; Yanagisawa *et al.*, 1988). Many of the triggering substances are transmitters which, when released from nerves, produce vasoconstriction via smooth muscle receptors, but cause vasodilatation via endothelial receptors.

It is considered unlikely that the same agent, released from perivascular nerves, could diffuse through the media without degradation to produce the opposite effect on vascular tone by its action on the endothelium. Therefore, in our laboratory, considerable work has been carried out recently to determine the source of the vasoactive substances which act on endothelial receptors. This has provided evidence that one source is the endothelial cell itself and subpopulations of endothelial cells have been shown to store and/or release ACh, ATP, VP, AgII and 5-HT (Parnavelas, Kelly and Burnstock, 1985; Burnstock *et al.*, 1988; Loesch and Burnstock, 1988; Lincoln, Loesch and Burnstock, 1990; Milner *et al.*, 1989, 1990a, b; Lincoln and Burnstock, 1990; Ralevic *et al.*, 1990).

The walls of the cavernous spaces as well as the penile vessels are lined with endothelial cells (Benson *et al.*, 1980; Juenemann *et al.*, 1987; de Tejada, Goldstein and Krane, 1988; Schmalbruch and Wagner, 1989). Despite this the endothelium has received little consideration with respect to the regulation of blood flow in erection. One group of workers has demonstrated that ACh-induced relaxation of the corpus cavernosum requires the presence of an intact endothelium and has speculated that the endothelium may have an active role in local haemodynamics in the penis (de Tejada, Goldstein and Krane, 1988). In addition an ultrastructural study has reported the possible direct innervation of endothelial cells in the corpus cavernosum of the monkey (Schmalbruch and Wagner, 1989). Two aspects of penile erection suggest that it is a physiological situation where the contribution by the endothelium to the regulation of blood flow could be of particular significance; these are the dramatic changes in flow required to produce tumescence, and the stretching that occurs as a consequence of increased volume.

Like the helicine arteries, the intracavernous nerves are coiled and undulating, which allows their elongation and adjustment to expansion of the corpus cavernosum. These nerves are surrounded by specialized fibrous sheaths which have been proposed to protect the nerves from compression during erection. However, where the nerves innervate the trabecular smooth muscle, the fibrous sheath is absent and it has proved difficult to explain how nerve impulses are preserved at this site in erection (Goldstein *et al.*, 1984). Similarly, the major vessels and nerves of the penis pursue a straight course from the pubis to the glans. It has been observed that the stretching they are subject to during erection would be disastrous to other peipheral nerves and arteries (Newman and Northup, 1983). It can be speculated that, after autonomic nerves have initiated vasodilatation and increased flow, an additional mechanism, mediated by the endothelium, is required to maintain tumescence once it has been achieved. It is possible that it is the very increase in flow that provides the stimulus for this mechanism to come into effect.

Increased flow has been shown to induce endothelium-dependent relaxation in a variety of vessels (Holtz *et al.*, 1984; Hull *et al.*, 1986; Rubanyi, Romero and Vanhoutte, 1986). Further we have demonstrated that SP, 5-HT, ATP and ACh are released from several vascular beds and/or endothelial cells in culture under hypoxia-induced vasodilatation or during shear stress due to increased flow (Burnstock *et al.*, 1988; Milner *et al.*, 1989, 1990a, b; Ralevic *et al.*, 1990). In this context, it is worth noting that membrane-limited dense granules, which are morphologically different from typical Wiebel-Palade bodies, have been observed in endothelial cells in the corpus cavernosum and have been speculated to contain a vasoactive agent (Schmalbruch and Wagner, 1989). VIP has been reported to be present in endothelium protruding into the sinusoidal spaces (Juenemann *et al.*, 1987). In addition, VIP has been shown to be released into the venous effluent during erection induced by intracavernosal injection of papaverine in man (Virag *et al.*, 1982). Since papaverine acts directly on the smooth muscle, this could imply a non-neuronal source for the VIP that was released. Clearly the part that the endothelium and its stores of vasoactive agents plays in erectile vasodilatation cannot be ignored and requires further investigation. It needs to be established whether endothelial cells are the source of VP in the penis and thus provide evidence that the powerful vasoconstrictor effect of VP could have some physiological role. ET, a potent vasoconstrictor, has been localized in endothelial cells, and the vasoconstrictor response to ET is reported to be greater in veins than arteries (de Nucci *et al.*, 1988; Le Monnier de Gouville *et al.*, 1989). It would be of interest to investigate whether ET is released from the endothelium of the deep dorsal vein by increased venous outflow in the initial stages of tumescence, thus contributing to venous constriction on full erection.

## Neuropeptides in impotence

Since neuropeptides have only recently been investigated with regard to the control of erection, there have been relatively few studies that directly investigate changes occurring in impotence. It is well known that erectile dysfunction can be due to a variety of causes including psychogenic impotence, spinal cord injury, multiple sclerosis, diabetes, vascular disease and radical surgery (see Weiss (1972) for review). Human tissue obtained from surgery for the implantation of penile prostheses as treatment for impotence, therefore, represents a heterogeneous population of patients which cannot be expected to reveal a single pattern of change in their autonomic innervation. Further, all studies in man are hampered by the difficulty in obtaining appropriate control material.

Gu *et al.*, (1984) reported a decrease in VIP-containing nerves and VIP levels in the corpus cavernosum from all impotent patients, regardless of cause of impotence, when compared with transsexuals. The decrease was, however, related to the degree of erectile dysfunction. We have studied patients with erectile dysfunction and attempted to determine whether different causes of impotence could reveal different patterns of change in autonomic innervation. One group consisted of patients in which damage to autonomic nerves was not indicated clinically as a factor in the development of dysfunction. A similar pattern of VIP- (Figure 1.2a, b) and AChE-containing nerves were observed in the corpus cavernosum, tunica albuginea and penile blood vessels from all these patients. In a patient with a cauda equina lesion there was a complete absence of VIP-containing nerves. Five out of six diabetic patients studied showed a marked reduction in VIP-containing nerves (Figure 1.2c) and a similar reduction in AChE-positive nerves (Lincoln *et al.*, 1987). A clinical trial of intracavernous injection of VIP has already been carried out in patients with erectile dysfunction due to a variety of causes. While VIP signifcantly increased both penile length and diameter in these patients, the response was not sufficient to produce penile rigidity adequate for intromission (Roy, Petrone and Said, 1990).

Of the diabetic patients with reduced VIP-containing nerves that we studied, two had symptoms of autonomic neuropathy (e.g. postural hypotension), one had evidence of peripheral neuropathy and in two there was no clinical evidence of peripheral or autonomic neuropathy (Lincoln *et al.*, 1987). It has been recognized for some time that there is a greatly increased incidence of impotence in diabetic patients (Kolodny *et al.*, 1974). The complications of atherosclerosis (Herman, Adar and Rubinstein, 1978; Jevtich *et al.*, 1982; Lehman and Jacobs, 1982) and autonomic neuropathy (Faermann *et al.*, 1974; Ellenberg, 1980; Karacan, 1980; Lin and Bradley, 1985) have both been implicated as the major aetiological factor in the development of impotence in diabetes. Since current evidence favours dual nervous/endothelial control of vascular tone, it is probable that these two complications cannot be considered separately. Indeed, in a recent study it has been shown that both nerve-mediated and endothelium-dependent relaxation of cavernous smooth muscle are attenuated in diabetic patients. In contrast, direct relaxation of the smooth muscle by papaverine or sodium nitroprusside was unaffected in diabetes (de Tejada and Goldstein, 1988; de Tejada *et al.*, 1989a). Interestingly, in the same study, nerve-mediated contraction of cavernous smooth muscle was not impaired. It has been shown, by ourselves and others, that NA levels of the corpus cavernosum are reduced in diabetes (Melman *et al.*, 1980; Lincoln *et al.*, 1987). Whether the preservation of nerve-mediated contraction, when NA levels are reduced, reflects a loss of the cholinergic or VIPergic inhibitory effects on adrenergic transmission in diabetes is not known (see p. 10). We have carried out preliminary experiments on the effect of diabetes on NPY in human corpus cavernosum which have revealed inconclusive results. While there was a tendency for reduced density of NPY-containing nerves, NPY levels were, if anything, increased in diabetes (unpublished observations).

Little is known of the state of other neuropeptides in penile vessels and erectile tissue in impotence, whether due to diabetes or other disorders. It is probable that animal models of disease will prove useful in elucidating the nature of the changes in the autonomic and endothelial control of erection in impotence. We have already shown that VIP-containing nerves are reduced in penile vessels of the streptozotocin-diabetic rat as has been observed in human diabetics (Crowe *et al.*, 1983; Lincoln *et al.*, 1987).

## Conclusions

Superficially, penile erection may appear to be a relatively simple haemodynamic phenomenon. However, the changes that occur in the rate of blood flow, intracavernosal pressure and penile volume in the erectile process are extreme in physiological terms. Review of the literature demonstrates the complexity of the process and the high degree of coordinated control that is required for normal function. This coordination is reflected at many peripheral levels in addition to those occurring in the higher centres in the brain and spinal cord: from (1) the interconnecting pathways of the extrinsic nerves and the local ganglia supplying the penis; (2) the differing responses in the appropriate vasculature within the penis to direct the blood flow; to (3) the multiplicity of transmitters present in penile

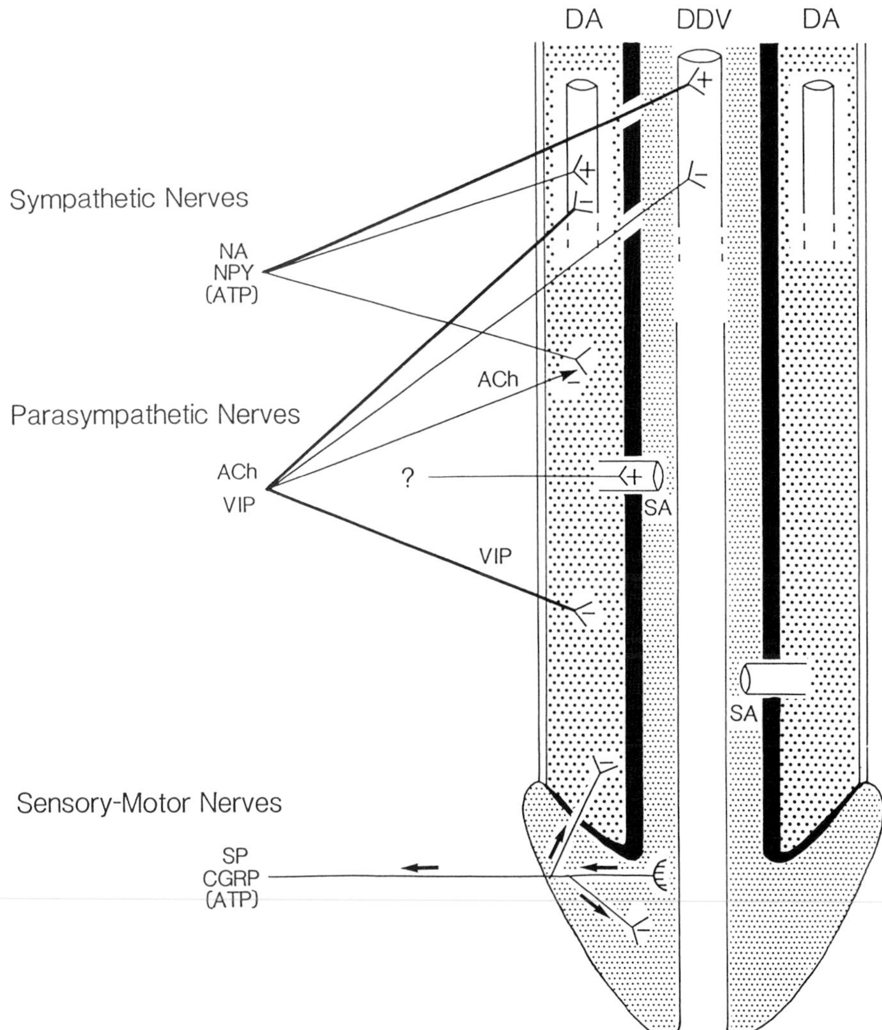


**Figure 1.3** Schematic representation of the main nerves controlling the erectile tissues and blood vessels of the penis: DDV, deep dorsal vein, DA, dorsal artery; SA, shunt artery; [dotted symbol], corpus cavernosum; ■, tunica albuginea; [dotted symbol], corpus spongiosum. The nerve supply has been divided into the sympathetic, parasympathetic, sensory and motor components. The most likely combination of neurotransmitters and/or neuromodulators, derived from direct investigation of both the penis and other vascular systems, are shown: NA, noradrenaline; NPY, neuropeptide Y; ATP, adenosine 5′-triphosphate; ACh, acetycholine; VIP, vasoactive intestinal polypeptide; SP, substance P; CGRP, calcitonin gene-related peptide. Brackets indicate that the presence of the transmitter has been postulated from studies of vascular systems other than the penis. The thickness of the lines represents the relative density of innervation. The diagram demonstrates the possible interactions in the nervous control of vascular tone: +, excitatory mechanism resulting in vasoconstriction; –, inhibitory mechanism resulting in vasodilatation. The arrowhead together with the minus sign indicate the neuromodulation by ACh of sympathetic vasoconstriction. Arrows on the sensory and motor nerve supply show the direction of nerve impulses following stimulation of the sensory nerve ending during hypothetical axon reflex vasodilatation.

perivascular nerves; (4) the interactions of transmitters and neuromodulators at the neuromuscular junction, both within the same nerves and between different nerve types; and (5) the interaction between the neural and endothelial control of vascular tone. Schematic representations are provided in Figures 1.3 and 1.4. We have emphasized the role of neuropeptides and vasoactive endothelial peptides as these are increasingly being implicated in current research on the regulation of blood flow. In view of their relatively recent discovery, suggestions as to their contribution to erection are inevitably speculative; nevertheless they may well be important since there is already evidence for similar mechanisms in other vascular systems. The scheme highlights the need for further research to elucidate the precise mechanisms of control of the erectile process and thereafter define the changes that are significant in the development of impotence.

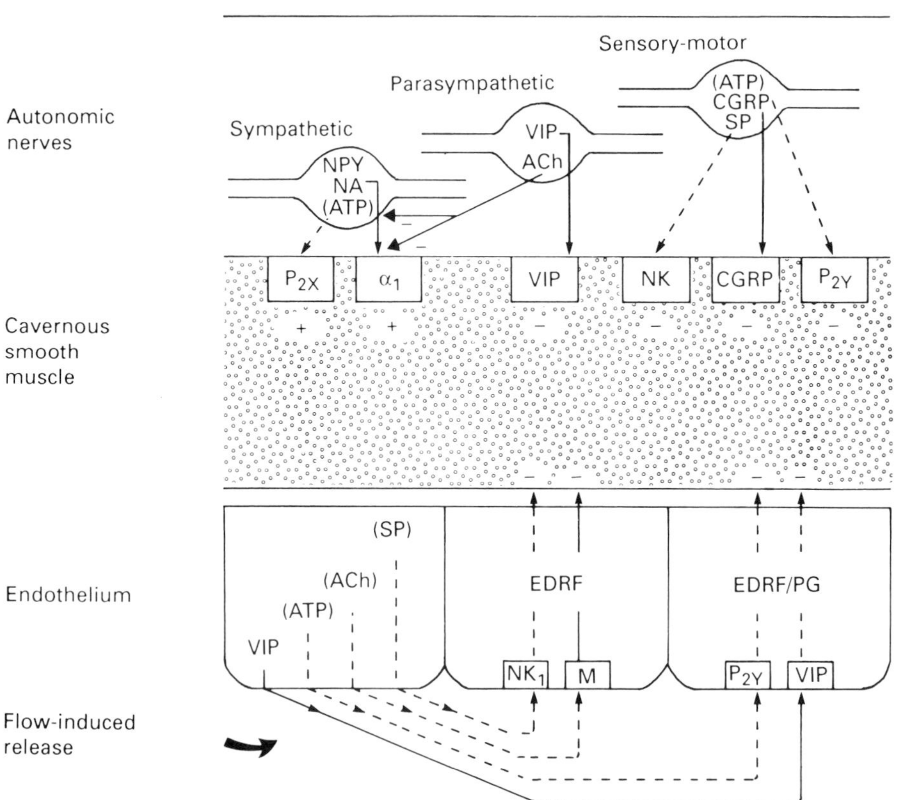


**Figure 1.4** Schematic representation of possible neural–endothelial interactions in the control of cavernous smooth muscle tone. Vasoactive substances are localized within the lining of the endothelial cells and the sympathetic, parasympathetic, sensory and motor nerves supplying the corpus cavernosum: NA, noradrenaline; NPY, neuropeptide Y; ATP, adenosine 5′-triphosphate; ACh, acetylcholine; VIP, vasoactive intestinal polypeptide; SP, substance P; CGRP, calcitonin gene-related peptide. Small arrows indicate release of vasoactive substances from nerve varicosities and endothelial cells following nerve stimulation and flow-induced shear stress, respectively, together with their action on receptors located on the cavernous smooth muscle or the endothelium. Endothelium-dependent responses are shown to be mediated by either endothelium-derived relaxing factor (EDRF) or prostaglandins (PG). +, contractile response; –, relaxation response. Brackets indicate that the presence of these vasoactive substances has been inferred from studies of vascular systems other than the penis. Similarly, dotted lines indicate that the release or subsequent action of the vasoactive substance has not been demonstrated by direct investigation of the penis but is known to occur in other vascular tissues. Large arrowheads together with minus signs indicate pre- and postjunctional neuromodulation of adrenergic mechanisms by ACh. Note that the cavernous smooth muscle and endothelium may have different populations of receptors providing dual control of vascular tone. Where possible, the likely subtypes of the receptors have been shown: $\alpha_1$, $\alpha_1$ adrenoceptor; $P_{2X}$, $P_{2X}$-purinoceptor; $P_{2Y}$, $P_{2Y}$-purinoceptor; NK, neurokinin receptor; $NK_1$, neurokinin$_1$ receptor; M, muscarinic receptor

## References


Aboseif, S. R. and Lue, T. F. (1988) Hemodynamics of penile erection. *Urologic Clinics of North America*, **15**, 1–7

Adaikan, P. G., Kottegoda, S. R. and Ratnam, S. S. (1986) Is vasoactive intestinal polypeptide the principal transmitter involved in human penile erection? *Journal of Urology*, **135**, 638–640

Adrian, T. E., Gu, J., Allen, J. M. *et al.* (1984) Neuropeptide Y in the human male genital tract. *Life Sciences*, **35**, 2643–2648

Alaranta, S., Uusitalo, H., Hautamäki, A.-M. and Klinge, E. (1990) Calcitonin gene-related peptide: immunohistochemical localization in and effects on bovine penile artery. *European Journal of Pharmacology*, **183**, 547

Andersson, P.-O., Björnberg, J., Bloom, S. R. and Mellander, S. (1987) Vasoactive intestinal polypeptide in relation to penile erection in the cat evoked by pelvic and by hypogastric nerve stimulation. *Journal of Urology*, **138**, 419–422

Andersson, P.-O., Bloom, S. R. and Mellander, S. (1984) Haemodynamics of pelvic nerve induced penile erection in the dog: possible mediation by vasoactive intestinal polypeptide. *Journal of Physiology*, **350**, 209–224

Andersson, K.-E., Hedlund, H., Mattiasson, A. *et al.* (1983) Relaxation of isolated human corpus spongiosum induced by vasoactive intestinal polypeptide, substance P, carbachol and electrical field stimulation. *World Journal of Urology*, **1**, 203–208

Aoki, H., Takagane, H., Banya, Y. *et al.* (1986) Human penile hemodynamics studied by a polarographic method. *Journal of Urology*, **135**, 872–876

Benson, G. S. (1983) Penile erection: in search of a neurotransmitter. *World Journal of Urology*, **1**, 209–212

Benson, G. S., McConnell, J., Lipshultz, L. I. *et al.* (1980) Neuromorphology and neuropharmacology of the human penis: and *in vitro* study. *Journal of Clinical Investigation*, **65**, 506–513

Blanco, R., de Tejada, I. S., Goldstein, I. *et al.* (1988) Cholinergic neurotransmission in human corpus cavernosum. II. Acetylcholine synthesis. *American Journal of Physiology*, **254**, H468–H472

Bowman, A. and Gillespie, J. S. (1983) Neurogenic vasodilatation in isolated bovine and canine penile arteries. *Journal of Physiology*, **341**, 603–616

Brindley, G. S. (1986a) Sacral and hypogastric plexus stimulators and what these models tell us about autonomic actions on the bladder and urethra. *Clinical Sciences*, **70**, (Suppl. 14), 41s–44s

Brindley, G. S. (1986b) Pilot experiments on the actions of drugs injected into the human corpus cavernosum penis. *British Journal of Pharmacology*, **87**, 495–500

Brindley, G. S. (1988) Autonomic control of the pelvic organs. In *Autonomic Failure: A Textbook of Clinical Disorders of the Autonomic Nervous System* (ed. R. Bannister), Oxford University Press, Oxford, pp. 223–237

Burnstock, G. (1987) Mechanisms of interaction of peptide and nonpeptide vascular systems. *Journal of Cardiovascular Pharmacology*, **10**, (Suppl. 12), S74–S81

Burnstock, G. (1988a) Nonadrenergic innervation of blood vessels – some historical perspectives and future directions. In *Nonadrenergic Innervation of Blood Vessels*, Vol.I (eds. G. Burnstock and S. G. Griffith), CRC Press, Boca Raton, Florida, pp. 1–14

Burnstock, G. (1988b) Regulation of local blood flow by neurohumoral substances released from perivascular nerves and endothelial cells. *Acta Physiologica Scandinavica*, **133**, (Suppl. 571), 53–59

Burnstock, G. (1990) Cotransmission. The Fifth Heymans Lecture, Ghent, February 17, 1990: Co-transmission. *Archives Internationales de Pharmacodynamie et de Therapie*, **304**, 7–33

Burnstock, G., Lincoln, J., Fehér, E. *et al.* (1988) Serotonin is localized in endothelial cells of coronary arteries and released during hypoxia: a possible new mechanism for hypoxia-induced vasodilatation of the rat heart. *Experientia*, **44**, 705–707

Carati, C.J., Goldie, R.G., Warton, A. and Henry, P.J. (1985) Pharmacology of the erectile tissue of the canine penis. *Pharmacological Research Communications*, **17**, 951–966

Carrillo, Y., Fernandez, E., Dail, W. G. and Walton, G. D. (1989) Neuropeptide Y innervation of penile erectile tissue. *Society for Neuroscience Abstracts*, **15**, 631

Casey, W. C. and Woods, R. W. (1982) Anatomy and histology of penile deep dorsal vein: venous cushions and proximal 'sphincter'. *Urology*, **19**,284–286

Crowe, R., Lincoln, J., Blacklay, P. F. *et al.* (1983) Vasoactive intestinal polypeptide-like immunoreactive nerves in diabetic penis. *Diabetes*, **32**, 1075–1077

Dail, W. G. Jr. and Evan, A. P. Jr. (1974) Experimental evidence indicating that the penis of the rat is innervated by short adrenergic neurons. *American Journal of Anatomy*, **141**, 203–218

Dail, W. G. and Hamill, R. W. (1989) Parasympathetic nerves in penile erectile tissue of the rat contain choline acetyltransferase. *Brain Research*, **487**, 165–170

Dail, W. G., Minorsky, N., Moll, M. A. and Manzanares, K. (1986) The hypogastric nerve pathway to penile erectile tissue: histochemical evidence supporting a vasodilator role. *Journal of the Autonomic Nervous System*, **15**, 341–349

Dail, W. G., Trujillo, D., de la Rosa, D. and Walton, G. (1989) Autonomic innervation of reproductive organs: analysis of the neurons whose axons project in the main penile nerve in the pelvic plexus of the rat. *Anatomical Record*, **224**, 94–101

Dail, W. G., Walton, G. and Olmsted, M. P. (1989) Penile erection in the rat: stimulation of the hypogastric nerve elicits increases in penile pressure after chronic interruption of the sacral parasympathetic outflow. *Journal of the Autonomic Nervous System*, **28**, 251–258

de Groat, W. C. (1987) Neuropeptides in pelvic afferent pathways. *Experientia*, **43**, 801–813

de Groat, W. C. and Kawatani, M. (1989) Reorganization of sympathetic preganglionic connections in cat bladder following denervation. *Journal of Physiology*, **409**, 431–449

de Groat, W. C. and Steers, W. D. (1988) Neural control of the urinary bladder and sexual organs: experimental studies in animals. In *Autonomic Failure: A Textbook of Clinical Disorders of the Autonomic Nervous System* (ed. R. Bannister), Oxford University Press, Oxford, pp. 196–222

de Nucci, G., Thomas, R., d'Orleans-Juste, P. *et al.* (1988) Pressor effects of circulating endothelin are limited by its removal in the pulmonary circulation and by the release of prostacyclin and endothelium-derived relaxing factor. *Proceedings of the National Academy of Sciences, USA*, **85**, 9797–9800

de Tejada, I. S., Blanco, R., Goldstein, I. *et al.* (1988) Cholinergic neurotransmission in human corpus cavernosum. I. Responses of isolated tissue. *American Journal of Physiology*, **254**, H459–H467

de Tejada, I. S. and Goldstein, I. (1988) Diabetic penile neuropathy. *Urologic Clinics of North America*, **15**, 17–22

de Tejada, I. S., Goldstein, I., Azadzoi, K. *et al.* (1989a) Impaired neurogenic and endothelium-mediated relaxation of penile smooth muscle from diabetic men with impotence. *New England Journal of Medicine*, **320**, 1025–1030

de Tejada, I. S., Goldstein, I. and Krane, R. J. (1988) Local control of penile erection: nerves, smooth muscle and endothelium. *Urologic Clinics of North America*, **15**, 9–15

de Tejada, I. S., Kim, N., Lagan, I. *et al.* (1989b) Regulation of adrenergic activity in penile corpus cavernosum. *Journal of Urology*, **142**, 1117–1121

Domer, F. R., Wessler, G., Brown, R. L. and Charles, H.C. (1978) Involvement of the sympathetic nervous system in the urinary bladder internal sphincter and in penile erection in the anesthetized cat. *Investigative Urology*, **15**, 404–407

Dorr, L. D. and Brody, M. J. (1967) Hemodynamic mechanisms of erection in the canine penis. *American Journal of Physiology*, **213**, 1526–1531

Ellenberg, M. (1980) Sexual function in diabetic patients. *Annals of Internal Medicine*, **92**, 331–333

Faerman, I., Glocer, L., Fox, D. *et al.* (1974) Impotence and diabetes: histological studies of autonomic nervous fibers of the corpora cavernosa in impotent diabetic males. *Diabetes*, **23**, 971–976

Furchgott, R. F. and Zawadzki, J. V. (1980) The obligatory role of endothelial cells in the relaxation of arterial smooth muscle by acetylcholine. *Nature*, **288**, 373–376

Goldstein, A. M. B., Morrow, J. W., Meehan, J. P. *et al.* (1984) Special microanatomical features surrounding the intracorpora cavernosa nerves and their probable function during erection. *Journal of Urology*, **132**, 44–46

Gu, J., Polak, J. M., Lazarides, M. *et al.* (1984) Decrease of vasoactive intestinal polypeptide (VIP) in the penises from impotent men. *Lancet*, **ii**, 315–318

Gu, J., Polak, J. M., Probert, L. *et al.* (1983) Peptidergic innervation of the human male genital tract. *Journal of Urology*, **130**, 386–391

Hedlund, H. and Andersson, K.-E. (1985a) Comparison of the responses to drugs acting on adrenoreceptors and muscarinic receptors in human isolated corpus cavernosum and cavernous artery. *Journal of Autonomic Pharmacology*, **5**, 81–88

Hedlund, H. and Andersson, K.-E. (1985b) Contraction and relaxation induced by some prostanoids in isolated human penile erectile tissue and cavernous artery. *Journal of Urology*, **134**, 1245–1250

Hedlund, H. and Andersson, K.-E. (1985c) Effects of some peptides on isolated human penile erectile tissue and cavernous artery. *Acta Physiologica Scandinavica*, **124**, 413–419

Hedlund, H., Andersson, K.-E. and Mattiasson, A. (1984) Pre- and postjunctional adreno- and muscarinic receptor functions in the isolated human corpus spongiosum urethrae. *Journal of Autonomic Pharmacology*, **4**, 241–249

Herman, A., Adar, R. and Rubinstein, Z. (1978) Vascular lesions associated with impotence in diabetic and non-diabetic arterial occlusive disease. *Diabetes*, **27**, 975–981

Holtz, J., Förstermann, U., Pohl, U. *et al.* (1984) Flow-dependent, endothelium-mediated dilation of epicardial coronary arteries in conscious dogs: effects of cyclooxygenase inhibition. *Journal of Cardiovascular Pharmacology*, **6**, 1161–1169

Hull, S. S., Kaiser, L., Jaffe, M. D. and Sparks, H. V. (1986) Endothelium-dependent flow-induced dilation in canine femoral and saphenous arteries. *Blood Vessels*, **23**, 183–198

Ignarro, L. J., Byrns, R. E. and Wood, K. S. (1986) Pharmacological and biochemical properties of endothelium-derived relaxing factor (EDRF): evidence that it is closely related to nitric oxide (NO) radical. *Circulation*, **74**, (Suppl. II), 287

Jevtich, M. J., Edson, M., Jarman, W. D. and Herrera, H. H. (1982) Vascular factor in erectile failure among diabetics. *Urology*, **19**, 163–168

Juenemann, K.-P., Lue, T. F., Fournier, G. R. Jr. and Tanagho, E. A. (1986) Hemodynamics of a papaverine- and phentolamine-induced penile erection. *Journal of Urology*, **136**, 158–161

Juenemann, K.-P., Lue, T. F., Luo, J.-A. *et al.* (1987) The role of vasoactive intestinal polypeptide as a neurotransmitter in canine penile erection: a combined *in vivo* and immunohistochemical study. *Journal of Urology*, **138**, 871–877

Juenemann, K.-P., Lue, T. F. and Tanagho, E. A. (1986) Further evidence of venous outflow restriction during erection. *British Journal of Urology*, **58**, 320–324

Juenemann, K.-P., Persson-Jünemann, C., Tanagho, E. A. and Alken, P. (1989) Neurophysiology of penile erection. *Urological Research*, **17**, 213–217

Karacan, I. (1980) Diagnosis of erectile impotence in diabetes mellitus. *Annals of Internal Medicine*, **92**, 334–337

Kimoto, Y. and Ito, Y. (1987) Autonomic innervation of the canine penile artery and vein in relation to neural mechanisms involved in erection. *British Journal of Urology*, **59**, 463–472

Kolodny, R. C., Kahn, C. B., Goldstein, H. H. and Barrett, D. M. (1974) Sexual dysfunction in diabetic men. *Diabetes*, **23**, 306–309

Lehman, T. P. and Jacobs. J. A. (1982) Etiology of diabetic impotence. *Journal of Urology*, **129**, 291–294

Le Monnier de Gouville, A.-C., Lippton, H. L., Cavero, I. *et al.* (1989) Endothelin – a new family of endothelium-derived peptides with widespread biological properties. *Life Sciences*, **45**, 1499–1513

Lin, J. T. and Bradley, W. E. (1985) Penile neuropathy in insulin-dependent diabetes mellitus. *Journal of Urology*, **133**, 213–215

Lincoln, J. and Burnstock, G. (1990) Neural–endothelial interactions in control of local blood flow. In *The Endothelium: An Introduction to Current Research* (ed. J. Warren), Wiley-Liss Inc., New York, pp. 21–32

Lincoln, J., Crowe, R., Blacklay, P. F. *et al.* (1987) Changes in VIPergic, cholinergic and adrenergic innervation of human penile tissue in diabetic and non-diabectic impotent males. *Journal of Urology*, **137**, 1053–1059

Lincoln, J., Loesch, A. and Burnstock, G. (1990) Localization of vasopressin, serotonin and angiotensin II in endothelial cells of the renal and mesenteric arteries of the rat. *Cell and Tissue Research*, **259**, 341–344

Loesch, A. and Burnstock, G. (1988) Ultrastructural localisation of serotonin and substance P in vascular endothelial cells of rat femoral and mesenteric arteries. *Anatomy and Embryology*, **178**, 137–142

Luduena, F. P. and Grigas, E. O. (1966) Pharmacological study of autonomic innervation of dog retractor penis. *American Journal of Physiology*, **210**, 435–444

Lue, T. F. and Tanagho, E. A. (1987) Physiology of erection and pharmacological management of impotence. *Journal of Urology*, **137**, 829–836

Lue, T. F., Zeineh, S. J., Schmidt, R. A. and Tanagho, E. A. (1984) Neuroanatomy of penile erection: its relevance to iatrogenic impotence. *Journal of Urology*, **131**, 273–280

Lundberg, J. M. (1981) Evidence for coexistence of vasoactive intestinal polypeptide (VIP) and acetylcholine in neurons of cat exocrine glands. Morphological, biochemical and functional studies. *Acta Physiologica Scandinavica*, Suppl. 496, 1–57

Maggi, C. A. and Meli, A. (1988) The sensory-efferent function of capsaicin-sensitive sensory neurons. *General Pharmacology*, **19**, 1–43

McConnell, J. and Benson, G. S. (1982) Innervation of human penile blood vessels. *Neurourology and Urodynamics*, **1**, 199–210

McConnell, J., Benson, G. S. and Wood, J. (1979) Autonomic innervation of the mammalian penis: a histochemical and physiological study. *Journal of Neural Transmission*, **45**, 227–238

Melman, A., Henry, D. P., Felten, D. L. and O'Connor, B. (1980) Effect of diabetes upon penile sympathetic nerves in impotent patients. *Southern Medical Journal*, **73**, 307–309

Merighi, A., Polak, J. M., Gibson, S. J. *et al.* (1988) Ultrastructural studies on calcitonin gene-related peptide-, tachykinin- and somatostatin-immunoreactive neurones in rat dorsal root ganglia: evidence for the colocalization of different peptides in single secretory granules. *Cell and Tissue Research*, **254**, 101–109

Milner, P., Bodin, P., Loesch, A. and Burnstock, G. (1990a) Endothelin and ATP: rapid release from isolated aortic endothelial cells exposed to increased flow. *Biochemical and Biophysical Research Communications*, **170**, 649–656

Milner, P., Kirkpatrick, K., Ralevic, V. *et al.* (1990b) Endothelial cells cultured from human umbilical vein release ATP, substance P and acetylcholine in response to altered shear stress. *Proceedings of the Royal Society, Series B*, **241**, 245–248

Milner, P., Ralevic, V., Hopwood, A. M. *et al.* (1989) Ultrastructural localisation of substance P and choline acetyltransferase in endothelial cells of rat coronary artery and release of substance P and acetylcholine during hypoxia. *Experientia*, **45**, 121–125

Newman, H. F. and Northup, J. D. (1981) Mechanism of human penile erection: an overview. *Urology*, **17**, 399–408

Newman, H. F. and Northup, J. D. (1983) Problems in male organic sexual physiology. *Urology*, **21**, 443–450

Palmer, R. M. J., Ferrige, A. G. and Moncada, S. (1987) Nitric oxide release accounts for the biological activity of endothelium-derived relaxing factor. *Nature*, **327**, 524–526

Parnavelas, J. G., Kelly, W. and Burnstock, G. (1985) Ultrastructural localization of choline acetyltransferase in vascular endothelial cells in rat brain. *Nature*, **316**, 724–725

Polak, J. M. and Bloom, S. R. (1984) Localisation and measurement of VIP in the genitourinary system of man and animals. *Peptides*, **5**, 225–230

Polak, J. M., Gu, J., Mina, S. and Bloom, S. R. (1981) VIPergic nerves in the penis. *Lancet*, **ii**, 217–219

Quinlan, D. M., Nelson, R. J., Partin, A. W. *et al.* (1989) The rat as a model for the study of penile erection. *Journal of Urology*, **141**, 656–661

Ralevic, V., Milner, P., Hudlická, O. *et al.* (1990) Substance P is released from the endothelium of normal and capsaicin-treated rat hindlimb vasculature *in vivo* by increased flow. *Circulation Research*, **66**, 1178–1183

Roy, J. B., Petrone, R. L. and Said, S. I. (1990) A clinical trial of intracavernous vasoactive intestinal peptide to induce penile erection. *Journal of Urology*, **143**, 302–304

Rubanyi, G. M., Romero, J. C. and Vanhoutte, P. M. (1986) Flow-induced release of endothelium-derived relaxing factor. *American Journal of Physiology*, **250**, H1145–H1149

Ruzbarsky, V. and Michal, V. (1977) Morphological changes in the arterial bed of the penis with aging: relationship to the pathogenesis of impotence. *Investiga-*

*tive Urology*, **15**, 194–199

Schmalbruch, H. and Wagner, G. (1989) Vasoactive intestinal polypeptide (VIP)- and neuropeptide Y (NPY)-containing nerve fibres in the penile cavernous tissue of green monkeys (*Cercopithecus aethiops*). *Cell and Tissue Research*, **256**, 529–541

Sjöstrand, N. O. and Klinge, E. (1979) Principal mechanisms controlling penile retraction and protrusion in rabbits. *Acta Physiologica Scandinavica*, **106**, 199–214

Sjöstrand, N. O., Klinge, E. and Himberg, J.-J. (1981) Effects of VIP and other putative neurotransmitters on smooth muscle effectors of penile erection. *Acta Physiologica Scandinavica*, **113**, 403–405

Steers, W. D., McConnell, J. and Benson, G. S. (1984) Anatomical localization and some pharmacological effects of vasoactive intestinal polypeptide in human and monkey corpus cavernosum. *Journal of Urology*, **132**, 1048–1053

Stief, C. G., Benard, F., Bosch, R. *et al.* (1989) Acetylcholine as a possible neurotransmitter in penile erection. *Journal of Urology*, **141**, 1444–1448

Stief, C. G., Benard, F., Bosch, R. J. L. H. *et al.* (1990) A possible role for calcitonin gene-related peptide in the regulation of the smooth muscle tone of the bladder and penis. *Journal of Urology*, **143**, 392–397

Virag, R., Ottesen, B., Fahrenkrug, J. *et al.* (1982) Vasoactive intestinal polypeptide release during penile erection in man. *Lancet*, **ii**, 1166

Wagner, G. and Gerstenberg, T. (1987) Intracavernosal injection of vasoactive intestinal polypeptide (VIP) does not induce erection in man *per se*. *World Journal of Urology*, **5**, 171–177

Wagner, G., Willis, E. A., Bro-Rasmussen, F. and Nielsen, M. H. (1982) New theory on the mechanism of erection involving hitherto undescribed vessels. *Lancet*, **i**, 416–418

Weiss, H.D. (1972) The physiology of human penile erection. *Annals of Internal Medicine*, **76**, 793–799

Wespes, E., Delcour, C., Struyven, J. and Schulman, C. C. (1984) Cavernometry-cavernography: its role in organic impotence. *European Urology*, **10** 229–232

Wespes, E., Depierreux, M. and Schulman, C. C. (1987) Penile deep dorsal vein cushions and erection. *British Journal of Urology*, **60**, 174–177

Wespes, E., Schiffman, S., Gilloteaux, J. *et al.* (1988) Study of neuropeptide Y-containing nerve fibers in the human penis. *Cell and Tissue Research*, **254**, 69–74

Willis, E. A., Ottesen, B., Wagner, G. *et al.* (1981) Vasoactive intestinal polypeptide as a possible neurotransmitter involved in penile erection. *Acta Physiologica Scandinavica*, **113**, 545–547

Willis, E. A., Ottesen, B., Wagner, G. *et al.* (1983) Vasoactive intestinal polypeptide (VIP) as a neurotransmitter in penile erection. *Life Sciences*, **33**, 383–391

Wimalawansa, S. J., Emson, P. C. and MacIntyre, I. (1987) Regional distribution of calcitonin-gene-related peptide and its specific binding sites in rats with particular reference to the nervous system. *Neuroendocrinology*, **46**, 131

Yanagisawa, M., Kurihara, H., Kimura, S. *et al.* (1988) A novel potent vasoconstrictor peptide produced by vascular endothelial cells. *Nature*, **332**, 411–415

# 2

# Penile erection: circulatory physiology

A. K. Batra and T. F. Lue

The last decade has seen much innovative research on the penile circulatory physiology of experimental animals and man, leading to a better understanding of penile physiology and pathophysiology. Accurate and precise clinical tests of penile neurovascular function and more physiological treatments are now available. This chapter summarizes the current understanding of the circulatory physiology of the penis.

## Anatomy of the penis

The penis consists of three corporeal bodies: the paired corpora cavernosa dorsally and corpus spongiosum ventrally. At the root of the penis, the corpora cavernosa diverge and form the crura, which are attached to the ipsilateral ischiopubic ramus. The corpus spongiosum encloses the urethra and expands distally to form the glans penis. A thick fibrous sheath, the tunica albuginea, surrounds the three corpora. It is made up of bundles of collagen and elastin fibres woven in different directions. This appears thinner when stretched during erection and is important in maintaining the structural integrity of the penis (Goldstein *et al.*, 1982). The tunica albuginea of the corpus spongiosum is much thinner and it is absent in the glans penis.

The erectile tissue is composed of a meshwork of interconnected sinusoidal spaces separated by trabeculae which contain bundles of smooth muscle in a framework of collagen, elastin and fibroblasts and helicine branches of the cavernous arteries and terminal branches of the cavernous nerves. The cavernous tissue is capable of considerable stretching. The sinusoidal spaces of the spongiosum are larger and there is less smooth muscle than in the corpus cavernosum. Branches of the dorsal arteries, dorsal nerves, and tributaries of the dorsal vein travel on the surface of the tunica albuginea and are covered by a fibrous sheath, Buck's fascia, the subcutaneous tissue and the skin. At the base of the penis, the ischiocavernosus and bulbocavernosus muscles surround and attach to the undersurface of the crura and urethral bulb respectively.

### **Arterial supply** (Figure 2.1)

The penile artery gives three terminal branches on each side: (1) spongiosal, bulbar or bulbourethral; (2) dorsal; and (3) deep or cavernosal arteries. The penile artery is usually the temination of the internal pudendal artery. However, it is not uncommon to have accessory internal pudendal arteries from the obturator, external iliac or other arteries giving supplemental branches to the dorsal or cavernous artery. In some instances, the accessory pudendal artery may become the only blood supply to the corpus cavernosum (Breza *et al.*, 1989) and injury to these accessory arteries may result in arteriogenic impotence. The cavernosus artery penetrates the tunica albuginea and gives off the terminal helicine arterioles, which open directly into the endothelium-lined sinusoidal spaces. The dorsal artery travels in the plane between the tunica albuginea and Buck's fascia accompanied by the deep dorsal vein. Distally, just proximal to the glans, the dorsal artery joins the spongiosal artery to form a vascular arch which gives off small branches to supply the glans. Anastomosis among the three branches is common and sometimes branches of the dorsal artery may become the major source of blood supply to the corpus cavernosum.

Most researchers now agree that the relaxation of the smooth muscle of the trabeculae and the arterioles results in erection. The exact mechanism that regulates the tone of the end arteriolar and sinusoidal smooth muscle is still under investigation.

### **Venous drainage** (Figure 2.2)

Venules that drain peripheral sinusoidal spaces form subtunical plexuses between the sinusoidal wall and the tunica albuginea. Several of these plexuses coalesce to become the emissary veins which pierce the tunica albuginea (Lue and Tanagho, 1988). In the distal one-half to two-thirds of the penis, these emissary veins drain into the circumflex veins laterally, dorsal veins dorsally, and urethral veins ventrally. Most of these veins empty into the deep

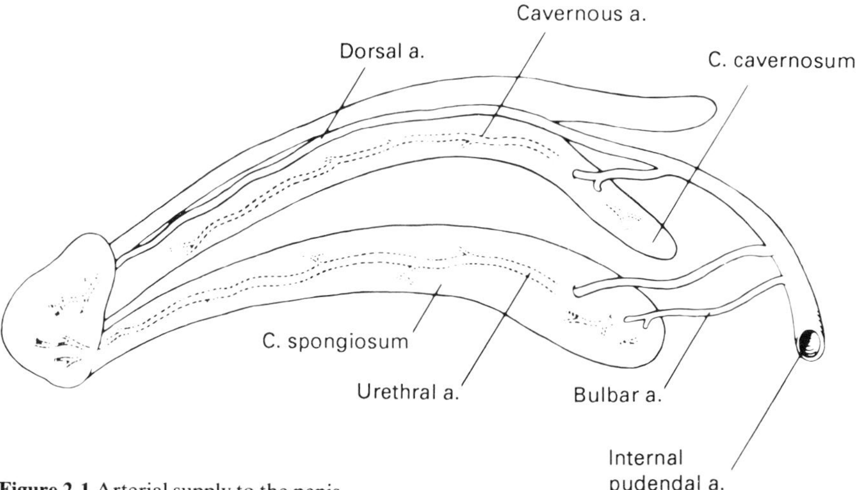


**Figure 2.1** Arterial supply to the penis

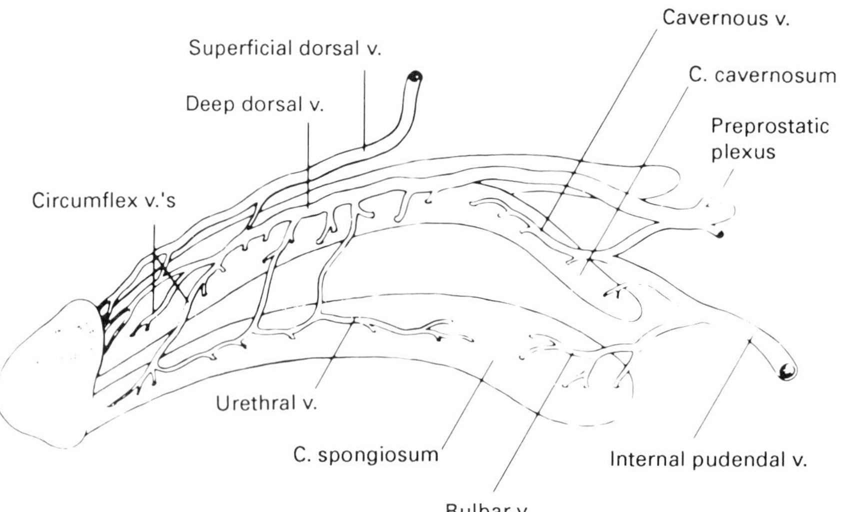


**Figure 2.2** Venous drainage of the penis

dorsal vein which in turn drains into the periprostatic veins. In the proximal portion of the penis, the emissary veins drain into the cavernous and crural veins, which eventually join the internal pudendal vein. The glans penis is drained by many large and small veins which are the origin of the deep dorsal vein. The corpus spongiosum is drained by the spongiosal and bulbar veins to the deep dorsal or the internal pudendal veins.

## Haemodynamics

The mechanism of penile erection and its haemodynamics have been controversial. In the early nineteenth century erection was thought to be due to venous occlusion; later it was thought to be a result of increased arterial inflow (Wagner and Uhrenholdt, 1980; Newman and Northup, 1981; Shirai and Ishii, 1981). Conti, (1952) 'polster' theory was based on his work on human cadavers. He showed the existence of cushions or muscular polsters in the afferent and efferent penile vessels and proposed that the relaxation of arterial polsters and the contraction of venous polsters result in erection. A recent histological study suggested that these so-called polsters may represent areas of intimal damage and myoepithelial proliferation, which may be a part of the ageing process (Newman and Tchertkoff, 1980; Benson, McConnell and Schmidt, 1981).

Numerous innovative investigations in animals and humans during the past two decades have finally clarified the haemodynamics of penile erection. The following discussion is a summary of these works.

### Arterial dynamics

In the flaccid state sympathetic influence dominates, the terminal arterioles and sinusoidal smooth muscles are contracted and a minimal amount of blood flows through the sinusoidal spaces mainly for nutritional purposes. This flow through cavernous tissue is estimated to be 2.5–8 ml/min/100 g of tissue (Wagner and Uhrenholdt, 1980). Following sexual stimulation there is a parasympathetic overdrive which decreases the peripheral resistance due to relaxation of the smooth muscle in the terminal arterioles and the trabeculae. This markedly increases the flow into the corpus cavernosum without any change in the systemic blood pressure. The relaxed trabecular smooth musculature markedly increases the compliance of the sinusoids which are then able to retain the incoming blood and cause the elongation, expansion and erection of the penis. When full erection is reached, the flow through the cavernous artery decreases as the intracavernous pressure rises to about 10–20 mmHg below the systolic blood pressure. In the glans and corpus spongiosum, the blood flow continues to be much higher than that of the flaccid state (Newman and Northup, 1981).

### Venous dynamics

Recent research by Wagner, Lue and others (Wagner and Uhrenholdt, 1980; Lue *et al.*, 1983; Fournier *et al.*, 1987; Lue and Tanagho, 1987) has settled some of the controversy regarding the vascular physiology. Our scanning electron microscopic study of canine and simian penile casts showed that in the flaccid state the sinusoids and arterioles are constricted while the subtunical venules flow freely to the emissary veins. During erection the arterioles are dilated, the sinusoids are distended, and the subtunical venules are compressed between the distended sinusoidal wall and the relatively indistensible tunica albuginea, thus effectively reducing the outflow (Figure 2.3a and b) (Lue, 1988). With further engorgement during the rigid phase of erection, the uneven stretching of the layers of the tunica albuginea further closes off most of the emissary veins and changes the corpus cavernosum to an almost completely closed system.

## Phases of penile erection

The state of erection and detumescence can be divided into seven phases (Figure 2.4):

0. Flaccid phase: minimal flow through the cavernous artery to the sinusoids for nutritional purposes. The intracorporeal blood gas values are identical to those of venous blood. Duplex ultrasonography shows an average inner diameter of 0.05 cm in the proximal cavernous artery and peak flow velocity of 15 cm/s or less.
1. Latent or filling phase: the blood flow is highest in this phase. There is increased blood flow through the internal pudendal and cavernous arteries during the systolic and diastolic phases. The penis elongates without change in the intracavernous pressure. In a healthy potent man, the inner diameter of the proximal cavernous artery dilates to 0.1 cm with a peak flow velocity of over 30 cm/s and forceful pulsation of the cavernous arteries.
2. Tumescence phase: the intracavernous pressure increases rapidly and the blood flow starts to decrease. The penis expands and elongates to its maximal capacity. After the intracavernous pressure rises above the diastolic pressure, inflow occurs only during the systolic phase. Duplex ultrasound shows a decreased inner diameter, sharper and shorter systolic wave form and absence of diastolic flow.
3. Full erection phase: the intracavernous pressure becomes steady and reaches about 90% of the systolic pressure. The flow in the pudendal artery is lower than in the tumescence phase, but higher than in the flaccid phase. Duplex ultrasound shows that the systolic wave form is lower than earlier phases with reverse of diastolic wave form. In men with healthy arteries, concentric pulsation with noticeable change of arterial diameter between the systolic and diastolic phases can be seen clearly. Intracavernous blood gases now reach the arterial blood gas values.
4. Rigid or skeletal erection phase: owing to the contraction of the ischiocavernosus muscle, the intracavernous pressure rises well above the systolic pressure, resulting in rigid erection. During this phase there is no inflow of blood. Its short duration due to skeletal muscle fatigue prevents ischaemia and tissue damage.
5. Initial detumescence phase: a small and transient increase of intracavernous pressure is common in the initial detumescence phase. This phase is abolished by clamping of the aorta, yet enhanced by stimulation of the sympathetic trunk, indicating continuing arterial flow as in the full erection phase and beginning smooth muscle contraction against a closed venous system.
6. Slow detumescence phase: this phase is noted by a slow decline of intracavernous pressure indicating slow reopening of the venous channels with decreasing arterial flow. This phase is abolished by sympathetic stimulation.
7. Fast detumescence phase: there is a fast decline

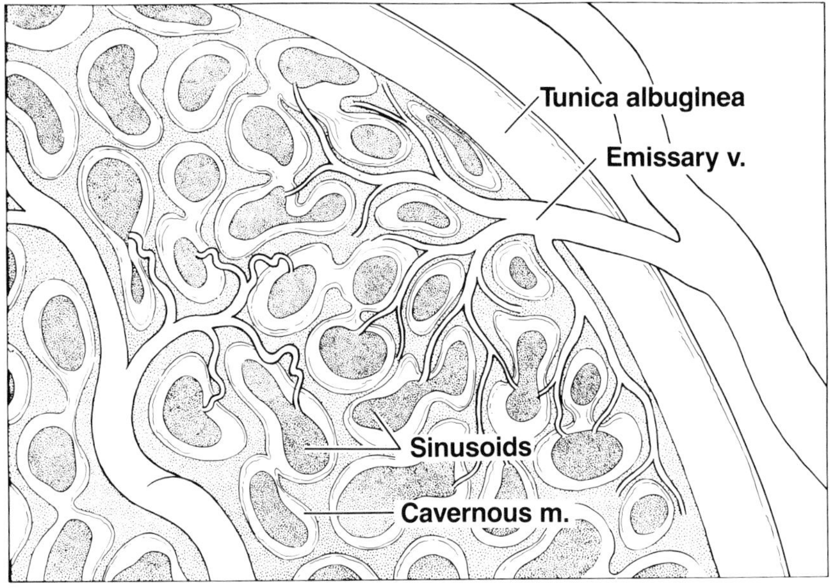


(a)

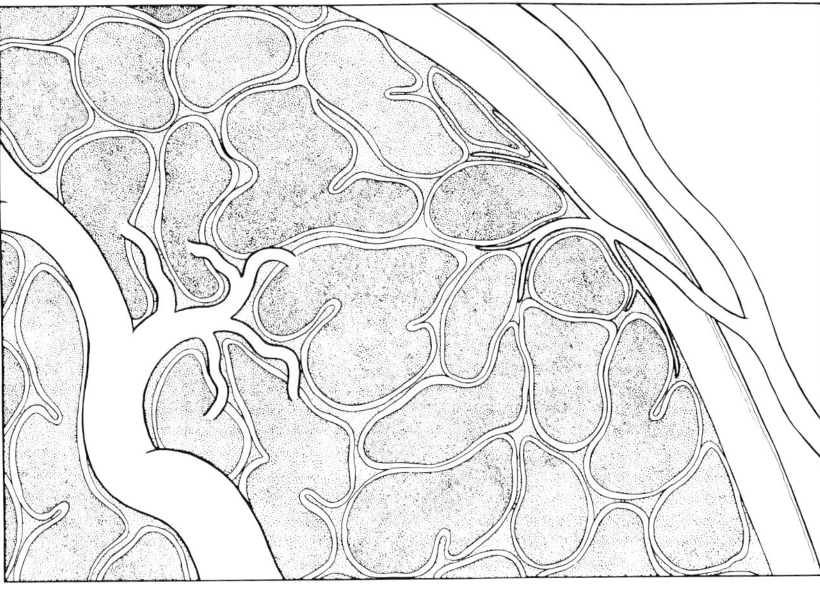

(b)

**Figure 2.3** The mechanism of erection: (a) in the flaccid state the arteries, arterioles and sinusoids are contracted. The intersinusoidal and subtunical venular plexuses are open with free flow to the emissary veins; (b) in the erect state the muscles of the trabeculae and the arterioles relax, allowing maximal flow to fill the non-compliant sinusoidal spaces. The small venules are compressed between the sinusoids. The larger intermediary venules are sandwiched and compressed between the distended sinusoidal wall and the now-compliant tunica albuginea thus restricting the venous flow to a minimum. (Reprinted from Lue (1988) with permission of the publisher)

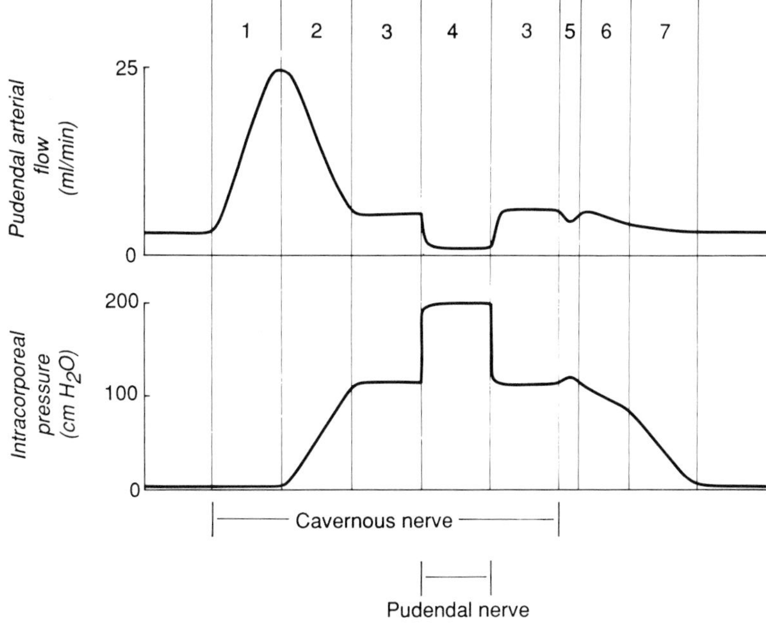


**Figure 2.4** Seven phases of penile erection: (0) flaccid, (1) latent, (2) tumescence, (3) full erection, (4) rigid erection, (5) initial detumescence, (6) slow detumescence and (7) fast detumescence. The upper graph shows the change of the arterial flow in the internal pudendal artery, and the lower graph demonstrates the change of intracavernous pressure during these phases

of intracavernous pressure with fully restored venous outflow capacity. The arterial flow returns to its prestimulation level.

In summary, penile erection is a result of relaxation of the intracorporeal smooth muscle and increases in (1) arterial flow, (2) venous resistance, and (3) compliance of sinusoids, whereas detumescence occurs when these processes are reversed.

## Neurophysiological control of penile vascular events

Various neurological and endocrinological factors in the control of circulatory physiology are described elsewhere in the book. Therefore only a brief summary of the central and peripheral mechanisms responsible for the vascular changes during erection and detumescence will be discussed.

It is generally agreed that sympathetic impulses contract and parasympathetic impulses relax the intracorporeal smooth muscles. However, the precise central and peripheral mechanism and the transmitters are yet to be clarified. The medial preoptic area (MPOA) of the hypothalamus is probably the most important central area involved in penile erection and libido. The spinal T10–12 and S2–4 are responsible for the vascular events of the penis. Various sexual stimuli, e.g. visual, auditory, imaginative and tactile, cause the release of neurotransmitters. In turn, these transmitters relax the intracorporeal smooth muscles and trigger the vascular event of erection. The possible transmitters responsible for erection include prostaglandins, acetylcholine, vasoactive intestinal polypeptide (VIP), calcitonin gene-related peptide (CGRP) (Stief *et al.*, 1990), endothelium-derived relaxing factor (EDRF) and others (de Tejada *et al.*, 1989a, b). The possible detumescence neurotransmitters are noradrenaline, neuropeptide Y and endothelin. A combination of neurotransmitter release and inhibition of the adrenergic influence has also been proposed (Benson, 1983; Willis *et al.*, 1983; Adrian *et al.*, 1984; Steers, McConnell and Benson, 1984; Hedlund and Andersson, 1985; Adaikan, Kottegoda and Ratnam, 1986).

## Alterations in circulatory physiology

The circulation through the penis depends on the integrity of the cavernous tissue, the state of health of the penile vessels, the state of mind and finally the nerve impulses to the penis. These impulses require a healthy brain and spinal cord and intact and properly functioning peripheral nerves. Pathology of any of the above-mentioned systems can result in changes in the blood flow through the penis causing: (1) dysfunction of the tumescence mechanism (erectile impotence); and (2) abnormalities of the detumescence mechanism (priapism).

## Erectile impotence

A variety of diseases are known to cause erectile dysfunction. In some cases the cause and effect association is established and in others it is not. Various processes are known to cause impotence:

1. Psychogenic erectile dysfunction.
2. Neurological disorders.
3. Endocrine disorders.
4. Arterial insufficiency.
5. Venous incompetence.
6. Sinusoidal disorders.
7. Others (iatrogenic, drug-associated causes, etc.).

The psychogenic, neurogenic, endocrinological disorders as well as pharmacological causes of impotence are discussed elsewhere in the book. We will concentrate on the arterial, venous and sinusoidal, as well as traumatic causes that affect the penile circulation leading to erectile dysfuntion.

### Arterial insufficiency

Thrombotic and thromboembolic occlusion at the aortic bifurcation, such as in Leriche's syndrome, results in pain, claudication of the hips and thighs and impotence in men (Leriche and Moral, 1948). Arteriosclerosis, fibrosis, calcification, obliteration and injury of the aortoiliac and pudendal vessels decrease blood flow through the penile arteries and result in erectile dysfunction. Penile arterial insufficiency is also frequently seen in patients with diabetes mellitus. Pelvic steal syndrome is seen in large vessel arteriosclerosis in the pelvis (Michal, Kramer and Popsichal, 1978; Goldstein, 1987) due to diversion of blood from the internal to the external iliac arteries associated with increased pelvic muscle activity; erection is achieved but cannot be sustained during intercourse.

### Venous incompetence and sinusoidal disorders

The venous occlusion mechanism depends on: (1) a normal tunica albuginea; (2) compliant trabeculae (a normal smooth muscle:collagen ratio); (3) intact neuromuscular function; and (4) normal endothelial function. Therefore, venous incompetence can result from dysfunction of any of the above factors such as a thin tunica, a tunical defect (penile fracture, shunting procedure for priapism), replacement of smooth muscle by fibrotic tissue (scleroderma, priapism), smooth muscle atrophy (diabetes, atherosclerosis), insufficient neurotransmitter release (neurological disorder, psychogenic inhibition, alcoholism, cigarette smoking) and poor function of the endothelial cells in diabetes and atherosclerosis (de Tejada *et al.*, 1989b). Our recent electron microscopic study of the human cavernous erectile tissue shows a good correlation of vascular insufficiency (by Duplex ultrasonography) with disorders of the cavernous erectile tissues (Persson *et al.*, 1989).

### Surgical and traumatic causes

Various surgical procedures such as transplant surgery, vascular surgery, radical pelvic surgery, surgery for priapism and pelvic irradiation are known to cause changes in the circulation to the penis leading to erectile dysfunction. Trauma to the lower urinary tract causes impotence in a high percentage of cases. For instance, the incidence of impotence in patients with a fractured pelvis with multisystem injury may be 50%. Walsh and Donker (1982) concluded that impotence can result from injury to autonomic innervation of the corpora cavernosa, most commonly during dissection of the prostatic apex and division of the urethra.

Renal transplantation may cause impotence if a second contralateral transplant is performed with an end-to-side anastomosis (Gittes and Waters, 1979). A similar situation may occur when both hypogastric arteries are ligated during a radical pelvic procedure.

The reported incidence of impotence after external beam irradiation to the pelvis in patients with prostatic malignancy is 22–84% (Bagshaw *et al.*, 1975).

## Abnormalities of the detumescence mechanism (priapism)

Alteration in the circulatory physiology can result in priapism. We propose that any erection that persists beyond 4–6 h be considered priapism. Priapism can be classified into spontaneous versus iatrogenic and ischaemic versus non-ischaemic as determined by intracavernous blood gas analysis (Lue *et al.*, 1986).

Pohl, Pott and Kleihans (1986), in their review of the world literature found that about one-third of all cases were idiopathic and 21% were related to drug or alcohol abuse. Other causes included perineal trauma (12%), sickle cell disease (11%) and inflammatory disorders of the urogenital tract (8%). However, the aetiological distribution varies with geography and age in various reports.

Based on our current knowledge, the cause of priapism appears to be in the detumescence mechanism owing to vascular or neurological dysfunction. This impairment can result from any of the following causes:

1. Thromboembolic factors: sickle cell disease or trait, leukaemia, anticoagulant therapy, penile trauma, neoplasm of the penis, haematological disorders and local inflammatory diseases.
2. Neurogenic factors: many CNS and spinal cord disorders, diabetic autonomic neuropathy and sexual overactivity. Impairment of the detumescence mechanism results in persistent closure of the veins and low-flow priapism.
3. Oral medications and chemicals: trazodone, chlorpromazine, alcohol and other drugs affect the tumescence and detumescence mechanisms centrally and peripherally.
4. Intracavernous vasoactive agents: papaverine (Virag, 1982), phenoxybenzamine (Brindley, 1983), phentolamine with papaverine (Zorgniotti and Lefleur, 1985), prostaglandin $E_1$ (Stackl, Hasun and Marberger, 1988) and other vasodilators are known to cause erection in man when injected into the corpus cavernosum. In high doses they effectively paralyse all the smooth muscle in the corpora cavernosa, thus blocking the drainage venules. If the patient's own detumescence mechanism cannot override these effects, priapism will result.

The changes in the corporeal tissue are progressive, depending on the pre-existing penile haemodynamics. Some patients completely regain erectile function after resolution of the priapism, while many do not. The outcome is determined by (1) the penile circulation before the event; (2) the duration of the ischaemia; and (3) the remaining penile circulation and erectile tissue. Younger petients have a better prognosis as far as potency is concerned (Pohl, Pott and Kleihans, 1986).

Spycher and Hauri (1986), in their ultrastructural and histological studies of tissue in high-flow priapism, found no discernible histological changes. On the other hand, in low-flow priapism the first reaction is trabecular interstitial oedema. About 12 h after onset, only a few minor cavernosal endothelial defects could be seen without evidence of smooth muscle damage. After 24–48 h, destruction of the endothelial tissue and exposure of the basement membrane were widespread, with subsequent thrombocyte adherence. Necrosis of smooth muscle cells was observed. When priapism persisted for more than 48 h, microthrombi were found in most of the sinusoidal spaces with destruction of the endothelial lining. The tissue is infiltrated by inflammatory cells with associated destruction of the smooth muscle and replacement by fibroblasts. In the end, the nerve fibres and their varicosities and capillaries are also destroyed by this prolonged ischaemia. After some days to weeks, fibrosis starts to take place (Hinman, 1960).

In conclusion, penile erection involves psychological, neurological, hormonal, arterial, venous and sinusoidal factors. The haemodynamics and anatomical mechanism of erection and detumescence have been clarified: relaxation of the intracorporeal smooth muscle from sexual stimulation results in sinusoidal relaxation, arterial dilation and venous compression culminating in penile erection. Cessation of sexual stimulation causes contraction of the smooth muscle and reverses the vascular events. Continuing research in the pathophysiology is urgently needed to improve the diagnosis and treatment of vasculogenic impotence.

## References

Adaikan, P. G., Kottegoda, S. R. and Ratnam, S. S. (1986) Is vasoactive intestinal polypeptide the principal transmitter involved in human penile erection? *Journal of Urology*, **135**, 638

Adrian, T. E., Gu, J., Allen, J. M. *et al.* (1984) Neuropeptide Y in the human genital tract. *Life Sciences*, **35**, 2643

Bagshaw, M.A., Ray, G. R., Pistenma, D. A. *et al.* (1975) External beam radiation therapy of primary carcinoma of prostate. *Cancer*, **36**, 723

Benson, G. S. (1983) Penile erection: in search of a neurotransmitter. *World Journal of Urology*, **1**, 209

Benson, G. S., McConnell, J. A. and Schmidt, W. A. (1981) Penile polsters: functional structures or atherosclerotic changes? *Journal of Urology*, **125**, 800

Breza, J., Aboseif, S. R., Orvis, B. R. *et al.* (1989) Detailed anatomy of penile neurovascular structures: surgical significance. *Journal of Urology*, **141**, 437–443

Brindley, G. S. (1983) Cavernosal alpha-blockade: a new technique for investigating and treating erectile impotence. *British Journal of Psychiatry*, **143**, 332

Conti, G. (1952) L'erection du penis humain et ses bases morphologico-vasculaires. *Acta Anatomica*, **14**, 217

de Tejada, I. S., Carson, M. P., Tarish, A. *et al.* (1989a) Role of endothelin in the local control of penile smooth muscle tone (Abstract). *Journal of Vascular Medicine and Biology*, **1**, 112

de Tejada, I. S., Goldstein, I., Azadzoi, K. *et al.* (1989b) Impaired neurogenic and endothelium-mediated relaxation of penile smooth muscle from diabetic men with impotence. *New England Journal of Medicine*, **320**, 1025–1030

Fournier, G. R. Jr., Juenemann, K. P., Lue, T. F. and Tanagho, E. A. (1987) Mechanism of venous occlusion during canine penile erection: anatomic demonstration. *Journal of Urology*, **137**, 163

Gittes, R. F. and Waters, W. B. (1979) Sexual impotence: the overlooked complication of a second renal transplant. *Journal of Urology*, **121**, 719

Goldstein, I. (1987) Vasculogenic impotence: its diagnosis and treatment. In *Problems in Urology: Sexual Function* (ed. R. M. de Vere White), J. B. Lippincott, Philadelphia, pp. 547–563

Goldstein, A. M. B., Meehan, J. P., Zakhary, R. *et al.*

(1982) New observations on the microarchitecture of the corpora cavernosa in man and possible relationship to mechanism of erection. *Urology*, **20**, 259–266

Hedlund, H. and Andersson, K. E. (1985) Contraction and relaxation induced by some prostanoids in isolated human penile erectile tissue and cavernous artery. *Journal of Urology*, **134**, 1245

Hinman, F. Jr. (1960) Priapism, reasons for failure. *Journal of Urology*, **83**, 420

Leriche, A. and Moral, A. (1948) Syndrome of thrombotic obliteration of aortic bifurcation. *Annals of Surgery*, **127**, 193

Lue, T. F. (1988) Male sexual dysfunction. In *Smith's General Urology*, 12th edn (eds. E. A. Tanagho and J. W. McAninch), Appleton and Lange, Norwalk, Conneticut, pp. 663–678

Lue, T. F., Hellstrom, W., McAninch, J. W. and Tanagho, E. A. (1986) Priapism: a refined approach to diagnosis and treatment *Journal of Urology*, **136**, 104

Lue, T. F., Takamura, T., Schmidt, R. A. *et al.* (1983) Hemodynamics of erection in the monkey. *Journal of Urology*, **130**, 1237–1241

Lue, T. F. and Tanagho, E. A. (1987) Physiology of erection and pharmacological management of impotence. *Journal of Urology*, **137**, 829

Lue, T. F. and Tanagho, E. A. (1988) Functional anatomy and mechanism of penile erection. In *Contemporary Management of Impotence and Infertility*, (eds E. A. Tanagho, T. F. Lue and R. D. McClure), Williams and Wilkins, Baltimore, pp. 39–50

Michal, V., Kramer, R. and Popsichal, J. (1978) External iliac steal syndrome. *Journal of Cardiovascular Surgery*, **19**, 255

Newman, H. F. and Northup, J. D. (1981) Mechanism of human penile erection: an overview. *Urology*, **17**, 399

Newman, H.F. and Tchertkoff, V. (1980) Penile vascular cushions and erection. *Investigative Urology*, **18**, 43

Persson, C., Lue, T. F., Yen, S. B. and Tanagho, E. A. (1989) Correlation of altered penile ultrastructure with clinical arterial evaluation. *Journal of Urology*, **142**, 1462–1468

Pohl, J., Pott, B. and Kleihans, G. (1986) Priapism: a three-phase concept of management according to aetiology and prognosis. *British Journal of Urology*, **58**, 113–118

Shirai, M. and Ishii, N. (1981) Hemodynamics of erection in man. *Archives of Andrology*, **6**, 27

Spycher, M.A. and Hauri, D. (1986) The ultrastructure of the erectile tissue in priapism. *Journal of Urology*, **135**, 142–147

Stackl, W., Hasun, R. and Marberger, M. (1988) Intracavernous injection of prostaglandin $E_1$ in impotent men. *Journal of Urology* **140**, 66–68

Steers, W. D., McConnell, J. and Benson, G. S. (1984) Anatomical localization and some pharmacological effects of vasoactive intestinal polypeptide in human and monkey corpus cavernosum. *Journal of Urology*, **132**, 1048

Stief, C. G., Benard, F., Bosch, R. J. L. H. *et al.* (1990) A possible role for calcitonin-gene-related peptide in the regulation of the smooth muscle tone of the bladder and penis. *Journal of Urology*, **143**, 392–397

Virag, R. (1982) Intracavernous injection of papaverine for erectile failure. *Lancet*, **ii**, 938

Wagner, G. and Uhrenholdt, A. (1980) Blood flow measurement by the clearance methods in the human corpus cavernosum in the flaccid and erect states. In *Vasculogenic Impotence* (Proceedings of the First International Conference on the Corpus Cavernosum Revascularization) (eds. A. W. Zorgniotti and G. Rossi) Charles C. Thomas, Springfield, Illinois, pp. 41–46

Walsh, P. C. and Donker, P. (1982) Impotence following radical prostatectomy: insight into etiology and prevention. *Journal of Urology*, **128**, 492–497

Willis, E. A., Ottesen, B., Wagner, G. *et al.* (1983) Vasoactive intestinal polypeptide (VIP) as a putative neurotransmitter in penile erection. *Life Sciences*, **33**, 383

Zorgniotti, A. W. and Lefleur, R. S. (1985) Autoinjection of the corpus cavernosum with a vasoactive drug combination for vasculogenic impotence. *Journal of Urology*, **133**, 39

# 3

# Neurophysiology

**G. S. Brindley**

## Peripheral nervous pathways

### Parasympathetic erectile

The classic erectile pathway is that discovered by Eckhardt (1863) in the dog. Eckhardt found that on the rostromedial surface of the levator ani muscle there runs a nerve or plexus (nervus erigens, pelvic nerve, pelvic splanchnic nerve), electrical stimulation of which causes erection. This was later found to hold for many other mammalin species, and it was shown that the erectile nerve fibres of the nervus erigens are in sacral anterior roots, their cells of origin lying in the corresponding segments of the spinal cord, probably in the intermediolateral cell column. The segments of origin vary from species to species, but are always sacral. In man the principal erectile root is usually S2 but sometimes S3 (Brindley *et al.*, 1986).

This classic erectile pathway belongs to the parasympathetic system and has (at least mainly) the usual anatomical properties of that system: small myelinated preganglionic fibres, a ganglionic relay close to the target organ, and unmyelinated postganglionic fibres. Pharmacologically, however, it is unusual. Most other parasympathetic pathways have acetylcholine as their postganglionic transmitter and are blocked by atropine, but erection is unaffected by large doses of atropine in all mammals that have been studied. The atropine resistance is shown by psychogenic and reflex erection in man, and equally by erections driven by electrical stimualtion of the nervi erigentes in other species (Henderson and Roepke, 1933; Sjöstrand and Klinge, 1979; Wagner and Brindley, 1980; Carati, Creed and Keogh, 1987). The postganglionic transmitter for erection is unknown. It may be vasoactive intestinal polypeptide (Polak *et al.*, 1981), but this is unproven (Andersson, Bloom and Mellander, 1984).

### Sympathetic erectile

There is evidence that the hypogastric plexus contains, at least in the rabbit, cat and man, efferent nerve fibres, impulses in which cause erection or partial erection. For the rabbit (Sjöstrand and Klinge, 1979) the existence of such fibres is certain: electrical stimulation of the hypogastric plexus, cut centrally, consistently causes erection. For man (Brindley, Sauerwein and Hendry, 1989) the evidence is almost as clear: electrical stimulation of the intact hypogastric plexus by a surgically implanted device consistently causes full erection in two of nine patients who have such implants, and conspicuous swelling of the penis in the other seven. The alternative hypothesis that this effect could be reflex is very unlikely since, in those patients in whom the relevant sensory pathways survive, the stimulation causes abdominal pain and no genital sensation whatever.

Lesions of the hypogastric plexus, though they regularly cause failure of ejaculation, do not usually cause complete erectile impotence. It thus seems that when the sympathetic erectile pathway is lost, the parasympathetic alone may suffice for erectile function. The reverse situation – loss of the parasympathetic erectile pathway with survival of the sympathetic – is seen in men with complete lesions of the cauda equina or conus medullaris. Many such men, though not all, are capable of full erection.

### Sympathetic anti-erectile

For this pathway also, the clearest evidence comes from the experiments of Sjöstrand and Klinge on rabbits. Electrical stimulation of the lowest parts of the sympathetic trunks in the rabbit causes shrinkage of the penis, even if all connections of these sympathetic trunks with the central nervous system are cut.

In man, the only evidence for an anti-erectile nervous pathway comes from experiments on the action of drugs given by intracavernosal injection. This evidence (Brindley, 1986) makes it almost certain that man, like the rabbit, has an anti-erectile nervous pathway which is continuously active when the penis is flaccid. The peripheral endings of this pathway release noradrenaline, which acts on α-adrenoceptors on smooth muscle cells. Nothing is known about the anatomy of the pathway, but it is likely to be roughly similar to its counterpart in the rabbit.

## Central mechanisms

Animal experiments provide little information about these; our knowledge comes mainly from observations on patients with anatomically well-defined lesions of the central nervous system.

### Reflex erection

This is seen in pure form in men with complete transections of the spinal cord at levels above T9. In these men, sexual thoughts have no influence on the penis, but in most of them erection occurs if the penis is stimulated mechanically. Though the penis is the chief receptive field, stimulation of other skin areas often modifies the response to penile stimulation and may sometimes cause erection in the absence of penile stimulation.

Mechanical stimulation of the penis in the complete absence of sexual thoughts (for example, while solving arithmetical problems) causes erection in some neurologically intact men, but not in the majority. However, in nearly all men sexual thoughts cause erection more easily and more quickly if the penis is stimulated mechanically at the same time than if it is not. It seems that the erection reflex that is consistently present after high transection of the spinal cord is partly or wholly inhibited in intact men when thoughts are non-sexual. One of the effects of sexual thoughts is to release the reflex from this inhibition.

Reflex erection can be mediated by the sacral cord and parasympathetic pathway alone. The proof of this is that it occurs in a minority of patients with complete transections of the spinal cord at lumbar segmental levels. In the majority of such patients there is no reflex erection, probably because of ischaemic damage to the isolated sacral segments of the cord, but its occurrence in a minority proves that the mechanism exists. It is not known whether, in men with thoracic or cervical cord lesions or in neurologically intact men, reflex erection uses the sympathetic pathways in addition to the parasympathetic.

It would be natural to suppose that the peripheral afferent pathways for reflex erection are the same as those involved in erotically coloured genital sensations. It seems that impulses in some sensory fibres from the penis (for example, those that end in the skin of the shaft) are not perceived as erotically coloured except by learned association, whereas impulses in other sensory fibres (for example, those fibres that respond to stretching of the fraenum, and those that are well excited by vibrations in the range 40–80 Hz) usually cause sensations with an erotic element, which seem not to require learning.

This natural supposition gains some support from the similarity in the masturbatory techniques that paraplegic men find effective in causing reflex erection and that neurologically intact men find pleasant. There is a related similarity in favourable vibrator frequencies: frequencies between 40 and 70 Hz are perceived by neurologically intact men as pleasant, and frequencies between 90 and 140 Hz as unpleasant. In men with complete transections of the spinal cord, a vibrator running at 40–70 Hz will usually cause erection and one running at 90–140 Hz will usually fail.

### Sleep erection

Sleep erection occurs in nearly all men during about a third of the time spent asleep, chiefly during the phases with rapid eye movements and relatively high dominant frequencies in the electroencephalogram. It is often called 'nocturnal penile tumescence', a bad name because the erections occur as much in the daytime sleep as in night-time sleep, and the penis is not tumescent (becoming swollen) but tumid (swollen, and in most men fully stiff). It is not known whether sleep erection uses both the parasympathetic and the sympathetic pathways or only one of these. Its mechanisms within the brain and spinal cord are entirely unknown.

### Psychogenic erection

Psychogenic erection i.e. erection resulting from sexual thoughts, occurs in nearly all young neurologically intact men. In some men without any known disease of the central nervous system it becomes inefficient or even disappears altogether as they become older, sleep erection remaining intact. Such erectile impotence is commonly ascribed to psychological causes. In some cases this may be correct, but it should not be assumed dogmatically. The normal sleep erections of these men prove that their peripheral mechanisms, both neural and vascular, are intact, but do not prove the absence of a relevant organic disorder within the central nervous system. The central mechanisms must be different for sleep erection and psychogenic erection, so it is possible that genetic, toxic or infective factors could damage the central mechanisms by which sexual thoughts cause erection, and yet cause no impairment of sleep erection.

Psychogenic erection can certainly use the sympathetic erectile pathway. The proof is that many men with complete lesions of the cauda equina or conus medullaris have intact psychogenic erection, despite complete loss of penile sensation and reflex erection (Comarr, 1979). Almost certainly psychogenic erection can also use the parasympathetic pathway. The evidence is that some men retain good psychogenic erection after radical sympathectomy (Whitelaw and Smithwick, 1951) or after lesions of the hypogastric plexus that appear to be complete, in that they cause complete failure of ejaculation. This evidence is not absolutely compelling, because of the difficulty of proving that the sympathetic lesions are complete.

It is noteworthy that though a complete parasympathetic lesion or a probably complete sympathetic lesion may leave psychogenic erection intact, more commonly such lesions impair it. Though psychological factors may contribute to this impairment, and may diminish with time, it would be rash to assume for any man that his erectile performance can be as good with only one erectile pathway as with both.

## Central nervous structures concerned in erection

The course of the spinal tracts concerned in sexual responses can in principle be investigated by studying patients with incomplete cord lesions. The best studied lesions are bilateral anterolateral cordotomies done, usually at an upper thoracic level, for the relief of pain. After these operations many patients say that they have lost erection and ejaculation. Some, however, retain erection and ejaculation but lose the orgasmic sensations that should accompany ejaculation, and probably also the lesser erotic sensations that ordinarily accompany erection (Foerster and Gagel, 1932; White and Sweet, 1969). The tactile threshold of the penis is unchanged and so, probably, are two-point discrimination and the ability to detect vibration.

From these observations and from analogous ones on women there seems to be little doubt that the afferent pathway for erotically coloured genital sensations in both sexes runs with or close to the spinothalamic pathways for pain and temperature, at least at the upper thoracic level. It is unknown whether the downgoing pathways for psychogenic erection are interrupted by anterolateral cordotomy. We can suppose that they run in other parts of the cord and are spared in anterolateral cordotomy; the loss of erection that many cordotomized men report would on that supposition be a consequence of the loss of erotic sensations. Alternatively, we can suppose that they are interrupted; on this supposition the preserved erection that a minority of cordotomized men report must be reflex in nature.

The sexual responses of men with incomplete spinal injuries have been described in several publications, but the responses have not been correlated with the kind of incompleteness of the lesion. We are still very ignorant of the course of the tracts involved.

Within the brain many sites have been found at which electrical stimulation causes erection in the unanaesthetized monkey (Robinson and Mishkin, 1968). Regions that are often effective include the anterior part of the cingulate gyrus, preoptic region, lateral hypothalamus and tegmentum. In these regions ineffective sites are found, mixed up among the effective ones. Regions of the brain that are consistently ineffective include the hippocampus, fornix, mammillary bodies, posterior cingulate gyrus, caudate nucleus, ansa lenticularis and the genital receiving area of the post-central gyrus. In man, among the many published accounts of effects of stimulation in the course of stereotaxic operations under local anaesthesia, no report has been found of erection being produced; although reference 24 of Weiss (1972) is said to be such a report, it is not. Sem-Jacobsen (1966) states definitely that in 429 electrode placements near the third ventricle in 82 patients, the responses to electrical stimulation, though they included movements, changes in tremor or rigidity, speech arrest, sensations of many kinds, mood changes, loss of consciousness and cardiovascular effects, were never sexual.

Genital sensations can be produced by electrical stimulation of the upper end of the post-central gyrus, but these sensations are not erotically coloured, according to Penfield and Jasper (1954).

There is one clear and convincing report of lasting impotence produced, similarly in two patients, by a small destructive surgical procedure in the brain (Meyers, 1962). The purpose of the operation was to cut the ansa lenticularis by an open procedure from the third ventricle. The approach was through the corpus callosum, and a piece of the fornix was sacrificed bilaterally to gain access to the third ventricle. Lesions of the corpus callosum and of the fornix have not caused impotence in other patients, nor have stereotaxic lesions that were intended to interrupt the ansa lenticularis bilaterally. Probably the impotence in the two patients of Meyers depended on damage to some neighbouring structure, but we have little knowledge to help us speculate on what structure it was.

## The pharmacology of central mechanisms of erection

Many drugs have a reputation for causing erectile impotence as a side effect (Barnes, 1984). Noteworthy among these are the antihypertensive drugs propranolol, labetolol and nifedipine, for all of which a small anti-erectile action of single doses has been confirmed in double-blind experiments on a normal volunteer. The same double-blind experiments show anti-erectile actions of the amine re-uptake blockers desipramine and clomipramine and the α-adrenoceptor agonist ephedrine. Desipramine and ephedrine are much more powerful inhibitors of erection than the antihypertensives. It is not entirely clear whether these six drugs, and the many other drugs for which anti-erectile actions are strongly suspected, act locally on the penis and its blood vessels or on the central nervous system, but some at least of their actions must surely be on the central nervous system, since if given by intracavernosal injection propranolol has no detectable effect on the penis, and the effects of α-adrenoceptor blockers (including labetolol) and α-adrenoceptor agonists (like ephedrine) are opposite, the former swelling the penis and the latter shrinking it (Brindley, 1986).

A few drugs are known to improve erectile function. They belong to three groups: dopamine agonists (apomorphine (Lal *et al.*, 1984), bromocriptine); α-adrenoceptor blockers (yohimbine, idazoxan); and cholinesterase inhibitors (physostigmine, neostigmine, the latter only if given intrathecally).

The relevant actions of all of these must be on the central nervous system, since at least one member of each group has been shown to be ineffective when given intracavernosally. The cholinesterase inhibitors certainly facilitate erectile mechanisms (and more conspicuously ejaculatory mechanisms) in the spinal cord, as is proved by their effectiveness in men with complete transections of the spinal cord at mid-thoracic and higher levels (Chapelle, 1984). The proven action on the spinal cord does not exclude the possibility that they may activate erectile and/or ejaculatory mechanisms in the brain also.

The rapid metabolic alteration of yohimbine in the body (Owen *et al.*, 1987) contrasts with its (in part) slowly cumulative action in improving erectile response (Morales *et al.*, 1987). The products of its metabolism therefore deserve pharmacological investigation.

The dopamine agonists and cholinesterase inhibitors are useless in treating erectile impotence, because the emetic dose exceeds the sexually helpful dose only very slightly, and sometimes not at all. The α-adrenoceptor blocker yohimbine is used to treat erectile impotence. Its action has been proved to be real (Morales *et al.*, 1987) but is not large, and it is doubtful whether very many impotent men are sufficiently helped to justify their taking it.

All the above pharmacological observations are likely to be clues that will help in answering scientific questions about the central mechanisms of erection. But at present, like the observations on effects of brain and spinal cord lesions on erectile performance in men and those on erection produced by deep brain stimulation in animals, they do not fit together to make a useful picture of what the brain and spinal cord are doing when the penis becomes erect.

## References

Andersson, P. O., Bloom, S. R. and Mellander, S. (1984) Haemodynamics of pelvic nerve induced penile erection in the dog: possible mediation by vasoactive intestinal polypeptide. *Journal of Physiology*, **350**, 209–224

Barnes, T. R. E. (1984) Drugs and sexual dysfunction. In *Current Themes in Psychiatry*, Vol. 3 (ed. R. N. Gaind), Spectrum, London, pp. 51–92

Brindley, G. S. (1986) Pilot experiments on the actions of drugs injected into the human corpus cavernosum penis. *British Journal of Pharmacology*, **87**, 495–500

Brindley, G. S., Polkey, C. E., Rushton, D. N. and Cardozo, L. (1986) Sacral anterior root stimulators for bladder control in paraplegia: the first 50 cases. *Journal of Neurology, Neurosurgery and Psychiatry*, **49**, 1104–1114

Brindley, G. S., Sauerwein, D. and Hendry, W. H. (1989) Hypogastric stimulators for obtaining semen from paraplegic men. *British Journal of Urology*, **64**, 72–77

Carati, C. J., Creed, K. E. and Keogh, E. J. (1987) Autonomic control of penile erection in the dog. *Journal of Physiology*, **384**, 525–538

Chapelle, P. A. (1984) Traitement de l'anéjaculation du paraplégique complet par association métoclopramide-ésérine. In *L'Ejaculation et ses Perturbations* (ed. J. Buvat and P. Jouannet), Simep, Lyon, pp. 54–55

Comarr, A. E. (1979) Sexual function among patients with spinal cord injury. *Urologia Internationalis*, **23**, 134–168

Eckhardt, C. (1863) Untersuchungen über die Erection des Penis beim Hunde. *Beiträge zur Anatomie und Physiologie*, **3**, 123–166

Foerster, O. and Gagel, O. (1932) Die Vorderseitenstrangdurchschneidung beim Menschen. *Zeitschrift für die Gesamte Neurologie und Psychiatrie*, **138**, 1–92

Henderson, V. E. and Roepke, M. H. (1933) On the mechanism of erection. *American Journal of Physiology*, **106**, 441–448

Lal, S., Ackman, D., Thavundayil, J. X. *et al.* (1984) Effect of apormorphine, a dopamine receptor agonist, on penile tumescence in normal subjects. *Progress in Neuropsychopharmacology and Biological Psychiatry*, **11**, 235–242

Meyers, R. (1962) Three cases of myoclonus alleviated by bilateral ansotomy, with a note on postoperative alibido and impotence. *Journal of Neurosurgery*, **19**, 71–81

Morales, A., Condra, M., Owen, J. A. *et al.* (1987) Is yohimbine effective in the treatment of erectile impotence? Results of a controlled trial. *Journal of Urology*, **137**, 1168–1172

Owen, J. A., Nakatsu, S. L., Fenemore, J. *et al.* (1987) The pharmacokinetics of yohimbine in man. *European Journal of Clinical Pharmacology*, **32**, 577–582

Penfield, W. and Jasper, H. (1954) *Epilepsy and the Functional Anatomy of the Human Brain*, Churchill, London.

Polak, J. M., Gu, J., Mina, S. and Bloom, S. R. (1981) Vipergic nerves in the penis. *Lancet*, **ii**, 217–219

Robinson, B. W. and Mishkin, M. (1968) Penile erection

evoked from forebrain structures in *Macaca mulatta*. *Archives of Neurology*, **19**, 184–198

Sem-Jacobsen, C. W. (1966) Depth-electrographic observations relating to Parkinson's disease. *Journal of Neurosurgery*, **24**, 388–402

Sjöstrand, N. O. and Klinge, E. (1979) Principal mechanisms controlling penile retraction and protrusion in rabbits. *Acta Physiologica Scandinavica*, **106**, 199–214

Wagner, G. and Brindley, G. A. (1980) Effect of atropine and alpha- and beta-blockers on human penile erection. In *Vasculogenic Impotence* (eds. A. Zorgniotti and G. Rossi), Thomas, Springfield, Illinois, pp. 77–82

Weiss, H. D. (1972) The physiology of human penile erection. *Archives of Internal Medicine*, **76**, 793–799

White, J. C. and Sweet, W. H. (1969) *Pain and the Neurosurgeon: A Forty-year Experience*, Thomas, Springfield, Illinois

Whitelaw, G. P. and Smithwick, R. H. (1951) Some secondary effects of sypathectomy. *New England Journal of Medicine*, **245**, 121

# 4

# Pharmacology

K.-E. Andersson, H. Hedlund and F. Holmquist

## Current concepts of penile erection

In order to understand better the possible mechanisms which are the targets for drugs interfering with penile erectile function, a brief description of current concepts of penile erection is given below.

Local sensory stimulation of the genital organs may lead to penile erection (reflexogenic erection). Erection can also be a consequence of central psychogenic stimuli received by or generated within the brain (psychogenic erection). The mechanisms probably act synergistically (de Groat and Steers, 1988). In the detumescent state, penile smooth muscle is kept contracted, probably by release of noradrenaline (NA) acting on postjunctional α-adrenoceptors on the cavernous and helicine arteries, and on trabecular smooth muscle. A contribution of myogenic activity and additional contractant factors cannot be excluded. According to current concepts (Lue and Tanagho, 1987; Krane, Goldstein and de Tejada, 1989) erection follows when the sinusoids and the cavernosal and helicinal arteries dilate with subsequent increase in blood flow to the lacunar spaces of the corpora cavernosa. It is believed that this is achieved partly by a decrease in NA-mediated tone, but also through the release of relaxing non-adrenergic, non-cholinergic transmitter(s) from nerves and from the endothelium. As the trabecular smooth muscle relaxes, the sinusoids will be filled with blood and compress the plexus of subtunical venules against the tunica albuginea. This 'veno-occlusive mechanism' reduces venous outflow from the lacunar spaces, increases the pressure within the corpora and makes the penis rigid. When the penile erectile tissue resumes its contractile state, detumescence is produced. Thus, as tone of the helicine arteries and the trabeculae is increased, arterial inflow is reduced, the pressure within the lacunar spaces decreases, venous outflow increases, and the penis becomes flaccid.

## Mechanisms for contraction and relaxation of penile erectile tissue

The detailed mechanisms for keeping the penis in the flaccid state and for producing relaxation of the cavernosal and helicine arteries and the trabeculae, are still largely unknown. However, several local factors are known to cause contraction or relaxation of penile vessels and trabecular smooth muscle. The investigation of these factors may produce information of both diagnostic and therapeutic importance.

### Adrenoceptor functions

#### α-adrenoceptors

In isolated human penile erectile tissue, NA produces concentration-dependent contractions (Benson *et al.*, 1980; Adaikan and Karim, 1981; Andersson *et al.*, 1983; Hedlund *et al.*, 1984; Hedlund and Andersson, 1985a; Kimura *et al.*, 1989; Kirkeby *et al.*, 1989a). Phenylephrine, which is selective for $\alpha_1$-adrenoceptors, and clonidine, which has a preference for $\alpha_2$-adrenoceptors, both contract trabecular tissue. Clonidine was found to be less potent and to have less intrinsic activity than phenylephrine and NA (Hedlund, Andersson and Mattiasson, 1984; Hedlund and Andersson, 1985a; Kimura *et al.*, 1989). In segments of the cavernosal artery, clonidine was the more potent contractile agent. The $\alpha_1$-adrenoceptor blocker prazosin, but not rauwolscine, selective for $\alpha_2$-adrenoceptors, effectively counteracted contractions induced by NA. In cavernosal artery segments, prazosin and rauwolscine were about equieffective for relaxation of NA-induced contractions (Hedlund and Andersson, 1985a). Prazosin was more potent than rauwolscine for inhibition of contractions evoked by electrical stimulation of nerves in trabecular tissue (Hedlund and Andersson, 1985a; de Tejada *et al.*,

1989a), but in arterial segments rauwolscine was more potent than prazosin (Hedlund and Andersson, 1985a). These findings suggested a difference between the postjunctional α-adrenoceptors in the trabecular tissue and in the cavernosal artery: $\alpha_1$-adrenoceptors predominating in the former, and $\alpha_2$-adrenoceptors in the latter (Hedlund and Andersson, 1985a).

The importance of α-adrenoceptors in penile erection has been demonstrated by several investigators showing that intracavernosal injection of α-adrenoceptor blockers (phenoxybenzamine, phentolamine, thymoxamine) may cause tumescence and erection (Brindley, 1983, 1986; Blum *et al.*, 1985; Buvat *et al.*, 1989), and that α-adrenoceptor agonists (metaraminol) given by the same route cause detumescence (Brindley, 1984; de Meyer and De Sy, 1986). Brindley (1986) found that intracavernosal injection of the selective $\alpha_2$-adrenoceptor blocker idazoxan had no effect, supporting the view that the $\alpha_1$-adrenoceptor is the functionally dominant subtype.

### β-adrenoceptors

Adaikan and Karim (1981) demonstrated relaxant effects of the β-adrenoceptor agonists isoprenaline and salbutamol in isolated human corpus cavernosum. The functional data of Hedlund and Andersson (1985a) and the radioligand binding studies of Dhabuwala, Ramakrishna and Anderson (1985) strongly suggest that the β-adrenoceptors of the human corpus cavernosum are of $\beta_2$-type. In isolated segments of the cavernosal artery, isoprenaline had no contractant or relaxant effect (Hedlund and Andersson, 1985a).

The role of β-adrenoceptors in human penile erection is unclear and disputed. Since the density of β-adrenoceptors was found to be only one-tenth of the density of α-adrenoceptors in human penile tissue (Levin and Wein, 1980), the physiological role of β-adrenoceptors within the corpora seems to be minor. Supporting this, Brindley (1986) found that salbutamol caused tumidity but no erection, and that the β-adrenoceptor antagonist propranolol had no effects when injected intracavernosally.

## Muscarinic receptor functions

Acetylcholinesterase positive nerve fibres have been demonstrated in human corpus cavernosum (Shirai, Sasaki and Rikimaru, 1972; Benson *et al.*, 1980), as have muscarinic receptors (Godec and Bates, 1984). Furthermore, transmural electrical field stimulation was shown to cause release of $^3$H-acetylcholine, synthesized in corporeal tissue after incubation with $^3$H-choline (Blanco *et al.*, 1988). In contrast to Adaikan *et al.* (1983) who found that in corpus cavernosum preparations acetylcholine produced contraction, relaxation, or contraction followed by relaxation, several investigators have demonstrated that carbachol and acetylcholine, while having no effect at basal tension, concentration-dependently relaxed NA-contracted corpus cavernosum and spongiosum preparations (Andersson *et al.*, 1983; Hedlund, Andersson and Mattiasson, 1984; Hedlund and Andersson, 1985a; de Tejada *et al.*, 1988). As this relaxant effect was blocked by the muscarinic receptor antagonist scopolamine, it seemed to be mediated by muscarinic receptors. It has been claimed that destruction of the endothelium eliminates or greatly attenuates relaxation produced by acetylcholine (de Tejada *et al.*, 1988), suggesting that the effect is mediated by release of a relaxation mediating factor from the endothelium. In isolated segments of the cavernosal artery contracted by NA, carbachol was less effective than in corporeal tissue, and induced relaxation only at high concentrations (Hedlund and Andersson, 1985a).

Since stimulation of the parasympathetic nerves innervating the penis leads to erection (Langley and Anderson, 1895), it was suggested that the peripheral nervous control of tumescence is dependent on an interaction between adrenergic and cholinergic nerves (Klinge and Sjöstrand, 1977; de Tejada *et al.*, 1988). Thus, tumescence may be the result of relaxation of erectile smooth muscle caused by cholinergic nerves suppressing excitatory adrenergic neurotransmission. In support of this suggestion, Hedlund, Andersson and Mattiasson (1984), studying the effect of carbachol on electrically-induced release of $^3$H-NA from adrenergic nerves in corpus spongiosum preparations, found a concentration-related inhibition of the electrically elicited efflux of $^3$H. Furthermore, it was shown that scopolamine concentration-dependently increased the $^3$H efflux.

Taken together, these findings suggest that parasympathetic activity may contribute to penile tumescence and erection by at least two mechanisms, both decreasing the effects of NA. Stimulation of muscarinic receptors on adrenergic nerve terminals may inhibit the release of NA. In addition, the postjunctional effects of NA may be counteracted by muscarinic receptor-mediated release of a relaxant factor from the endothelium.

## Non-adrenergic, non-cholinergic functions

### Peptides

Vasoactive intestinal polypeptide (VIP)-containing nerves have been demonstrated in human erectile tissues by several investigators (Polak *et al.*, 1981; Gu *et al.*, 1983; Willis *et al.*, 1983; Steers, McConnell and Benson, 1984; Shirai *et al.*, 1990), as have several other peptides including substance P, somatostatin (Gu *et al.*, 1983), and neuropeptide Y

(NPY; Adrian *et al.*, 1984). The localization of these peptides to penile erectile tissues has led to speculations about their functional roles as inhibitory or excitatory transmitters and/or modulators of neurotransmission in the penis.

### *Endothelin-1*

As mentioned previously, the state of contraction of the penile arteries and of sinusoidal smooth muscle necessary to maintain detumescence is believed to be mediated mainly by the sympathetic nervous system, stimulating $\alpha_1$-adrenoceptors through continuous release of NA into the synaptic cleft (Andersson, Hedlund and Fovaeus, 1987). Even if myogenic activity may contribute to tone, it is possible that additional mechanisms take part in keeping the penis in its flaccid state. The 21-amino acid peptide endothelin-1, first isolated and identified in porcine aortic endothelial cells by Yanagisawa *et al.* (1988), has been suggested to be involved in such a mechanism (de Tejada *et al.*, 1989b; Holmquist, Andersson and Hedlund, 1990; Holmquist, *et al.*, 1990). Endothelin-1 mRNA is expressed in cultured endothelial cells from the human corpus cavernosum (de Tejada *et al.*, 1989b), and binding sites for the peptide can be demonstrated in cavernosal smooth muscle (Holmquist *et al.*, 1990). Endothelin-1 potently contracts isolated human corpus cavernosum and enhances contractions induced by NA. Furthermore endothelin-1-induced contractions could be effectively counteracted by muscarinic receptor stimulation and by VIP (Holmquist, Andersson and Hedlund, 1990).

### *Neuropeptide Y (NPY)*

Nerve fibres containing NPY have been demonstrated in the human penis (Adrian *et al.*, 1984; Wespes *et al.*, 1988). Wespes *et al.* (1988) studied by immunohistochemical techniques the distribution of NPY-containing nerves in the human penis and found an accumulation of fibres in the inner part of the adventitia close to the media of the arterial and venous vessels, and among the intracavernous smooth muscle cells. They speculated that the peptide could act as a neurotransmitter or neuromodulator in the mechanisms of penile erection, especially during detumescence. Adrian *et al.* (1984) found moderately high concentrations of NPY in the human corpus cavernosum, and they suggested that NPY, 'as a potent vasoconstrictor locally present in high concentrations', could be intimately involved in the control of erection. If so, a contractile effect on erectile tissues would be expected.

Hedlund and Andersson (1985b) studied the effects of NPY on isolated human erectile tissues. They found that neither in corpus cavernosum nor in segments of the cavernosal artery had NPY any effects on preparations studied at basal tension level, or contracted by NA. NPY did not affect electrically-induced contractions in cavernosal tissue. Thus, these results did not support the view that NPY is of importance in the control of smooth muscles involved in penile erection.

### *Arginine vasopressin (AVP)*

It is generally held that AVP is a circulating hormone. However, AVP-like immunoreactivity was demonstrated to be widely distributed in the sympathetic nervous system of mammals (Hanley *et al.*, 1984). This AVP-like activity was found in both ganglionic neurones and in nerve fibres innervating peripheral tissues. Hedlund and Andersson (1985b) found AVP to contract isolated human corpus cavernosum and spongiosum and preparations of the cavernosal artery in a concentration-dependent way. By radioimmunoassay, AVP could be demonstrated in cavernous tissue in concentrations up to ten times those circulating in plasma (Andersson *et al.*, 1987). This suggested that the peptide was either taken up and stored, and/or synthesized locally. However, AVP antagonists found to almost completely suppress the contractions induced by exogenous AVP, had no effect on electrically-induced contractions in corpus cavernosum preparations (Andersson *et al.*, 1987). Therefore, it did not seem plausible that AVP was released on electrical stimulation in amounts which could affect the smooth muscle directly and/or influence the response to released NA.

### *Somatostatin*

Gu *et al.* (1983) localized by immunocytochemistry somatostatin-containing nerves in the male genital tract, mainly associated with the smooth muscle of the seminal vesicle and the vas deferens. However, by radioimmunoassay, the concentrations of somatostatin in these structures were shown to be only slightly higher than those found in corpus cavernosum. Somatostatin was found to have no contractant effects on cavernosal tissue *in vitro* (Hedlund and Andersson, 1985b), except at high concentrations ($10^{-5}$ M). Preparations of the cavernosal artery responded with a contraction at lower concentrations ($10^{-7}$ M), but the maximum effect was approximately 25% of that induced by 124 mM potassium. These effects do not suggest that somatostatin has any direct effects on smooth muscle structures of importance for penile erection

### *Vasoactive intestinal polypeptide (VIP)*

VIP has been found in high concentrations in the erectile tissue of the human penis (Polak *et al.*, 1981; Gu *et al.*, 1983; Willis *et al.*, 1983; Shirai *et al.*, 1990). It is present in nerve fibres with nerve endings around cavernous smooth muscle and blood vessels, mainly arteries and arterioles (Polak *et al.*, 1981; Gu *et al.*, 1983; Willis *et al.*, 1983). A role for VIP as a neurotransmitter or neuromodulator has been postulated by several investigators. Thus, for example, Shirai *et al.* (1990) speculated that the peptide controlled a valvular structure in the helicine arteries adjusting the blood flow into the cavernous spaces of the penis.

VIP was found to have a relaxant action on human erectile tissue (Larsen *et al.*, 1981; Andersson *et al.*, 1983; Willis *et al.*, 1983; Steers, McConnell and Benson, 1984; Hedlund and Andersson 1985b; Adaikan, Kottegoda and Ratnam, 1986a). In isolated corpus cavernosum strips, the effect on spontaneous (myogenic) contractile activity and on electrically-induced contractions was pronounced, but that on NA-contracted preparations was poor (Hedlund and Andersson 1985b; Adaikan, Kottegoda and Ratnam, 1986a). The effects of VIP on electrically-induced contractions in segments of the cavernosal artery were small, as were its relaxant actions on NA-contracted arterial preparations (Hedlund and Andersson, 1985b).

A marked release of VIP during tumescence and erection produced by visual sexual stimulation, by intracavernous injection of papaverine, or by intracavernous infusion of saline has been demonstrated in pilot studies (Virag *et al.*, 1982; Ottesen *et al.*, 1984). However, Kiely *et al.* (1987) measuring cavernosal and peripheral VIP concentrations during erection induced by a variety of vasoactive compounds in patients with either predominantly organic or predominantly psychogenic impotence, found no increase in cavernosal VIP concentration.

It cannot be excluded that VIP has a role in penile erectile responses, but how it is involved remains to be established. Its inability to produce erection when injected intracavernosally in impotent men (Adaikan, Kottegoda and Ratnam, 1986a; Kiely, Bloom and Williams, 1989; Roy, Petrone and Said, 1990) suggests that it cannot be the only non-adrenergic, non-cholinergic mediator for relaxation of penile erectile tissues.

### *Calcitonin gene-related peptide (CGRP)*

CGRP is a 37-amino acid peptide shown to be present in both the central and peripheral nervous system (Ishida-Yamamoto and Tohyama, 1989). It is known to be a potent vasodilator in a variety of human blood vessels, where it is believed to produce an endothelium-dependent relaxation (Hughes *et al.*, 1986; Crossman *et al.*, 1987). Stief *et al.* (1990) demonstrated CGRP in nerves of the canine corpus cavernosum.

When given intracavernosally to impotent patients in combination with prostaglandin (PG) $E_1$, CGRP produced erection. The combination was more effective and had fewer side effects than $PGE_1$ alone or a combination of papaverine and phentolamine (Stief, personal communication). *In vitro*, CGRP had little relaxant effect on strips of human corpus cavernosum contracted by NA or by electrical field stimulation (Holmquist, unpublished results). Whether the peptide has a role in normal penile physiology remains to be established. Nevertheless, even in the absence of such a role, this does not exclude the possibility that CGRP may be useful for therapeutic purposes.

### *Substance P*

Few substance P-immunoreactive nerves were found in cavernosal tissue (Andersson *et al.*, 1983; Gu *et al.*, 1983). Substance P was more concentrated in groups of nerve fibres underneath the epithelium of the glans penis (Gu *et al.*, 1983). *In vitro* investigations of strips of human corpus cavernosum (Andersson *et al.*, 1983; Hedlund and Andersson, 1985b) showed contractile effects of substance P at resting tension, while no effects were observed in segments of the cavernosal artery. The contractant response in isolated human erectile tissue proper is in contrast to the vasodilator effects produced by substance P *in vivo* in the dog penis (Andersson, Bloom and Mellander, 1984). It cannot be excluded that substance P is involved in the sensory innervation of the penis. However, available information does not suggest that the peptide has any direct effects on penile erectile smooth muscle.

## Prostanoids

Several studies have shown that the human penis has the ability to synthesize various prostanoids (Roy *et al.*, 1984, 1989; Bornman *et al.*, 1986; Jeremy *et al.*, 1986), and it has been suggested that arachidonate cascade products may be involved in the control of penile erection. Thus, Hedlund and Andersson (1985c) demonstrated that $PGF_{2\alpha}$, $PGI_2$, high concentrations of $PGE_2$, and, most potently among the prostanoids tested, the thromboxane (TX) $A_2$ analogues U46619 and U44069 contracted corpus cavernosum and arterial preparations at baseline tension. The contraction-mediating prostanoid receptor in the human corpora is most probably a $TXA_2$-sensitive receptor, even if the presence of more than one contraction-mediating prostanoid receptor cannot be excluded (Hedlund *et al.*, 1989a, b). Whether or not tone in penile erectile tissues is maintained by stimulation of the $TXA_2$-sensitive receptor remains to be established.

Carbachol completely relaxed $PGF_{2\alpha}$-contracted trabecular preparations, but the arterial segments remained contracted. Both corpus cavernosum and arterial preparations contracted by $PGF_{2\alpha}$ could be relaxed to baseline by VIP (Hedlund and Andersson, 1985c). This is of particular interest with respect to the suggestion that both acetylcholine and VIP may be involved in the mechanisms leading to penile smooth muscle relaxation and erection.

Hedlund and Andersson (1985c) found no contractile effect of $PGE_1$, but the prostanoid was effective in relaxing human trabecular tissue, and also segments of the cavernous artery contracted by NA or $PGF_{2\alpha}$. Furthermore, contributing to a direct smooth muscle effect of $PGE_1$, the prostanoid has been claimed to inhibit release of NA from penile adrenergic nerves (Adaikan, Kottegoda and Ratnam, 1986b; Porst, 1989). Also $PGE_2$ at low concentrations was shown to have a certain relaxant action in the corpus cavernosum preparations, but was without any obvious effects in NA-contracted arterial segments.

Jeremy *et al.* (1986) reported that muscarinic receptor stimulation caused synthesis and release of $PGI_2$ in human penile corpus cavernosum tissue. In isolated preparations of the cavernosal artery, $PGI_2$ was found to be highly effective as a relaxant agent in both NA- and $PGF_{2\alpha}$-contracted preparations, which was in contrast to its effects on trabecular tissue. The findings that $PGI_2$ caused contraction and had no relaxant action when added to isolated corpus cavernosum preparations contracted by NA or $PGF_{2\alpha}$ (Hedlund and Andersson, 1985c) do not support the suggestion that $PGI_2$ mediates relaxation of trabecular tissue. However, it cannot be excluded that this prostanoid may serve as a vasodilator in the initial phase of penile erection (Hedlund and Andersson, 1985c). Furthermore, during penile enlargement and blood stasis, $PGI_2$ synthesized from the endothelium in vessels as well as from the sinusoids may counteract local thrombosis induced by $TXA_2$ and other endogenous platelet aggregators.

Thus, if any of the prostaglandins plays a physiological role in the processes leading to penile erection, $PGE_1$ seems to have the most appropriate profile of action (Hedlund and Andersson, 1985c). Supporting this, intracorporeal injection of $PGE_1$ was shown to be effective for production of penile erection (see below).

### Endothelium-derived relaxing factors (EDRFs)

Relaxing factors produced by the endothelium have been shown to mediate the relaxant responses of vascular smooth muscle not only to acetylcholine, but to several other agents (Furchgott, 1984). One of the EDRFs has been identified as nitric oxide (Palmer, Ferrige and Moncada, 1987; Moncada Radomski and Palmer, 1988). This factor is believed to cause smooth muscle relaxation by stimulating soluble guanylate cyclase, thereby increasing the content of the cyclic GMP in the smooth muscle cells, a mechanism of action similar to that of, for example, nitroglycerin. In contracted penile erectile tissue, muscarinic receptor stimulation by carbachol and acetylcholine causes relaxation (Andersson *et al.*, 1983; Hedlund, Andersson and Mattiasson, 1984; Hedlund and Andersson, 1985a; de Tejada *et al.*, 1988). This relaxation seems to require an intact endothelium (de Tejada *et al.*, 1988). Furthermore, relaxation of pre-contracted human cavenous tissue, induced by electrical stimulation of nerves, could be inhibited by $N^G$-nitro-L-arginine, which inhibits the synthetics of nitric oxide (Holmquist, Hedlund and Andersson, 1991). However, the role of nitric oxide and/or other EDRFs in penile physiology remains to be established.

## Causes of impotence

Impotence seems to be an age-related disorder with an incidence of 1.9% at the age of 40 and 25% at the age of 65 (Krane, Goldstein and de Tejada, 1989). In diabetic patients the prevalence of impotence is particularly high, between 50 and 75% (Kaiser and Korenman, 1988). The most common causes of impotence are generally classified as being of vascular, endocrine, neurological and psychogenic nature, but most often the exact mechanisms involved are not known. There is frequently an overlap between aetiologies, such as in diabetic patients who may have both vascular and neurological complications contributing to impotence. Furthermore, there is often a psychogenic component in patients with a distinct organic cause of impotence.

In patients with impotence, Gu *et al.* (1984) found that VIP-containing nerves were depleted, and that the extent of the depletion broadly reflected the severity of erectile dysfunction irrespective of its aetiology. They suggested that VIP not only was the principal neurotransmitter involved in penile erection, but also that depletion of the peptide may play a key role in the development of impotence. Lincoln *et al.* (1987) arrived at a similar conclusion, finding that five out of six diabetic patients with impotence had a marked reduction of VIP-like immunoreactivity in nerves associated with the cavernous smooth muscle.

Adrenergic and cholinergic nerves were shown to be affected in impotent diabetics (Lincoln *et al.*, 1987). Furthermore, Melman *et al.* (1980) reported statistically significant reductions of the NA content in corpus cavernosum taken from men with erectile dysfunction due to, for example, diabetes or Peyronie's disease. A change in α-adrenoceptor function in impotent patients would therefore not be unexpected. However, no differences were found between tissues taken from impotent men with diabetes, alcoholism, Peyronie's disease, or men with no obvious condition causing the impotence (Creed *et al.*, 1989). Likewise, Kirkeby *et al.* (1989b) found no difference in penile α-receptor function between potent and impotent men (venous leakage), at least not in isolated penile circumflex veins.

de Tejada *et al.* (1989c) found that in diabetic patients with impotence, endothelium-dependent relaxation of corpus cavernosum smooth muscle was impaired. They suggested that vasodilators producing endothelium-independent relaxation would be preferable in diabetic patients treated with intracavernosal injections. Whether this prediction is clinically valid remains to be tested.

Drug-induced erectile dysfunction seems to be an increasing problem (Nelson, 1988; Wein and Van Arsdalen, 1988). The mechanisms by which most drugs cause impotence are unknown, but both central and peripheral structures may be involved. Many of the data on drug-induced erectile dysfunction are based on case records only, and controlled studies on the effects of a particular drug on erectile functions are rare.

Interference with central mechanisms is the most probable cause of impotence associated with the use of major tranquillizers or antipsychotic drugs, antidepressants and minor tranquillizers or anti-anxiety agents. Centrally, major tranquillizers like phenothiazines (e.g. chlorpromazine) and butyrophenones (e.g. haloperidol) produce sedation, have a central antidopamine effect and cause release of prolactin, all actions that may be of importance for erectile functions. Peripherally, these drugs have many effects including anticholinergic and α-adrenoceptor antagonistic actions. At least the latter action would not be expected to produce erectile dysfunction, but may rather be involved in rare cases of priapism (Wein and Van Arsdalen, 1988). Among antidepressants, imipramine, clomipramine and other tricyclic drugs have been reported to be associated with erectile failure. On the other hand, trazodone is a newer antidepressant reported to produce erection, probably by an α-adrenoceptor blocking action (Abber *et al.*, 1987), and to improve erectile function (Lal, Rios and Thavundayil, 1990). The minor tranquillizers, e.g. the benzodiazepines, are frequently assumed to interfere with sexual function but there is little actual evidence of a cause–effect relationship (Wein and Van Arsdalen, 1988).

Several antihypertensive agents have been reported to cause erectile dysfunction (Wein and Van Arsdalen, 1988), e.g. sympatholytics like methyldopa and guanethidine, α-adrenoceptor blockers (prazosin), β-adrenoceptor blockers (e.g. propranolol), and diuretics (e.g. thiazides). However, it is still a matter of dispute whether or not there is a change of prevalence of sexual dysfunction in treated hypertensive men (Bansal, 1988). The decrease in systemic blood pressure induced by antihypertensive agents may reduce perfusion pressure of the sinusoids leading to reduced penile rigidity. This is probably a dominating factor since agents leading to a decreased adrenergic tone in penile smooth muscle like sympatholytics and α-adrenoceptor blockers would rather be expected to facilitate erection. In line with this, treatment with prazosin has been reported to cause priapism (Bhalla *et al.*, 1979; Adams and Soucheray, 1984).

The anti-androgenic effects of cimetidine, blocking histamine ($H_2$) receptors, may be important for impotence reported during treatment with this drug (Peden *et al.*, 1979).

## Effects and mechanisms of action of drugs used for treatment of erectile dysfunction

Endocrinological causes of impotence can be successfully treated by medical therapy, but otherwise drug therapy for erectile dysfunction has not been satisfactory. However, intracavernosal injections of vasoactive drugs has proved an important therapeutic advance. Several agents have been used for this purpose, but only three drugs and/or drug combinations have gained clinical acceptance, namely papaverine, papaverine and phentolamine in combination and $PGE_1$ (alprostadil) (Jünemann and Alken, 1989). In addition, there is reported preliminary clinical experience with some other drugs.

### Papaverine

Papaverine is often characterized as a non-specific vasodilator, and its cellular mechanism of action is unclear. Its effect pattern includes phosphodiesterase inhibition, calcium influx inhibition and possibly also calcium efflux increase, all mechanisms whereby the intracellular concentration of calcium can be decreased and smooth muscle relaxed (Huddart, Langton and Saad, 1984; Sunagane *et al.*, 1985; Krall, Fittingoff and Rajfer, 1988). At the high concentrations obtained at intracavernosal injection, which are in the mM range (Kirkeby, Forman and Andersson, 1990), it is difficult to establish which of these mechanisms is dominating. Additional actions of a more non-specific nature exerted directly on the muscle membrane may also contribute. Papaverine relaxes all components of the penile erectile system: the deep artery, the cavernous sinusoids and the penile veins (Kirkeby, Forman and Andersson, 1990). The enhanced venous resistance found after intracavernous papaverine injections may therefore be created by passive compression of the venous outflow by the dilated sinusoids.

It is well known that an intracavernosal injection of papaverine can produce side effects, both locally and systemically. A main local side effect is intracavernous fibrosis (see Jünemann and Alken, 1990). A 2% solution of papaverine in water has a pH of 3–4 and the importance of this for production of intracavernous fibrosis has been discussed (Seidmon and Samaha, 1989). Attempts have been made to buffer the papaverine solution used for intracavernosal injection, but this resulted in a precipitate at a pH equal to or greater than 5. It was suggested that on intracavernosal injection, buffering by blood will lead to precipitation of the drug which may cause primary intracorporeal scarring (Seidmon and Samaha, 1989). Another main side effect of papaverine is prolonged erection and priapism (Jünemann and Alken, 1990). This is most probably due to a relative overdosage, and seems to be possible to avoid by careful titration of the lowest possible dose, or by combination therapy. Available pharmacokinetic data for papaverine are scarce, but it is known that the drug has a relatively short plasma half-life (1–2 h) and that it is extensively metabolized in the liver. It is predictable that when the drug is injected intracavernosally, some of it may reach the systemic circulation and produce adverse circulatory reactions. Less predictable is the known hepatotoxicity of the drug which may manifest itself either as an increase in liver transaminases which is common (>1/100), or as a drug-induced hepatitis which is rare (<1/1000).

## α-adrenoceptor blockers

As mentioned previously, the importance of sympathetic nervous activity and α-adrenoceptor function for keeping the penis in the flaccid state is generally accepted. What would then be the most suitable effect profile in an α-adrenoceptor blocker to be used for intracavernosal injection? Brindley (1986) showed that intracavernosal injection of the selective $\alpha_2$-adrenoceptor blocker idazoxan had no effect, which means that $\alpha_1$-adrenoceptor blockade is required. Should the most effective drug be selective for $\alpha_1$-adrenoceptors or are non-selective blockers preferable? Clinical experience is available for the non-selective agents phentolamine and phenoxybenzamine, and to a limited extent for the $\alpha_1$-adrenoceptor selective blocker thymoxamine (moxisylyte).

### Phentolamine

A single phentolamine injection does not result in a satisfactory erectile response in most cases, possibly because the drug has no effect on venous return (Wespes, Rondeux and Schulman, 1989). The drug is widely used in combination with papaverine (Zorgniotti and Lefleur, 1985; Jünemann and Alken, 1989). Despite, or maybe because of, the long time phentolamine has been available, there is a general lack of information about its pharmacokinetics. It is known that the drug has a short plasma half-life and that it is extensively metabolized before excretion. It is also known that the most common side effects encountered after injection of phentolamine are hypotension and tachycardia. It should be mentioned that cardiac arrhythmias and myocardial infarction have been reported when the drug has been injected intravenously, but these are very rare events.

### Phenoxybenzamine

Phenoxybenzamine injected intracavernosally was introduced for diagnosis and treatment of erectile dysfuntion in 1983 (Brindley, 1983). The drug has some characteristics which theoretically should be disadvantageous. It has an irreversible receptor blocking effect (alkylates the receptor) which should make it difficult to reverse its actions. It has also a very long plasma half-life, which may exceed 24 h, and a long duration of action with demonstrable effects persisting for 3–4 days (Weiner, 1985).

The drug is effective for treatment of erectile dysfunction as documented in double-blind placebo-controlled trials (Szasz *et al.*, 1987; Keogh *et al.*, 1989), but has disadvantages when administered intracavernosally, including pain at the injection site, slow onset of effect, prolonged erections and a tendency to produce cavernous fibrosis (Jünemann and Alken, 1989). This and the side effect pattern including postural hypotension, and also its carcinogenic effect in rodents (Flind, 1984), make phenoxybenzamine unattractive as a treatment alternative.

### Thymoxamine

Thymoxamine (moxisylyte) is a drug with a relatively selective action on $\alpha_1$-adrenoceptors. Brindley (1986) showed this drug to produce erection when injected intracavernosally. Buvat *et al.* (1989) reported on the experiences of intracavernous injections of thymoxamine in 170 patients with impotence. Although thymoxamine in a double-blind crossover study was shown to be more active than saline, it was less active than papaverine. In most cases, thymoxamine was said only to facilitate erection by inducing prolonged tumescence. Buvat *et al.* (1989) stressed that the main advantage of the drug was its safety; only two out of the 170 patients injected had prolonged erections (1.2%).

## Prostaglandin $E_1$

Many studies have confirmed the finding of Ishii *et al.* (1986) that intracavernosally administered $PGE_1$ is effective for treatment of impotence of various aetiologies (see Jünemann and Alken, 1989). Open as well as controlled studies have shown $PGE_1$ to be at least as effective as papaverine or the papaverine/phentolamine combination (Jünemann and Alken, 1989; Earle *et al.*, 1990). Little is known about its pharmacokinetics. It is of interest that $PGE_1$ is extensively metabolized in the lungs (Hamberg and Samuelsson, 1971), which may explain why it seldom causes circulatory side effects when injected intracavernosally. The principal side effect of intracavernosal injection of $PGE_1$ is local pain, whereas prolonged erection seems to be a rare complication (Jünemann and Alken, 1989), possibly because $PGE_1$ can be metabolized in the penis (Roy *et al.*, 1989). The pH of the $PGE_1$ solution can easily be buffered (Seidmon and Samaha, 1989) which means that the potentially negative effects of a low pH can be avoided.

## Other drugs

### VIP

Adaikan, Kottegoda and Ratnam (1986a) injected VIP intracavernously in seven subjects. In five of these some degree of penile enlargement was evident, but none had an erection. Roy, Petrone and Said (1990) performed a double-blind, placebo-controlled trial of intracavernous injection of VIP in 24 men with erectile dysfunction of diabetic, neurogenic and psychogenic aetiology. None of the patients achieved penile rigidity adequate for intromission. Negative experiences were also reported by Wagner and Gerstenberg (1987) who found that even in high doses (20 μg), VIP was unable to induce erection on intracavernous injection. On the other hand, when used in conjunction with visual or vibratory stimulation, intracavernous VIP facilitated normal erection. In 12 men with impotence of varying aetiology, Kiely, Bloom and Williams (1989) injected VIP, papaverine or phentolamine, as well as combinations of these drugs. They confirmed that VIP alone is poor at inducing human penile erections. However, in combination with papaverine, VIP produced penile rigidity similar to that with papaverine/phentolamine. It is interesting to note that patients receiving intracavernosal injection of VIP in combination with phentolamine experienced the erection as more 'natural' than the erection induced by, for example papaverine/phentolamine or $PGE_1$ (Gerstenberg, personal communication).

It may be concluded that, on intracavernous injection, VIP alone may act as a facilitating drug in combination with visual or vibratory stimulation. In combination with other drugs the peptide may also be useful.

### Nitroglycerin

Intracorporeal administration of vasoactive drugs has inevitable drawbacks, reflected by the relatively large number of drop-outs from therapy. Other non-invasive ways of drug administration may, when possible, be preferable. Nitroglycerin, a well known vasodilator that can be given transcutaneously, and isosorbide dinitrate were both found to relax isolated strips of human corpus cavernosum (Heaton, 1989). The drugs are believed to produce vasodilation through stimulation of soluble guanylate cyclase, increasing the intracellular concentration of cGMP.

Under laboratory conditions, Owen *et al.* (1989) performed a placebo-controlled, double-blind study on the effect of penile application of nitroglycerin ointment in impotent patients diagnosed as organic, psychogenic or mixed. They found that nitroglycerin increased penile circumference better than placebo (18 out of 26) as well as increasing blood flow in the cavernous arteries (seven out of 20). One patient had systemic side effects (hypotension and headache). Claes and Baert (1989) treated 26 impotent men with transcutaneous nitroglycerin (patches) in a double-blind, randomized, placebo-controlled trial. A positive response was reported by 21 patients. Of these, complete response was reported by 12, and partial response (not sufficient to restore satisfactory sexual performance) in nine. Twelve patients reported mild to moderate headache during nitroglycerin treatment.

It seems that transcutaneous nitroglycerin may be of benefit for some patients, and a non-invasive way of administration may have advantages.

### Yohimbine

Many drugs have been tried as an oral treatment of impotence, including yohimbine which for a long time has been considered as an aphrodisiac. Good responses to treatment of impotent patients with a yohimbine-containing combination product (Margolis *et al.*, 1971) were reported. Controlled trials have been performed on patients with organic (Morales *et al.*, 1987), psychogenic (Reid *et al.*, 1987) and mixed (Riley *et al.*, 1989; Susset *et al.*, 1989) aetiology to their impotence. These trials revealed a marginal, non-significant effect of yohimbine in organically impotent patients, i.e. 43% responded (complete or partial response) to yohimbine and 28% to placebo (Morales *et al.*, 1987). Similar figures (now significantly different) were obtained in a study of the same design in patients with psychogenic impotence (Reid *et al.*, 1987). In the studies on patients with mixed aetiologies, positive responses were reported in approximately one-third of the patients (Riley *et al.*, 1989; Susset *et al.*, 1989). Owing to the ease of administration of yohimbine and the relatively few and benign side effects with the doses used, these results were considered encouraging. Yohimbine has a relative selective effect on $\alpha_2$-adrenoceptors, and even if other effects have been demonstrated (Goldberg and Robertson, 1983), these only occur in concentrations unlikely to be obtained in man. Its mode of action is most probably not peripheral, since the predominant subtype of α-adrenoceptors in penile erectile tissue is of $\alpha_1$-type (see above), and since intracavernosal injection of another $\alpha_2$-adrenoceptor blocker, idazoxan, had no effect (Brindley, 1986).

It cannot be excluded that the principle of blockade of a central $\alpha_2$-adrenoceptor may represent a therapeutically interesting approach to the treatment of some cases of impotence.

## Treatment of prolonged erection

Production of prolonged erection may occur with any of the vasodilators in clinical use. In turn this may necessitate the use of various operative procedures as well as of pharmacological antidotes. Most of the drugs recommended are α-adrenoceptor agonists and include adrenaline, NA, phenylephrine, dopamine and metaraminol. Clonidine may also be used (Lin *et al.*, 1989). It has been reported that the $\beta_2$-receptor agonist terbutaline given orally can be used with success (Shantha, Finnerty and Rodriquez, 1989). Theoretically this vasodilator would be expected to produce erection, and the mechanism behind the effect remains unclear.

## Concluding remarks

Intracorporeal injections of vasoactive substances as a treatment of impotence have gained wide acceptance over the last few years. However, the fact that as many as 45% of the patients drop out from this kind of therapy cannot be overlooked. One common reason for this is lack of effect of the injected substances, but quite a significant number of patients discontinue the treatment because of side effects, lack of spontaneity, partner resistance and difficulties in handling the injection equipment (Kromann-Andersen, personal communication). Considering these circumstances, it is desirable to develop both new drugs and new techniques by which they can be administered. Thus, future drugs for intracorporeal injection should be cheap to manufacture, easy to handle and store, devoid of side effects such as pain, prolonged erection and local fibrosis, and they should induce a 'normal' erection with detumescence occurring shortly after ejaculation. Furthermore, the drugs should be suitable for a non-invasive route of administration, e.g. transdermally, with preserved efficacy and a possibility to regulate the onset and time of erection.

Continued basic research on the mechanisms of erection and clinical exploration of promising drug effects found, for example *in vitro*, should result in further progress in this field.

## References


Abber, J. C., Lue, T. F., Luo, J.-A. *et al.* (1987) Priapism induced by chlorpromazine and trazodone: mechanism of action *Journal of Urology*, **137**, 1039–1042

Adaikan, P. G. and Karim, S. M. M. (1981) Adrenoreceptors in the human penis. *Journal of Autonomic Pharmacology*, **1**, 199–203

Adaikan, P. G., Karim, S. M. M., Kottegoda, S. R. and Ratnam, S. S. (1983) Cholinoreceptors in the corpus cavernosum muscle of the human penis. *Journal of Autonomic Pharmacology*, **3**, 107–111

Adaikan, P. G., Kottegoda, S. R. and Ratnam, S. S. (1986a) Is vasoactive intestinal polypeptide the principal transmitter involved in human penile erection? *Journal of Urology*, **135**, 638–640

Adaikan, P. G., Kottegoda, S. R. and Ratnam, S. S. (1986b) A possible role for prostaglandin $E_1$ in human penile erection. In *Proceedings of the Fifth Conference on Vasculogenic Impotence and Corpus Cavernosum Revascularization* (Second World Meeting on Impotence), International Society for Impotence Research (ISIR), Prague, 2.6

Adams, J. W. and Soucheray, J. A. (1984) Prazosin-induced priapism in a diabetic. *Journal of Urology*, **132**, 1208

Adrian, T. E., Gu, J., Allen, J. M. *et al.* (1984) Neuropeptide Y in the human male genital tract. *Life Sciences*, **35**, 2643–2648

Andersson, K.-E., Fovaeus, M. Hedlund, H. and Lundin, S. (1987) Characterization of immunoreactive arginine vasopressin (AVP) and effects of AVP on isolated human penile erectile tissues. *Journal of Urology*, **137**, 1278–1282

Andersson, K.-E., Hedlund, H. and Fovaeus, M. (1987) Interactions between classical neurotransmitters and some neuropeptides in human penile erectile tissues. In *Neuronal Messengers in Vascular Function* (eds A. Nobin, C. Owman and B. Arneklo-Nobin), Elsevier Science Publishers, Amsterdam, pp. 505–524

Andersson, K.-E., Hedlund, H., Mattiasson, A. *et al.* (1983) Relaxation of isolated human corpus spongiosum induced by vasoactive intestinal polypeptide, substance P, carbachol and electrical field stimulation. *World Journal of Urology*, **1**, 203–208

Andersson, P.-O., Bloom, S. R. and Mellander, S. (1984) Haemodynamics of pelvic nerve induced penile erection in the dog: possible mediation by vasoactive intestinal polypeptide. *Journal of Physiology*, **350**, 209–224

Bansal, S. (1988) Sexual dysfunction in hypertensive men. A critical review of the literature. *Hypertension*, **12**, 1–10

Benson, G. S., McConnell, J., Lipshultz, L. I. *et al.* (1980) Neuromorphology and neuropharmacology of the human penis. *Journal of Clinical Investigation*, **65**, 506–513

Bhalla, A. K., Hoffbrand, B. I., Phatak, P. S. and Reuben, S. R. (1979) Prazosin and priapism. *British Medical Journal*, **ii**, 1039

Blanco, R., de Tejada, I. S., Goldstein, I. *et al.* (1988)

Cholinergic neurotransmission in human corpus cavernosum. II. Acetylcholine synthesis. *American Journal of Physiology*, **254**, H468–H472

Blum, M. D., Bahnson, R. R., Porter, T. N. and Carter, M. F. (1985) Effect of local alpha-adrenergic blockade on human penile erection. *Journal of Urology*, **134**, 479–481

Bornman, M. S., Franz, R. C., Jacobs, D. J., and Du Plessis, D. J. (1986) Thromboxane $B_2$ production during erection. *Andrologia*, **18**, 220–223

Brindley, G. S. (1983) Cavernosal alpha-blockade: a new technique for investigating and treating erectile impotence. *British Journal of Psychiatry*, **143**, 332–337

Brindley, G. S. (1984) New treatment for priapism. *Lancet*, **ii**, 220–221

Brindley, G. S. (1986) Pilot experiments on the actions of drugs injected into the human corpus cavernosum penis. *British Journal of Pharmacology*, **87**, 495–500

Buvat, J., Lemaire, A., Buvat-Herbaut, M. and Marcolin, G. (1989) Safety of intracavernous injections using an alpha-blocking agent. *Journal of Urology*, **141**, 1364–1367

Claes, H. and Baert, L. (1989) Transcutaneous nitroglycerin therapy in the treatment of impotence. *Urologia Internationalis*, **44**, 309–312

Creed, K. E., Carati, C. J., Adamson, G. M. and Callahan, S. M. (1989) Responses of erectile tissue from impotent men to pharmacological agents *British Journal of Urology*, **63**, 428–431

Crossman, D., McEwan, J., MacDermot, J. *et al.* (1987) Human calcitonin gene-related peptide activates adenylate cyclase and releases prostacyclin from human umbilical vein endothelial cells. *British Journal of Pharmacology*, **92**, 695–701

de Groat, W. C. and Steers, W. D. (1988) Neuroanatomy and neurophysiology of penile erection. In *Contemporary Management of Impotence and Infertility* (eds E.A. Tanagho, T. F. Lue and R. D. McClure), Williams and Wilkins, Baltimore, pp. 3–27

de Meyer, J. M. and De Sy, W. A. (1986) Intracavernous injection of noradrenaline to interrupt erections during surgical interventions. *European Urology*, **12**, 169–170

de Tejada, I. S., Blanco, R., Goldstein, I. *et al.* (1988) Cholinergic neurotransmission in human corpus cavernosum. I. Responses of isolated tissue. *American Journal of Physiology*, **254**, H459–H467

de Tejada, I. S., Carson, M. P., Traish, A. *et al.* (1989b) Role of endothelin, a novel vasoconstrictor peptide, in the local control of penile smooth muscle. *Proceedings of the Journal of Urology*, **141**, 222A

de Tejada, I. S., Goldstein, I., Azadzoi, K. *et al.* (1989c) Impaired neurogenic and endothelium-mediated relaxation of penile smooth muscle from diabetic men with impotence. *New England Journal of Medicine*, **320**, 1025–1030

de Tejada, I. S., Kim, N., Lagan, I. *et al.* (1989a) Regulation of adrenergic activity in penile corpus cavernosum. *Journal of Urology*, **142**, 1117–1121

Dhabuwala, C. B., Ramakrishna, V. R. and Anderson, G. F. (1985) Beta adrenergic receptors in human cavernous tissue. *Journal of Urology*, **133**, 721–723

Earle, C. M., Keogh, E. J. Wisniewski, Z. S. *et al.* (1990) Prostaglandin $E_1$ therapy for impotence, comparison with papaverine. *Journal of Urology*, **143**, 57–59

Flind, A. C. (1984) Cavernosal alpha-blockade: a warning. *British Journal of Psychiatry*, **144**, 329–330

Furchgott, R. F. (1984) The role of endothelium in the responses of vascular smooth muscle to drugs. *Annual Review of Pharmacology and Toxicology*, **24**, 175–197

Godec, C. J. and Bates, H. (1984) Cholinergic receptors in corpora cavernosa. *Investigative Urology*, **24**, 31–33

Goldberg, M. R. and Robertson, D. (1983) Yohimbine: a pharmacological probe for study of the $\alpha_2$-adrenoceptor. *Pharmacological Reviews*, **35**, 143–180

Gu, J., Polak, J. M., Lazarides, M. *et al.* (1984) Decrease of vasoactive intestinal polypeptide (VIP) in the penises from impotent men. *Lancet*, **ii**, 315–317

Gu, J., Polak, J. M., Probert, L. *et al.* (1983) Peptidergic innervation of the human male genital tract. *Journal of Urology*, **130**, 386–391

Hamberg, M. and Samuelsson, B. (1971) On the metabolism of prostaglandins $E_1$ and $E_2$ in man. *Journal of Biological Chemistry*, **246**, 6713–6721

Hanley, M. R., Benton, H. P., Lightman, S. L. *et al.* (1984) A vasopressin-like peptide in the mammalian sympathetic nervous system. *Nature*, **309**, 258–261

Heaton, J. P. W. (1989) Synthetic nitrovasodilators are effective, *in vitro*, in relaxing penile tissue from impotent men: the findings and their implications. *Canadian Journal of Physiology and Pharmacology*, **67**, 78–81

Hedlund, H. and Andersson, K.-E. (1985a) Comparison of the responses to drugs acting on adrenoceptors and muscarinic receptors in human isolated corpus cavernosum and cavernous artery. *Journal of Autonomic Pharmacology*, **5**, 81–88

Hedlund, H. and Andersson, K.-E. (1985b) Effects of some peptides on isolated human penile erectile tissue and cavernous artery. *Acta Physiologica Scandinavica*, **124**, 413–419

Hedlund, H. and Andersson, K-E. (1985c) Contraction and relaxation induced by some prostanoids in isolated human penile erectile tissue and cavernous artery. *Journal of Urology*, **134**, 1245–1250

Hedlund, H., Andersson, K.-E., Fovaeus, M. *et al.* (1989a) Characterization of contraction-mediating prostanoid receptors in human penile erectile tissues. *Journal of Urology*, **141**, 182–186

Hedlund, H., Andersson, K.-E., Holmquist, F. and Uski, T. (1989b) Effects of the thromboxane receptor antagonist AH 23848 on human isolated corpus cavernosum *International Journal of Impotence Research*, **1**, 19–25

Hedlund, H., Andersson, K.-E. and Mattiasson, A. (1984) Pre- and postjunctional adreno- and muscarinic receptor functions in the isolated human corpus spongiosum urethrae. *Journal of Autonomic Pharmacology*, **4**, 241–249

Holmquist, F., Andersson, K.-E. and Hedlund, H. (1990)

Actions of endothelin on isolated corpus cavernosum from rabbit and man. *Acta Physiologica Scandinavica*, **139**, 113–122

Holmquist, F., Hedlund, H. and Andersson, K.-E. (1990) L-N$^G$-nitro arginine inhibits non-adrenergic, non-cholinergic relaxation of human isolated corpus cavernosum. *Acta Physiologica Scandinavica*, **141**, 441–442

Holmquist, F., Larsson, B., Hedlund, H. and Andersson, K.-E. (1990) Studies on endothelin-1 in isolated rabbit and human penile erectile tissues. *European Journal of Pharmacology*, **183**, 2407–2408

Huddart, H., Langton, P. D. and Saad, K. H. M. (1984) Inhibition by papaverine of calcium movements and tension in the smooth muscles of rat vas deferens and urinary bladder. *Journal of Physiology*, **349**, 189–194

Hughes, A., Thom, S., Martin, G. and Sever, P. (1986) Endothelial dependent relaxation of human arteries by peptide hormones. *Clinical Science*, **70**, Suppl. 13, 88P

Ishida-Yamamoto, A. and Tohyama, M. (1989) Calcitonin gene-related peptide in the nervous tissue. *Progress in Neurobiology*, **33**, 335–386

Ishii, N., Watanabe, H., Irisawa, C. and Kikuchi, Y. (1986) Therapeutic trial with prostaglandin $E_1$ for organic impotence. In *Proceedings of the Fifth Conference on Vasculogenic Impotence and Corpus Cavernosum Revascularization* (Second World Meeting on Impotence), International Society for Impotence Research (ISIR), Prague, 11.2

Jeremy, J. Y., Morgan, R. J., Mikhailidis, D. P. and Dandona, P. (1986) Prostacyclin synthesis by the corpora cavernosa of the human penis: evidence for muscarinic control and pathological implications. *Prostaglandins, Leukotrienes and Medicine*, **23**, 211–216

Jünemann, K.-P. and Alken, P. (1989) Pharmacotherapy of erectile dysfunction: a review *International Journal of Impotence Research*, **1**, 71–93

Kaiser, F. E. and Korenman, S. G. (1988) Impotence in diabetic men. *American Journal of Medicine*, **85**, 147–152

Keogh, E. J., Tulloch, A. G. S., Earle, C. M. *et al.* (1989) Treatment of impotence by intrapenile injections of papaverine and phenoxybenzamine: a double blind, controlled trial. *Australian and New Zealand Journal of Medicine*, **19**, 108–112

Kiely, E. A., Blank, M. A., Bloom, S. R. and Williams, G. (1987) Studies on intracavernosal VIP levels during pharmacologically induced penile erections. *British Journal of Urology*, **59**, 334–339

Kiely, E. A., Bloom, S. R. and Williams, G. (1989) Penile response to intracavernosal vasoactive intestinal polypeptide alone and in combination with other vasoactive agents. *British Journal of Urology*, **64**, 191–194

Kimura, K., Kawanishi, Y., Tamura, M. and Imagawa, A. (1989) Assessment of the alpha-adrenergic receptors in isolated human and canine corpus cavernosum tissue. *International Journal of Impotence Research*, **1**, 189–195

Kirkeby, H. J., Forman, A. and Andersson, K.-E. (1990) Comparison of the papaverine effects on isolated human penile circumflex veins and corpus cavernosum. *International Journal of Impotence Research* **2**, 49–54

Kirkeby, H. J., Forman, A., Sørensen, S. and Andersson, K.-E. (1989a) Effects of noradrenaline, 5-hydroxytryptamine and histamine on human penile cavernous tissue and circumflex veins. *International Journal of Impotence Research*, **1**, 181–188

Kirkeby, H. J., Forman, A. Sørensen, S. and Andersson, K.-E. (1989b) Alpha-adrenoceptor function in isolated penile circumflex veins from potent and impotent men. *Journal of Urology*, **142**, 1369–1371

Klinge, E. and Sjöstrand, N. O. (1977) Suppression of the excitatory adrenergic neurotransmission; a possible role of cholinergic nerves in the retractor penis muscle. *Acta Physiologica Scandinavica*, **100**, 368–376

Krall, J. F., Fittingoff, M. and Rajfer, J. (1988) Characterization of cyclic nucleotide and inositol 1,4,5-trisphoshate-sensitive calcium-exchange activity of smooth muscle cells cultured from the human corpora cavernosa. *Biology of Reproduction*, **39**, 913–922

Krane, R. J., Goldstein, I. and de Tejada, I. S. (1989) Impotence. *New England Journal of Medicine*, **321**, 1648–1659

Lal, S., Rios, O. and Thavundayil, J. X. (1990) Treatment of impotence with trazodone: a case report. *Journal of Urology*, **143**, 819–820

Langley, J. N. and Anderson, H. K. (1895) The innervation of the pelvic and adjoining viscera. Part III. The external generative organs. *Journal of Physiology*, **19**, 85–121

Larsen, J.-J., Ottesen, B., Fahrenkrug, J. and Fahrenkrug, L. (1981) Vasoactive intestinal polypeptide (VIP) in the male genitourinary tract. Concentration and motor effect. *Investigative Urology*, **19**, 211–213

Levin, R. M. and Wein, A. J. (1980) Adrenergic alpha receptors outnumber beta receptors in human penile corpus cavernosum. *Investigative Urology*, **18**, 225–226

Lin, J., S.-N., Yu, P.-C., Yang, M. C. M. and Kuo, J.-S. (1989) Detumescent effect of clonidine on penile erection. *International Journal of Impotence Research*, **1**, 201–210

Lincoln, J., Crowe, R., Blacklay, P. F. *et al.* (1987) Changes in the vipergic, cholinergic and adrenergic innervation of human penile tissue in diabetic and non-diabetic impotent males. *Journal of Urology*, **137**, 1053–1059

Lue, T. F. and Tanagho, E. A. (1987) Physiology of erection and pharmacological management of impotence. *Journal of Urology*, **137**, 829–836

Margolis, R., Prieto, P., Stein, L. and Chinn, S. (1971) Statistical summary of 10 000 male cases using Afrodex in treatment of impotence. *Current Therapeutic Research*, **13**, 616–622

Melman, A., Henry, D. P., Felten, D. L. and O'Connor, B. L. (1980) Alteration of the penile corpora in patients with erectile impotence. *Investigative Urology*, **17**, 474–477

Moncada, S., Radomski, M. W. and Palmer, R. M. J. (1988) Endothelium-derived relaxing factor. Identification as nitric oxide and role in the control of vascular tone and platelet function. *Biochemical Pharmacology*, **37**, 2495–2501

Morales, A., Condra, M., Owen, J. A. *et al.* (1987) Is yohimbine effective in the treatment of organic impotence? Results of a controlled trial. *Journal of Urology*, **137**, 1168–1172

Nelson, R. P. (1988) Nonoperative management of impotence. *Journal of Urology*, **139**, 2–5

Ottesen, B., Wagner, G., Virag, R. and Fahrenkrug. J. (1984) Penile erection: possible role for vasoactive intestinal polypeptide as a neurotransmitter. *British Medical Journal*, **288**, 9–11

Owen, J. A., Saunders, F., Harris, C. *et al.* (1989) Topical nitroglycerin: a potential treatment for impotence. *Journal of Urology*, **141**, 546–548

Palmer, R. M. J., Ferrige, A. G. and Moncada, S. (1987) Nitric oxide release accounts for the biological activity of endothelium-derived relaxing factor. *Nature*, **327**, 524–526

Peden, N. R., Cargill, J. M., Browning, M. C. K. *et al.* (1979) Male sexual dysfunction during treatment with cimetidine. *British Medical Journal*, **i**, 659

Polak, J. M., Gu, J., Mina, S. and Bloom, S. R. (1981) Vipergic nerves in the penis. *Lancet*, **ii**, 217–219

Porst, H. (1989) Prostaglandin $E_1$ bei erektiler dysfunktion. *Urologe*, **28**, 94–98

Reid, K., Morales, A., Harris, C. *et al.* (1987) Double-blind trial of yohimbine in treatment of psychogenic impotence. *Lancet*, **ii**, 421–423

Riley, A. J., Goodman, R. E., Kellett, J. M. and Orr, R. (1989) Double blind trial of yohimbine hydrochloride in the treatment of erection inadequacy. *Sexual and Marital Therapy*, **4**, 17–26

Roy, A. C., Adaikan, P. G., Sen, D. K. and Ratnam, S. S. (1989) Prostaglandin 15-hydroxydehydrogenase activity in human penile corpora cavernosa and its significance in prostaglandin-mediated penile erection. *British Journal of Urology*, **64**, 180–182

Roy, J. B., Petrone, R. L. and Said, S. I. (1990) A clinical trial of intracavernous vasoactive intestinal peptide to induce penile erection. *Journal of Urology*, **143**, 302–304

Roy, A. C., Tan, S. M., Kottegoda, S. R. and Ratnam, S. S. (1984) Ability of human corpora cavernosa muscle to generate prostaglandins and thromboxanes *in vitro*. *IRCS Journal of Medical Science*, **12**, 608–609

Seidmon, E. J. and Samaha, A. M. Jr. (1989) The pH analysis of papaverine-phentolamine and prostaglandin $E_1$ for pharmacologic erection. *Journal of Urology*, **141**, 1458–1459

Shantha, T. R., Finnerty, D. P. and Rodriquez, A. P. (1989) Treatment of persistent penile erection and priapism using terbutaline. *Journal of Urology*, **141**, 1427–1429

Shirai, M., Sasaki, K. and Rikimaru, A. (1972) Histochemical investigation on the distribution of adrenergic and cholinergic nerves in human penis. *Tohoku Journal of Experimental Medicine*, **107**, 403–404

Shirai, M., Yanaihara, N., Maki, A. *et al.* (1990) Content and distribution of vasoactive intestinal polypeptide (VIP) in cavernous tissue of human penis. *Investigative Urology*, **35**, 360–363

Steers, W. D., McConnell, J. and Benson, G. S. (1984) Anatomical localization and some pharmacological effects of vasoactive intestinal polypeptide in human and monkey corpus cavernosum. *Journal of Urology*, **132**, 1048–1053

Stief, C. G., Benard, F., Bosch, R. J. L. H. *et al.* (1990) A possible role for calcitonin gene-related peptide in the regulation of the smooth muscle tone of the bladder and penis. *Journal of Urology*, **143**, 392–397

Sunagane, N., Ogawa, T., Uruno, T. and Kubota, K. (1985) Mechanism of relaxant action of papaverine. VI. Sodium ion dependence of its effect on $^{45}Ca$-efflux in guinea-pig *Taenia coli*. *Japanese Journal of Pharmacology*, **38**, 133–139

Susset, J. G., Tessier, C. D., Wincze, J. *et al.* (1989) Effect of yohimbine hydrochloride on erectile impotence: a double-blind study. *Journal of Urology*, **141**, 1360–1363

Szasz, G., Stevenson, R. W. D., Lee, L. and Sanders, H. D. (1987) Induction of penile erection by intracavernosal injection: a double-blind comparison of phenoxybenzamine *versus* papaverine-phentolamine *versus* saline. *Archives of Sexual Behavior*, **16**, 371–378

Virag, R., Ottesen, B., Fahrenkrug, J., Levy, C. and Wagner, G. (1982) Vasoactive intestinal polypeptide release during penile erection in man. *Lancet*, **ii**, 1166

Wagner, G. and Gerstenberg, T. (1987) Intracavernosal injection of vasoactive intestinal polypeptide (VIP) does not induce erection in man *per se*. *World Journal of Urology*, **5**, 171–177

Wein, A. J. and Van Arsdalen, K. N. (1988) Drug-induced male sexual dysfunction. *Urologic Clinics of North America*, **15**, 23–31

Weiner, N. (1985) Drugs that inhibit adrenergic nerves and block adrenergic receptors. In *Goodman and Gilman's The Pharmacological Basis of Therapeutics*, 7th edn (eds A. Gilman, L. S. Goodman, T. W. Rall and F. Murad), Macmillan, New York, pp. 183–187

Wespes, E., Rondeux, C. and Schulman, C. C. (1989) Effect of phentolamine on venous return in human erection. *British Journal of Urology*, **63**, 95-97

Wespes, E., Schiffman, S., Gilloteaux, J. *et al.* (1988) Study of neuropeptide Y-containing nerve fibers in the human penis. *Cell and Tissue Research*, **254**, 69–74

Willis, E. A., Ottesen, B., Wagner, G. *et al.* (1983) Vasoactive intestinal polypeptide (VIP) as a putative neurotransmitter in penile erection. *Life Sciences*, **33**, 383–391

Yanagisawa, M., Kurihara, H., Kimura, S. *et al.* (1988) A novel potent vasoconstrictor peptide produced by vascular endothelial cells. *Nature*, **332**, 411–415

Zorgniotti, A. W. and Lefleur, R. S. (1985) Auto-injection of the corpus cavernosum with a vasoactive drug combination for vasculogenic impotence. *Journal of Urology*, **133**, 39–41

# 5

# Endocrinology


## P.-M. G. Bouloux and J. A. H. Wass


Optimal male sexual and reproductive capability depends upon a complex interrelationship between psychological, emotional, neurological, vascular and endocrine factors. Endocrine disturbances are an important and potentially treatable cause of sexual dysfunction, and include disorders of the hypothalamo–pituitary–testicular (HPT) axis, hyperprolactinaemia (both associated with hypogonadism) and diabetes mellitus. Disturbances of thyroid, adrenal and calcium disorders may also result in subtle but adverse disturbances of sexual function. The commonest endocrinopathy causing impotence is diabetes mellitus, prevalence studies suggesting that up to 50% of patients with both insulin-dependent and non-insulin-dependent diabetes mellitus suffer from sexual dysfunction (McCulloch *et al.*, 1980).

Endocrinopathies have been estimated to account for 5–35% of cases of impotence. If diabetes mellitus is included, the higher figure is probably accurate. The predominant focus of this chapter will be on the physiology and pathophysiology of the HPT axis and prolactin secretion in so far as they are relevant to the understanding of sexual dysfunction. We will also review recent advances in the pathophysiology of diabetic impotence.

## The hypothalamo–pituitary–testicular (HPT) axis

### Endocrinology of the HPT axis

The endocrine function of the testicle involves a complex finely regulated interaction between the central nervous system, the anterior pituitary and the testis. The hypothalamus forms the most important part of the axis in the CNS, secreting gonadotrophin releasing hormone (GnRH) which stimulates pituitary production of luteinizing and follicle stimulating hormones (LH and FSH), which in turn stimulate the testes. The latter contain two functionally distinct compartments each of which subserves a different role:

1. The seminiferous tubules which house the Sertoli cells and spermatogonia, and their function is to produce spermatozoa.
2. The Leydig or interstitial cells produce and secrete sex steroids, notably testosterone and to a lesser extent oestradiol. Testosterone is responsible for the initiation, development and maintenance of primary and secondary sexual characteristics as well displaying a role in normal male sexual behaviour and potency. Testosterone also has an intratesticular paracrine (local) role in the initiation and maintenance of spermatogenesis.

Testicular function is regulated by the pituitary gonadotrophins, luteinizing hormone (LH) and follicle stimulating hormone (FSH). These glycoprotein hormones are made up of an alpha and beta subunit. The alpha subunit is common to all glycoprotein hormones (thyroid stimulating hormone, human chorionic gonadotrophin), biological activity and specificity being conferred by the beta subunit. LH acts on a specific Leydig cell receptor which is coupled to the adenyl cyclase enzyme. The ensuing intracellular cAMP generation initiates the cascade of effects leading to testosterone and to a much lesser extent oestradiol biosynthesis and secretion. Testosterone feeds back to the hypothalamus and pituitary to regulate LH secretion. Hypothalamic feedback on GnRH secretion is thought to be via the intermediary oestradiol, which is formed from CNS testosterone aromatization. FSH stimulates Sertoli cells predominantly, and possibly the developing spermatogonia. Stimulation also results in intracellular cAMP generation leading to the synthesis of proteins important in spermatogenesis. These include androgen binding protein (ABP) and transferrin. Inhibin production is also stimulated; this is a protein made up of A and B subunits involved in the negative feedback control of FSH secretion. Both testosterone and FSH are responsible for the production of ABP. The latter ensures a high local concentration of intratesticular testosterone, essential for spermatogenesis.

### Regulation of gonadotrophin secretion

Both LH and FSH are released in a pulsatile manner from pituitary gonadotrophs. The periodicity of pulsatility for LH is about 90 min. Pulsatile gonadotrophin secretion is secondary to pulsatile secretion of hypothalamic gonadotrophin releasing hormone (GnRH). GnRH is produced in the hypothalamic arcuate nucleus and reaches the anterior pituitary via portal vessels in the pituitary stalk. GnRH interacts with specific gonadotroph receptors which are coupled to adenyl cyclase. Generation of intracellular cAMP is necessary both for synthesis and secretion of gonadotrophins. Continuous exposure of these receptors to GnRH is associated with a desensitization process (down-regulation) and loss of responsivity to GnRH. A similar process follows administration of superactive analogues of GnRH. Therapeutic suppression of GnRH secretion by such analogues to produce medical castration is in current use in the management of androgen-dependent prostatic cancers and in the suppression of precocious puberty.

Secretion of GnRH is under the influence of central catecholamines and neuropeptides, including opioids.

## Biological actions of testosterone

In most androgen-responsive tissues testosterone is reduced to its active metabolite dihydrotestosterone (DHT) by the enzyme 5α-reductase. In other tissues (hypothalamus and some peripheral tissues) it may also be converted to oestradiol. Testosterone has both paracrine (local actions) and systemic effects. In the circulation it is bound to the plasma beta-globulin, sex hormone binding globulin (SHBG, derived from the liver) and, to a lesser extent, albumin. SHBG has one androgen binding site per molecule and also binds oestradiol. It binds dihydrotestosterone (DHT) with 2–3 times greater affinity than testosterone. However, androstenedione and oestrogen binding are only about 40% that of testosterone. In the blood about 42% testosterone is bound to SHBG (low capacity, high affinity) and 54% bound to albumin and other proteins (high capacity, low affinity). SHBG production is depressed by pharmacological doses of androgens and stimulated by pharmacological doses of oestrogens. Insulin may also play a role in its control. Only the non-protein bound steroid (3%) is biologically active. Factors that determine the SHBG concentration and hence the total testosterone level are listed in Table 5.1. In men with an intact HPT axis the consequence of alteration in SHBG levels and hence free testosterone are few, since the system merely resets to establish a normal steady state level of free testosterone. In disturbances of HPT function, alterations in SHBG can have a profound effect on the level of free sex steroids, particularly the free testosterone/oestrogen ratio.

**Table 5.1 Factors influencing circulating levels of SHBG**

| *Causes of raised SHBG* | *Causes of reduced SHBG* |
|---|---|
| Thyrotoxicosis | Androgens |
| Oestrogens | Acromegaly |
| Cirrhosis of the liver | Obesity |
| Hypogonadism | Hypothyroidism |
| Pre-puberty | Chronic liver failure |
| Alcohol | Insulin-like growth factor 1 (IGF1) |
| Anticonvulsants | |
| Any liver enzyme-inducing drug | |
| Free fatty acids | |

### Androgen action

In androgen-dependent tissues, testosterone and DHT bind to androgen receptors to produce the androgen–receptor complex within which the nucleus interacts with regulatory elements of the genome. This leads to androgen-dependent transcription, translation and protein synthesis. Qualitative or quantitative changes in the androgen receptors are one cause of male pseudohermaphrodism.

The effects of testosterone deficiency differ depending on the stage of development at which it occurs. *In utero*, it leads to the development of varying degrees of ambiguous genitalia, ranging from phenotypic females to near normal males. Testosterone deficiency before puberty causes failure of secondary sexual development, with infantile genitalia, eunuchoidism, lack of androgen-dependent hair growth, high pitched voice and persistence of prepubertal body fat distribution. In adults, testosterone deficiency is associated with reduced libido and potency, infertility, lethargy, fatigue and a number of behavioural changes. The hypogonadal male characteristically also has smooth youthful looking skin, lack of temporal hair recession and sparse facial and corporal hair (Figure 5.1). A decrease in ejaculatory volume (or absence thereof) is an early feature of loss of libido caused by hypogonadism. This is because stimulation of prostatic and seminal vesicular secretions requires high levels of testosterone. In general, the presence of a normal seminal volume is unlikely to indicate a hormonal cause for the sexual dysfunction.

### Actions of testosterone on sexual behaviour

Three lines of evidence support the importance of androgens in male sexual activity:

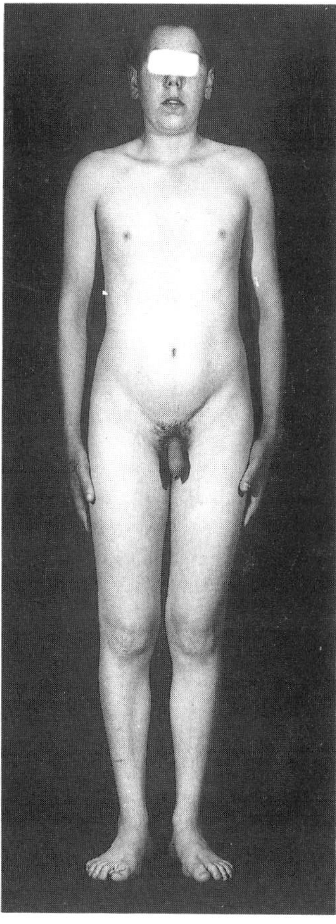

**Figure 5.1** Appearance of a 21-year-old hypogonadal male. Note the bilateral inguinal scars, female hair line and habitus, paucity of body hair and eunuchoid segments

1. Male castrates report a decline in sexual interest and ability, though potency is not lost in all (Bremer, 1959).
2. Hypogonadal males have decreased sexual interest which is reversed by androgen administration (Davidson, Camargo and Smith, 1979).
3. Both the anti-androgen cyproterone acetate and the superactive GnRH agonists will suppress sexuality in man. In the case of GnRH superactive agonists, impotence may become complete although sexual awareness and interest may persist.

Although it is recognized that low circulating testosterone levels adversely affect the whole gamut of male sexual behaviour (libido, sexual thoughts and fantasies, potency), the precise mechanisms whereby androgens exert these effects are largely unknown. In the human male, prepubertal castration uniformly prevents the development of normal sexual behaviour; orchidectomy in adults causes a decline in sexual activity, with only occasional castrated males continuing to have intercourse over a period of years (Beach, 1977; Bremer, 1959). In such individuals it is possible that the small quantities of testosterone and oestrogen formed by the adrenal may be adequate to sustain libido and potency. Androgen replacement to physiological levels in such men rapidly and reliably restores male sexual activity (Davidson, Camargo and Smith, 1979; Shakkebeak *et al.*, 1981). In men, raising the circulating testosterone level above the normal range by exogenous testosterone administration has little effect on sexual function, although pharmacological doses of androgens – as, for example, taken by body builders – are associated with an increase in aggressive behaviour.

The latency from administration of androgen to onset of sexual effect in the treatment of the hypogonadal male, particularly between the different components of sexual behaviour (sexual thoughts, fantasies, the capacity to respond to sexual stimuli, potency, orgasm and ejaculation frequency) has been poorly investigated. However, hypogonadal males receiving replacement treatment with intramuscular testosterone preparations usually describe peak erectile responsiveness as occurring 2–6 days after injection. Priapism not infrequently results in the androgen 'naive' individual; for this reason testosterone replacement should be gradually built up to the full dose over a number of months.

### Effect of age

There is a tendency for testosterone to fall slightly with advancing age in the male, although true male 'climacteric' is exceedingly rare. However, by the age of 65 years, 25% of males experience erectile failure (Federman, 1982). Low testosterone levels are associated with decreased sexual activity, and studies have shown that older men with high testosterone levels tend to be sexually more active compared with men with lower values. However, the association is modest and does not support a causal relationship, and testosterone therapy in this age group is rarely followed by improved sexual function.

## Clinical and laboratory evaluation of the impotent male

In the younger patient the history should focus on developmental milestones, progression through puberty and development of secondary sexual characteristics. This will include questions on axillary, pubic, facial hair and shaving frequency, growth, change in voice and body habitus and phallic enlargement, frequency of morning erections and masturbation. A complaint of reduced libido or potency after puberty may be the earliest clue to hypogonadism, antedating changes in shaving habits, loss of axillary or pubic hair, or development of gynaecomastia or galactorrhoea. Clinical examination may reveal anosmia, suggesting Kallmann's syndrome (olfactogenital dysplasia), and eunuchoidism (defined as an arm span of 5 cm or more in excess of height, or sole to pubis length exceeding crown to pubis length by more than 2 cm) indicative of delayed fusion of the long bone epiphyses. Regression of secondary sexual characteristics may be present, as well as gynaecomastia and galactorrhoea. The latter is characterized by increased retroareolar glandular tissue rather than adipose tissue and is often seen in primary testicular failure secondary to a fall in testosterone/oestradiol ratios. Testicular size should be measured using a Prader orchidometer and the testes carefully examined for evidence of nodularity suggesting a possible Leydig cell oestrogen secreting tumour (gynaecomastia and loss of libido are invariably present in such cases). In Klinefelter's syndrome the testes are pea-sized, the patients tall and eunuchoid; gynaecomastia is usually present and the buccal smear positive with an XXY karyotype. Other signs of systemic illness should be sought. In suspected prolactinoma, visual field and fundal examination should be carried out, and galactorrhoea sought. A classification of hypogonadism is given in Table 5.2.

**Table 5.2 Causes of hypogonadism**

GnRH deficiency:
- Hypothalamic lesions (tumours; encephalitis; granulomas; craniopharyngioma)
- Isolated GnRH deficiency (idiopathic; associated with Kallmann's)
- Prader–Willi syndrome (massive obesity, neonatal hypotonia, hyperphagia, mental retardation)
- Laurence–Moon–Biedl syndrome (growth retardation, obesity, syndactyly, retinitis pigmentosa)
- Alström's syndrome (obesity, nephropathy, hypertriglyceridaemia, hyperuricaemia, acanthosis nigricans and hypogonadotrophic hypogonadism)
- Familial cerebellar syndrome (cerebellar ataxia, nerve deafness, short fourth metacarpal)
- Hyperprolactinaemia (functional)
- Haemochromatosis
- Neurosarcoid

Pituitary disorders (gonadotrophin deficiency):
- Isolated LH deficiency (Pasqualini syndrome; eunuchoidism, absent secondary sexual characteristics, oligospermia)
- Tumours (functioning and non-functioning)
- Pituitary infarction
- Pituitary apoplexy
- Empty sella syndrome
- Haemochromatosis

Testicular disorders (primary gonadal failure):
- Undescended testes
- Bilateral torsion of testes
- Orchitis
- Seminiferous tubule dysgenesis (Klinefelter's syndrome)
- Haemochromatosis
- Impaired Leydig cell activity:
  - (a) Inborn errors of testosterone biosynthesis:
    - (i) 3β-hydroxysteroid dehydrogenase
    - (ii) 17α-hydroxylase
    - (iii) 17, 20-desmolase
    - (iv) 17β-hydroxysteroid dehydrogenase
  - (b) Leydig cell hypoplasia

Androgen-resistant states and enzyme defects:
- Testicular feminization (absence of androgen receptors)
- Incomplete androgen insensitivity
- 5α-reductase deficiency

## Biochemical evaluation

If hypogonadism is present, an attempt should be made to determine whether it is due to testicular or hypothalamopituitary disease. A 09.00 a.m. total testosterone level, SHBG, LH, FSH, oestradiol and prolactin levels should be measured. Low testosterone levels associated with high gonadotrophin levels and elevated oestrogen levels suggest primary gonadal failure. Provocative testing with human chorionic gonadotrophin (LH-like) in a dose of 4000 units intramuscularly for 4 days will fail to give the normal 2.5-fold increase in testosterone level in this situation. It is, however, rarely necessary to perform this test as it does not usually add information to the basal studies. Low gonadotrophin and testosterone levels but elevated oestradiol levels suggest the presence of an oestrogen-secreting testicular tumour. The finding of low gonadotrophin levels associated with low testosterone levels should prompt a search for hypothalamopituitary disease. A skull radiograph should be performed to detect an abnormal pituitary fossa or suprasellar calcification (this may signify the presence of a craniopharyngioma) and measurement of other basal hormones (thyroxine, cortisol), plasma and urine osmolality performed. A GnRH test (100 μg GnRH i.v.) with measurement of LH and FSH at 0, 30 and 60 min will evaluate the pituitary gonadotrophin reserve. The clomiphene test (50 mg clomiphene twice daily for 10 days: normal response is a doubling or more of the basal LH level) will test the integrity of the hypothalamic–pituitary axis. A positive response to GnRH but non-response of LH and FSH to clomiphene suggests GnRH deficiency (hypothalamic disease). A high gonadotrophin level with elevated testosterone level is compatible with an androgen insensitivity state, or alternatively a gonadotrophin-secreting pituitary tumour.

## Hyperprolactinaemia

Unlike other anterior pituitary hormones, the dominant regulation of prolactin secretion in man is inhibitory, mediated by hypothalamic dopamine originating in the tuberoinfundibular neurones of the arcuate nucleus. Minor prolactin secretagogues are thyrotrophin releasing hormone (TRH), vasoactive intestinal peptide (VIP) and peptide histidine isoleucine (PHI). Hyperprolactinaemia ensues if for any reason hypothalamic dopamine fails to reach the pituitary lactotroph and bind to the lactotroph membrane receptor, where it acts to suppress both cAMP generation and the phosphoinositide pathways. These actions of dopamine form the basis for the therapeutic effect of the longer acting dopamine agonist bromocriptine in hyperprolactinaemic disorders. Hypothalamic disturbances with destruction of dopaminergic neurones, stalk lesions with impaired dopamine transport to the anterior pituitary, and compression of portal vessels by a pituitary tumour impairing the delivery of dopamine (pseudoprolactinoma) are all associated with hyperprolactinaemia. Drugs that block the dopamine receptor have a similar effect, e.g. metoclopramide and phenothiazines. Prolactin-secreting tumours (prolactinomas) are among the commonest pituitary tumours seen in females, but are more rare in men. There are a number of medical conditions that may also lead to hyperprolactinaemia (Table 5.3).

### Hyperprolactinaemia and sexual dysfunction in man

Severe hyperprolactinaemia (prolactin >2000 mu/l may cause hypogonadism and is almost invariably associated with sexual dysfunction in the male.

#### Incidence of hyperprolactinaemia as a cause of sexual dysfunction

In one cohort of 850 impotent males screened systematically for hyperprolactinaemia there were ten with hyperprolactinaemia (prolactin >700 mu/l; 1.1%) of whom six showed evidence of a pituitary adenoma. Seventeen patients with mild hyperprolactinaemia (360–700 mu/l) were also found (Buvat *et al.*, 1985). Of 124 patients with premature ejaculation, 10% had mild hyperprolactinaemia. However, it is unlikely that the association is causal. Friedman *et al.* (1986) have reported a cohort of 49 unselected males (age range 19–69 years) presenting with erectile failure of one year's duration, and in whom other endocrinopathy and hepatic dysfunction had been excluded. The prolactin level was raised in only one, and that only mildly. Although hyperprolactinaemia is a rare cause of impotence, it remains a remediable cause and therefore estimation of prolactin level should feature in the investigative work-up of all impotent males.

**Table 5.3 Causes of hyperprolactinaemia**

| *Disorders of dopamine synthesis* |
|---|
| Hypothalamic disease: |
| Tumours (craniopharyngioma; third ventricular tumour; glioma; hamartoma; metastases) |
| Granulomas (sarcoidosis; histiocytosis X; tuberculoma) |
| Pituitary disorders: |
| Tumours (prolactinoma; acromegaly; non-functioning tumours (pseudoprolactinomas)) |
| Stalk section (surgical; traumatic; meningioma) |
| Drugs (dopamine antagonists, e.g. phenothiazines and metoclopramide; methyldopa; reserpine; oestrogens; opiates; intravenous cimetidine) |
| Miscellaneous disorders: |
| Primary hypothyroidism |
| Chronic renal failure |
| Cirrhosis |
| Chest wall lesions (neurogenic mechanisms) |
| Stress |
| Idiopathic |

#### Clinical features

Men with hyperprolactinaemia usually have gonadal dysfunction of gradual onset and, unless impotence is complete, patients may minimize symptoms attributing them to ageing or stresses. Similarly, the physician may easily invoke a psychogenic cause in a 40–50-year-old man with declining libido and elect to treat empirically with testosterone. The mean age for men at diagnosis of hyperprolactinaemia is about ten years greater than women (Franks and Jacobs, 1983). This delay in diagnosis may account for the greater incidence of macroadenomas, visual field defects and hypopituitarism in males at the time of presentation. The level of hyperprolactinaemia does not always correlate with the presence of symptoms.

About 40% of males with a prolactinoma have a visual field defect of some sort and headache is not infrequent. Men with hyperprolactinaemia tend to have not only reduced libido and erectile dysfunction but also a small ejaculatory volume. Some 14–33% of men with hyperprolactinaemia have galactorrhoea (Carter, Tyson and Tolis, 1978), and this important physical sign has to be carefuly sought in the impotent male although its absence does not rule out hyperprolactinaemia. Hyperprolactinaemia is also a cause of infertility (Segal *et al.*, 1979). In a survey of 171 infertile men, seven (4%) had hyperprolactinaemia which was reversed by bromocriptine.

### Measurement of serum prolactin

Because of the pulsatile nature of prolactin release and the rise which may follow stress (fear, pain, venepuncture), a minimum of three measurements are required before confirming the presence of hyperprolactinaemia. Once drugs and systemic disease (see Table 5.3) have been excluded, prolactin-secreting pituitary micro- or macroadenomas are the usual underlying cause, although levels of up to 2000 mu/l are often seen in apparently functionless tumours due to interference with dopamine delivery to the lactotroph. The patient should then be referred to an endocrinologist for further workup. This will include skull radiography, computed tomographic (CT) scanning, formal plotting of visual fields, and full basal and dynamic anterior pituitary function tests.

## Mechanism of hyperprolactinaemic hypogonadism

Hyperprolactinaemia may lead to hypogonadism, as well as exerting behavioural effects. The mechanism of hypogonadism is complex.

### Actions of prolactin on the hypothalamus

In the rat, hyperprolactinaemia causes increase in tuberoinfundibular dopamine content, leading to disruption of the normal pulsatility of GnRH and hence LH and FSH secretion. Similar mechanisms are believed to operate in the hyperprolactinaemic male where levels of LH and testosterone tend to be lower as a group than in normals. As the LH and FSH response to exogenous GnRH is frequently normal or frankly excessive in these patients – suggesting a normal pituitary gonadotrophin reserve – the defect is likely to reside in the hypothalamus and is generally thought to be a functional and potentially reversible alteration in GnRH secretion.

Increased hypothalamic dopamine content is thought to cause inhibition of LH and FSH release in man (Yen, 1977). A defect in GnRH pulsatility in hyperprolactinaemia has been suggested by some studies. A rise in portal vein dopamine has been inferred from the excessive response of thyroid stimulating hormone to dopamine receptor blockade in this situation (Scanlon *et al.*, 1980) as well as stimulation of LH and FSH secretion following dopamine antagonists reported in some but not all studies (Quigley *et al.*, 1979). Failure of LH pulsatility (Bouchard *et al.*, 1985) with a decreased 24 h urinary LH secretion has been recorded in male prolactinoma patients. In these studies, pulsatile administration of GnRH restored LH pulsatility and normal testosterone levels in four males with hyperprolactinaemia.

Prolactin-induced increases in hypothalamic opioid tone may also contribute to the decrease in amplitude and pulsatility of GnRH secretion.

### Pituitary actions

A destructive or invasive pituitary tumour may not only impair GnRH delivery to the gonadotroph, but may compress or destroy the gonadotrophs leading to hypogonadotrophic hypogonadism. In such situations, gonadotrophins and testosterone levels are low, and the LH/FSH response to exogenous GnRH is impaired.

### Peripheral actions of hyperprolactinaemia

Several abnormalities of testosterone metabolism have been demonstrated in hyperprolactinaemia. A direct effect of prolactin on the gonad was suggested in two studies demonstrating a blunted testosterone response to exogenous human chorionic gonadotrophin (HCG) in hyperprolactinaemia (Besser and Thorner, 1976; Faglia *et al.*, 1977). In contrast, Ambrosi *et al.* (1976) reported an enhanced testosterone response to HCG stimulation in males with drug-induced hyperprolactinaemia. Martikainen and Vinko (1982) found a blunted response of plasma 17β-oestradiol to HCG stimulation in hyperprolactinaemia, suggesting an inhibition of testicular aromatase activity. Magrini *et al.* (1976) failed to demonstrate an alteration in testosterone response to HCG, but found a diminshed rise in the testosterone metabolite 5α-dihydrotestosterone, suggesting an inhibitory effect of hyperprolactinaemia on 5α-reductase activity in peripheral tissues.

In general, therefore, it seems likely that the hypogonadism of hyperprolactinaemia is both central and peripheral in origin.

### Prolactin and libido

Diminished testosterone levels in themselves appear to be rather less important in the mechanism of sexual dysfunction than hyperprolactinaemia *per se*. Thus increasing plasma testosterone by intramuscular injections does not appear to improve potency consistently in hyperprolactinaemic patients. In contrast, administration of the dopamine agonist bromocriptine which rapidly lowers prolactin, produces a rapid improvement in potency even when the testosterone level remains subnormal (Nagulesparen, Ang and Jenkins, 1978; Prescott *et al.*, 1982). The suggestion implicit in this finding is that hyperprolactinaemia in some way acts centrally to depress the mechanisms responsible for libido and potency.

## Thyroid dysfunction and impotence

Both hyper- and hypothyroidism may be associated with decreased potency. Hyperthyroidism has been associated with decreased libido in 71% of affected men (Kidd, Glass and Vigersky, 1979). Gynaecomastia is present in 10–40% and is probably due to increased circulating oestrogens and SHBG, which may reflect increased peripheral conversion of androgen to oestrogen (Chopra and Tulchinsky, 1974). Patients with hypothyroidism frequently complain of lethargy, loss of libido and erectile failure. Testosterone secretion is decreased in hypothyroidism and the metabolic transformation of testosterone is shifted towards aetiocholanolone rather than androsterone (Hellman and Bradlow 1970). Hyperprolactinaemia may also contribute to impotence in such individuals. Thyroid function should be evaluated in cases of unexplained impotence.

## Adrenal and calcium disorders

These can produce sexual dysfunction by non-specific effects. Impotence is usually restored on correction of the underlying defect.

## Diabetes mellitus and impotence

Diabetes mellitus is among one of the most common causes of organic impotence. Some 15% of diabetic men below the age of 35 years and 55% of diabetic men aged 60 years or above are impotent. Libido is usually preserved, and testosterone and gonadotrophine levels are almost invariably within the normal range. Both vasculogenic and neurogenic causes have been considered among the major aetiological factors in diabetic impotence.

### Clinical features

Erectile dysfunction in diabetics is usually gradual in onset. A decrease in penile rigidity is followed by a decline in the frequency of morning erections and nocturnal, masturbatory and coital erections become similarly impaired. Psychological stress may occur secondarily or reactively in patients with organic impotence, complicating the clinical picture and exacerbating the impairment. Thus men with partial erectile failure may achieve sufficient rigidity to permit penetration and coitus when unstressed, but experience total erectile failure under stress, presumably due to increased sympathetic anti-erectile activity.

Ejaculatory disturbances also occur in diabetes, particularly retrograde ejaculation, whereby the patient experiences the rhythmic pumping action associated with ejaculation without semen emerging from the penis. A similar problem may arise following guanethidine and phenoxybenzamine therapy, and in diabetes it is thought that the competence of the $\alpha$-adrenergically innervated internal sphincter of the bladder is compromised.

### Recent insights into the mechanism of diabetic impotence

Studies in animal models of diabetes as well as in humans have revealed pathological changes in penile arteries, morphological alterations in penile nerves and neurotransmitter depletion within the corpus cavernosum. These are likely to relate to the effects of atherosclerosis, hypertension and hyperlipidaemia associated with diabetes mellitus. Somatic and autonomic nerve dysfunction can be demonstrated in these patients, and the sacral arc reflex may be abnormal (Campbell, 1976; Jevitch *et al.*, 1982). The noradrenaline content of the corpora cavernosa is decreased in diabetic impotent males as compared with males whose impotence has a non-neurological cause (Melman *et al.*, 1980), presumably reflecting some degree of autonomic nerve dysfunction.

Further, several studies have reported that in the cardiovascular system parasympathetic fibres are damaged before sympathetic nerves (Ewing *et al.*, 1981), and it is possible that the long parasympathetic nerves to the pelvic organs are the most vulnerable of the autonomic nerves, perhaps explaining why erectile failure may be the earliest and most common feature of diabetic autonomic neuropathy. Because of the lack of sensitivity of current investigative techniques for early diagnosis of autonomic neuropathy, it is uncertain to what extent neurogenic factors may contribute to sexual impairment in diabetics; macro and microvascular complications of diabetes are also likely to contribute significantly to diabetic impotence.

### Aetiology of diabetic neuropathy

This is either metabolic or vascular in origin, or both.

#### Metabolic sequelae of hyperglycaemia

Much of what is known is derived from observations in experimental diabetes mellitus. It is presently envisaged that the peripheral nerves of diabetic patients take up glucose from blood, this being converted to sorbitol by aldose reductase. Sorbitol is in turn converted to fructose by the enzyme sorbitol dehydrogenase, the whole reaction being in direct relationship to blood glucose level. Fructose accumulation leads to inhibition of sodium-dependent myoinositol uptake, depressed intraneural myoinositol, and consequently reduced membrane phospholipid. $Na^+/K^+$ ATPase activity is thereby depressed, and this sets up a vicious circle further inhibiting sodium-dependent myoinositol uptake. In experimental diabetes the administration of aldose reductase inhibitors can reverse these metabolic changes with restoration of $Na^+/K^+$ ATPase activity and normalization of conduction velocities. In man, the administration of aldose reductase inhibitors has led to slight improvements in electrical conduction velocities and in clinical sensory symptoms. No beneficial effects of these agents on impotence have as yet been reported.

### Vascular effects

In man, the insertion of glass platinum microelectrodes into peripheral nerve fascicles has demonstrated the *in vivo* ischaemic nature of peripheral nerve damage in subjects with clinical neuropathy. Microscopically, the vasa nervorum of these patients are occluded (Dyck *et al.*, 1987).

### Tissue glycosylation

The pathophysiological effects of tissue protein glycosylation (advanced glycosylation products) are poorly understood, but may contribute to neuronal malfunction in diabetes.

### Endothelium-dependent abnormalities in diabetes

Recent studies have shown impaired neural and endothelium-dependent mechanisms of corporeal smooth muscle relaxation in specimens of tissue from diabetic patients with impotence (de Tejada *et al.*, 1989). Autonomic nerve relaxation of corporeal smooth muscle is impaired (Figure 5.2a), although autonomic mediated contractions are maintained, suggesting dysfunction of vasodilator nerves. Further, reduced endothelium-dependent relaxation of the trabecular smooth muscle in response to acetylcholine has been demonstrated (Figure 5.2b). Acetylcholine acts by releasing nitric oxide (endothelial-derived relaxing factor; EDRF) from endothelial cells, and this causes smooth muscle relaxation via an increase in intracellular 3′5′-cyclic guanosine monophosphate content. The *in vitro* relaxation response to sodium nitroprusside and papaverine is normal in this tissue (Figure 5.2c), suggesting that diabetic men have a decreased synthesis or release of EDRF rather then insensitivity of smooth muscle to its actions. These observations suggest that diabetes can fundamentally alter the properties of the trabeculae, thereby impairing their relaxation and thus the erectile process. These findings also form a rational basis for the use of intracavernosal smooth muscle relaxant drugs (phentolamine, papaverine) in the management of the diabetic impotent male.

## Treatment of endocrine causes of impotence

Hypothalamopituitary disorders require referral to an endocrinologist for assessment and treatment. The underlying condition will require investigation and treatment in its own right. Prolactinomas may be treated medically or surgically with or without radiotherapy. The response of this tumour to the dopamine agonist bromocriptine can be dramatic with significant shrinkage of the tumour and resumption of normal pituitary function where this had previously been defective (Figure 5.3). Visual field defects due to suprasellar extensions and potency may be rapidly restored to normal on treatment. However, the benefits of dopamine agonists are usually only maintained so long as the patient remains on treatment. Definitive therapy in the form of surgery and radiotherapy (or the combination) is usually required. When residual hypogonadism persists, long-term androgen replacement is indicated. This may be accomplished by administering the orally active compound testosterone undecanoate (Restandol) at a dose of 40–80 mg t.d.s. or testosterone enanthate (Primoteston Depot) i.m. 3–4-weekly at a dose of 250–500 mg. The same doses are usually effective in the treatment of hypogonadism due to Leydig cell failure.

Endocrinologists are frequently referred patients with sexual dysfunction and mild hyperprolactinaemia (360–800 mu/l). In these instances it is customary to repeat the measurements on two or more occasions to confirm the abnormality. In the absence of drug or other ‘secondary’ causes of hyperprolactinaemia (see Table 5.3), investigation with sellar X-rays and CT scanning rarely reveals a tumour. A therapeutic trial of bromocriptine should be given in such instances, although this is rarely successful.

## Treatment of diabetic impotence

Diabetic impotence poses an altogether greater management problem. Even with optimal glycaemic control, impotence is seldom improved. The only treatments currently are intracavernosal pharmacotherapy (with papaverine, phentolamine and prostaglandin $E_1$, alone or in combination), the use of vacuum erection aids or penile implants. An insulin syringe with a 27–30 gauge needle is used for intracavernosal pharmacotherapy and this minimizes pain and bleeding. Following an optimal dose of vasorelaxant drug, the erection should last 30 min or so. About 70% of diabetic patients experience a satisfactory erection with this treatment. The follow-up of a large number of patients treated by this method has now been published (Zentgraf, Baccouche and Juenemann, 1988). Local complications of therapy include fibrotic nodules (1.5–60%), infection and priapism (2.5–15%) which, if not treated, urgently may lead to pancavernosal scarring. The painless nodules can lead to penile

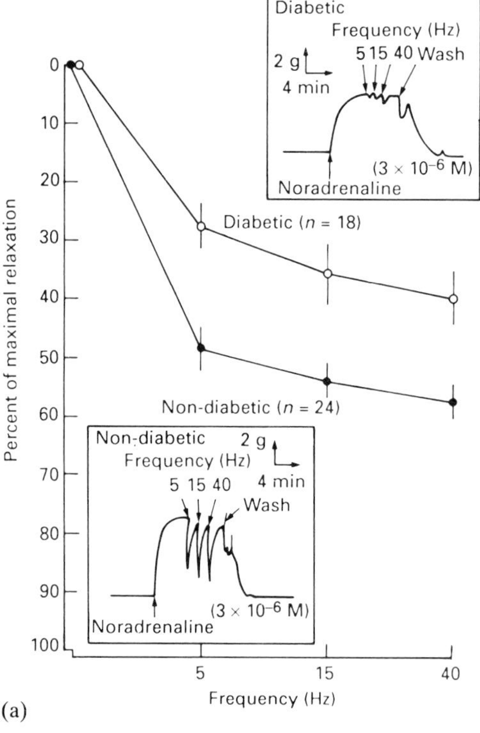


(a)

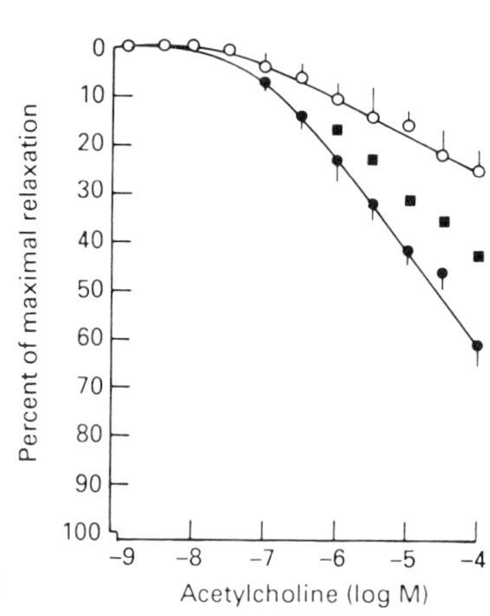


(b)

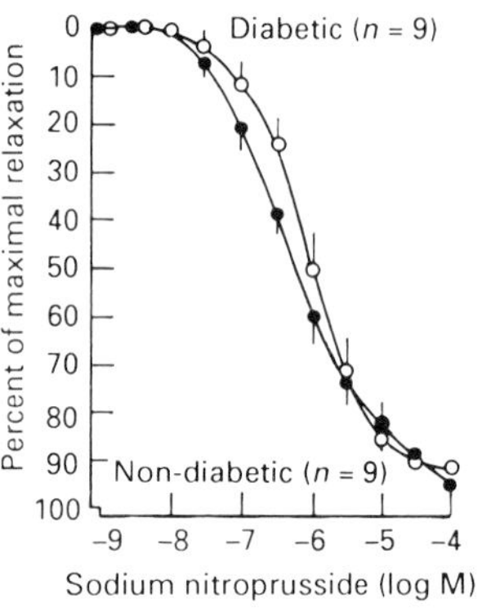


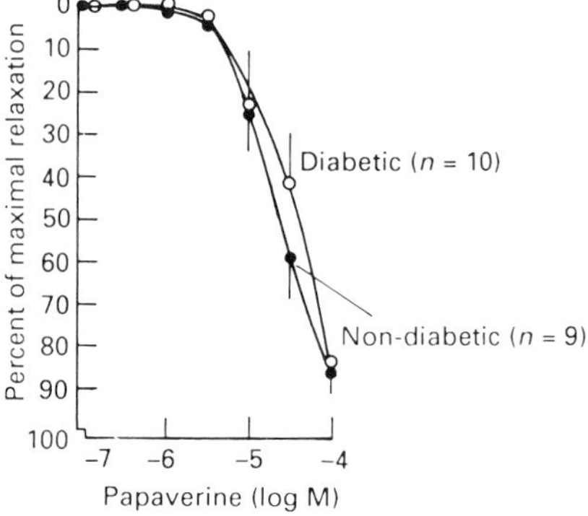


(c)

**Figure 5.2** (a) Relaxation of smooth muscle from the corpora cavernosa of diabetic and non-diabetic men, induced by transmural electrical stimulation of autonomic nerves. The asterisks indicate significant differences in relaxation between diabetic and non-diabetic patients; (b) relaxation of smooth muscle from the corpora cavernosa of 16 diabetic (○) and 22 non-diabetic (●) men induced by acetylcholine (results given as mean + s.e.m.). Asterisks indicate statistically significant differences in relaxation at each concentration of acetylcholine between corporal muscle strips from diabetic and non-diabetic patients; (c) relaxation of smooth muscle from the corpora cavernosa of diabetic and non-diabetic patients induced by sodium nitroprusside and papaverine. Tone was induced in each muscle strip by noradrenaline ($3 \times 10^{-6}$ M). There were no significant differences in the contraction caused by noradenaline or in the relaxation induced by either endothelium independent diabetic and non-diabetic tissue. (Reproduced from de Tejada *et al.* (1989) with kind permission of the editor)

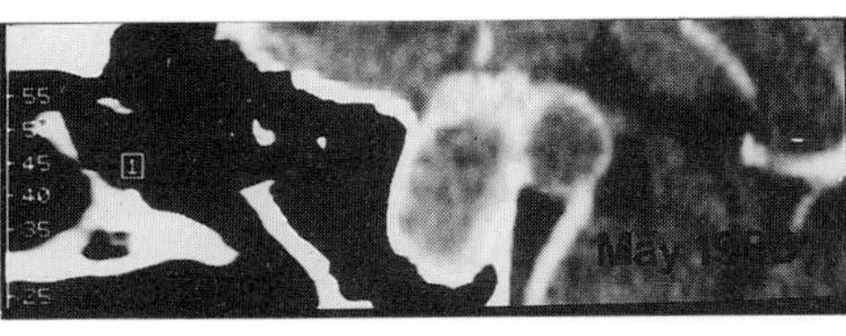


(a)

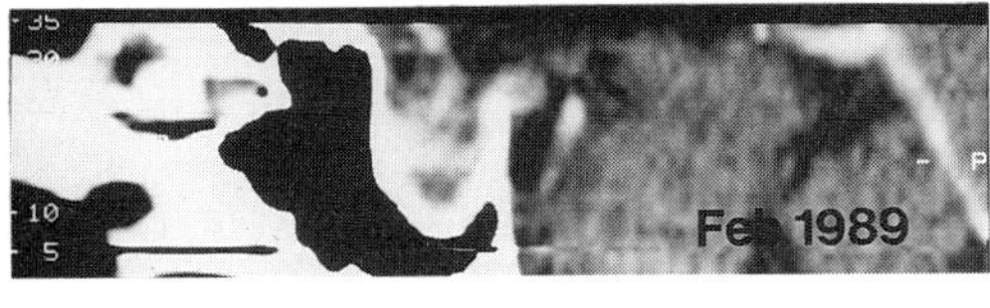


(b)

**Figure 5.3** Contrast enhanced sagittal reconstructed CT scan showing macroadenoma (a) before and (b) after bromocriptine-induced shrinkage

curvature. Systemic side effects of treatment include vasovagal attacks and hepatotoxicity (associated with papaverine but reversible after cessation of therapy). The prostanoid prostaglandin $E_1$ is not associated with prolonged erections or corporeal fibrosis, although penile pain after injection is frequent.

## References


Ambrosi, B., Traraglini, P., Beck-Peccoz, P. *et al.* (1976) Effect of sulpiride-induced hyperprolactinaemia on serum testosterone response to HCG in normal men. *Journal of Clinical Endocrinology and Metabolism*, **43**, 700–703

Beach, F. A. (1977) Hormonal control of sex-related behaviour. In *Human Sexuality in Four Perspectives*, John Hopkins Press, Baltimore, pp.247–267

Besser, G. M. and Thorner, M. O. (1976) Bromocriptine in the treatment of the hyperprolactinaemia-hypogonadism syndromes. *Postgraduate Medical Journal* **52**, (Suppl. 1), 64–70

Bouchard, P., Lagoguey, M., Brailly, S. and Schaison, G. (1985) Gonadotrophin releasing hormone pulsatile administration restores luteinising hormone pulsatility and normal testosterone levels in males with hyperprolactinaemia. *Journal of Clinical Endocrinology and Metabolism*, **60**, 258–262

Bremer, J. (1959) Asexualization: a follow-up study of 244 cases. Macmillan, New York, pp. 63–117

Buvat, J., Lemaire, A., Buvat-Herbaut, M. *et al.* (1985) Hyperprolactinaemia and sexual function in males. *Hormone Research*, **22**, 196–203

Campbell, I. W. (1976) Diabetic autonomic neuropathy. *British Journal of Hospital Practice*, **30**, 153–156

Carter, J. N., Tyson, J. E. and Tolis, G. (1978) Prolactin secreting tumours and hypogonadism in 22 men. *New England Journal of Medicine*, **299**, 847–852

Chopra, I. J. and Tulchinsky, D. (1974) Status of estrogen–androgen balance in hyperthyroid men with Graves' disease. *Journal of Clinical Endocrinology amd Metabolism*, **38**, 297–301

Davidson, J. M., Camargo, C. A. and Smith, E. R. (1979) Effect of androgens on sexual behaviour in hypogonadal men. *Journal of Clinical Endrocrinology and Metabolism*, **48**, 955–958

de Tejada, I. S., Goldstein, I., Azadzoi, K. *et al.* (1989) Impaired neurogenic and endothelium-mediated relaxation of penile smooth muscle from diabetic men with impotence. *New England Journal of Medicine*, **320**, 1025–1030

Dyck, P. J., Thomas, P. K., Asbury, A. K. *et al.* (eds) (1987) *Diabetic Neuropathy*, W.B. Saunders, Philadelphia

Faglia, G., Beck-Peccoz, P., Travaglini, P. *et al.* (1977) Functional studies in hyperprolactinaemic states. In *Prolactin and Human Reproduction* (eds P. G. Crosignani and C. Robyn), Academic Press, New York, pp. 225–238

Federman, D. D. (1982) Impotence: etiology and management. *Hospital Practice*, **17**, 155–159

Franks, A. and Jacobs, H. S. (1983) Hyperprolactinaemia. *Clinical Endocrinology and Metabolism*, **12**, 641–668

Friedman, D. E., Clare, A. W. *et al.* (1986) Should impotent males who have no clinical evidence of hypogonadism have routine endocrine screening? *Lancet*, **(i)**, 1041

Hellman, L. and Bradlow, H. L. (1970) Recent advances in human steriod metabolism. *Advances in Clinical Chemistry*, **13**, 1–25

Jevitch, M. J., Edson, M., Jarman, W. D. *et al.* (1982) Vascular factors in erectile failure among diabetics. *Urology*, **19**, 163–168

Kidd, G. S., Glass, A. R. and Vigersky, R. A. (1979) The hypothalamo–pituitary–testicular axis in thyrotoxicosis. *Journal of Clinical Endocrinology and Metabolism*, **48**, 798–801

Magrini, G., Ebiner, J. R., Burchardt, P. and Felber, J. P. (1976) Study on the relationship between plasma prolactin levels and androgen metabolism in man. *Journal of Clinical Endocrinology and Metabolism*, **43**, 944–947

Martikainen, H. and Vinko, F. (1982) HCG stimulation of testicular steroidogenesis during induced hyper and hypoprolactinaemia in man. *Clinical Endocrinology*, **16**, 227–234

McCulloch, D. K., Campbell, I. W., Wu, F. C. *et al.* (1980) The presence of diabetic impotence. *Diabetologia*, **18**, 279–283

Melman, A., Henry, D. P., Felten, D. L. *et al.* (1980) Alteration of the penile corpora in patients with erectile impotence. *Investigative Urology*, **17**, 474–477

Nagulesparen, M., Ang, V. and Jenkins, J. S. (1978) Bromocriptine treatment of males with pituitary tumours, hyperprolactinaemia and hypogonadism. *Clincal Endocrinology*, **9**, 73–79

Prescott, R. W. G., Kendall Taylor, P., Hall, K. *et al.* (1982) Hyperprolactinaemia in men – response to bromocriptine therapy. *Lancet*, **i**, 245–249

Quigley, M. E., Judd, S. J., Gililand, G. B. and Yen, S. C. C. (1979) Effects of dopamine antagonist on the release of gonadotropin and prolactin in normal women and women with hyperprolactinaemic anovulation. *Journal of Clinical Endocrinology and Metabolism*, **48**, 718–720

Scanlon, M. F., Rodriguez-Arnao, M. D., McGregor, A. M. *et al.* (1980) Altered dopaminergic regulation of thyrotropin release in patients with prolactinomas: comparison with other tests of hypothalamic pituitary function. *Journal of Clinical Endocrinology and Metabolism*, **14**, 133–143

Segal, S., Jaffe, H., Laufer, N. *et al.* (1979) Male hyperprolactinaemic effects on infertility. *Fertility and Sterility*, **32**, 556–559

Shakkebeak, N. E., Bancroft, J., Davidson, D. W. *et al.* (1981) Androgen replacement with oral testosterone undecanoate in hypogonadal men: a double blind controlled study. *Clinical Endocrinology*, **14**, 49–61

Yen, S. C. C. (1977) Neuroendocrine aspects of the regulation of cyclic gonadotrophin release in women. In *Clinical Neuroendocrinology* (eds L. Martini and G.M. Besser), Academic Press, New York, pp. 27–34

Zentgraf, M., Baccouche, M. and Juenemann, K. P. (1988) Diagnosis and therapy of erectile dysfunction using papaverine and phentolamine. *Urologia Internationalis*, **43**, 65–75

# Section Two

# Evaluation of the impotent male

# 6

# Initial assessment of patients with erectile dysfunction

R. S. Kirby and I. Eardley

As our knowledge of the pathogenesis of erectile dysfunction has expanded there has been a parallel increase in the variety and complexity of investigations employed to establish the cause of the disorder. However, despite the highly technological diagnostic modalities we now have at our means, we must not forget – and this is especially important in the evaluation of the impotent male – the basic principle taught to all medical students that accurate diagnosis depends on history and examination which are supplemented by special investigations. Subsequent chapters dwell in some depth on the still developing and increasingly sophisticated modalities of diagnosis used in erectile impotence, but in this chapter we shall consider how the patient should be assessed initially.

## History

Because of the sensitive nature of the complaint of impotence it is of paramount importance to establish early an amicable relationship of trust between patient and clinician. Building this rapport requires more time and patience than is usually required in, for example, the assessment of a patient with benign prostatic enlargement, and appointment schedules need to be adjusted accordingly. Some clinicians find it helpful to send the patient and his partner a questionnaire to complete (Nowinski and LoPiccolo, 1979) before the first visit, but in our experience the relevant questions can usually be covered in a half-hour interview with more flexibility than can be achieved in a questionnaire.

By far the most common presenting complaint is that of reduced rigidity and duration of erections; less commonly the patient complains of a total absence of erectile activity. Enquiry should concentrate initially on this element of the symptoms and their duration, as well as the rapidity and particular circumstances of onset. A key question is obviously whether the impairment of erections is consistent rather than 'situational' with preservation of nocturnal and early morning erections. Although the majority of physicians are now acquainted with the association between preservation of the latter and psychogenic impotence, most patients do not make this connection. A useful guide to the severity of the problem is to enquire when intercourse was last possible – one not uncommonly receives the surprising reply that this was accomplished only a few days ago! Discreet enquiry should also be made as to whether the problem is confined to sexual encounters with one partner or whether present with other partners. The partner's attitude to the potency problem should also be established. Enquiry about deviant sexual behaviour or taboo practices at this early stage, although relevant, may be unhelpful because they risk compromising the developing relationship between interviewer and patient. While libido is usually preserved in patients with erectile impotence, inevitably increasing the psychological frustrations of the patient, a decline of libido may suggest an endocrinological cause of the problem and should be documented. Ejaculation is much less commonly affected than erection itself, but enquiry should be made as to whether ejaculation is premature, delayed or dry (as commonly occurs following transurethral resection of the prostate).

The previous medical history should include a brief survey of sexual history which may provide a clue to a congenital problem due perhaps to a veno-occlusive disorder or congenital chordee. Previous surgery, especially pelvic surgery for bowel, bladder or prostatic malignancy, reconstructive vascular surgery or renal transplantation, may obviously be relevant. Multisystem disorders may result in impotence and can sometimes present with this symptom. Hypertension and diabetes are by far the most common of these and the family history may provide a clue, but alcoholism, thyroid dysfunction, haemochromatosis and other systemic disorders should be borne in mind (Table 6.1).

**Table 6.1 Organic causes of erectile dysfunction**

| | |
|---|---|
| Congenital deformities:<br>Epispadias<br>Hypospadias<br>Congenial chordee<br>Microphallus | Metabolic disorders:<br>Diabetes<br>Haemochromatosis<br>Alcoholism<br>Sickle cell disease<br>Hepatic/renal failure<br>Scleroderma |
| Mechanical:<br>Morbid obesity<br>Peyronie's disease<br>Bilateral hydrocele<br>Phimosis<br>Tethered frenulum<br>Carcinoma of penis | Neurogenic disorders:<br>Multiple system atrophy<br>Spinal cord lesions<br>Multiple sclerosis<br>Tabes dorsalis<br>Peripheral neuropathies<br>Spina bifida<br>Amyotrophic lateral sclerosis |
| Post-surgical:<br>Cystectomy, urethrectomy<br>Radical prostatectomy<br>Abdominoperineal resection of rectum<br>Low anterior resection of rectum<br>Rectal pull-through procedures<br>Transurethral resection of prostate<br>External sphincterotomy | Abnormalities of hypothalamopituitary function:<br>1. Congenital: LH-FSH deficiency (Kallmann's syndrome)<br>Congenital hypogonadotrophic hypogonadism<br>Panhypopituitarism<br>2. Acquired:<br>Trauma, infiltrative disease, tumours of pituitary, etc.<br>Exogenous hormones<br>Hyperprolactinaemia |
| Vascular insuffiency:<br>Aorto-iliac disease (Leriche syndrome)<br>Internal iliac atheroma<br>Atheroma of pudendal vessels<br>Distal vessel disease<br>Post-priapism<br>Smoking<br>Anaemia<br>Venous leakage<br>Post-pelvic fracture | Primary gonadal abnormalities:<br>Chromosomal abnormalities (e.g. Klinefelter's syndrome)<br>Bilateral anorchia<br>Gonadal toxins<br>Drug-induced gonadal damage (chemotherapeutic agents)<br>Gonadal injury (trauma/mumps) |

Of the neurological disorders which may cause impotence multiple sclerosis (MS) is the most common, but this is seldom a presenting feature of the disorder. Another diffuse disease affecting the central nervous system, however, may produce impotence as its earliest presenting manifestation. This disease, originally known as the Shy–Drager syndrome but now more commonly termed multiple system atrophy (MSA), is characterized by selective degeneration of autonomic neurones in the CNS. There is progressive selective cell loss from the pons, medulla and cerebellum, as well as degeneration of the neurones of the intermediolateral cell column of the thoracolumbar sympathetic outflow and sacral parasympathetic outflow. The condition affects patients in their middle age with a male to female ratio of 2:1. In the male, erectile impotence is accompanied by frequency and urgency of micturition which may be confused with bladder outflow obstruction due to benign prostatic enlargement. An important symptom which may provide a clue to this often elusive diagnosis is postural (orthostatic) hypotension due to impaired sympathetic vasoconstrictor tone, and this can usually be demonstrated on measuring blood pressure in the standing and lying positions (Bannister, 1988).

## Drug history

A detailed history of all medications is essential in the evaluation of patients with impotence since many pharmacological agents may be associated with problems of potency (Table 6.2). Often it is difficult to decide whether it is the drug itself or the condition for which it is being administered (i.e. hypertension) which has caused the symptom.

Antihypertensive agents have most often been cited as the most common medication-related cause of impotence (Slag *et al.*, 1983). Clonidine, methyldopa and reserpine, all of which share a centrally acting sympatholytic effect, are associated with an incidence of impotence in about one-third to

**Table 6.2 Drugs associated with erectile dysfunction**

| | |
|---|---|
| Major tranquillizers:<br>Phenothiazines, e.g. fluphenazine, chorpromazine, promazine, mesoridazine<br>Butyrophenones, e.g. haloperidol<br>Thiozanthines, e.g. thiothixene, chorprothixine | Antihypertensives:<br>Diuretics, e.g. thiazides, spironolactone<br>Vasodilators, e.g. hydralazine<br>Central sympatholytics, e.g. methyldopa, clonidine, reserpine<br>Ganglion blockers, e.g. guanethidine, bethanidine<br>Alpha-blockers, e.g. phentolamine, phenoxybenzamine, prazosin etc.<br>Beta-blockers, e.g. propranolol, metoprolol, atenolol, etc. |
| Antidepressants:<br>Tricyclics, e.g. nortryptyline, amitriptyline, desipramine, doxepin<br>MAO inhibitors, e.g. isocarboxazide, phenelzine, tranylcypromine, pargylene, procarbazine | Recreational drugs:<br>Alcohol<br>Marijuana<br>Amphetamines<br>Barbiturates<br>Nicotine<br>Opiates |
| Anxiolytics:<br>Benzodiazepines, e.g. chlordiazepoxide, diazepam, chorazepate | |
| Anticholinergics:<br>Atropine<br>Propantheline<br>Benztrophine<br>Dimenhydrinate<br>Diphenhydramine | Miscellaneous:<br>Cimetidine<br>Clofibrate<br>Cyproterone acetate<br>Digoxin<br>Oestrogens<br>Indomethacin<br>+ many others |

one-quarter of patients treated, but are seldom used therapeutically now. The precise mechanism by which they impair potency is unclear, but probably they directly reduce libido by a central effect and they may also elevate serum prolactin levels. Peripherally acting α-adrenoceptor blockers such as phenoxybenzamine (mixed $\alpha_1$ and $\alpha_2$ blockade) and the newer $\alpha_1$ selective adrenoceptor blockers prazosin, doxazosin and terazosin are less commonly associated with impotence – indeed from their vasodilatory action on cavernosal vessels one might expect their effect to be mildly beneficial – but by blocking the sympathetically-mediated closure of the bladder neck at the time of ejaculation they may occasionally produce retrograde ejaculation; phenoxybenzamine has also been shown to decrease LH production.

By contrast, β-adrenoceptor blockers have often been reported to cause impotence especially at higher doses, either directly by a peripheral action on the corporeal tissue and also by a central effect on libido (Papadopoulous, 1980). Their ability to penetrate the central nervous system and induce a sympatholytic effect depends on their lipid solubility. Newer beta-blockers such as atenolol are water soluble and seem to cause less impairment of sexual function. Spironolactone has been reported to induce gynaecomastia, erectile dysfunction and reduced libido in some patients and vasodilators such as hydralazine as well as diuretics, including hydrochlorothiazide and frusemide, have also been cited in this context. However, the newer angiotensin converting enzyme (ACE) inhibitors do not as yet seem to produce this result.

It must be remembered that in some patients with partial vasculogenic impotence high systolic arterial pressures may be required to achieve sufficient cavernosal artery flow for erection. Lowering blood pressure into the normal range in itself may therefore to some extent compromise penile blood flow and induce impotence.

Many major and minor tranquillizers and hypnotics have been reported to cause both diminished libido and erectile impotence. Antidepressants such as monoamine oxidase (MAO) inhibitors and tricyclic compounds may cause impotence, probably by decreasing libido. The minor tranquillizers or anxiolytic agents, particularly the benzodiazepines, exert a depressive effect on the brainstem, limbic system and septal region. Libido can also be reduced and impotence may follow. Meprobamate, barbiturates and other sedative hypnotics all exert a central effect similar to the benzodiazepines with similar effects.

Drugs with anti-androgenic activity such as ketoconazole, cyproterone acetate and the histamine receptor blocker cimetidine (Pedan *et al.*, 1979) are known to cause diminished potency although interestingly flutamide, which is also an anti-androgen, seems to spare both potency and libido while still effectively blocking androgen receptors.

Recreational drugs such as marijuana (Horowitz and Gobel, 1979) and cocaine and heroin (Mirin *et al.*, 1980) may also cause impotence and reduce libido and are associated with a reduction of testosterone levels. Cigarette smoking, probably by virtue of its vasoconstricting effect, has also been reported to cause impaired potency (Forsberg *et al.*, 1979). Alcoholism may induce impotence by several mechanisms: peripheral neuropathy, testicular dysfunction, an effect on the hypothalamopituitary axis as well as impaired hepatic function resulting in increased serum oestrogen levels. Even moderate doses of alcohol may impair erectile function (though paradoxically increase libido) and all patients with potency problems should be advised to reduce their alcohol consumption, as well as refrain from cigarette, cigar and pipe smoking.

## Physical examination

A thorough physical examination is essential and care should be taken to look for signs of either thyroid under-activity or over-activity as well as stigmata of liver failure or anaemia. Hypertension must obviously be excluded. All peripheral pulses should be palpated and any cardiac murmurs or arrhythmias excluded. A full neurological examination is important, with special attention being paid to the sacral spinal outflow. Saddle anaesthesia with loss of bulbocavernosus reflex in combination with a lax anal sphincter may suggest the presence of an occult cauda equina lesion. These may occasionally present with impotence due to a central prolapse of an intervertebral disc or a slow-growing lumbar or sacral intraspinal tumour.

Examination of the external genitalia must exclude congenital or acquired abnormalities of the penis itself. Peyronie's plaques should be sought along the palpable length of the corpora and the patient questioned about the presence of any erectile deformity. Preputial abnormalities such as tethering of the frenulum or phimosis may occasionally present with impotence as well as a spectrum of other genital abnormalities including microphallus, epispadias and squamous cell carcinoma of the penis. The presence of small testes and reduced secondary sexual characteristics may suggest hypogonadism and it is worth enquiring about the frequency of facial shaving as this declines with androgen insufficiency. The anterior chest wall should be examined to exclude gynaecomastia and enquiry made concerning galactorrhoea. The causes of primary hypogonadism and testicular failure are listed in Table 6.1 and when present are an indication for referral for specialist endocrine opinion.

Rectal examination should be carefully performed in every case of erectile dysfunction to assess prostatic size and consistency. If the presence of benign prostatic enlargement is detected a flow rate should be determined and the patient warned that androgen therapy may cause further bladder outflow obstruction. The presence of prostatic nodules should raise the possibility of early prostatic cancer and a prostate specific antigen (PSA) value measured. A prostatic biopsy under transrectal ultrasound control may be necessary – in these circumstances androgen therapy is contraindicated.

Investigation of the impotent male must obviously be tailored to the individual concerned and any leads given by the history or examination. Baseline haematological and biochemical screens are necessary which will include importantly a random plasma glucose to exclude diabetes mellitus. Also included are liver function tests to exclude hepatic impairment which may be associated with increased serum oestrogen levels and a reduced plasma testosterone. The baseline values are also useful if papaverine therapy is subsequently employed because of the occasional hepatotoxicity with this treatment.

Estimation of serum hormone levels are expensive and some investigators suggest that a single measurement of serum testosterone is all that is required. In occasional cases of hyperprolactinaemia, however, serum testosterone may be just within normal limits and a space-occupying lesion of the pituitary fossa is obviously something that must not remain undetected. In our laboratory we routinely measure testosterone, prolactin, follicle stimulating hormone and luteinizing hormone and have detected a number of patients with significant abnormalities; these patients have often responded well to treatment.

Often the most valuable information obtained in an outpatient or office setting is the degree of response to intracorporeal papaverine (or papaverine/phentolamine combination) together with Doppler scan. Although some clinicians withhold this diagnostic test until the second visit, we usually employ a small test dose (20–40 mg of papaverine plus 2 mg phentolamine) on the first attendance. Prior to administration of this compound the patient must be warned about the possibilities of bruising (which is of little significance) and a prolonged response (which must be treated by corporeal aspiration or intracorporeal phenylephrine or other α-adrenergic injection within 6–8 h). A signed consent form is useful as well as a detailed description of whom to contact and what to do should the erection fail to go down. We regard an absent or impaired response as an indication for colour Doppler scanning of the cavernosal and dorsal penile artieries with higher dosage of papaverine and phentolamine to exclude arterial insufficiency or venous leakage and this can be arranged before the second consultation.

Further details of this and other special techniques for elucidating the cause of impaired erectile potency will be discussed in greater detail in subsequent chapters.

## References

Bannister, R. (1988) Clinical features of progressive autonomic failure. In *Autonomic Failure. A Textbook of Clinical Disorders of the Autonomic Nervous System,* 2nd edn (ed. R. Bannister), Oxford University Press, Oxford, 267–288

Forsberg, L., Gustavii, B., Hojerback, T. and Olsson, A. M. (1979) Impotence, smoking and orgasmic–ejaculatory response in human males. *Fertility and Sterility,* **31**, 589

Horowitz, J. D. and Gobel, A. J. (1979) Drugs and impaired male sexual function. *Drugs,* **18**, 206

Mirin, S. M., Meyer, R. E., Mendelsohn, J. H. and Ellingboe, J. (1980) Opiate use and sexual function. *American Journal of Psychiatry,* **137**, 909

Nowinski, J. and LoPiccolo, J. (1979) Assessing sexual behaviour in couples. *Journal of Sex and Marital Therapy,* **5**, 225–243

Papadopoulos, C. (1980) Cardiovascular drugs and sexuality. *Archives of Internal Medicine,* **140**, 1341

Pedan, N. R., Cargill, J. M., Browning, M. C. K. *et al.* (1979) Male sexual dysfunction during treatment with cimetidine. *British Medical Journal,* **i**, 659

Slag, M. T., Morley, J. E., Elson, M. K. *et al.* (1983) Impotence in medical clinic outpatients. *Journal of the American Medical Association,* **249**, 1736–1740

# 7

# NPT/Rigidometry

**M. Hirshkowitz, C. A. Moore and I. Karacan**

## Background

The presence of naturally occurring, sleep-related penile erections has long been known. In the 1800s, spermatorrhoea rings were marketed for the purpose of inhibiting sleep erections in young boys. These devices were worn around the penis and had spike-like protrusions that would awaken the sleeper when erections occurred. The nature and cycle of sleep-related erections in adults were not reported in the scientific literature until Ohlmeyer and associates (1944) described a regular, repetitive cycle of erections occurring during sleep. Subsequent studies confirmed this finding and added some detail about the phenomenon. The next major advance occurred in 1965 when Karacan and Fisher, working independently, both demonstrated that sleep-related erections were principally associated with rapid eye movement (REM) sleep. This confirmed Aserinsky and Kleitman's (1953) speculation that the erection cycle was related to their newly discovered REM cycle.

The discovery of REM sleep, and in particular its association with dreaming, revived discussion of the underlying psychosexual nature of dreams. Karacan (1965) investigated dream content and sleep-related erections. He adopted the term nocturnal penile tumescence (NPT) in deference to his advisors' suggestion that 'penile erections in sleep' was too explicit in those pre-sexual revolution, more restrained times. He found that erotic dream content did not typically accompany NPT. Fisher (1966) also investigated the relationship between sleep erections and erotic dream content. In a four-case series he described sudden NPT increases related to overtly erotic dream content. Subsequent research, however, demonstrated that erotic dream content is rare (Snyder, 1970; Gaillard and Moneme, 1977). In fact, McCarley and Hoffman (1981) found no erotic content in 104 dreams from 14 subjects they studied.

## Sleep laboratory quantification of sleep-related erections

In the early NPT studies, investigators recorded electroencephalographic and electro-oculographic activity in conjunction with penile circumference increase. The tracings were scored for sleep stages (stages 1, 2, 3, 4 or REM) and wakefulness (stage 0). The fact that NPT was a sleep phenomenon, and in particular principally a REM sleep phenomenon, was not lost on these pioneer researchers. Contemporary sleep laboratory studies usually include monitoring of breathing patterns and leg movement activity.

The traditional laboratory technique for recording penile circumference increase involved placing mercury-filled strain gauges around the penis. The distension of the gauges during erection increases the gauges' electrical resistance. A bridge amplifier transduces the change in resistance to voltage. This signal is calibrated and interfaced to the polygraph to provide a continuous tracing of circumference change. The placement of two gauges, one at the penile base and one at the coronal sulcus, offers improved reliability and sensitivity. Penile musculovascular and haemodynamic measures, including bulbocavernosus–ischiocavernosus activity and penile blood flow, may also provide useful information concerning sleep-related erections (Karacan, Salis and Williams, 1978; Karacan, Aslan and Hirshkowitz, 1983; Allen and Smolev, 1984; Karacan *et al.*, 1987, 1989).

Tracings are either manually or computer scored to provide quantitative information about the nocturnal erections. Quantitative dimensions of NPT include frequency (the number of tumescence episodes), magnitude (maximum circumference increase) and duration (total tumescence time). Measures of erectile architecture can also be tabulated, including slopes of ascending tumes-

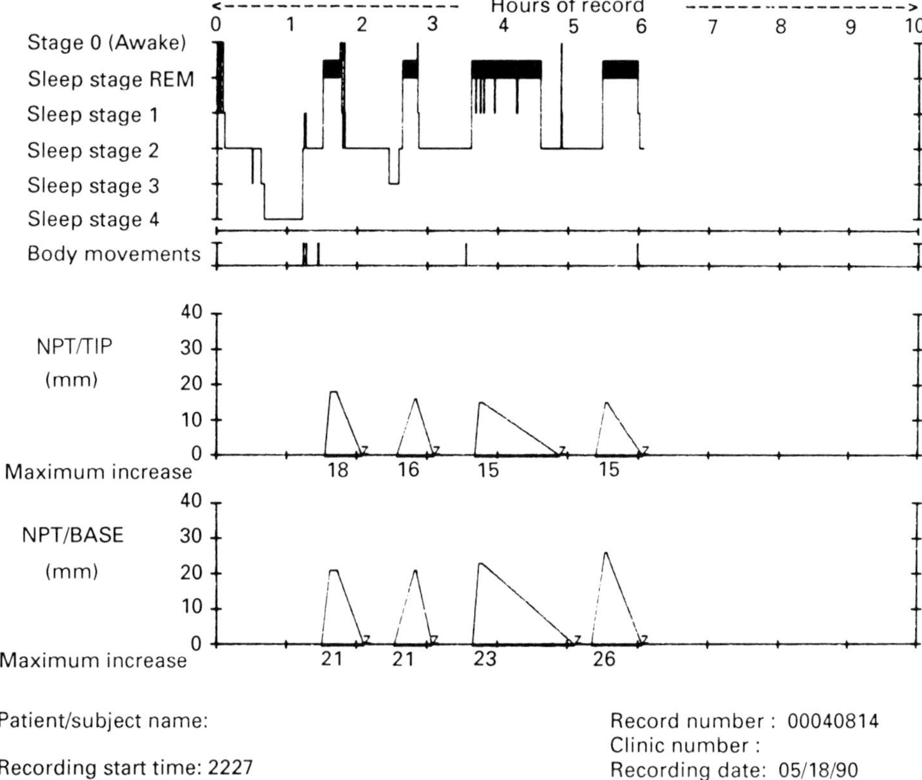


**Figure 7.1** Sleep stage histogram and nocturnal penile tumescence for a 34-year-old patient with psychogenic impotence

cence, duration of sustained maximal erections and the swiftness of detumescence. Data concerning the coordination between NPT and the REM sleep state, the periodicity of NPT, and concordance between expansion at the penile base and at the coronal sulcus help complete the picture.

Figure 7.1 illustrates sleep stages and NPT recorded in a 34-year-old man recently evaluated at our laboratory for erectile dysfunction. The patient had four normal sleep-related erections, with magnitude and duration within normal limits. The architecture of the NPT episodes was normal and coordination with REM sleep was good. Penile rigidity measured by buckling resistance was within normal limits. Clinical interviews and psychometric testing revealed mild depression, somatization and sexual performance anxiety.

## NPT and the diagnosis of erectile dysfunction

It occurred to Karacan (1970) that assessment of NPT might be useful in the diagnosis of male impotence. Karacan and his research group proceeded to compile normative descriptions of the NPT cycle in young boys, young adults, middle-aged men and the elderly (Karacan *et al.*, 1972a, 1972b, 1975, 1976; Hursch, Karacan and Williams, 1972; Karacan, Hursch and Williams, 1972). Age-related changes in NPT have recently been replicated by Reynolds and associates (1989). With these data, the sleep-related erections in men with erectile problems could be compared to those of non-impaired men. The search for biological markers of impotence was motivated by the desire for an objective basis for distinguishing psychogenic from organic impotence. Thus, the use and validation of NPT criteria for the differential diagnosis of erectile failure became a focus of numerous investigations. Painstaking and methodical scientific approach to this task produced a number of advances.

Investigators used three general strategies to test the diagnostic utility of NPT assessment. In the first approach, criterion groups were devised consisting of men with conditions presumably associated with organic impotence. Investigators compared the sleep-related erections in these groups to NPT in men with no sexual complaint or with impotence of presumably psychogenic origin. NPT has been assessed in men with diabetes (Karacan *et al.*, 1977a, 1978a; Karacan, 1980; Hirshkowitz *et al.*, 1990a), hypogonadism (Cunningham *et al.*, 1982, 1990), chronic obstructive pulmonary disease (Fletcher and Martin, 1982), alcoholism (Snyder and Karacan, 1981; Karacan and Moore, 1983), spinal lesions (Karacan *et al.*, 1977b, 1978b; Halstead *et al.*, 1984), end-stage renal disease (Karacan *et al.*, 1978c) and hypertension (Karacan *et al.*, 1989; Hirshkowitz *et al.*, 1989a).

Another paradigm popular in validation studies is to explore concordance between NPT values and other measures that reputedly detect organic or psychogenic erectile failure. These studies characteristically compare a selected parameter of NPT, pick a 'cutting score' value for that parameter, and compare diagnostic agreement based on that score with some other diagnostic procedure. Several problems inherent in the design of such studies, however, need to be addressed.

One problem involves the frequent use of circumference increase as the NPT criterion parameter. Circumference increase is the most variable of NPT measures because of individual differences in penile morphology. We have seen full, firm erections with as little as 5 mm circumference increase and non-rigid erections with circumference increases exceeding 25 mm. Another obstacle in concordance-type validation studies is selection of the measure against which NPT results will be 'validated'. The impetus for developing NPT testing procedures was precisely because objective standards were unavailable. Therefore, when NPT measures disagree with other indices, it is sometimes difficult to determine whether the NPT data or the other data are faulty. Finally comparisons of NPT data with psychometric results have a unique complexity. First, it is incorrect to assume psychiatric scale elevations will accompany psychogenic impotence. Psychogenic impotence may arise from specific behavioural or relationship problems in the absence of psychopathology. Likewise, men with organic impotence are not immune to psychological and psychiatric conditions. The stress, frustration and interpersonal problems that can result from organic impotence may produce psychiatric disturbance.

Finally, some validation studies have assessed the effect of behavioural and psychological factors on sleep-related erections. In general, the notion is that if psychologically-related diminutions occur in NPT, the usefulness of the technique is compromised. We have shown that sexual activity and sexual arousal before sleep do not alter NPT patterns. Also, NPT is unchanged by sexual abstinence in healthy volunteer subjects (Karacan, Williams and Salis, 1970; Karacan *et al.*, 1979).

Karacan and colleagues (1966) reported dream anxiety diminished NPT, a finding reiterated in subsequent reports (Karacan, 1970). This result is frequently cited as evidence for the unreliability of NPT. What we actually studied were dream report content analyses and anxiety descriptor index scores. Dreams were either associated with normal erections, irregular erections, or no erections. The content analysis for anxiety but not the anxiety index scores were statistically higher in dreams with irregular or no erections (samples were mostly derived from irregular erections). It must be emphasized that, in this study, irregular erections were those in which circumference fluctuated or detumescence began before the dream gathering awakening. Irregular erection in this study did not mean that subjects had abnormal NPT test results (Kaya, Moore and Karacan, 1979).

In the past, conventional wisdom ascribed impotence associated with depression to loss of libido. Recent evidence demonstrates that significantly reduced NPT can occur during episodes of depression (Thase *et al.*, 1987a). Some authors contend that this is evidence that psychological factors can alter NPT. In contrast, NPT reduction during episodes of depression can be viewed as evidence that major depression is truly endogenous or organic (as it used to be labelled). The leading researchers in this area state: 'Whether or not these observations lead to the conclusion that depression is a cause of "false positive" NPT studies depends on whether one construes an abnormal NPT profile as indicative of an irreversible lesion and/or whether depression is viewed as, at least in part, involving organic process' (Thase *et al.*, 1988).

## Penile buckling resistance

Researchers and clinicians using NPT testing procedures noticed that sleep-related circumference increase was not always associated with penile rigidification. We first remarked on the importance of penile rigidity as a crucial measure of erectile function in 1977 (Karacan, 1977). Other investigators soon followed with documentation of dissociation between nocturnal penile enlargement and rigidity (Wein *et al.*, 1981).

In 1978 we published a description of our standard technique for evaluating penile rigidity during nocturnal erections. This procedure involves awakening the patient during a representative sleep erection, applying a calibrated force to the tip of the penis, and recording the force at which the shaft of the penis buckles. Our original recording device was a large syringe modified with a rubber cap on one end and a sphygmomanometer on the other. Buckling was measured in pressure (0–300 mmHg). Some confusion has arisen because our later improved devices measured the force applied in grams. When the buckling rigidity is measured, we also photograph the erect penis and ask the patient to estimate what percentage of a full erection he has. The technician performing the procedure also rates the erection. We find the photograph useful for validation and for documenting any abnormality in the size or shape of the penis. Visual inspection and the photograph document penile curvature associated with Peyronie's disease. In patients who elect prosthetic implantation, the photograph may help the surgeon to select the proper size device (Karacan, Salis and Williams, 1978).

To better understand the relationship between penile rigidity and erectile function we conducted several studies. In one study (Karacan, Moore, and Sahmay, 1985), female volunteers performed vaginal insertions with lucite rods, varying in size, with and without lubrication. They recorded the force needed to achieve penetration under these conditions. We found that with lubrication the average minimum force needed to achieve penetration was 500 g. Without lubrication and with varying circumference rods, insertion forces of up to 1500 g were needed. Another source of information about the relationship between rigidity and erectile functionality derives from patient and volunteer subject self-reports. During rigidity measurement we asked men if their erection was adequate for sexual intercourse. As in vaginal insertion studies, we found that erections with buckling forces of 500 g or more were usually rated as sufficient to achieve penetration.

## Non-laboratory techniques for measuring NPT

The dire need to objectify diagnostic techniques contributed to the enthusiasm for using NPT in clinical practice. Because of its intuitive appeal for demonstrating erectile capacity, NPT was adopted by many as the 'gold standard' in the differential diagnosis of impotence. DSM-III recommended the use of NPT in diagnostic practice. Critics of NPT testing often comment on the expense of the evaluation. However, since NPT refers specifically to the phenomenon of sleep-related erections and not to the traditional assessment technique that includes all-night laboratory polygraphic recordings, non-laboratory techniques were developed as inexpensive alternatives to sleep studies (Kenepp and Gonick, 1979; Barry, Blank and Boileau, 1980; Procci and Martin, 1984; Bradley *et al.*, 1985; Virag, Virag and Lajujie, 1985; Bertini and Boileau, 1986; Bradley, 1987; Kessler, 1988; Slob, Blom and van der Werff ten Bosch, 1990).

The use of postage-type stamps encircling the penis during sleep was one of the earliest shortcut techniques developed to detect NPT (Barry, Blank and Boileau, 1980). In this approach, a ring of stamps is placed by the patient around the penis at bedtime and the patient is asked to note in the morning whether separation occurred at the perforations. Breakage of the ring is attributed to nocturnal erections and conversely an intact ring is thought to verify organic impotence. In the original study, 22 potent men broke the stamp ring on 58 of 62 nights. In contrast, only one stamp breakage was observed among 11 impotent patients tested for 30 nights. Less consistent results have been reported in subsequent studies by other research groups (Imagawa and Kawanishi, 1986; Morales *et al.*, 1983; Morales, Condra and Reid, 1990).

Based on the same principle, more elaborate devices have been developed. These include snap gauges, felt gauges and expandable telescoping tubes placed around the penis at night. Again, initial success in validating some of these procedures was followed by mixed results (Allen and Brendler, 1990). It should be emphasized that these approaches only detect the presence of an erection and provide no information about NPT frequency and duration. Morales and colleagues (1990) suggested that sleep-related movements might be responsible for artefactual detection of erections with some of these devices, including one developed at their own laboratory. Therefore, false negative tests (the finding of normal NPT when the patient is organically impaired) represent a serious shortcoming of the technique.

Several devices are available for continuous monitoring of penile circumference or circumference change during the sleep period. This approach models technology used in sleep centres, but does not entail recording brain or eye movement activity. Strain gauges or penile loops are worn on the penis and data are recorded. The number of erections, their duration and circumference increase can be visualized. Information concerning the extent to which sleep is disturbed, the presence or absence of REM sleep, sleep quality, and the coordination between penile circumference increase and sleep states are not available with these devices. However, the presence of repetitive, periodic, sleep erections obtained with these machines may provide useful diagnostic information. The absence of an erection cycle can result from a variety of factors only one of which is organic impotence; therefore, cautious interpretation is warranted especially when considering surgical treatment. False positive tests (a finding of reduced NPT that is not produced by organic impotence) represent a major concern.

## Penile buckling resistance versus penile compressibility

Felt gauges, snap gauges and the RigiScan device all attempt to provide information about penile rigidity. Most of the original literature emphasizing the importance of penile rigidity referred to penile buckling resistance (axial rigidity). The use of the term rigidity with respect to these recording devices refers to penile tissue compressibility. In fact, in an advertisement for snap gauges the headline statement is: 'For complete impotence evaluation . . . think rigidity'. RigiScan advertisement quotes our work and states: 'relying solely on the NPT data could result in incorrect conclusions' and goes on to cite Allen (1981) indicating that NPT misdiagnosis with only NPT data is as high as 42%. These statements are correct but the context in which they were made was a discussion of penile buckling resistance, not compressibility.

Snap gauges have embedded filaments that will break under certain outward pressures. If the penis engorges and reaches a level of non-compressible expansion, one or several calibrated filaments will break. Similarly, a felt gauge will expand when a specified non-compressible expansion is exceeded, if it is not twisted on the penile shaft. The RigiScan device periodically tightens its penile loops and measures the resistance to compression exerted by the penis. Some attempts have been made to correlate penile engorgement, buckling resistance and penile compressibility.

## Comparison of sleep laboratory and non-laboratory NPT testing

Laboratory NPT sleep studies offer a number of advantages over non-laboratory procedures. Table 7.1 summarizes the type of information available using various recording devices.

In summary, the simple, most inexpensive devices shown in the first two columns indicate whether any erection has occurred and may provide a crude index of compressibility. Bedside NPT monitors and RigiScan supply most of the parametric information about the penile circumference increase. However, they do not attempt to assess the sleep state that is a prerequisite for NPT. Of these two techniques, only RigiScan provides data about compressibility. Because these are unattended procedures, no visual inspection or buckling resistance data are available. Attended, laboratory sleep studies provide all parameters of penile circumference and sleep state. Because visual observations and buckling resistance measures are available, compressibility measures are omitted. Thase and associates (1987b) assessed the effect of NPT monitoring procedures on sleep continuity and architecture. They found negligible differences in multi-night laboratory tests. By contrast, it is assumed, not demonstrated, that the other procedures do not disrupt sleep.

Table 7.2 summarizes the susceptibility of the various NPT recording procedures to false positive and false negative interpretations. A positive NPT test indicates organic impotence while a negative test suggests psychogenic causes. As previously mentioned, devices providing discrete information about the presence of an erection are prone to false negative test results when body movements occur. Reflex erections, as seen in spinal injury and neurogenic patients, may also cause stamp rings and snap gauges to break, and telescoping and felt gauges to expand, even though the erectile pattern is grossly abnormal. False negative test results from equipment providing continuous NPT tracings (bedside monitors and RigiScan) can usually be avoided if tracings are carefully reviewed by experienced scorers. An erroneous diagnosis of psychogenic impotence can lead to ineffective behavioural or psychological treatment. This unfortunately may increase the patient's and spouse's frustration level, exacerbate guilt, provoke additional marital discord, or promote conversion reactions.

False positive tests leading to incorrect diagnosis of organic impotence represent another, equally

**Table 7.1 NPT recording devices and what they measure**

| | *Stamp rings* | *Telescoping, snap and felt gauges* | *Bedside NPT monitor* | *RigiScan* | *Sleep studies* |
|---|---|---|---|---|---|
| Presence/absence | Yes | Yes | Yes | Yes | Yes |
| NPT frequency | No | No | Yes | Yes | Yes |
| NPT magnitude | No | Yes | Yes | Yes | Yes |
| NPT duration | No | No | Yes | Yes | Yes |
| NPT architecture | No | No | Yes | Yes | Yes |
| REM sleep coordination | No | No | No | No | Yes |
| Sleep disruptions | No | No | No | No | Yes |
| Abnormal penile curvature | No | No | No | No | Yes |
| Buckling resistance | No | No | No | No | Yes |
| Penile compressibility | No | Yes* | No | Yes | No |

* Not measured with telescoping gauges.

**Table 7.2 Comparison of non-laboratory and laboratory recording procedures for susceptibility to artefact and tampering. A false positive (+) NPT test erroneously supports the diagnosis of organic impotence**

| | *Stamp rings* | *Telescoping, snap and felt gauges* | *Bedside NPT monitor* | *RigiScan* | *Sleep studies* |
|---|---|---|---|---|---|
| Body movement artefact | False – | False – | OK* | OK* | OK |
| Reflex spasm erection | False – | False – | OK* | OK* | OK |
| Short sleep period | False + | False + | OK | OK | OK |
| Disrupted sleep | False + | False + | False + | False + | OK |
| Disrupted REM sleep | False + | False + | False + | False + | OK |
| Sleep apnoea | False + | False + | False + | False + | OK |
| Nocturnal myoclonus | False + | False + | False + | False + | OK |
| Tampering/faking good | False – | False – | OK* | OK* | OK |
| Tampering/faking bad | False + | False + | False + | False + | OK |

* Very careful inspection of tracings by an experienced scorer looking for sudden baseline changes can help avoid false negative conclusions. However, it has been shown that the addition of simultaneous EMG tracing improves overall accuracy (Marshall, McGrath and Schillinger, 1983).

serious, problem. This situation may arise from the presence of concomitant sleep disorders. We and others have found that many sleep pathologies occur occultly (Schmidt and Wise, 1981; Pressman *et al.*, 1986; Hirshkowitz *et al.*, 1989a, 1989b, 1990b). These undiagnosed sleep disorders are frequently masked by patient adaptation, denial or impaired introspective ability. Reasonably intact sleep continuity and consolidated REM sleep are key ingredients for a normal sleep-related erection cycle. If sleep or REM sleep is disrupted, NPT parameters must be interpolated given the sleep milieu. In some cases, NPT recordings may be deemed uninterpretable because of sleep disruption. The sleep data, even if used only to invalidate a procedure, serve an important role in avoiding false positive NPT tests.

Two additional clinical concerns involve patients who attempt to manipulate the test outcome. The motivation behind these attempts vary from psychopathology to calculated intent to defraud. Men with Munchausen's syndrome seeking surgical procedures can produce a false positive NPT test by not using the stamp ring, snap or felt gauge, or misreporting the results of the telescoping gauge. Similarly, we have evaluated men with psychogenic impotence who wanted prosthetic implantation because they 'didn't have time for therapy' or were uninterested in marital counselling. Data from bedside NPT monitors and RigiScan can be manipulated by avoiding sleep, either through external stimulation or use of stimulants. In legal cases where sexual assault accusation or injury compensation is at stake, these manoeuvres to produce false positive tests would probably succeed in non-laboratory assessments. In contrast, some patients have been known to 'fake good', that is intentionally produce a false negative psychogenic profile to avoid surgery, obtain vasodilator injection, or be prescribed anxiolytics or other psychotherapeutic medications. Discrete devices are easily manipulated by tampering but equipment that continuously measures circumference is difficult to fool.

## NPT and sleep disorders

The most common sleep pathologies encountered in the population of men with impotence are nocturnal myoclonus and sleep apnoea. Nocturnal myoclonus is marked by periodic leg movements in sleep (PLMS) that are 'stereotyped, repetitive movements of the lower extremities' (Coleman, 1982). PLMS are often associated with arousals from sleep. Sleep apnoea is a cessation of breathing for ten or more seconds during sleep (Guilleminault, van den Hoed and Mitler, 1978). These episodes may result from airway obstruction, cessation of diaphragmatic movement, or both. There is a strong male predominance for sleep apnoea.

Our tabulation of PLMS in 768 consecutively evaluated impotent men revealed 54% had 15 or more leg movements per hour of sleep (Hirshkowitz *et al.*, 1989b). Many of these patients had disrupted sleep. In another recent study (Hirshkowitz *et al.*, 1990b) we reviewed the sleep-related respiratory status of 1025 men referred for evaluation of erectile dysfunction. We found that 44% of patients had significant sleep apnoea (five or more episodes per hour of sleep) and 20% had moderate to severe sleep apnoea (15 or more apnoeas per hour). Our prevalence estimates for PLMS and sleep apnoea confirm previous findings (Schmidt and Wise, 1981; Pressman *et al.*, 1986). Pressman and colleagues (1986) provide evidence that occult sleep disorders can distort recordings of penile circumference increase. The polysomnographic data collected in laboratory NPT studies provide valuable information that contributes to the interpretation process.

An important contribution that sleep laboratory procedures can make to NPT-based diagnostic procedures relates specifically to sleep apnoea. Nasal continuous positive air pressure (CPAP) therapy represents a recent advance in the management of sleep apnoea syndrome (Sullivan *et al.*, 1981; Guilleminault and Partinen, 1990). The patient with apnoea is provided with air at constant pressure through a mask. This positive air pressure acts as a pneumatic splint and thus maintains airway patency. CPAP therapy effectively remediates sleep apnoea in most patients and is considered by many the preferred treatment. As already mentioned, we find significant sleep apnoea in 20–44% of men with erectile dysfunction. In many cases we titrate CPAP pressure levels on the second or third night of evaluation. Patients with apnoea-related reductions in REM sleep characteristically have high percentages of REM sleep after CPAP is applied. This REM-rebound sometimes unmasks REM-disrupted reduced NPT. The net effect is that a night with reduced NPT concomitant with evidence of significant sleep apnoea may be followed by a CPAP trial in which NPT is normalized.

To illustrate the relationship between apnoea, CPAP and NPT, we present the following case data.

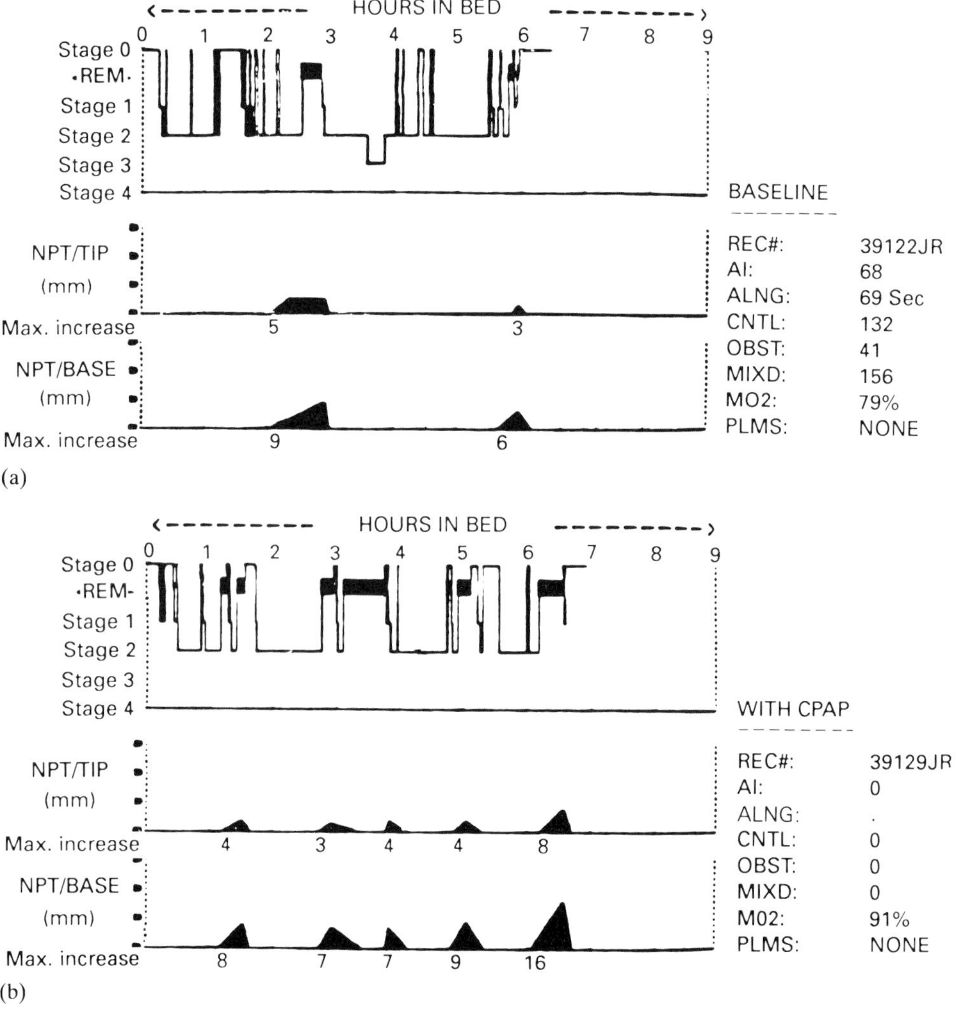


**Figure 7.2** Sleep stage and NPT histograms for an impotent patient with sleep apnoea: (a) data from the baseline (untreated) night and (b) the CPAP titration night. REC#, recording number; AI, apnoea index (number apnoea episodes per hour of sleep); ALNG, longest apnoea episode (seconds); CNTL, number of central apnoeas; OBST, number of obstructive apnoeas; MIXD, number of mixed apnoeas; $MO_2$, lowest oxygen saturation; PLMS, periodic leg movements in sleep.

Figure 7.2 shows the sleep and NPT histograms for two nights from a patient we recently evaluated at our centre. On the first night he had 68 apnoea episodes per hour, the longest episode lasting 69 s, and a minimum oxygen saturation of 79%. On this night we observed two NPT episodes with a maximum buckling resistance of 30 g. This NPT pattern, if the sleep-related respiratory impairment were not detected, would be interpreted as indicative of organic impotence. We administered CPAP on the following night and effectively eliminated the patient's sleep apnoea. Oxygen saturation was maintained at a high level, never dropping below 90%. With CPAP, the patient's REM sleep cycle was restored and he had five NPT episodes, with a penile buckling rigidity of 1000 g during the final erection. This case demonstrates the value of sleep laboratory NPT studies in the diagnosis of impotence. In cases such as the one presented, the mechanism of the apnoea-related impotence is not known. Several explanations exist; among them are speculations that erectile failure is secondary to excessive daytime sleepiness associated with sleep apnoea or that sleep apnoea represents a reversible organic impotence with impairment of mechanisms needed to meet the oxygen demand of sexual activity. Alternatively, apnoea and its associated extreme increases in blood pressure may produce neurogenic dysfunction, vascular damage, or both. Finally, apnoea-related declines in testosterone levels have been reported (Grunstein *et al.*, 1987). At present, we are conducting studies designed to investigate the underlying interrelationship between sleep apnoea and erectile dysfunction.

## Usefulness of NPT testing in the diagnosis of impotence

Confusion often abounds in discussions of NPT because laboratory polysomnographic evaluations and non-laboratory, non-polygraphic techniques are considered together. This is especially true when the reliability and validity of NPT results versus other diagnostic techniques are debated.

Those whose intent is to detract from the value of NPT testing frequently cite publications concerned with improvement of NPT recording procedures or practices. Investigators concerned with methodological refinement of NPT technique underscore the weakness of the then current practice. These didactic discussions find their way into portrayals of NPT testing as an unreliable procedure. Thus the proverbial baby is thrown out with the bath water.

Another common argument against the use of NPT is based on cost containment. This is a complex issue; however, the wellbeing of the patient must always be considered. To our minds, accurate diagnostic assessment is crucial before an expensive surgical procedure that destroys the normal penile physiology is performed. Though some consider this a 'purist' attitude, placing oneself in the 'patient's shoes' makes 'purists' out of many of our pragmatic colleagues.

As the popularity of non-laboratory techniques increases, we have noticed a shift in the type of patients referred for NPT evaluation. The built-in selection bias in referrals may subtly reflect what our colleagues really think about the value of NPT testing. Our routine assessment workload has increasingly shifted toward four special types of evaluations. The first are those complicated and difficult cases where the history is confusing. The second type consists of physicians or other health care workers needing differential diagnosis of impotence. Legal cases where the status of erectile capacity is crucial are frequently referred for comprehensive assessment. Finally, foreign dignitaries, celebrities and other VIP patients virtually always undergo thorough multi-night laboratory NPT sleep studies before a surgical or alternative treatment plan is finalized.

In summary, NPT testing provides objective, diagnostically useful information about erectile capacity. Laboratory sleep studies produce more complete information than non-laboratory procedures, but at greater expense. In some cases the data from sleep studies are needed for correct diagnostic interpretation. Non-laboratory methods need further study, validation and improvement. If these techniques can be extended to include information about sleep, most of the false positive test liabilities can be avoided. Non-laboratory techniques for recording sleep state are already under development. NPT data, as always, will need careful interpretation. In the hands of a skilled clinician, NPT test information is very valuable; in naïve hands it can be misleading and dangerous.

## References


Allen, R. P. (1981) Erectile impotence: objective diagnosis from sleep-related erections (nocturnal penile tumescence). *Journal of Urology*, **126**, 353

Allen, R. P. and Brendler, C. B. (1990) Snap-gauge compared to a full nocturnal penile tumescence study for evaluation of patients with erectile impotence. *Journal of Urology*, **143**, 51–54

Allen, R. P. and Smolev, J. K. (1984) Bulbo-ischio-cavernosus muscle activity in determining etiology for organic impotence. In *Proceedings of the First World Meeting on Impotence* (Paris, 1984), (eds R. Virag and H. Virag-Lappas), Editions du CERI, Paris, pp. 95–99

Barry, J. M., Blank, B. and Boileau, M. (1980) Nocturnal penile tumescence monitoring with stamps. *Urology*, **15**, 171–172

Bertini, J. and Boileau, M. A. (1986) Evaluation of

nocturnal penile tumescence with Potentest. *Urology,* **27**, 492–494

Bradley, W. E. (1987) New techniques in evaluation of impotence. *Urology,* **29**, 383–388

Bradley, W. E., Timm, G. W., Gallagher, J. M. and Johnson, B. K. (1985) New method for continuous measurement of nocturnal penile tumescence and rigidity. *Urology,* **26**, 4–9

Coleman, R. M. (1982) Periodic movements in sleep (nocturnal myoclonus) and restless legs syndrome. In *Sleeping and Waking Disorders: Indications and Techniques* (ed. C. Guilleminault). Addison-Wesley, Menlo Park, California, pp. 265–295

Cunningham, G. R., Hirshkowitz, M., Korenman, S. G. and Karacan, I. (1990) Testosterone replacement therapy and sleep-related erections in hypogonadal men. *Journal of Clinical Endocrinology and Metabolism,* **70**, 792–797

Cunningham, G. R., Karacan, I., Ware, J. C. *et al.* (1982) The relationships between serum testosterone and prolactin levels and nocturnal penile tumescence (NPT) in impotent men. *Journal of Andrology,* **3**, 241–247

Fisher, C. (1966) Dreaming and sexuality. In *Psychoanalysis – A General Psychology* (eds R. M. Loewenstein, L. M. Newman, M. Schur and A. J. Solnit). International Universities Press, New York, pp. 537–569

Fisher, C., Gross, J. and Zuch, J. (1965) Cycle of penile erection synchronous with dreaming (REM) sleep. *Archives of General Psychiatry,* **12**, 29–45

Fletcher, E. C. and Martin, R. J. (1982) Sexual dysfunction and erectile impotence in chronic obstructive pulmonary disease. *Chest,* **81**, 413–421

Gaillard, J. M. and Moneme, A. (1977) Modification of dream content after preferential blockade of mesolimbic and mesocortical dopaminergic systems. *Journal of Psychiatric Research,* **13**, 247–256

Grunstein, R. R., Lawrence, S., Handelsman, D. J. *et al.* (1987) Endocrine dysfunction in obstructive sleep apnea – changes with nasal CPAP. *Sleep Research,* **16**, 340

Guilleminault, C. and Partinen, M. (eds) (1990) *Obstructive Sleep Apnea Syndrome: Clinical Research and Treatment,* Raven Press, New York

Guilleminault, C., van den Hoed, J. and Mitler, M. M. (1978) Clinical overview of the sleep apnea syndromes. In *Sleep Apnea Syndromes* (eds C. Guilleminault and W. C. Dement), Alan R. Liss, New York, pp. 1–12

Halstead, L. S., Dimitrijevic, M., Karacan, I. and Aslan, C. (1984) Impotence in spinal cord injury: neurophysiological assessment of diminished tumescence and its relation to supraspinal influences. *Current Concepts in Rehabilitative Medicine,* **1**, 8–14

Hirshkowitz, M., Karacan, I., Arcasoy, M. O. *et al.* (1989b) The prevalence of periodic limb movements during sleep in men with erectile dysfunction. *Biological Psychiatry,* **26**, 541–544

Hirshkowitz, M., Karacan, I., Arcasoy, M. O. *et al.* (1990b) Prevalence of sleep apnea in men with erectile dysfunction. *Urology,* **36**, 232–234

Hirshkowitz, M., Karacan, I., Gurakar, A. and Williams, R. L. (1989a) Hypertension, erectile dysfunction, and occult sleep apnea. *Sleep,* **12**, 223–232

Hirshkowitz, M., Karacan, I., Rando, K. C. *et al.* (1990a) Diabetes, erectile dysfunction, and sleep-related erections. *Sleep,* **13**, 53–68

Hursch, C. J., Karacan, I. and Williams, R. L. (1972) Some characteristics of nocturnal penile tumescence in early middle-aged males. *Comparative Psychiatry,* **13**, 539–548

Imagawa, A. and Kawanishi, Y. (1986) NPT monitoring with stamps: actual intracavernous pressure at separation. *Impotence,* **1**, 64

Karacan, I. (1965) The effect of exciting presleep events on dream reporting and penile erections during sleep. *ScD Thesis,* State University of New York, Downstate Medical Center, Brooklyn

Karacan, I. (1970) Clinical value of nocturnal erection in the prognosis and diagnosis of impotence. *Medical Aspects of Human Sexuality,* **4**, 27–34

Karacan, I. (1977) Advances in the psychophysiological evaluation of male erectile impotence. In *Weekly Psychiatry Update Series,* No. 43 (ed. F. F. Flach), Biomedia, New York, pp. 1–6

Karacan, I. (1980) Diagnosis of erectile impotence in diabetes mellitus. An objective and specific method. *Annals of Internal Medicine,* **92**, 334–337

Karacan, I., Aslan, C. and Hirshkowitz, M. (1983) Erectile mechanisms in man. *Science,* **220**, 1080–1082

Karacan, I., Dervent, A., Cunningham, G. *et al.* (1987c) Assessment of nocturnal penile tumescence as an objective method for evaluating sexual functioning in ESRD patients. *Dialysis Transplant,* **7**, 872–876, 890

Karacan, I., Dervent, A., Salis, P. J. *et al.* (1978b) Spinal cord injuries and NPT. *Sleep Research,* **7**, 261

Karacan, I., Dimitrijevic, M., Lauber, A. *et al.* (1977b) Nocturnal penile tumescence (NPT) and sleep stages in patients with spinal cord injuries. *Sleep Research,* **6**, 52

Karacan, I., Goodenough, D. R., Shapiro, A. and Starker, S. (1966) Erection cycle during sleep in relation to dream anxiety. *Archives of General Psychiatry,* **15**, 183–189

Karacan, I., Hirshkowitz, M., Salis, P. J. *et al.* (1987) Penile blood flow and musculovascular events during sleep-related erections of middle-aged men. *Journal of Urology,* **138**, 177–181

Karacan, I., Hursch, C. J. and Williams, R. L. (1972) Some characteristics of nocturnal penile tumescence in elderly males. *Journal of Gerontology,* **27**, 39–45

Karacan, I., Hursch, C. J., Williams, R. L. and Littell, R. C. (1972a) Some characteristics of nocturnal penile tumescence during puberty. *Pediatric Research,* **6**, 529–537

Karacan, I., Hursch, C. J., Williams, R. L. and Thornby, J. I. (1972b) Some characteristics of nocturnal penile tumescence in young adults. *Archives of General Psychiatry,* **26**, 351–356

Karacan, I. and Moore, C. A. (1983) Sexual dysfunction in alcoholic men. In *Psychopharmacology and Sexual Disorders,* British Association for Psychopharmacology

Monograph No. 4, (ed. D. Wheatley), Oxford University Press, Oxford, pp. 113–122

Karacan I., Moore, C. A. and Sahmay, S. (1985) Measurement of pressure necessary for vaginal penetration. *Sleep Research,* **14**, 269

Karacan, I., Salis, P. J., Hirshkowitz, M. *et al.* (1989) Erectile dysfunction in hypertensive men: sleep-related erections, penile blood flow and musculovascular events. *Journal of Urology,* **142**, 56–61

Karacan, I., Salis, P. J., Thornby, J. I. and Williams, R. L. (1976) The ontogeny of nocturnal penile tumescence. *Waking and Sleeping,* **1**, 27–44

Karacan, I., Salis, P. J., Ware, J. C. *et al.* (1978a) Nocturnal penile tumescence and diagnosis in diabetic impotence. *American Journal of Psychiatry,* **135**, 191–197

Karacan, I., Salis, P. J. and Williams, R. L. (1978) The role of the sleep laboratory in the diagnosis and treatment of impotence. In *Sleep Disorders. Diagnosis and Treatment* (eds R. L. Williams and I. Karacan), Wiley, New York, pp. 353–382

Karacan, I., Scott, F. B., Salis, P. J. *et al.* (1977a) Nocturnal erections, differential diagnosis of impotence and diabetes. *Biological Psychiatry,* **12**, 373–380

Karacan, I., Ware, J. C., Salis, P. J. *et al.* (1979) Sexual arousal and activity: effect on subsequent nocturnal penile tumescence patterns. *Sleep Research,* **8**, 61

Karacan, I., Williams, R. L. and Salis, P. J. (1970) The effect of sexual intercourse on sleep patterns and nocturnal penile erections. *Psychophysiology,* **7**, 338–339

Karacan, I., Williams, R. L., Thornby, J. I. and Salis, P. J. (1975) Sleep-related penile tumescence as a function of age. *American Journal of Psychiatry,* **132**, 932–937

Kaya, N., Moore, C. and Karacan, I. (1979) Nocturnal penile tumescence and its role in impotence. *Psychiatric Annals,* **9**, 426–431

Kenepp, D. and Gonick, P. (1979) Home monitoring of penile tumescence for erectile dysfunction. Initial experience. *Urology,* **14**, 261–264

Kessler, W. O. (1988) Nocturnal penile tumescence. *Urologic Clinics of North America,* **15**, 81–86

Marshall, P., McGrath, P. and Schillinger, J. (1983) Importance of electromyographic data in interpreting nocturnal penile tumescence. *Urology,* **22**, 153–156

McCarley, R. W. and Hoffman, E. (1981) REM sleep dreams and the activation-synthesis hypothesis. *American Journal of Psychiatry,* **138**, 904–912

Morales, A., Condra, M., Reid, K. (1990) The role of nocturnal penile tumescence monitoring in the diagnosis of impotence: a review. *Journal of Urology,* **143**, 441–446

Morales, A., Marshall, P. G., Surridge, D. H. and Fenemore, J. (1983) A new device for diagnostic screening of nocturnal penile tumescence. *Journal of Urology,* **129**, 288–290

Ohlmeyer, P., Brilmayer, H. and Hullstrung, H. (1944) Periodische vorgange im Schlaf. *Pflueger Archiv,* **248**, 559–560

Pressman, M. R., DiPhillipo, M. A., Kendrick, J. I. *et al.* (1986) Problems in the interpretation of nocturnal penile tumescence studies: disruption of sleep by occult sleep disorders. *Journal of Urology,* **136**, 595–598

Procci, W. R. and Martin, D. J. (1984) Preliminary observations of the utility of portable NPT. *Archives of Sexual Behavior,* **13**, 569–580

Schmidt, H. S. and Wise, H. A. II (1981) Significance of impaired penile tumescence and associated polysomnographic abnormalities in the impotent patient. *Journal of Urology,* **126**, 348–352

Reynolds, C. F., Thase, M. E., Jennings, J. R. *et al.*, (1989). Nocturnal penile tumescence in healthy 20–59-year-olds: a revisit. *Sleep,* **12**, 368–373

Slob, A. K., Blom, J. H. M. and van der Werff ten Bosch, J. J. (1990) Erection problems in medical practice: differential diagnosis with relatively simple method. *Journal of Urology,* **143**, 46–50

Snyder, F. (1970) The phenomenology of dreaming. In *The Psychodynamic Implications of the Physiological Studies on Dreams* (eds L. Madow and L. H. Snow), Charles C. Thomas, Springfield, Illinois, pp. 124–151

Snyder, F. and Karacan, I. (1981) Effects of chronic alcoholism on nocturnal penile tumescence. *Psychosomatic Medicine,* **43**, 423–429

Sullivan, C. E., Issa, F. G., Berthon-Jones, M. and Eves, L. (1981) Reversal of obstructive sleep apnoea by continuous positive airway pressure applied through the nares. *Lancet,* **i**, 862–865

Thase, M. E., Reynolds, C. F. III, Glanz, L. M. *et al.* (1987a) Nocturnal penile tumescence in depressed men. *American Journal of Psychiatry,* **144**, 89–92

Thase, M. E., Reynolds, C. F. III, Jennings, J. R. *et al.* (1987b) Do nocturnal penile tumescence recordings alter electroencephalographic sleep? *Sleep,* **10**, 486–490

Thase, M. E., Reynolds, C. F. III, Jennings, J. R. *et al.* (1988) Nocturnal penile tumescence is diminished in depressed men. *Biological Psychiatry,* **24**, 33–46

Virag, R., Virag, H. and Lajujie, J. (1985) A new device for measuring penile rigidity. *Urology,* **25**, 80–81

Wein, A. J., Fishkin, R., Carpiniello, V. L. and Mallory, T. B. (1981) Expansion without significant rigidity during nocturnal penile tumescence: a potential source of misinterpretation. *Journal of Urology,* **126**, 343–344

# 8

# Diagnostic pharmacotherapy and cavernosography

C. C. Carson

To produce a normal erection there must be a normal hormonal milieu, adequate sensory, sympathetic and parasympathetic nerve activity and a vascular system with adequate arterial inflow and controlled venous outflow. Vascular function for normal human erections therefore depends not only upon arterial inflow to the penis and active arteriolar dilatation with sinusoidal opening due to corpus cavernosum smooth muscle relaxation, but also upon passive venous constriction. The importance of venous constriction to produce storage of blood within the penis during erection has only recently been extensively studied. The basic physiology of erection is now more clearly understood and allows clinical investigation and treatment of disorders of the penile venous system.

In order for a normal erection to occur, stimulation of the cavernosal nerve must produce a neurotransmitter and endothelial substances to allow relaxation of smooth muscles controlling the lacunar and helicine vessels of the penis. An increase in cavernosal artery inflow then occurs, increasing the pressure within the corporeal bodies from less than 10 mmHg to pressures equalling the mean arterial pressure. As this inflow increases and corporeal body pressure rises, small emissary veins are compressed against the rigid tunica albuginea of the corpora cavernosa. This decreased venous outflow in the presence of marked increase in arterial inflow produces the storage phase of erection. Abnormalities of either arterial inflow or venous outflow systems may produce erectile dysfunction.

The venous anatomy of the penis begins in the corporeal body with the small venules which drain the lacunar spaces of the corpora cavernosa. These small emissary veins form larger veins which pass obliquely through the tunica albuginea. This oblique exit of emissary veins allows the increased pressure within the corpus cavernosum during the initiation phase of erections to inhibit venous otuflow and thus a rise in pressure within the corporeal bodies. The emissary veins are the beginning of the deep venous drainage system of the penis. These emissary veins of the corpora cavernosum and the corpora spongiosum drain by way of circumflex branches around the tunica albuginea beneath Buck's fascia into the deep venous system of the penis. This deep venous system consists of the urethral veins, deep dorsal veins, and bulbar veins. Small, short veins drain the proximal portion of the corpora cavernosa at the crura directly into the pelvic plexus. The deep dorsal vein passes within the neurovascular bundle beneath Buck's fascia and lies between the dorsal arteries of the penis. This deep dorsal venous system which is anatomically variable drains the glans penis, the corpora spongiosum, and the corpora cavernosa. There are connections between the deep and superficial dorsal veins. The superficial venous system is above Buck's fascia and is drained through the superficial dorsal vein which lies in the midline of the penis and empties into the saphenous, scrotal and epigastric veins (Fuchs, Mehringer and Rajfer, 1989).

Dysfunction of the occlusive mechanism in the venous circulation has been demonstrated to decrease the ability to store blood in the corpora cavernosa and result in erectile dysfunction. Venous abnormalities have been demonstrated in patients with primary impotence, Peyronie's disease, post-traumatic erectile dysfunction, and as a result of some neurological diseases (Fitzpatrick, 1973; Delcour, Vandenbosch and Struyven, 1988; Rajfer, Rosciszewski and Mehringer, 1988). Thus inadequate emissary vein compression and venous leakage may result from abnormal tunica albuginea venous compression in such conditions as Peyronie's disease, in patients with inadequate filling and thus decreased initiation pressure within the corpora cavernosa limiting venous occlusion pressure in such conditions as vascular disease, diabetes mellitus and cigarette smoking. Similarly, neurological diseases may produce inadequate blood flow to the corpus cavernosum and limit initiation pressure and a failure to decrease venous outflow. Finally, these abnormal veins may occur as a primary, possibly congenital, malformation producing venous leakage from the onset of erectile function.

Investigation of the venous system can be done with invasive or non-invasive testing; however, pharmacological stimulation provides the baseline for the best estimate of venous occlusive function.

## Venous diagnostic studies

### Non-invasive evaluation

Initial vascular studies must include an assessment of arterial inflow as well as investigations of the venous occlusive system. Non-invasive arterial testing is discussed in Chapter 9. Initially, however, Doppler ultrasonography and penile blood pressure as well as hormone profile and nocturnal penile tumescence studies may sugggest venous abnormalities. A nocturnal penile tumescence monitoring study performed with rigidity monitoring using instruments such as the RigiScan may demonstrate erections of short-lived duration with reasonable turgidity and increase in size (Figure 8.1). These 'spike' erections demonstrated in some nocturnal tumescence monitoring studies will strongly suggest the possibility of venous occlusive abnormalities. Confirmation of a suspected 'venous leak' should then be performed using cavernosography and cavernosometry associated with pharmacological erectile stimulation.

Duplex ultrasonography and colour Doppler evaluation may provide an excellent non-invasive method for estimating venous function in patients with adequate arterial inflow (Figure 8.2a and b) (Lue *et al.*, 1985). By measuring increased diastolic velocity after administration of pharmacologically active agents to the penis, one can visualize the drainage from the deep dorsal vein before initiation of erection, during the initiation phase, and after erection has occurred. If diastolic velocity is adequate and maximal arterial inflow is obtained, one can use colour Doppler studies to visualize the initial increase in venous outflow followed by rapid loss of venous outflow and decrease in deep dorsal vein diameter (Figure 8.2c). While the specificity of these studies continues to demonstrate mixed results, many patients with venous abnormalities can be differentiated from patients with arterial abnormalities using this study in combination with pharmacological injection therapy with papaverine, papaverine/phentolamine or prostaglandin $E_1$.

Colour Doppler examinations are performed 10–20 min after injection of 60 mg papaverine and 1 mg phentolamine into the corpus cavernosum using a 25 gauge needle. Initial observation demonstrates and quantitates an increase in systolic velocity as well as a decrease in venous outflow. The sonographic probe is placed on the patient at the

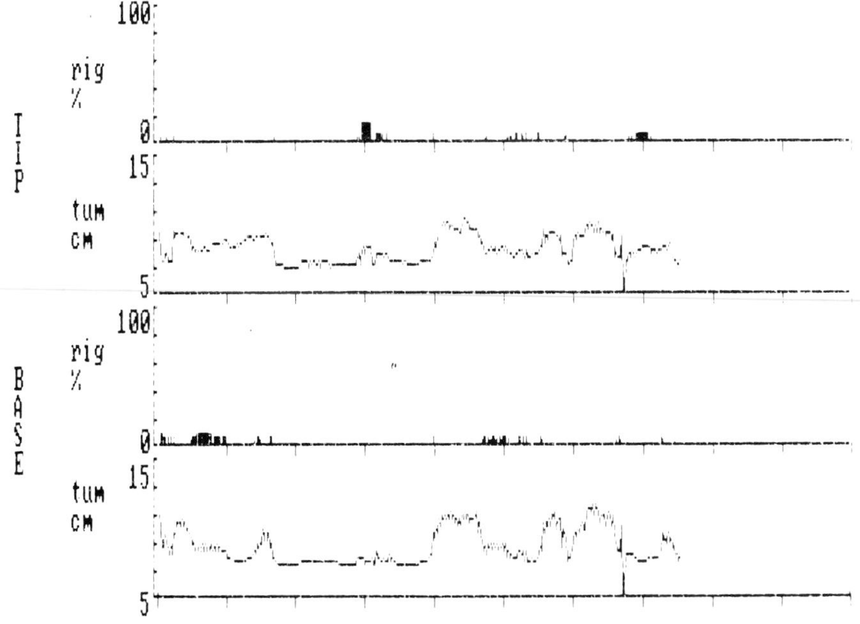


**Figure 8.1** Nocturnal penile tumescence (RigiScan) monitoring in a patient with venous leak. Note increased penile girth at the tip and base of the penis without a significant change in penile rigidity

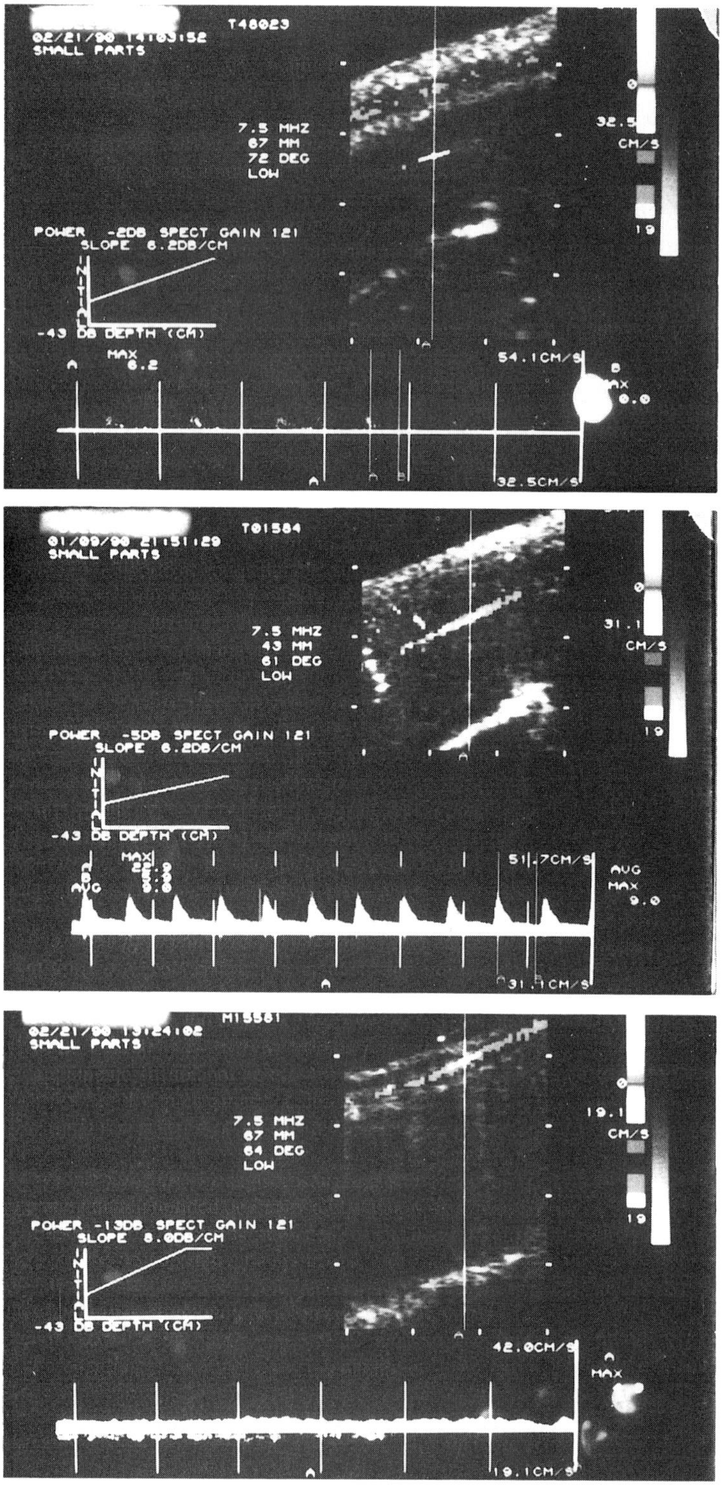

(a)

(b)

(c)

**Figure 8.2** Colour Doppler studies: (a) poor arterial inflow after papaverine/phentolamine injection (less than 25 ml $s^{-1}$; (b) normal arterial inflow after papaverine and phentolamine; (c) abnormal deep dorsal vein flow in a patient with normal arterial inflow 20 min after papaverine/phentolamine injection

base of the penis on the ventral surface. The anatomy of the corpora cavernosa, corporeal arteries and venous structures are detailed using high-resolution real-time imaging. Any gross abnormalities such as Peyronie's plaques are identified with this initial examination. The cavernosal arteries and deep dorsal vein are identified and measured using electronic cursors. Blood flow is evaluated using colour Doppler imaging of both the arterial and venous systems. Flow access correction during real-time monitoring optimizes measurement of systolic blood flow. The angle corrected velocity wave form is displayed and measured on the ultrasound monitor identifying peak systolic and end diastolic velocities. During response to papaverine and phentolamine, changes in the cavernosal arteries and deep dorsal veins can be measured accurately. For normal venous function to occur, mean peak systolic velocity must exceed 25 cm $s^{-1}$ with an end diastolic velocity of approximately 5 cm $s^{-1}$ (Guam *et al.*, 1989).

This non-invasive study will demonstrate the ability of the relaxed cavernosal spaces to recruit blood flow from the pudendal arteries. If recruitment is inadequate, the venous system cannot function and erection cannot occur. If recruitment is adequate but veins are abnormal, a marked increase in arterial velocity will be identified without a concomitant decrease in venous outflow. This combination is strongly suggestive of a venous leak phenomenon.

## Invasive studies

The injection of pharmacoactive agents and infusion of the corpora cavernosa have allowed accurate and physiological testing of the venous system of the penis (Brindley, 1983; Stief *et al.*, 1988). Initial attempts at cavernosography began with infusion of normal saline and dilute contrast without neuropharmacological activation of the erectile mechanism of the penis. These studies, while helpful, were not physiological (Newman and Reisch, 1984). Wagner introduced the method of infusion to evaluate the corpora cavernosa (Ebdhoj and Wagner, 1979; Wagner and Uhrenhold, 1980). His studies were refined by Virag and Wespes and his associates to evolve to the current studies described as dynamic cavernosography or dynamic infusion cavernosometry and cavernosography (Fitzpatrick, 1973; Virag *et al.*, 1984; Wespes *et al.*, 1984, 1986). Initial studies without pharmacological activation measured the rate that normal saline could be perfused into the cavernous bodies to achieve and maintain an artificial erection (Wespes *et al.*, 1984). Demonstration of erection was by observation of flow or by measurement of intracavernosal pressure. Differentiation between initiation flows and maintenance flows could be measured and cavernosography could be performed if an artificial erection was inadequate. By producing a more physiological erection through the injection of papaverine or other vasoactive agents, a more physiological study was developed (Lue *et al.*, 1986; Stief *et al.*, 1988; Goldstein and Padma-Nathan (1990). Wespes and associates clearly showed that the flow rate needed to initiate and maintain an erection in patients with psychogenic erectile dysfunction was markedly diminished when papaverine was instilled (Wespes *et al.*, 1986). Without papaverine, 110 ml $min^{-1}$ of normal saline infusion was necessary to initiate an erection in normal patients while only 35 ml $min^{-1}$ was necessary after the injection of 60 mg papaverine. Similarly, maintenance flows were significantly reduced when patients were pretreated with papaverine injection. Penile resistance and intracavernous pressure can also be measured to further quantitate erectile venous function. Goldstein and Padma-Nathan (1990) demonstrated that normal venous function could be defined by a decrease in intracavernous pressure of less than 25 mmHg per 30 s after a satisfactory erection had been stimulated. At normal saline infusion rates of 120 ml $min^{-1}$ after papaverine pretreatment, venous leakage will not occur if pressures rise above 110 mmHg. While the cavernosometry and cavernosography studies have added a great deal to evaluation of erectile dysfunction, they continue to be lacking in total phsyiological reproduction of the erectile event. The pharmacological substances used including papaverine, phentolamine and prostaglandin $E_1$ are probably not the natural neurotransmitter substances used to initiate erectile function. Pericavernosal structures such as the cavernous muscle and perineal muscles are not activated during these studies. Despite these limitations, however, cavernosography and cavernosometry are quite useful in the clinical evaluation and diagnosis of the penile venous system.

### Dynamic cavernosography technique

Initially the penis is cleansed with antiseptic solution and sterile towels are placed around the site of injection. A tourniquet or rubber band may be placed at the base of the penis. A 21 gauge scalp vein needle is inserted into one corpus cavernosum and connected to a constant infusion pump. One may then use an additional 21 gauge scalp vein needle in the opposite corpus cavernosum for pressure monitoring or a Y-connector can be used if a single needle technique is preferred; 30–60 mg papaverine with 1 mg phentolamine per 30 mg of papaverine is injected via the corpus cavernosum needle. If a tourniquet has been used, it is removed in approximately 90 s. Observation of the penis will identify normal erectile function as a palpably firm, complete erection. Pressure measurement demonstrates an intracavernous pressure in excess of 80 mmHg if arterial and venous mechanisms are intact. During this time, duplex ultrasonography can be carried out. A firm erection or intracavernous pressure above 80 mmHg indicates that continuing with the study is not necessary as arterial and venous mechanisms are quite normal. If erection is not adequate, normal saline is infused beginning at a rate of approximately 5 ml $min^{-1}$ and is gradually increased until erection occurs. If infusion rates exceed 110 ml $min^{-1}$ without adequate erection, further infusion is not necessary. If a painful

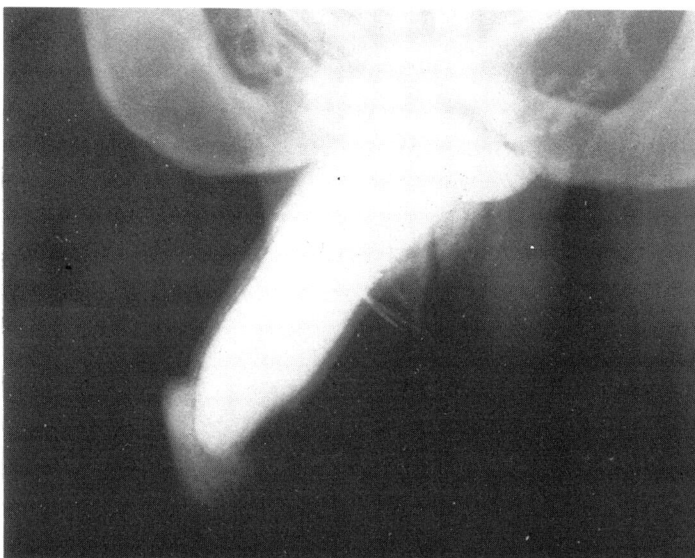

**Figure 8.3** Corpus cavernosogram in a patient with venous leak. Note poor opacification of glans penis suggesting absence of spongiosal leakage

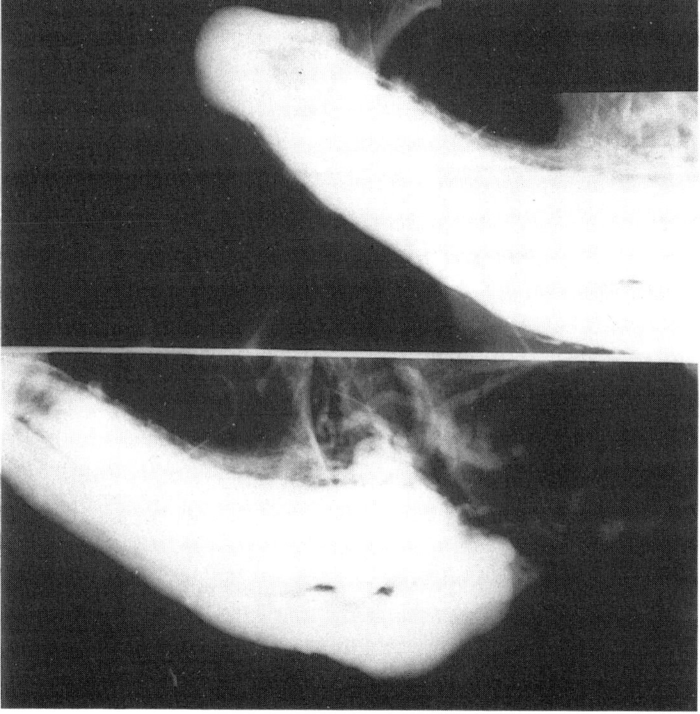

**Figure 8.4** Corpus cavernosogram in a patient with venous leak and spongiosal leakage. Note glans penis opacification in top film and spongiosal filling in lower film

erection or pressures above 80 mmHg are measured, infusion is slowed until a constant rate for maintenance of erection is determined. Erection should be maintained at infusion rates below 60 ml $min^{-1}$. If erection or intracavernous pressures above 80 mmHg cannot be maintained at infusions below 60 ml $min^{-1}$, venous incompetence is highly probable. Once this maintenance infusion rate is identified, infusion can be discontinued to watch for cavernosal pressure of turgidity decay. Dilute contrast medium is instilled through the same pump and infusion needle with fluoroscopic monitoring. Films are obtained in the supine and oblique positions to identify the course of abnormally draining veins. It is especially important to evaluate the corpus spongiosum and glans penis fluoroscopically to identify venous leakage through the spongiosum (Figures 8.3 and 8.4) (Delcour *et al.*, 1988). This drainage is critical in those patients in whom surgery is contemplated as venous leak with corpus cavernosum connection to spongiosum or glans is difficult to treat surgically and the success rate is markedly diminished (Figure 8.5a and b).

A simple outpatient method for recreating cavernosometry is to administer papaverine and phentolamine or prostaglandin $E_1$. After approximately 10–12 min, 60 ml of normal saline is infused using a 60 ml syringe by hand at a rapid rate. If an excellent and turgid erection ensues with slow decay of the erectile event, the venous system is most probably intact and pressure determinations and contrast medium infusion are unnecessary.

The complications of this study are few; however, the majority of patients who have normal arterial and venous systems will have prolonged erections at the conclusion of the study. One must be prepared, therefore, to treat these patients appropriately with pharmacological therapy and aspiration to prevent later priapism. In most cases, however, simple aspiration and lavage of the corpus cavernosum with normal saline will result in immediate detumescence without recurrence of the prolonged erection. Care must be taken in infusing normal saline in patients with marginal cardiac status as large amounts of normal saline may be infused during a study in patients with a significant venous leak. The potential for the production of cardiac failure, while rare, must be considered.

Since many impotence evaluation centres perform cavernosography and cavernosometry using different methods, comparison of results and techniques is difficult. There has thus far been no standardization with regard to dosage of pharmacological agents used, pressure recording methods, X-ray techniques, or the exact normal values associated with marginal venous incompetence. It will require additional study and experience before standardization can be achieved and appropriate surgical candidates successfully chosen.

## Pharmacological testing

The evaluation of normal erectile function, especially for arterial disease, has presented a problem to investigators of erectile dysfunction. Attempts to use visual sexual stimulation by some investigators have been successful in a few patients. Our own experience has indicated that the psychological overlay and cultural difficulties with sexually explicit stimulatory material inhibits the use of this study as a widespread screening procedure for evaluating penile arterial disease.

Simple arterial screening in the office setting can be carried out using a Doppler stethoscope and 2 cm infant blood pressure cuff. Penile blood pressures can be effectively measured, after some practice, over each cavernosal artery. By comparing penile blood pressure and brachial systolic blood pressure a ratio can be calculated termed the penile:brachial index (PBI) (Engel, Burnham and Carter, 1978). Normal values should exceed 0.95 and those below 0.65 are significantly impaired. The normal PBI varies greatly with age, smoking and in patients with diabetes mellitus. Measurements of PBI before and after exercise with a penile blood pressure decrease of more than 20 mmHg will suggest a pelvic steal syndrome (Goldwasser *et al.*, 1985). Exercise can be simply performed by 30–50 rises.

Doppler blood pressure testing the PBI determination and penile plethysmography, while helpful as a screening study in the office, is not effective or reproducible in all patients. An alternative and more physiological method for vascular testing is the use of intracavernous injection of vasoactive pharmacological agents to produce a normal erection. Simple office evaluation of erectile function can, therefore, be carried out using papaverine alone, papaverine combined with phentolamine, or prostaglandin $E_1$. Combining this injection with duplex ultrasonography and colour Doppler evaluation further adds to the precise diagnosis of vascular abnormalities of the penis. Without this equipment being available, however, a reasonable evaluation of erectile function can be carried out using the injection of these medications. Further objective information can be obtained by vasoactive injection with monitoring using a RigiScan nocturnal penile tumescence monitoring study.

The use of 60 mg papaverine, 30 mg papaverine mixed with 1 mg phentolamine, or 40 μg prostaglandin $E_1$ will provide adequate stimulation for most patients. Allowances must be made for patients with unusually large penises and the dosage may be increased for these individuals. Injection and observation may be sufficient for diagnosis in most patients. If a patient has a normal study, many of these patients will have prolonged erections which will require aspiration. If the patient continues to have a full erection 60–90 min after injection, aspiration using a 21 gauge butterfly needle usually results in rapid and continuous detumescence. If tumescence recurs or if detumescence is not effected by aspiration alone, other vasoactive agents can be used to lavage the corpora cavernosa as described in Chapter 25. Patients are carefully counselled to return if a prolonged erection is observed after discharge from the clinic. Patients are further counselled that sexual activity within 24 h of a large injection should be avoided in order to eliminate the possibility of prolonged erection.

Additional complications include systemic reactions to large doses of papaverine in those patients with severe venous leaks. These systemic complica-

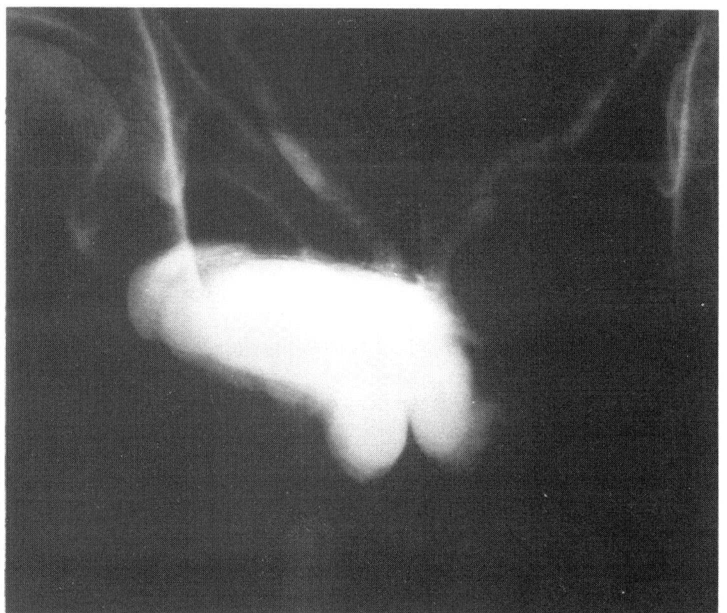

(a)

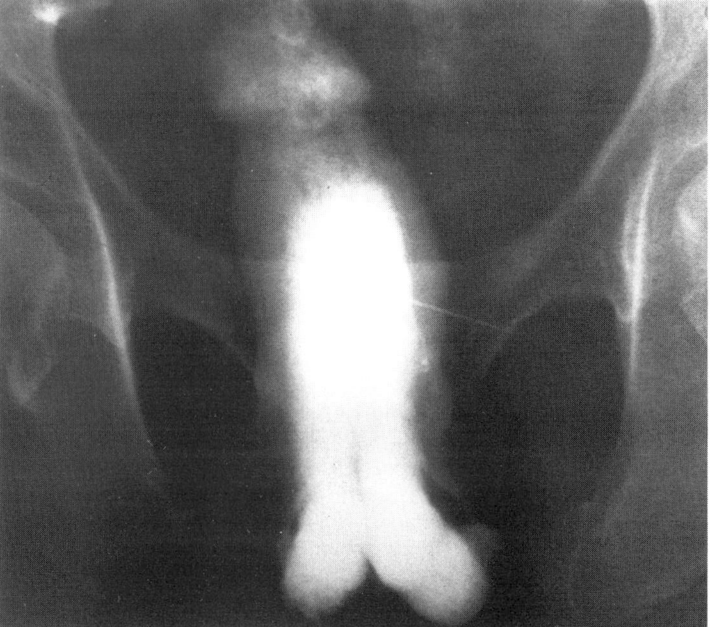

(b)

**Figure 8.5** (a) Preoperative cavernosography in a 32-year-old man with fleeting erections and abnormal RigiScan. Infusion cavernosometry suggested venous leak; (b) postoperative study. Infusion terminated following high intracavernosal pressures. No leak noted

tions include dizziness, occasional hypotension and lightheadedness. Local complications such as penile shaft haematoma and ecchymosis can be expected in 5–10% of patients.

**Table 8.1 Infusion rates in patients with impotence and venous leakage (after Lewis, 1990)**

| *Author* (Year) | *Infusion rates* (ml/min) | |
|---|---|---|
| | *Initiation* | *Maintenance* |
| Without pharmacological stimulation: | | |
| Virag (1982) | >200 | >100 |
| Payau and Lewis (1983) | >180 | |
| Wespes *et al.* (1986) | 200 | 110 |
| Delcour *et al.* (1988) | 215.5 | 145 |
| Lewis (1990) | | >100 |
| Carson (1990)* | >160 | >100 |
| Pharmacologic stimulation: | | |
| Wespes *et al.* (1986) | 103 | 43.5 |
| Delcour *et al.* (1988) | 124 | 73.4 |
| Lewis (1990) | | >50 |
| Carson (1990)* | >110 | >60 |

*Unpublished data

## Conclusion

The importance of the vascular system in erectile function has long been appreciated. The role of controlled venous outflow thought for many years to be under the active control of valves or 'polsters' is now recognized to be a more passive inhibition to venous flow. As many as 68% of impotent patients may have some component of venous leak contributing to erectile failure (Rajfer, Rosciszewski and Mehringer, 1988). Newer diagnostic studies, especially colour Doppler and cavernosography and cavernosometry, can provide accurate diagnostic information with low morbidity. It is essential, however, that neuropharmacological stimulation of the corpora cavernosa precedes any venous or arterial diagnostic study.

### References

Brindley, G. S. (1983) Cavernosal alpha-blockade: a new technique for investigating and treating erectile impotence. *British Journal of Psychiatry,* **143**, 332

Carson, ?

Delcour, C. P., Vandenbosch, G. A. and Struyven, J. L. (1988) Cavernosography and cavernosometry in the evaluation of impotence. *Urologic Radiology,* **10**, 144

Delcour, C. P., Wespes, E., Vandenbosch, G. A. *et al.* (1988) Opacification of the glans penis during cavernosography. *Journal of Urology,* **139**, 732

Ebehoj, J. and Wagner, G. (1979) Insufficient penile erection due to abnormal drainage of cavernous bodies. *Urology,* **13**, 507

Engel, G., Burnham, S. J. and Carter, M. F. (1978) Penile blood pressure in the evaluation of erectile impotence. *Fertility and Sterility,* **30**, 687

Fitzpatrick, T. J. (1973) Spongiosograms and cavernosograms: a study of their value in priapism. *Journal of Urology,* **109,** 843

Fuchs, A. M., Mehringer, C. M. and Rajfer, J. (1989) Anatomy of penile venous drainage in potent and impotent men during cavernosography. *Journal of Urology,* **141**, 1353

Goldstein, I. and Padma-Nathan, H. (1990) Venous evaluation of impotence. In *Infertility and Impotence* (ed. J. Rajfer), Yearbook Medical Publishers, Chicago, p. 268

Goldwasser, B., Carson, C. C., Braun, S. D. and McCann, R. L. (1985) Impotence due to the pelvic steal syndrome: treatment by transluminal angioplasty. *Journal of Urology,* **133**, 860

Guam, J. P., King, B. F., James, E. M. *et al.* (1989) Duplex and color Doppler sonographic evaluation of vasculogenic impotence. *American Journal of Radiology,* **153**, 1141

Lewis, R. W. (1990) Diagnosis and management of corporal veno-occlusive dysfunction. *Seminars in Urology,* **8**, 113

Lue, T. F., Hricak, H., Marich, K. W. and Tanagho, E. A. (1985) Vasculogenic impotence evaluated by high resolution ultrasonography and pulsed Doppler spectrum analysis. *Radiology,* **155**, 777

Lue, T. F., Hricak, H., Schmidt, R. A. and Tanagho, E. A. (1986) Functional evaluation of penile veins by cavernosography in papaverine induced erection. *Journal of Urology,* **135**, 479

Newman, H. F. and Reish, H. (1984) Artifical perfusion in impotence. *Urology,* **24**, 469

Payau, F. A. and Lewis, R. W. (1983) Corpus cavernosography – pressure flow and radiography. *Investigative Radiology,* **18**, 517

Rajfer, J., Rosciszewski, A. and Mehringer, C. M. (1988) Prevalence of corporal venous leakage in impotent men. *Journal of Urology,* **140**, 69

Stief, C. G., Bernard, F., Diederichs, W. *et al.* (1988) The rationale for pharmacologic cavernosography. *Journal of Urology,* **140**, 1564

Virag, R. (1982) Intracavernous injection of papaverine for erectile failure. *Lancet,* **ii**, 938

Virag, R., Frydman, D., Legman, M. and Virag, H. (1984) Intracavernous injection of papaverine as a diagnostic and therapeutic method in erectile failure. *Angiology,* **35**, 79

Wagner, G. and Uhrenholdt, T. A. (1980) Blood flow

measurement by the clearance methods in the human corpus cavernosum in the flaccid and erect states. In *Vasculogenic Impotence* (Proceedings of the 1st International Conference on the Corpus Cavernosum Revascularization) (eds A. W. Zorgniotti and G. Rossi), Charles C. Thomas, Springfield, Illinois, pp. 41–46

Wespes, E., Delcour, C., Struyven, J. and Schulmann, C. C. (1984) Cavernosometry–cavernosography, its role in organic impotence. *European Urology,* **10**, 229

Wespes, E., Delcour, C., Struyven, J. and Schulmann, C. C. (1986) Pharmacocavernosometry cavernosography in impotence. *British Journal of Urology,* **58**, 429

# 9

# Non-invasive investigation of penile artery function

**K. M. Desai and H. G. Gilbert**

## Introduction

One of the principal haemodynamic events leading to erection is a pronounced increase in cavernosal arterial inflow in response to neurogenically mediated relaxation of the cavernosal sinusoids and arterial smooth muscle. It has been estimated by means of radioisotope studies in human subjects that whereas the blood flow through the flaccid penis is only 2.5–8.0 ml $min^{-1}$ 100 g tissue (Wagner and Uhrenholdt, 1980), the average flow into the erecting penis exceeds 90 ml $min^{-1}$ and in a potent young man approaches levels as high as 270 ml $min^{-1}$ during the rapid phase of tumescence (Shirai and Ishii, 1981). It is obvious, therefore, that any restriction in the arterial supply of the penis will interfere with the ability to achieve a rigid erection. This pathophysiological mechanism of impotence was recognized in the early part of this century by Hirsch (1930) and by Leriche (1940) and has subsequently been reiterated by many contemporary vascular surgeons (De Palma, Levine and Feldman, 1978; Queral *et al.*, 1979; Nath *et al.*, 1981; Virag *et al.*, 1981), all of whom reported a high incidence of impotence in groups of men with peripheral vascular disease. Penile arterial insufficiency constitutes one of the major causes of organic impotence, especially in men over the age of 50 years, and screening for this factor is of prime importance when exploring the aetiology of impotence in a particular individual.

From a practical standpoint, detailed haemodynamic investigation should nowadays be reserved for those patients who have failed to respond to a therapeutic trial of either intracavernosal vasoactive agents or vacuum constriction devices. Both of these treatment options can be tried without attempting to define the exact underlying cause of the erectile failure. Refined arterial assessment, therefore, is appropriate only when considering penile arterial reconstruction or venous ligation surgery, the results of which are directly influenced by the accuracy of this screening. Occasionally one may have to carry out such investigations purely to satisfy the patient's desire to discover whether the cause of his dysfunction is physical in nature.

Several methods have been described for the evaluation of penile arterial function but, as will be discussed, most have failed to meet the necessary criteria of an effective test: a high degree of sensitivity and specificity with reproducibility, minimal discomfort to the patient together with safety and ease of application. The investigations described may be termed non-dynamic or dynamic according to whether arterial function is assessed during flaccidity or whilst an erection is developing.

## Non-dynamic investigations

### Penile temperature

The temperature of a limb at rest is largely governed by the amount of blood passing through it; compromised circulation will produce a relative cooling. This principle has been used in an effort to identify men with arteriopathic impotence. Two methods have been used to measure penile temperature:

1. Ishii, Mitsukawa and Shirai (1977) used thermography to monitor changes in penile temperature in normal and impotent subjects during exposure to visual erotic stimulation. They found an appreciably lower rise in penile skin temperature in the organically impotent group compared with the group of men who were either normal or were psychogenically impotent.
2. Jevtich (1981) measured intra-urethral temperature using an electronic thermometer and showed a good correlation between this and penile blood pressure measurements, thereby concluding that his simple technique was an effective means of diagnosing arteriogenic impotence.

Neither technique, however, has gained wider acceptance. This is for two reasons. Firstly, although skin temperature may correlate with cavernosal artery flow, the arterial supply to the skin is distinct. Skin temperature is, therefore, at best an indirect measurement. Hence it is not surprising that Buvat *et al.* (1982) found thermography to be a poor diagnostic aid in separating non-arteriogenically impotent men from those with arteriogenic impotence as defined by arteriography. Secondly, even though intra-urethral temperature may approximate to the temperature of the cavernosal bodies more closely than skin temperature, it must be appreciated that the cavernosal arteries carry little blood in the flaccid state. This observation is of fundamental relevance when assessing the validity of any technique designed to measure penile blood flow in the resting or non-functional state. Such measurements are likely to represent flow through the dorsal and spongiosal rather than the cavernosal arteries which, as we know, are of greater and more crucial importance in the process of erection. One can therefore readily understand, and probably dismiss as having little practical significance, the close correlation observed by Jevtich (1981) between intra-urethral temperature and penile blood pressure. Although Ishii and colleagues (1977) were among the first to recognize the value of a dynamic assessment by introducing erotic stimulation during penile thermographic monitoring, the technique, whilst useful for distinguishing between psychogenic and organic impotence, could not really help in segregating neuropathic from arteriogenic cases.

## Isotope scanning

Radioisotopes have been used in two basic ways to study penile artery function: washout studies and perfusion studies.

### Washout studies

These involve the injection of xenon-133 directly into the corpus cavernosum. The rate of decline of radioactivity within the penis is directly dependent upon the rate of dilution by arterial inflow. This dilution can be monitored sequentially from flaccidity to erection thereby giving a functional index. Shirai and Ishii (1981), who originally used this technique to study the haemodynamics of normal erection, reported a rapid washout of the isotope following visual sexual stimulation, implying that erection was not accompanied by cavernosal venous occlusion. These findings were to be contradicted a few years later by Wagner and Uhrenholdt (1980) who found a delayed $^{133}$Xe washout from the cavernosal bodies during erection induced in a similar way. These conflicting findings can be explained by differences in methodology with regard to the duration of sexual stimulation and the timing of the monitoring of radioactivity; arterial flow, and hence washout, is increased during tumescence but as intracavernosal pressure rises, the venous outflow and with it the arterial inflow are dramatically reduced. Unfortunately the diagnostic potential of $^{133}$Xe washout has never been satisfactorily evaluated, presumably because of technical difficulties; the isotope is not readily available and the actual dosage delivered is difficult to determine due to adsorbance of $^{133}$Xe onto both glass and plastic surfaces of syringes. The few studies that have been performed are difficult to interpret and show inconsistent results. Haden *et al.* (1989) found no difference in intracavernosal $^{133}$Xe washout between potent and impotent men when measured in the flaccid state. However, it is not clear to what extent their impotent group constituted men with an arteriopathic aetiology defined by other criteria. On the other hand Lin *et al.* (1989), using a subcutaneous preputial injection of $^{133}$Xe – an approach described earlier by Nseyo *et al.* (1984) – found a close correlation between an abnormal isotope study and penile arterial insufficiency (demonstrated by selective arteriography) in ten patients who had a poor response to papaverine. Nevertheless, five patients who exhibited an abnormal washout curve had a normal response to the vasoactive agent which led the authors to concede that the subcutaneously injected $^{133}$Xe technique could not reliably detect cavernosal flow; a predictable conclusion.

### Perfusion studies

This technique involves the systemic injection of radiolabelled material. Shirai and Nakamura (1970) who pioneered the concept of measuring penile blood flow by this method initially used $^{131}$I-labelled human albumin. Radioactivity was counted over the penis in the flaccid as well as the tumescent state. Sequential counts were plotted against time in order to establish a curve which they termed the 'radioisotope penogram'. Although their small study proved the method to be valuable in distinguishing organic from psychogenic impotence, they had to abandon this particular isotope because of its unacceptably long half-life. Subsequently they employed technetium-99 labelled autologous red blood cells in conjunction with visual sexual stimulation which demonstrated an increase in intrapenile blood volume during tumescence (Shirai *et al.*, 1976). In order to simplify the investigation, Fanous *et al.* (1982) substituted an intravenous injection of a vasodilator (isoxsuprine hydrochloride) in the place of visual erotic stimulation to promote cavernosal vasodilatation, a technique with which they reported encouraging preliminary results. Townell *et al.* (1985), by modifying and improving the imaging and accuracy of counting, were able to reliably discriminate between psychogenic and vasculogenic impotence in a series of 12 patients, in all of whom there was concordance with the findings on arteriography. In a more recent study, Schwartz *et al.* (1989a) also found a close agreement between peak cavernosal flow measurements taken by the $^{99}$Tc-labelled autologous red blood cell method during papaverine-induced tumescence and penile artery patency revealed by arteriography. By using intracavernosal papaverine, they overcame the theoretical objection to the use of systemically administered vasodilators whose ability to induce penile vasodilatation may itself be influenced by more proximal occlusive disease of vessels.

Overall, therefore, although radioisotope penile 'plethysmography' is a rational and worthwhile means of assessing total penile blood flow, it is a method that has been underused and is likely to remain so, mainly because of logistical considerations. Furthermore the specificity of these techniques remains to be determined (see Chapter 10).

## Penile blood pressure

The measurement of perfusion pressure by detecting the return of blood flow following the release of an occluding pneumatic cuff is a well established technique in the assessment of the arterial supply to a limb. This principle has been applied to the penis and, by virtue of its simplicity, has become the most commonly used investigation of the penile arteries to date.

The first successful attempts at measuring penile blood pressure involved mercury strain gauge plethysmography (Britt, Kemmerer and Robison, 1971) and spectroscopic analysis of blood flow in the glans penis (Gaskell, 1971). In 1975, Abelson described a simple method utilizing a Doppler ultrasound probe. Use of the Doppler principle to detect blood flow was first described by Satomura in 1959, when he suggested that it might be of use in the assessment of arterio-occlusive disease. The ultrasound probe or 'stethoscope' contains two piezo-electric crystals. One crystal transmits low power ultrasound waves which are reflected by the target tissues. Interaction with moving particles, such as red blood cells, causes the waves to be reflected at a frequency different from that of the incident beam. This frequency change, or shift, is dependent on the velocity of the moving particles and can be detected by the second crystal. Electronic processing can allow these transducers to be used either qualitatively to determine the presence or absence of blood flow, or quantitatively to actually measure the precise characteristics of the flow.

However, although measurement of penile blood pressure is relatively easy, this information by itself does not assist in distinguishing between normal and abnormal arterial function. Various indices relating penile blood pressure to other parameters have therefore been proposed in order to define significant arterial compromise.

Britt, Kemmerer and Robison (1971) suggested that a penile blood pressure which was 20 mmHg or more below brachial systolic pressure represented impaired penile perfusion whereas Gaskell (1971) concluded that a pressure anything below mean brachial pressure was indicative of obstruction to flow in the main vessels of the penis. Abelson (1975), on the other hand, determined that a difference between penile and brachial pressures of more than 30 mmHg was suggestive of compromised arterial supply. The use of such absolute criteria was, however, considered unreliable because of their susceptibility to fluctuations in systolic blood pressure. In order to overcome this Engel, Burnham and Carter (1978) recommended that the calculation of a ratio relating penile to systolic brachial pressure would provide a more reproducible measurement. Since the maximum pressure transmitted from the arterial system to the cavernosal sinusoids approximates to systolic pressure, this ratio should normally be 1. In a study of 126 men, Metz and Bengtsson (1981) found that within a group of potent men aged between 35 and 70 years, the penile brachial index (PBI) ranged between 0.7 and 1.02 with a tendency for the value to diminish with age. In addition, it was found that although a PBI of less than 0.6 was 91% accurate in predicting arteriogenic impotence, values exceeding 0.6 did not necessarily exclude this diagnosis; 28% of arteriogenically impotent men registered a PBI value greater than 0.6. A smaller study undertaken by Desai (1988) found the PBI to be even less reliable than in the above report. In comparing a group of 28 patients with proven haemodynamic normality as shown by a rigid erectile response to a standard dose (30 mg) of intracavernosally injected papaverine, with a group of 15 arteriogenically impotent men all of whom had arteriographic evidence of significant aortoiliac disease, he found that almost two-thirds of the patients in the latter group exhibited PBI values above 0.6.

There have been several attempts at improving the discriminating ability of the PBI, either by changes in the analysis of the raw data or by modifications in the methodology. In an elegant statistical analysis of data derived from a study of 503 patients referred to a vascular surgery unit from a variety of sources and for a number of different indications, Chiu, Lidstone and Blundell (1989) found that the diagnostic value of the PBI could be improved in certain predetermined subgroups such as those with peripheral vascular disease or diabetes. This really only served to confirm the previous work of other investigators such as Metz and Bengtsson (1981) who found that a PBI of less than 0.6 correlated well with the presence of peripheral vascular disease.

Stress testing was developed in order to reveal haemodynamically significant disease not evident at rest. Initially this was done by comparing the PBI before and after a series of gluteal and thigh muscle exercises (Goldstein *et al.*, 1982), the test being based on the concept of an external iliac 'steal' syndrome first proposed by Michal, Kramar and Pospichal (1978). This phenomenon is associated with atheromatous narrowing of the common iliac arteries and results in the patient being unable to sustain a rigid erection once coital movement begins. It is a symptom analogous to angina; although the arterial supply may be adequate to initiate an erection, the presence of proximal large vessel disease leads to its gradual deterioration during pelvic thrusting due to the diversion of blood from the internal to the external iliac system in order to supply the demands of the gluteal and thigh muscles. In a study of 97 men, the pelvic steal test helped to confirm the arteriopathic nature of the erectile dysfunction in 17 (27%) out of 63 impotent men whose resting PBI values would otherwise have placed them within the equivocal range.

An alternative modification is the hyperaemic stress test. This is performed by measuring the PBI before and after a 5 min period of penile artery occlusion produced by inflating a pneumatic cuff, placed around the base of the penis, to a suprasystolic pressure. In normal men relief of the occlusion produces reactive hyperaemia and the resulting rise in penile blood pressure is reflected in an increase in the PBI. Those with an inadequate arterial supply respond with either no change or even a fall in the PBI. In the only study of its kind this test allowed the distinction between arteriogenic and other forms of impotence in 36% of men whose PBI values fell in the non-diagnostic range of 0.7–0.8 (Bell, Lewis and Kerstein, 1983). No further validation of this technique is available and therefore, although promising, the clinical usefulness of this test remains uncertain.

## Arterial waveform analysis

When blood passes through a diseased vessel, the pulse waveform becomes attenuated in a characteristic way; the amplitude decreases, the acceleration is reduced, the deceleration phase is prolonged and the dicrotic notch disappears. These changes can be measured and used to quantify the severity of arterial disease. The techniques of recording arterial waveforms were originally described for the assessment of lower limb perfusion and have subsequently been applied in the investigation of impotence. The first – pulse volume plethysmography (De Palma, Kedia and Persky, 1980; Kedia, 1984) – involves the use of a pneumatic cuff placed around the base of the penis and inflated to a level just below systolic pressure to detect volumetric changes with each cardiac cycle. Like isotope plethysmography, this method measures the total penile blood flow which, in the flaccid state, essentially represents flow in the dorsal and spongiosal arteries as previously described. The only real merit of this technique is that it is easy to perform. It cannot reliably differentiate between arteriogenic and non-arteriogenic impotence.

Penile arterial pulse waveforms can also be obtained using the Doppler ultrasound probe, with the advantage over plethysmography that the penile arteries can be individually examined. By eliminating the sources of error associated with the use of a pneumatic cuff, this method theoretically would seem more reliable than measurement of penile blood pressure. Firstly the arteries can be 'insonated' at the base of the penis where they are much less likely to have branched compared with the position distal to a pressure cuff. Secondly the variability caused by the size of the cuff and also the potential for incomplete compression of arteriosclerotic vessels are eliminated.

### Penile flow index

Earlier attempts at distinguishing normal from abnormal by simply 'eye-balling' the waveforms were replaced by a more scientific approach. Velcek *et al.* (1980) described a penile flow index which was derived as a ratio of the radial artery waveform acceleration to that of the averaged penile artery. In a study of 42 men he found that this index was highly accurate in detecting arteriogenic impotence, using arteriography as the gold standard. Furthermore, he claimed that by subtle manipulation of the Doppler probe he could distinguish between the deep and superficial penile arteries, i.e. the dorsal arteries responded to pressure by a decrease in the wave amplitude whereas the cavernosal arteries responded with an increase.

It may be argued that the close agreement between waveform analysis and penile arteriography found by Velcek was attributable more to the limitations of the latter rather than the reliability of the former. The need to induce cavernosal smooth muscle relaxation with vasoactive drugs as well as to employ magnification when performing penile arteriography has been recogonized only relatively recently (Bookstein and Lang, 1987; Bahren *et al.*, 1988). Such technical refinements are absolutely essential to avoid misinterpreting physiological non-filling of the cavernosal arteries during flaccidity as pathological occlusion.

### Penile acceleration ratio

The penile acceleration ratio, calculated as the ratio between the maximum tangent of acceleration of the brachial artery waveform to that of a penile artery, was described by Forsberg in 1980. In 1982, in a report of the technique applied to 20 patients before and after aortoiliac reconstructive surgery, Forsberg and colleagues found that as a diagnostic tool this version of waveform analysis was better than penile blood pressure measurements which were prone to underdiagnose arterial disease. However, in a comparative study of the two methods, Metz *et al.* (1983) found that waveform analysis did not offer any significant advantage over PBI measurements.

Whilst these various indices, including the PBI, may contribute some information on the state of the penile arterial supply, there are a number of theorectical objections to their validity. All the investigations described above may be described as non-dynamic, i.e. they provide data on the state of the penile arteries at rest and, hence, they are incapable of reliably assessing the functionally more important cavernosal arteries. The depth and tortuosity of these vessels, combined with the extremely low volume of blood flow through them in the flaccid state, makes it very difficult to consistently locate them with conventional 8–10 MHz Doppler equipment. A further potential pitfall is that they may be confused with the circumflex branches of the dorsal arteries which course over the lateral aspect of the penis. These arteries which are nearer to the skin surface have a more pronounced flow in the resting state and can be mistaken for the cavernosal arteries (Reiss, 1985). Lane, Appleberg and Williams (1982) have emphasized the diagnostic fallibility of some of these methods by demonstrating their inability to detect cavernosal artery patency even in normal men.

Because the penis is subject to tremendous haemodynamic changes, it seems only logical that its arterial inflow should be assessed by dynamic tests of arterial function.

## Dynamic investigations

### Use of intracavernosal vasoactive agents

The discovery that an intracavernosal injection of papaverine (ICP), a non-specific smooth muscle relaxant, could induce a full erection in man (Virag, 1982) introduced a new era in the diagnosis and treatment of erectile failure. However, the early expectations of ICP becoming a reliable test of penile haemodynamic integrity have only partly been realized. Although it is generally accepted that a fully rigid response occurring within a few minutes of the administration of ICP excludes any significant haemodynamic abnormality, the converse does not always apply. Thus equivocal responses have been observed in men with confirmed psychogenic impotence (Buvat *et al.*, 1986) presumably due to psychic inhibition in a clinical environment devoid of sexual stimulation. Furthermore, even if genuinely attributable to a disturbance of penile haemodynamics, an abnormal reponse to ICP cannot help to differentiate between arterial insufficiency and cavernosal veno-occlusive imcompetence as the cause of the impotence. Nevertheless the ability of ICP to enhance cavernosal artery inflow has proved to be a valuable adjunct in developing more sensitive Doppler techniques for the assessment of the arterial component of erection. This property of papaverine has been exploited in the following tests.

### Computerized Doppler waveform analysis

A straightforward method of combining ICP with penile artery Doppler waveform analysis was developed in this unit a few years ago by Desai *et al.* (1987). This type of dynamic assessment overcame two major disadvantages associated with the analysis of waveforms recorded during flaccidity. Firstly, the reproducible manner in which papaverine induces relaxation of the cavernosal sinusoidal and arterial smooth muscle eliminated a number of variables inherent in measurements of penile blood flow taken in the flaccid state, such as the ambient temperature and the patient's anxiety level. Secondly, because of the tortuosity of the cavernosal arteries at rest and the dependence of the Doppler signal on its angle of incidence on the blood stream, the latter is highly susceptible to observer variation; in the stimulated state the artery becomes straightened and the variation in signal response is consequently reduced.

In order to quantify the waveforms, Desai and colleagues chose Laplace Transform Analysis (LTA), a method previously applied to the study of lower limb arterial disease and proven to be a sensitive modality for the detection of minor stenoses of the aortoiliac segment, capable of differentiating between less than or greater than 50% occlusion (Skidmore and Woodcock, 1980a, b; Skidmore *et al.*, 1980). LTA is a complex mathematical procedure, originally described by Skidmore and Woodcock, which involves the digital conversion of the waveform allowing the calculation of the Fourier Transform and, consequently, the evaluation of the equivalent Laplace Transform by a curve-fitting manoeuvre. The reconstituted waveform is described by a three-pole mathematical model whose coefficients, $\delta$, $\omega_0$ and $\gamma$, are related to proximal lumen size, vessel elasticity and peripheral resistance respectively. A microcomputer linked to the continuous wave Doppler system allows the complicated analysis to be performed rapidly and easily. Although the system uses commercially available equipment, we have modified the Doppler probes in order to reduce the likelihood of confusing the dorsal and cavernosal arteries. We employ two purpose-built 10 MHz probes with their ultrasound beams accurately focused at 6 mm and 12 mm respectively, a refinement made possible by a unique optical system designed by Follett (1986). Commercial probes, which are not focused, will record all signals within the transmitted ultrasound beam's path to the limit of its penetrance through the tissues.

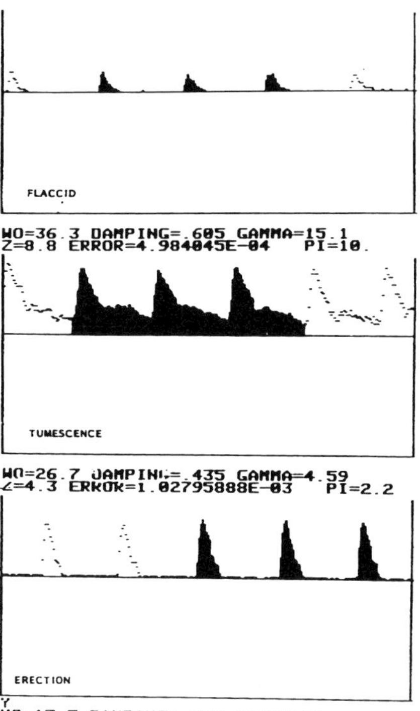


**Figure 9.1** Evolution of the cavernosal artery Doppler waveform during pharmacologically induced erection

## Practical procedure

The study is performed during the phase of tumescence induced by an intracavernosal injection of 15–30 mg papaverine followed by penile massage in the manner described by Brindley (1986). As soon as the penis is tumescent, each of the two dorsal arteries is separately located over the dorsum of the penis just distal to the symphysis pubis, using the 6 mm probe. The probe is moved at an angle of 45–60 degrees to the direction of the arteries until the optimal (maximum) Doppler signal is heard as well as observed on the video monitor which continuously displays the arterial waveforms. The optimal waveforms are 'frozen' on the screen and three are selected for analysis by moving an integral cursor. This information is stored for later analysis in an Apple II microcomputer. The procedure is repeated for the other dorsal artery and subsequently, after changing to the 12 mm probe, the cavernosal artery waveforms are recorded, this time placing the probe on the ventrolateral surface of the penis. Each study takes 20–30 min to complete with analysis of the stored data taking a further 5 min.

## Normal penile artery waveforms

The evolution of the dorsal and cavernosal artery waveforms during erection has been documented by Desai *et al.* (1987) who carefully monitored the shape of the waveforms in the flaccid, tumescent and rigid phases (Figure 9.1). The observed changes occur in a characteristic manner and are consistent with the proposed haemodynamic mechanism of erection in man. In the flaccid penis, the cavernosal artery waveform is of low amplitude and brief duration indicating a low volume of blood flow through these arteries in the resting state. The tumescent waveform is typified by a marked rise in amplitude during systole and an enhanced Doppler frequency shift throughout diastole, representing a greatly increased blood flow throughout the cardiac cycle. That this is due to a fall in impedance, ostensibly as a result of sinusoidal relaxation, is evident from the dramatic fall in the value of the $\gamma$ coefficient which, as will be recalled, is related to the peripheral resistance to blood flow in a vessel. At erection, blood flow in the cavernosal vessels can still be detected albeit at a much reduced level, the waveforms comprising of brief high amplitude systolic spurts with a sharp peak. The value of the $\gamma$ coefficient rises once again, reflecting the increased peripheral resistance. Cavernosal artery flow can, at this stage, be abolished by voluntary contraction of the bulbocavernosus muscles which causes the intracavernosal pressure to exceed systolic blood pressure.

These observations of the variation in penile artery waveform shape, and with it the changes in the Laplace coefficients relating to the particular phase of erection, had an important bearing on the actual technique of utilizing waveform analysis to quantify penile artery blood flow. In order to ensure uniformity, the waveforms had to be recorded during the same phase for all individuals. Since the cavernosal signals tended to be relatively more pronounced and easy to elicit during early tumescence, only these waveforms were recorded and analysed.

In a preliminary study comparing a group of 28 potent men with a group of 15 arteriogenically impotent patients, all of whom had arteriographically proven aortoiliac disease, it was demonstrated, by means of multivariant analysis, that the damping factor ($\delta$) relating to proximal lumen size best discriminated between the two groups (Desai, 1988). Although there was some overlap between

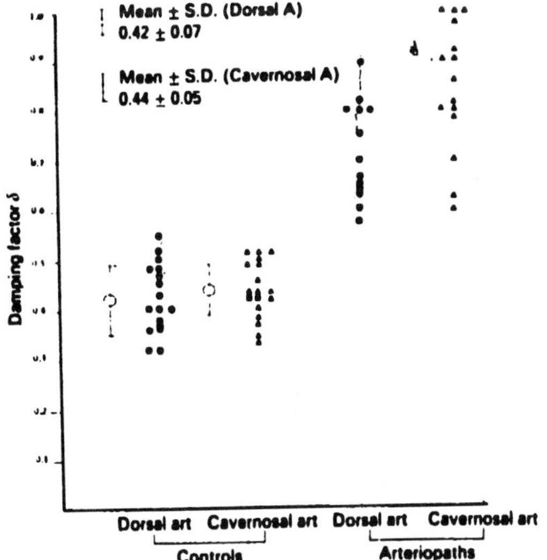


**Figure 9.2** Graph showing mean Laplace δ values obtained from the dorsal and cavernosal arteries for the two groups. Note the complete separation achieved for the cavernosal arteries

the values obtained from the dorsal arteries for the two groups, this was not so for the cavernosal arteries where complete separation was achieved (Figure 9.2). Interestingly, the dorsal artery δ values demonstrated a significant correlation with age, analagous to the findings reported by Metz and Bengtsson (1981) who obtained PBI values from the same arteries.

Though a significant advance, the technique of computerized Doppler waveform analysis as described above suffers from two potential drawbacks. Both of these relate to the use of continuous wave Doppler equipment. Firstly, because the waveform shape is dependent on the angle at which the probe insonates the artery, the method is prone to operator variability and can result in an appreciable loss of reproducibility. Whilst these problems can be reduced with experience, it also means that the technique cannot readily be used by an inexperienced or casual investigator. The second shortcoming concerns the uncertainty regarding the accurate localization of the cavernosal arteries. Even though one may be convinced that the Doppler signal is arising from the deep artery, it is not always easy to separate between the right and left arteries.

Despite these criticisms, it is the authors' view that this method is of practical value particularly when resources are limited. It provides information that is far more accurate and meaningful than the PBI. The system is now commercially available as a lap-top unit, and costs less than one-tenth of the price of the more sophisticated duplex scanners.

## Duplex scanning

Many of the difficulties inherent in the use of a continuous wave Doppler probe can be eliminated by duplex ultrasonography which combines a real-time image with pulsed Doppler spectral analysis. The assessment of the penile arteries by duplex scanning was introduced by Lue and his coworkers in 1985. The real-time image is provided by a 10 MHz transducer and allows the definition of any cavernosal or tunical pathology, for example Peyronie's disease, as well as the assessment of the arteries themselves. An integral 4.5 MHz range-gated pulsed Doppler probe enables the operator to measure blood flow velocity within the cavernosal and dorsal arteries. Using this system, Mueller and Lue (1988) were able to define the normal response of the penile arteries to intracorporeal papaverine and examine how those with arterial disease differed. It was suggested that following the injection of 60 mg papaverine the internal calibre of the cavernosal arteries should increase by at least 75% and that the peak flow velocity should exceed 25 cm $s^{-1}$ in those with adequate arterial function for erection.

There have been few corroborative studies of Lue's original work, mainly because the equipment needed for this investigation is expensive. Neither Collins and Lewandowski (1987) nor Shabsigh *et al.* (1989) were able to demonstrate a clear distinction between those with normal and those with abnormal penile haemodynamics. Benson and Vickers (1989) have suggested that conventional duplex ultrasonography can identify those patients with severe arteriopathy (peak flow velocity <30 cm $s^{-1}$) and those with normal arteries (>40 cm $s^{-1}$) but cannot confidently detect those with mild or moderate disease.

The reason for this is that duplex ultrasonography is a technique that requires considerable operator skill; if difficulties with the identification of the cavernosal arteries are encountered placement of the pulsed Doppler sample volume and correction of the Doppler angle are prevented or at best delayed. As discussed above, the timing of sampling is critical. The evolution of the arterial waveform, described originally by Desai *et al.* (1987), has recently been further defined by Schwartz *et al.* (1989b). These workers have confirmed that the peak flow velocities recorded in the cavernosal arteries vary considerably during erection in normal subjects and that the cavernosal arteries are at their functional maximum in early tumescence. Any delay in localizing the arteries may, therefore, lead to a falsely low estimation of peak flow velocity.

Schwartz *et al.* (1989b) were able to continuously monitor the response to intracavernosal papaverine because they had the benefit of colour-coded Doppler imaging, a recent innovation in ultrasono-

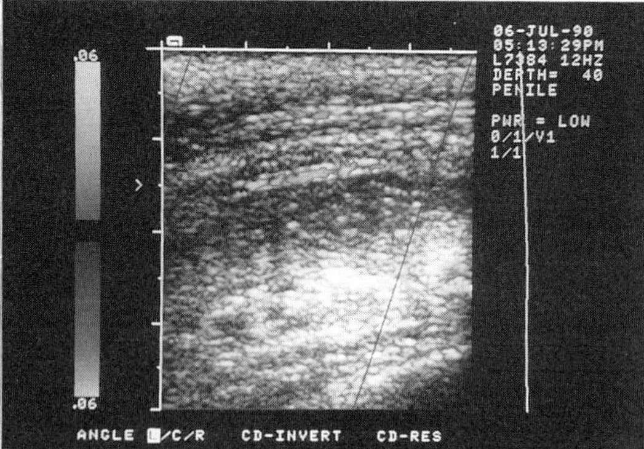


**Figure 9.3** Colour Doppler scan of tumescent penis showing the two cavernosal arteries with the septum in between

graphic technology. Most frequency shifts caused by blood flow are ignored by the conventional duplex scanner which only analyses the small area of the image contained within the sample gate. By dividing the whole real-time image into a large number of small areas each of these can be evaluated for frequency shifts. If each area is then ascribed a colour dependent on the direction (red or blue) and velocity of blood flow (intensity), and this information is continuously updated and superimposed on the real-time image, then a striking anatomical and functional 'ultrasound arteriogram' is produced (Figure 9.3). This, together with the advent of the far less cumbersome linear array tranducers, has facilitated the clinical application of duplex ultrasonography. Because of the ease and rapidity with which the cavernosal arteries are identified, their response to intracorporeal papaverine can be readily and instantly monitored. This in turn allows the selection of the most appropriate time for recording of the arterial waveform and dispenses with the arbitrary timing of recordings previously recommended. The direction of flow is obvious and therefore the placement of the angle correction guide is made more accurate. These facilities are particularly useful during the early stages of tumescence when the vessels are still tortuous and the changes in flow are rapid.

## Practical procedure

Duplex scanning is performed in those patients who have failed to respond to papaverine at initial screening. With the patient lying supine the flaccid penis is placed in the anatomical position and scanned with a 7 MHz linear array probe. Areas of calcification or Peyronie's plaques are noted and the internal calibre of the cavernosal arteries is determined using the electronic calipers. A tourniquet is then placed around the base of the penis and 60 mg papaverine is injected with a 25G needle into the right corpus cavernosum; the patient massages the penis to ensure complete distribution. The tourniquet is released after 2 min. With the penis lying along the inguinal groove and the transducer placed longitudinally along its ventrolateral aspect, the right cavernosal artery is identified using colour imaging and, having corrected for the Doppler angle, the response is monitored. When the maximal response is observed, which is characterized by maximal systolic and diastolic flow, the peak flow velocity is recorded. The left artery is then immediately imaged and the peak velocity is likewise recorded (Figure 9.4). The internal calibre of both the arteries is then re-estimated. In order to standardize this measurement, it is our practice to make this measurement at the systolic peak. The dorsal arteries can be imaged with the semi-erect penis in the anatomical position, with the transducer applied longitudinally or transversely in relation to the penis. The value of measurements taken from the dorsal artery in view of their minor contribution to erection is unclear (Lue *et al.*, 1985). The patient is allowed to return home at this stage but is warned that should an erection be present 6 h after the investigation he should return to the clinic for pharmacological detumescence.

A small number of studies have appeared which have investigated the use of colour imaging in the diagnosis of impotence. Most of these have been based upon Lue's pioneering work and have examined the ability of the increment in internal calibre of the cavernosal arteries and the peak flow velocity through them to identify those with arteriopathic impotence. Our own experience is that changes in the diameter of these arteries are not significantly different in those with and those

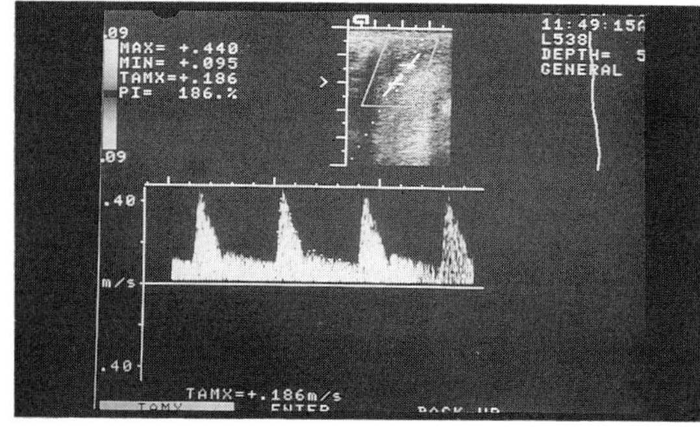


**Figure 9.4** A normal duplex Doppler scan depicting a cavernosal peak flow velocity of 44 cm/s

without arterial disease. These findings are in agreement with those of Quam *et al.* (1989). The reasons for this include variation in the resting state of the arteries due to psychological influence or arteriosclerotic disease; it is for this reason that Lue now uses the absolute value after injection (>0.8 mm) as the parameter of choice (personal communication).

In a study of 70 patients using colour duplex ultrasonography, we have established that mean cavernosal peak flow velocity is the single most useful parameter in distinguishing between arteriogenic and non-arteriogenic impotence. Based on statistical analysis using 95% confidence intervals, we found that all of our haemodynamically normal men (as defined by a full erection lasting more than 20 min in response to ICP) registered mean peak flow velocities equal to or greater than 28 cm $s^{-1}$, whereas all but six out of 50 papaverine non-responders (88%) were shown to have mean peak flow velocities below this value. Five out of these six men demonstrated venous leakage on subsequent pharmacocavernosometry.

Attempts have been made to determine the clinical accuracy of duplex scanning by comparing it with other more established methods of investigation. Quam *et al.* (1989), using colour imaging, investigated the accuracy of a cut-off value of 25 cm $s^{-1}$ cavernosal peak flow velocity to define arteriopathy, a value recommended by Lue *et al.* (1988). Twelve patients with arteriographically proven disease all had peak velocities less than 25 cm $s^{-1}$ whereas the normal subjects in their study all had values above this figure. These findings were confirmed by Mueller *et al.* (1990) in a series of 43 patients; they reported an excellent correlation with the findings of selective arteriography. However, such comparisons may not be entirely appropriate because, although arteriography can give excellent anatomical detail of the relevant arteries, it offers very limited functional information about these vessels. Furthermore, because of obvious ethical constraints, there is a paucity of normative data relating to arteriographic features in potent men. This dearth of knowledge as to what constitutes the limits of normality means that arteriography remains subject to observer interpretation and should not be considered an investigational 'gold standard'.

Duplex scanning has also been compared with nocturnal penile tumescence monitoring (NPT), another investigation which is perceived as a 'gold standard', in this case for the distinction of functional and organic impotence. Duplex scanning has been shown to correlate well with the results of NPT monitoring with the additional advantage that it is capable of successfully identifying those patients with the steal syndrome who would otherwise have been designated haemodynamically normal on the basis of NPT alone (Shabsigh *et al.*, 1990).

## Conclusion

Duplex ultrasonography does appear to improve the statistical end-points that define normal and abnormal arterial function, bearing in mind that the accuracy of any investigation, in the absence of corroborative date, is difficult to determine. Nevertheless, a mean peak flow velocity value of below 25 cm $s^{-1}$ unequivocally indicates the presence of significant arterial disease which can be confirmed by selective internal iliac arteriography. Internal calibre measurements are less reliable in identifying compromised vessels, but a post-injection value of greater than 0.8 mm is consistent with normal function.

There is no doubt that tests of penile artery function based on the flaccid penis should now be abandoned in favour of dynamic testing incorporating the simultaneous intracavernosal injection of a vasoactive agent. Accurate arterial assessment is essential when considering penile revascularization or venous ligation, and is critical to the outcome of such surgery. Though expensive, duplex ultrasonography with colour imaging is steadily acquiring a reputation as the investigation of choice for penile artery screening. Whilst it is generally accepted that cavernosal mean peak flow velocities of 25–28 cm $s^{-1}$ provide a reasonable cut-off level between normal and significantly abnormal arterial inflow, the search for other parameters continues. Computerized Doppler waveform analysis nevertheless remains an acceptable and much cheaper alternative in circumstances where economic constraints prohibit the use of duplex ultrasonography.

## References


Abelson, D. (1975) Diagnostic value of the penile pulse and blood pressure: a Doppler study of impotence in diabetics. *Journal of Urology*, **113**, 636–639

Bahren, W., Gall, H., Scherb, W. *et al.* (1988) Arterial anatomy and arteriographic diagnosis of arteriogenic impotence. *Cardiovascular and Interventional Radiology*, **11**, 195–210

Bell, D., Lewis, R. and Kerstein, M. D. (1983) Hyperaemic stress test in diagnosis of vasculogenic impotence. *Urology*, **22**, 611–613

Benson, C. B. and Vickers, M. A. (1989) Sexual impotence caused by vascular disease: diagnosis with duplex sonography. *American Journal of Roentgenology*, **153**, 1149–1153

Bookstein, J. J. and Lang, E. V. (1987) Penile magnification arteriography: details of intrapenile arterial anatomy. *American Journal of Roentgenology*, **148**, 883–888

Brindley, G. S. (1986) Maintenance treatment of erectile impotence by cavernosal unstriated muscle relaxant injection. *British Journal of Psychiatry*, **149**, 210–215

Britt, D. B., Kemmerer, W. T. and Robison, J. R. (1971) Penile blood flow determination by mercury strain gauge plethysmography. *Investigative Urology,* **8**, 673–678

Buvat, J. Buvat-Herbaut, M., Dehaene, J. L. and Lamaire, A. (1986) Is intracavernosal injection of papaverine a reliable screening test for vasculogenic impotence? *Journal of Urology,* **135**, 476–478

Buvat, J., Lemaire, A., Besson, P. *et al.* (1982) Lack of correlations between penile thermography and pelvic arteriography in 29 cases of erectile impotence. *Journal of Urology,* **128**, 298–299

Chiu, R. C. J., Lidstone, D. and Blundell, P. E. (1989) Predictive power of penile/brachial index in diagnosing male sexual impotence. *Journal of Vascular Surgery,* **4**, 251–256

Collins, J. P. and Lewandowski, B. J. (1987) Experience with intracorporeal injection of papaverine and duplex ultrasound scanning for the assessment of arteriogenic impotence. *British Journal of Urology,* **59**, 84–88

De Palma, R. G., Levine, S. B. and Feldman, S. (1978) Preservation of erectile function after aortoiliac reconstruction. *Archives of Surgery,* **113**, 958–962

De Palma, R. G., Kedia, K. and Persky, L. (1980) Surgical options in the correction of vasculogenic impotence. *Vascular Surgery,* **14**, 92–103

Desai, K. M. (1988) The investigation of diabetic impotence and the factors involved in its aetiology. *MCh Thesis*, University of Bristol

Desai, K. M., Gingwell, J. C. Skidmore, R. and Follett, D. H. (1987) Application of computerized penile arterial waveform analysis in the diagnosis of arteriogenic impotence: an initial study in potent and impotent men. *British Journal of Urology,* **60**, 450–456

Engel, G., Burnham, S. J. and Carter, M. F. (1978) Penile blood pressure in the evaluation of erectile impotence. *Fertility and Sterility,* **30**, 687–690

Fanous, H. N., Jevtich, M. J., Chen, D. C. P. and Edson, M. (1982) Radioisotope penogram in diagnosis of vasculogenic impotence. *Urology,* **20**, 499–502

Follett, D. H. (1986) A versatile schlieren system for beam and waveform visualization with quantitative real-time profiling capability. In *Physics in Medical Ultrasound*, The Institute of Physical Sciences in Medicine; Report No. 47

Forsberg, L., Olsson, A. M. and Neglen, P. (1982) Erectile function before and after aorto-iliac reconstruction: a comparison between measurements of Doppler acceleration ratio, blood pressure and angiography. *Journal of Urology,* **127**, 379–382

Gaskell, P. (1971) The importance of penile blood pressure in cases of impotence. *Canadian Medical Association Journal,* **105**, 1047–1051

Goldstein, I., Siroky, M. B., Nath, R. L. *et al.* (1982) Vasculogenic impotence: role of the pelvic steal test. *Journal of Urology,* **128**, 300–306

Haden, H. T., Katz, P. G., Mulligan, T. and Zasler, N. D. (1989) Penile blood flow by xenon-133 washout. *Journal of Nuclear Medicine,* **30**, 1032–1035

Hirsch, E. W. (1930) Sexual impotence of organic origin. *Clinical Medicine and Surgery,* **37**, 350–355

Ishii, N., Mitsukawa, S. and Shirai, M. (1977) Studies on male sexual impotence: differential diagnosis of organic and functional impotence by determining penile skin temperature. *Japanese Journal of Urology,* **68**, 136

Jevtich, M. J. (1981) Penile body temperature as a screening test for penile arterial obstruction in impotence. *Urology,* **17**, 132–135

Kedia, K. R. (1984) Vasculogenic impotence: diagnosis and objective evaluation using quantitative segmental pulse volume recorder. *British Journal of Urology,* **56**, 516–520

Lane, R. J., Appleberg, M. and Williams, W. (1982) A comparison of two techniques for the detection of the vasculogenic component of impotence. *Surgery, Gynaecology and Obstetrics,* **155**, 230–234

Leriche, R. (1940) Le syndrome de l'obliteration terminoaortique par arterite. *La Presse Medical,* **48**, 601–604

Lin, S. N., Chang, L. S., Liu, R. S. *et al.* (1989) Diagnosis of vasculogenic impotence: combination of penile xenon-133 washout and papaverine tests. *Urology,* **34**, 28–32

Lue, T. F., Hricak, H., Marich, K. W. and Tanagho, E. A. (1985) Vasculogenic impotence evaluated by high-resolution ultrasonography and pulsed Doppler spectrum analysis. *Radiology,* **155**, 777–781

Metz, P. and Bengtsson, J. (1981) Penile blood pressure. *Scandanavian Journal of Urology and Nephrology,* **15**, 161–164

Metz, P., Christiensen, V., Mathiesen, F. R. and Ostri, P. (1983) Ultrasonic Doppler pulse wave analysis versus penile blood pressure measurement in the evaluation of arteriogenic impotence. *Vasa,* **12**, 363–366

Michal, V., Kramar, R. and Pospichal, J. (1978) External iliac 'steal syndrome'. *Journal of Cardiovascular Surgery,* **19**, 355–357

Mueller, S. C. and Lue, T. F. (1988) Evaluation of vasculogenic impotence. *Urologic Clinics of North America,* **15**, 65–76

Mueller, S. C., Wallenberg-Pachaly, H., Voges, G. E. and Schild, H. H. (1990) Comparison of selective internal iliac pharmacoangiography, penile brachial index and duplex sonography with pulsed Doppler analysis for the evaluation of vasculogenic (arteriogenic) impotence. *Journal of Urology,* **143**, 928–932

Nath, R. L., Menzoian, J. O., Kaplan, K. H. *et al.* (1981) The multidisciplinary approach to vasculogenic impotence. *Surgery,* **89**, 124–133

Nseyo, U. O., Wilbur, H. J., Kang, S. C. *et al.* (1984) Penile xenon-133 washout: a rapid method of screening for vasculogenic impotence. *Urology,* **23**, 31–34

Quam, J. P., King, B. F., James, E. M. *et al.* (1989) Duplex and colour Doppler sonographic evaluation of vasculogenic impotence. *American Journal of Roentgenology,* **153**, 1141–1147

Queral, L. A., Whitehouse, W. M., Flinn, W. R. *et al.* (1979) Pelvic haemodynamics after aortoiliac reconstruction. *Surgery,* **86**, 799–809

Reiss, H. F. (1985) Difficulties in Doppler auscultation of

cavernous arteries of the penis. *Urology,* **26**, 222

Satomura, S. (1959) Study of the flow patterns in peripheral arteries by ultrasonics. *Journal of the Acoustical Society of America,* **15**, 151–158

Schwartz, A. N., Graham, M. M., Ferency, G. F. and Miura, R. S. (1989a) Radioisotope penile plethysmography: a technique for evaluating corpora cavernosal blood flow during early tumescence, *Journal of Nuclear Medicine,* **30**, 466–473

Schwartz, A. N., Wang, K. Y., Mack, L. A. *et al.* (1989b) Evaluation of normal erectile function with colour flow Doppler sonography. *American Journal of Roentgenology,* **153**, 1155–1160

Shabsigh, R., Fishman, J. J., Queseda, E. T. *et al.* (1989) Evaluation of vasculogenic erectile impotence using penile duplex ultrasonography. *Journal of Urology,* **142**, 1469–1474

Shabsigh, R., Fishman, I. J., Shotland, Y. *et al.* (1990) Comparison of penile duplex ultrasonography with nocturnal penile tumescence monitoring for the evaluation of erectile impotence. *Journal of Urology,* **143**, 924–927

Shirai, M. and Ishii, N. (1981) Haemodynamics of erection in man. *Archives of Andrology,* **6**, 27–32

Shirai, M. and Nakamura, M. (1970) Differential diagnosis of organic and functional impotence by the use of 131-iodine labelled human serum albumin. *Tohoku Journal of Experimental Medicine,* **101**, 317–324

Shirai, M., Nakamura, M., Ishii, N. *et al.* (1976) Determination of intrapenile blood volume using 99m-technetium labelled autologous red blood cells. *Tohoku Journal of Experimental Medicine,* **120**, 377–383

Skidmore, R. and Woodcock, J. P. (1980a) Physiological interpretation of Doppler-shift waveforms. I: Theoretical considerations. *Ultrasound in Medicine and Biology,* **6**, 7–10

Skidmore, R. and Woodcock, J. P. (1980b) Physiological interpretation of Doppler-shift waveforms. II: Validation of the Laplace transform method for characterization of the common femoral blood velocity/time waveform. *Ultrasound in Medicine and Biology,* **6**, 219–225

Skidmore, R., Woodcock, J. P., Wells, P. N. T. *et al.* (1980c) Physiological interpretation of Doppler-shift waveforms. III: Clinical results. *Ultrasound in Medicine and Biology,* **6**, 227–231

Townell, N. J., Siraj, Q. H., Hilson, A. J. *et al.* (1985) Isotope phallogram: preliminary communication. *Journal of the Royal Society of Medicine,* **78**, 562–566

Velcek, D., Sniderman, K. W., Vaughan, E. D. *et al.* (1980) Penile flow index utilising a Doppler pulse wave analysis to identify penile vascular insufficiency. *Journal of Urology,* **123**, 669–673

Virag, R. (1982) Intracavernous injection of papaverine for erectile failure. *Lancet,* **ii**, 938

Virag, R., Zwang, G., Dermange, H. and Legman, L. (1981) Vasculogenic impotence: a review of 92 cases with 54 surgical operations. *Vascular Surgery,* **15**, 9–17

Wagner, G. and Uhrenholdt, A. (1980) Blood flow measurement by the clearance method in the human corpus cavernosum in the flaccid and erect states. In *Vasculogenic Impotence* (eds A. W. Zorgniotti and G. Rossi), Charles C. Thomas, Springfield, Illinois, pp. 41–46

Zorgniotti, A. W., Rossi, G., Padula, G. and Makovsky, R. D. (1980) Diagnosis and therapy of vasculogenic impotence. *Journal of Urology,* **123**, 674–677

# 10

# Radionuclide evaluation

**P. Grech and R. O'N. Witherow**

## Introduction

The investigation of impotence by radionuclide methods has evolved gradually over the last 20 years with improvements in technique following the introduction of new radiopharmaceuticals and advances in the understanding of the physiology of normal erection and the mechanism of its failure. The radionuclide evaluation of venosinusoidal leakage, postoperative graft patency and priapism has been attempted (see below), yet radionuclide techniques are best suited to the assessment of penile arterial flow where the alternative forms of investigation are least satisfactory. It is, therefore, to this subject that the major part of this chapter is devoted.

Radionuclide techniques have theoretical advantages, not shared by other forms of imaging, which are particularly relevant to the investigation of impotence, the principal being the ability to obtain functional information. Arteriography can provide excellent anatomical detail and demonstrate the site of an arterial stenosis or occlusion, but radionuclide studies demonstrate the haemodynamic consequences, if any, of such an abnormality. Variations in arterial anatomy do not invalidate the technique, and disease in small vessels, beyond the resolution of arteriography or ultrasound, may be detected. In addition radionuclide methods are relatively non-invasive, do not require a high level of operator skill, remain valid after vascular surgery and result in a smaller gonadal radiation dose than arteriography or cavernosography. These potential advantages have long been recognized in the investigation of limb ischaemia and these methods have become accepted clinical practice alongside assessment by history, clinical examination and arteriography. Several groups of workers have transferred radionuclide techniques, developed primarily for the investigation of limb blood flow, to the investigation of impotence but the results have been confusing and often contradictory, prompting scepticism regarding the value of radionuclide methods in the evaluation of the penile vasculature (Melman, 1988). It is of value to consider the theoretical basis of these methods further before examining how they might be applied to the special case of penile blood flow.

## Radionuclide investigation of limb blood flow

### Xenon clearance

#### Muscle blood flow

One of the earliest attempt to develop a clinically applicable method for assessing limb blood flow by the use of radionuclides was reported by Lassen, Lindbjerg and Munck (1964). Xenon-133 was injected into the calf muscle and the rate of washout of activity from the injection site was measured. The xenon gas was prepared for injection by dissolving in a small volume of saline. Being highly lipid-soluble, the injected xenon rapidly diffuses out of the extravascular compartment into the local capillary network and is subsequently carried away from the injection site. Diffusion is so rapid that equilibrium between the extravascular and intravascular compartments is maintained even at high blood flow rates, so that the rate at which xenon is removed from the injection site is limited only by blood flow (Siegel and Stewart, 1984). In the limbs, where volume is constant, venous outflow and arterial inflow are equal so that measurement of washout provides a means of measuring arterial inflow. Xenon is cleared from the blood in its passage through the pulmonary circulation and for practical purposes recirculation is negligible. Blood flow is calculated from the Schmidt–Kety formula:

$$F = K \times \lambda \times 100$$

where $F$ = flow in ml min$^{-1}$ per 100 g, K = the slope constant of xenon-133 washout derived from the washout curve and $\lambda$ = the tissue:blood partition coefficient (0.7).

Since a large proportion of arterial blood flow to the limb supplies skeletal muscle, the measurement of muscle blood flow by xenon washout provides an approximate measurement of total limb blood flow.

### Skin blood flow

In the investigation of limb ischaemia blood flow to the skin is, in some circumstances, of greater relevance than total limb blood flow since this determines whether an ischaemic ulcer or an amputation stump will heal. The xenon washout technique has been used to determine skin blood flow by recording the rate of xenon-133 clearance from an intradermal injection (Daly and Henry, 1980). It should be noted that this method does not give an assessment of total limb flow and is influenced markedly by ambient temperature.

### Blood pool labelling

Total blood flow to the limbs may be assessed by blood pool imaging. The intravascular compartment is labelled by intravenously injected radionuclide. The ideal preparation remains confined to the intravascular compartment and has a sufficiently long biological and atomic half-life to enable the study to be completed with little loss of activity. Various radiopharmaceuticals have been tried but the currently used preparation of choice is $^{99m}$Tc-labelled red blood cells ($^{99m}$Tc-RBC).

### First-pass technique

Oshima *et al.* (1984) adminstered an intravenous bolus of $^{99m}$Tc-labelled human serum albumin ($^{99m}$Tc-HSA) and assessed flow in the lower limbs by recording the shape of the time–activity curve produced by arrival of tracer in the feet: the 'first-pass' technique. This method did not provide an absolute measurement of flow but the shape of the curve was abnormal in patients with arterial insufficiency and returned to normal following successful vascular surgery.

### Stimulated limb blood flow by limb isolation

Blood pool labelling was used by Parkin *et al.* (1986) to provide an absolute measurement of limb blood flow. A cuff was first applied to the proximal part of the limb and inflated to above arterial pressure. This had the effect of isolating the limb from the circulating blood pool and causing reactive hyperaemia in the limb on release of the cuff. The remaining blood pool was labelled by the intravenous injection of $^{99m}$Tc-RBC and the isolated limb positioned under the scintillation camera. Blood pool activity was measured by withdrawing a venous sample and then the cuff was released to allow labelled blood to enter the limb. The time–activity curve over the limb showed three phases:

1. Initial phase;
2. Exponential phase;
3. Equilibrium phase.

These phases are represented schematically in Figure 10.1. The initial phase occurs immediately after release of the cuff and is the result of labelled arterial blood flowing into the limb. The displaced blood is not labelled and therefore the increase in activity in the limb is linear and unaffected by venous outflow. As mixing of labelled and unlabelled blood occurs in the limb the displaced blood shows progressively increasing activity so that the shape of the exponential phase of the curve is influenced both by arterial and venous flow. The final phase results when there is complete mixing of activity in the circulation so that inflowing and outflowing blood is of the same activity. The activity in the limb during this phase is unaffected by flow and is proportional to the intravascular blood volume. The product of the gradient of the initial phase of the curve and blood pool activity provides an absolute measurement of flow to the limb.

The use of the above techniques of limb blood flow measurement cannot simply be transferred to the measurement of penile blood flow. Special features of penile structure and circulation must be considered if such studies are to remain valid.

## Penile circulation

### Arterial anatomy

The penile arterial supply can be considered to arise from two independent sources. The arterial supply to the penile skin is derived from the external iliac arterial system and plays no role in the process of erection. The arterial supply of interest in the investigation of impotence is that to the corpora cavernosa, which is derived from the internal iliac system. The dual supply is important in the correct interpretation of radionuclide measurements of penile perfusion but it has been disregarded in several of the studies described below. Measurement of penile skin perfusion by xenon washout may provide evidence of disease in the external iliac vessels but otherwise must be considered irrelevant to the investigation of impotence. Washout studies attempting to measure cavernosal arterial flow require intracavernosal injection of tracer.

### Venous system

The venous drainage of the penis plays an important role in the initiation and maintenance of erection and, unlike the situation in the limbs, has a

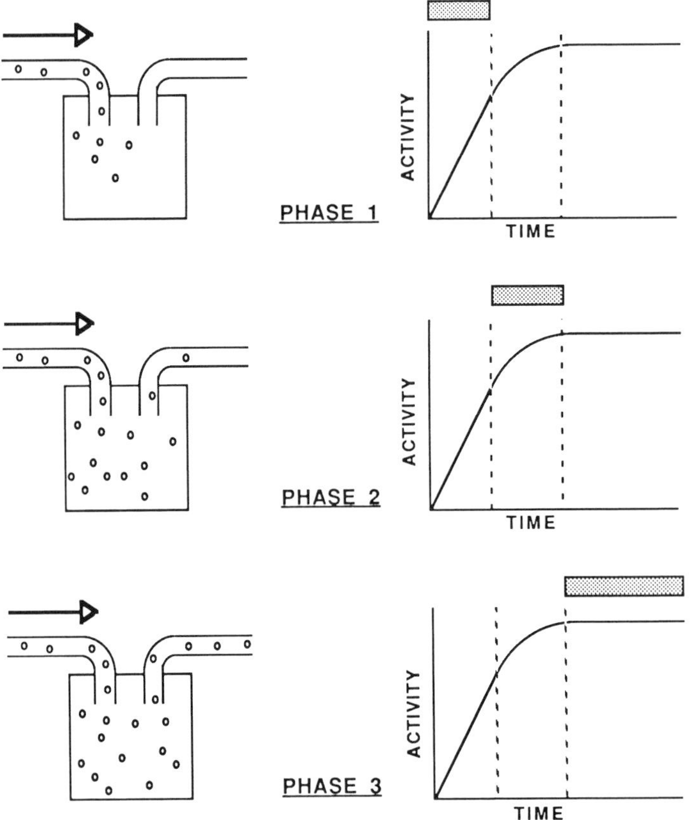


**Figure 10.1** Production of time–activity curve in blood flow studies using occlusion cuff

controlling effect on arterial inflow. The arrangement of the venous system is such that there is trapping of blood within the penis during erection. In addition to reducing venous outflow this trapping causes tamponade of the arterial supply during full erection and thus reduces arterial inflow (Aboseif and Lue, 1988). The consequences of this role of the venous circulation to the measurement of penile perfusion are two-fold. Firstly, methods based on the washout techniques are likely to give misleading results in the presence of a competent venous trapping mechanism since, for such studies to be valid, it is necessary to assume that arterial inflow and venous outflow are in equilibrium. This only occurs in the flaccid or fully erect state. During these periods penile blood flow is low and is of less interest to the study of impotence than the maximum flow that can be achieved during the initiation of erection. Secondly, arterial flow alters during erection and must be measured at the same point during the process for the results to be reproducible and comparable in different studies.

## Volume changes

During erection the changes in arterial inflow, venous outflow and sinusoidal compliance allow the erectile bodies to undergo large and rapid increases in volume. Such changes in volume cause difficulty in the interpretation of radionuclide studies.

Flow measurements by cavernosal xenon clearance are not valid indicators of arterial flow if the cavernosal volume is not fixed. Clearance in these circumstances reflects venous outflow and will thus underestimate arterial flow during initiation of erection and exceed arterial flow during detumescence.

Errors may also arise in the interpretation of labelled blood pool studies. If, following blood pool labelling, the rate of change of penile scintigraphic activity caused by erotic or pharmacological stimulation is measured, a value for arterial flow can be calculated. In some of the studies described below the changes in scintigraphic activity simply reflect the change in penile volume. It must be appreciated that changes in penile volume reflect not only changes in arterial inflow but also changes in venous outflow and erectile tissue compliance. This source of error would tend to cause underestimation of arterial inflow in a patient with severe venous leakage since, although arterial inflow may increase normally following stimulation, venous outflow would also increase and both the final volume and the rate of increase in volume would be less than in the subject with a competent venous system. Similarly a decrease in cavernosal compliance, such as may occur with fibrosis, may limit the increase in penile volume despite a normal arterial supply.

### Stimulation of arterial flow

The effects of arterial insufficiency on the penile circulation are manifest as impotence rather than the nutritional changes characteristic of arterial disease in the limbs. It is not clear whether the cause of arteriogenic impotence is due directly to critical narrowing of the major vessels that supply the corpora or due to the decreased compliance of the sinusoids which occurs in diabetes, following priapism, in heavy smokers and in the presence of penile arterial disease (Mueller and Lue, 1988), but the final result is the inability to increase penile arterial flow in response to appropriate neurological or pharmacological stimulation. In the absence of such stimuli, penile perfusion in the impotent arteriopath is probably no less than in the potent male (Haden *et al.*, 1989).

It is clear therefore that any non-invasive technique for detecting arteriogenic impotence must be performed under conditions which reproduce the physiological stimuli normally resulting in erection. Various stimuli have been used in conjunction with radionuclide studies in order to maximize arterial inflow. The uncritical use of such stimulation can introduce an additional source of error. Visual erotic stimulation is more physiological but the effectiveness of the stimulus requires a normal psychological state and intact neuronal pathways. The use of systemic vasodilators such as isoxsuprine may increase penile arterial flow in the normal patient but would also be expected to affect venous outflow and sinusoidal smooth muscle tone. Such stimulation does not usually induce erection in the potent male. Where these systemic vasodilators have been used in conjuction with flow measurements it has been difficult to ascribe their effects solely to changes in arterial flow. In animal experiments the effects of neurostimulation most closely simulated the normal physiological changes of erection (Lue *et al.*, 1983). Such stimuli cause an increase in arterial inflow, relaxation of smooth muscle in the sinusoids and passive occlusion of the draining veins of the corpora cavernosa. Once full erection is established the high intracavernosal pressure causes a reduction in arterial flow to a value sufficient only to replace venosinusoidal drainage.

Such methods have not been combined with blood flow estimation in man but similar effects can be achieved by the intracavernosal injection of vasodilators such as papaverine and phentolamine which provide a consistent means of inducing penile tumescence applicable to man (Juenemann *et al.*, 1985). Since the diagnostic value of intracavernosal papaverine was described by Virag in 1982 its use in the investigation and treatment of impotence has increased and it has been combined with radionuclide and other techniques in the evaluation of penile arterial flow. However, difficulties in its use have emerged. It appears that a proportion of otherwise normal potent males fail to respond to papaverine in the doses which normally cause erection. This may be due to antagonism by circulating adrenergic compounds in anxious individuals (Buvat *et al.*, 1986). Such antagonism may be overcome by the use of higher doses of papaverine or by the addition of phentolamine, but this increases the risk of inducing priapism in those with a normal response. Resistance to the effects of intracavernosal vasodilators results in the overdiagnosis of arterial disease when these agents are combined with arterial flow measurements by radionuclide or other techniques.

## Estimation of penile arterial supply

Both xenon clearance and blood pool labelling techniques have been used in the evaluation of penile arterial supply and advances in both methods continue to be made, particularly since the introduction of intracavernosal (i.c.) vasodilators (Table 10.1).

### Penile blood flow by xenon washout

The investigation of penile blood flow by xenon washout was reported by Wagner and Uhrenholdt (1980). Taking advantage of the rapid excretion of xenon from the body these authors attempted to measure blood flow by cavernosal clearance during different phases of erection in four normal subjects under the influence of visual erotic stimulation. The study revealed a flow of 3–8 ml $min^{-1}$ per 100 g in the flaccid penis, decreasing to 0–4 ml $min^{-1}$ per 100 g during established erection. The highest flow rates recorded were 20–75 ml $min^{-1}$ per 100 g during early detumescence. These results are surprising since current theories of erection would require the maximal arterial flow to occur during initiation of erection, and the flow to decrease during detumescence (Aboseif and Lue, 1988). The results can be explained if the effect of venous trapping in the

**Table 10.1 The radionuclide evaluation of penile perfusion**

| *Technique* | *Principal author* | *Method* | *Radiopharmaceutical* | *Stimulus* |
|---|---|---|---|---|
| Blood pool labelling | Shirai (1970) | Volume change | $^{131}$I-HSA | Yohimbine (s.c.) |
| | Shirai (1975) | Volume change | $^{99m}TcO_4^-$ | Visual |
| | Shirai (1976) | Volume change | $^{99m}$Tc-RBC | Visual |
| | Fanous (1982) | Volume change | $^{99m}TcO_4^-$ | Isoxsuprine (i.v.) |
| | Siraj (1986) | Rate of volume change | $^{99m}$Tc-RBC | Isoxsuprine (i.v.) |
| | Schwartz (1989) | Rate of volume change | $^{99m}$Tc-RBC | Papaverine (i.c.) |
| | Grech (in press) | Rate of activity entry on cuff release | $^{99m}$Tc-RBC | Papaverine (i.c.) |
| Xenon washout | Wagner (1980) | Cavernosal washout | $^{133}$Xe | Visual |
| | Nseyo (1984) | Skin washout | $^{133}$Xe | None |
| | Lin (1989) | Skin washout | $^{133}$Xe | None |
| | Haden (1989) | Cavernosal washout | $^{133}$Xe | None |

RBC, red blood cells; HSA, human serum albumin

corpora cavernosa is considered. In these normal subjects arterial flow increased and venous outflow decreased during the initiation of erection resulting in an increase in penile volume and a decrease in xenon washout. The reverse process occurred during detumescence and explains the high flow rate measured in the study. It is clear that since, in these circumstances, arterial and venous flow are not identical, the use of the washout technique is inappropriate for the assessment of penile arterial flow. While the method is not suitable for measuring stimulated flow in the potent male the measurement of flaccid state arterial flow is valid and the method may prove useful in those cases with known venosinusoidal leakage although, if partial trapping occurred, difficulties in interpretation would still result.

Haden *et al.* (1989) sought to establish a normal range for cavernosal xenon washout in the flaccid state. These workers found no difference in washout between young potent and elderly impotent subjects and concluded that the measurement of flow in the flaccid penis was unhelpful. Mean flow rates of only 0.7 ml $min^{-1}$ per 100 g were recorded.

Nseyo *et al.* (1984) attempted to use subcutaneous xenon washout to identify patients with penile vascular insufficiency. A flow rate of less than 7 ml $min^{-1}$ per 100 g was considered to indicate vascular insufficiency. Flow measurements were made only in the flaccid state. The study was repeated by Lin *et al.* (1989) who also measured xenon washout from the penile skin and compared the findings to the result of a papaverine test in the same patients. Skin flow greater than 6 ml $min^{-1}$ per 100 g was considered to be normal in the flaccid penis. Inexplicably, although intracavernosal papaverine was administered as part of the study, the flow after papaverine was not measured. Unfortunately both these studies only measured flow to the penile skin which, as explained above, is independent of that to the erectile tissues so the results are of doubtful relevance to the investigation of impotence.

## Penile blood flow by labelled blood pool studies

One of the earliest studies utilizing radionuclides in the investigation of impotence was reported by Shirai and Nakamura (1970). These workers sought to discriminate between organic and inorganic impotence by blood pool labelling with $^{131}$I-labelled human serum albumin ($^{131}$I-HSA). Following intravenous administration of the label, activity over the penis was monitored and once equilibration was attained a subcutaneous injection of a preparation containing yohimbine, a weak alpha-blocking alkaloid which has in the past been credited with aphrodisiac qualities (Morales *et al.*, 1988) and strychnine, a general CNS stimulant, was administered. Scintigraphic activity over the penis was recorded for a further 20 min and was claimed to show a rise in normal patients and in patients with functional impotence but no increase in patients with organic impotence. At the time of this study the vast majority of cases of impotence were considered to be psychogenic (Masters and Johnson, 1970) and the role of venosinusoidal leakage was not appreciated. These workers therefore did not distinguish between impotence caused by arterial disease and venosinusoidal leakage. It would seem most unlikely that the organic group consisted only of patients with arterial insufficiency and at least some, if not most of the patients in this group, would be expected to have a normal arterial supply. In addition no statistical analysis of the results was undertaken and the discrimination of the two types of impotence was based on a visual assessment of differences in the shape of the time–activity curves which, on the examples the authors provided, were unimpressive. Despite these limitations, and others discussed below, the study did establish the basic principles of the use of a radionuclide method in impotence and attempted pharmacological stimulation of penile blood flow.

The same workers later used $^{99m}$Tc pertechnetate to label the blood pool in a similar study and recorded the response to visual erotic stimulation (Shirai and Nakamura, 1975). This radioisotope has a 6 h half-life as opposed to 8 days for $^{131}$I and therefore provided higher count rates and exposed the patient to a much smaller radiation dose. In this form, however, the isotope leaves the intravascular compartment such that approximately 50% is lost within 30 min. The following year this problem was overcome and more reliable blood pool labelling was achieved using $^{99m}$Tc-RBC in a similar study (Shirai *et al.*, 1976). The studies produced various patterns of time–activity curve by which it was possible to discriminate between normal and impotent subjects.

$^{99m}$Tc pertechnetate blood pool labelling was used by Fanous *et al.* (1982), who monitored the change in scintigraphic activity over the penis following the administration of intravenous isoxsuprine, a sympathomimetic with largely α-adrenergic effects. No characteristic pattern of response emerged and it was not possible to discriminate between the control and impotent groups, though there was a tendency for the control group to show a greater increase in activity following isoxsuprine.

The technique used in the above four studies does not allow actual measurement of arterial flow. The studies measured the change in penile scintigraphic activity which occurred with erection and therefore, indirectly, measured the change in penile blood volume. Such studies represent the radionuclide equivalent of observing the change in penile size. It seems self-evident therefore that erection should result in an increase in activity but the studies do not help to determine the cause of failure to achieve erection. As previously explained, changes in volume cannot be attributed solely to changes in arterial inflow.

Siraj *et al.* (1986) used $^{99m}$Tc-RBC blood pool imaging and intravenous isoxsuprine in a study which attempted to measure the rate of change of penile activity rather than simply the change in activity. It was concluded that this measurement was abnormal in most patients with vasculogenic impotence. In this study it is likely that the impotent group contained cases due to arterial disease, venosinusoidal leakage or a combination of both. The study did not therefore discriminate between the various conditions.

A further refinement to the method was described by Schwartz *et al.* (1989). Again blood pool labelling was achieved with $^{99m}$Tc-RBC but the rate of change in penile activity was recorded after intracavernosal injection of 60 mg papaverine. The authors quote a range of peak corporeal penile flows of between 2.2 and 66.5 ml min$^{-1}$ with good correlation of measured flow to arteriographic appearance. By the use of papaverine this study achieved more reliable stimulation of arterial inflow than the previous examples, but it was still necessary to assume the absence of venosinusoidal outflow in order to calculate arterial flow from the change in penile activity. Such an assumption may not result in a large error in normal erection but, where impotence is related to venosinusoidal leakage, the authors admit that the method would underestimate arterial flow. In practice this group of patients is the most difficult to assess and the combination is not unusual since arterial insufficiency is thought to be a factor in venosinusoidal leakage (Lue *et al.*, 1986).

## Stimulated penile blood flow by penile isolation

We attempted to overcome the errors caused by venous outflow by modifying the limb blood flow method of Parkin *et al.* (1986) and used this to measure unstimulated and stimulated penile arterial flow (Grech *et al.*, in press). The principles of the technique have been described above where it was explained that flow is calculated from the gradient of the initial phase of the time–activity curve, following release of an occluding cuff. The isolation of the penile circulation by the use of a cuff is an important departure from previously described blood pool methods. The cuff isolates the penile circulation so that labelled blood enters the penis as a bolus and displaces only unlabelled blood; this removes the influence of venous outflow and changes in volume, making the method particularly suitable for use in the penile circulation. In addition the cuff allows time for the vasodilators to act on the smooth muscle of the penile vessels and sinusoids while maintaining the penis in the flaccid state so that when the cuff is released maximal arterial flow can occur. Any ischaemia caused by the inflated cuff causes a reactive hyperaemia which may increase this effect (Bell, Lewis and Kerstein, 1983). The cuff prevents dilution and washout of the vasodilators in the presence of venosinusoidal leakage so that a more consistent effect is achieved. The release of the cuff provides a single point at which blood flow can be measured thus avoiding any error due to changes in flow during the later phases of erection.

The flaccid penile dimensions were first measured to allow calculation of penile volume, assuming a cylindrical shape for ease of calculation. A 19 mm pneumatic cuff was then applied to the base of the penis and inflated to above arterial pressure. Intracavernosal vasodilator was administered and allowed to act for 10 min. During this period *in vivo* blood pool labelling with $^{99m}$Tc-RBC was undertaken and the flaccid penis positioned under the

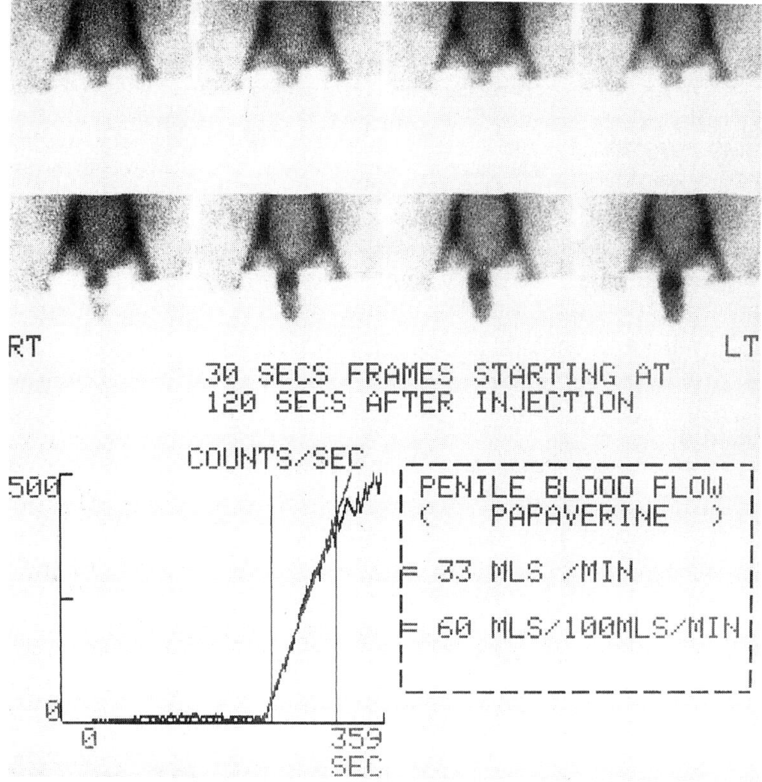


**Figure 10.2** Papaverine-stimulated penile blood flow in normal patient by blood pool labelling and cuff occlusion

gamma camera, with a lead rubber sheet beneath the penis to shield radiation from the thighs. Blood pool activity was measured in a venous blood sample and then the cuff released. A series of images of the penis and a time–activity curve were produced and, from the initial linear portion of the curve, penile arterial flow was calculated (Figure 10.2). Erection was assessed 20 min after cuff release.

In our initial studies 30 mg papaverine was used as a vasodilator and three groups of patients were studied. Patients who developed full erection following administration of papaverine were not considered to have vasogenic impotence and formed a control group. The remaining patients were classified as having arterial insufficiency or venous leakage by clinical examination, arteriography and/or cavernosography. Patients with both arterial disease and venous leakage were placed in the arterial disease group.

In the 23 patients studied, unstimulated penile blood flow varied over a range of 2.5–24.0 (mean: 9.1) ml $min^{-1}$ per 100 ml tissue, with no clear discrimination between the three groups, although the higher flow rates tended not to occur in patients with arterial disease (Figure 10.3). Following papaverine stimulation blood flow increased to between 8.3 and 81.3 (mean: 34.3) ml $min^{-1}$ per 100 ml. In the patients who achieved erection, stimulated flow rates were between 21.2 and 59.5 (mean 36.8) ml $min^{-1}$ per 100 ml. Stimulated flows in patients with venous leakage were not significantly different with a range of 23.2–81.3 (mean: 45.7) ml $min^{-1}$ per 100 ml. However patients with arterial disease had significantly lower flow rates, with a range of 8.3–19.0 (mean: 13.2) ml $min^{-1}$ per 100 ml. A cut-off value for stimulated flow of approximately 20 ml $min^{-1}$ per 100 ml appeared to discriminate between those with and without arterial disease. As would be expected, the presence of venosinusoidal leakage did not influence the result of the arterial flow measurement, provided there was no concomitant arterial disease, despite a similar failure to achieve erection.

Our values for flaccid state arterial flow were greater than those recorded by cavernosal xenon clearance (Wagner and Uhrenholdt, 1980; Haden *et al.*, 1989). Some of the difference may be accounted for by reactive hyperaemia caused by the cuff but,

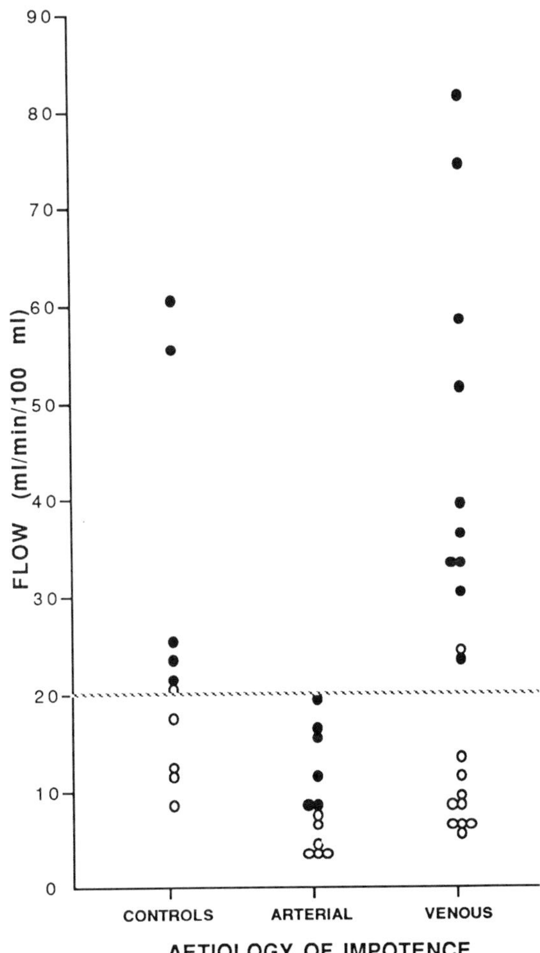


**Figure 10.3** Flaccid and stimulated penile perfusion in three study groups: ○, without papaverine; ●, with papaverine

allowing for the large errors inherent in the measurement of such low flow rates, the discrepancy is not large.

Approximate comparison of our stimulated penile arterial flow measurements with those of other workers is possible despite differences in methodology. Newman and Northup (1981) perfused the penile arteries in a cadaver and were able to induce erection with a flow of 25 ml min$^{-1}$. The same workers also perfused the corpora cavernosa directly in cadavers and induced erection at flow rates below 50 ml min$^{-1}$. Lue *et al.* (1986), by extrapolation from animal studies, stated that a perfusion rate of 60–80 ml min$^{-1}$ should be sufficient to induce erection in man. In the study by Schwartz *et al.* (1989) in which, as in our study, blood pool labelling and intracavernosal papaverine were used, mean cavernosal blood flow in angiographically normal subjects was 14.7 ml min$^{-1}$. By correcting for mean cavernosal volume, using the authors' own data, this corresponds to a flow rate of 50.7 ml min$^{-1}$ per 100 ml. In patients with severe arterial disease the mean cavernosal flow was 16.6 ml min$^{-1}$ per 100 ml. These results are broadly similar to our own measurements of total penile perfusion and appear to support our conclusion that a penile perfusion of less than 20 ml min$^{-1}$ per 100 ml indicates penile arterial insufficiency.

### Miscellaneous studies on penile arterial flow

Radionuclide imaging has been described for the assessment of graft patency following treatment for impotence by femorocavernous anastomosis (Casey and Zucker, 1979). In six postoperative patients with patent grafts it was possible to demonstrate graft patency in four cases by production of a scintigraphic angiogram following blood pool labelling with $^{99m}$Tc pertechnetate. The technique gave anatomical information by showing activity in the lumen of the patent graft but no measurement of flow was attempted. Nevertheless the authors felt that the method may obviate the need for arteriography in some patients.

Hashmat *et al.* (1989) attempted to categorize patients with priapism into high and low-flow subgroups. A scintigraphic penogram was obtained following blood pool labelling with $^{99m}$Tc pertechnetate and the images were visually assessed for activity in the corpora cavernosa and corpus spongiosum. The method again did not attempt to quantitate flow but suggested the diagnosis of low-flow priapism if the labelled blood failed to enter the erectile tissue. The use of the terms 'high-flow' and 'low-flow' was perhaps unjustified since, in this study, anatomical rather than functional information was obtained. Measurement of penile blood gases revealed hypoxia and acidosis in both 'low' and 'high' flow groups so that, while there is little doubt that the photopenic regions on the penogram represented sites of low or absent flow, it is probable that flow in the remaining regions was also decreased though perhaps to a lesser extent.

## Investigation of venosinusoidal leakage

There has been little attention paid to the use of radionuclides for the investigation of venosinusoidal leakage. Haden *et al.* (1989) suggested that xenon washout might be a promising method for quantitating venous outflow with stimulated or induced erection. Yeh *et al.* (1987) measured the rate of cavernosal xenon washout in eight normal and ten impotent subjects with known venous leakage. The study was done only in the flaccid state. A mean flow of 4.7 ml $min^{-1}$ per 100 g was recorded for the control group and 2.7 ml $min^{-1}$ per 100 g for the venous leak group. These values are of similar magnitude to flaccid state arterial flow recorded by other workers but approximately 10–100 times less than venous outflow measurements generally recorded during cavernosometry in subjects with venous leakage. Obviously xenon washout and therefore venous outflow in this study simply reflected flaccid state arterial flow.

The use of xenon washout for the assessment of venous leakage requires a normal and known value of arterial inflow since, in arterial insufficiency, xenon washout is low whatever the degree of venous leakage. Intracavernosal vasodilators or artificial erection by intracavernosal infusion would be required, since not only is the normal venous trapping mechanism not active in the flaccid state, but the arterial (and hence venous) blood flow rates are so low that a diagnosis of excessive venous outflow could not be made.

Conventional pharmacocavernosography is able to document the presence and degree of venous leakage, demonstrate its site and display structural abnormalities of the corpora cavernosa. It appears unlikely that radionuclide methods could quantitate the degree of venous leakage as effectively and the anatomical information would almost certainly be inferior. The technique would be no less invasive and it would appear that currently available radionuclide methods offer no advantage over pharmacocavernosography in the investigation of venous leakage.

## Conclusion

Further progress in the use of radionuclide methods for the evaluation of penile arterial supply will undoubtedly be made. We are currently attempting to increase the specificity of our test by the combined use of phentolamine and papaverine, since we have found that some normal subjects fail to respond to a dose of up to 60 mg papaverine alone, resulting in a false negative papaverine test and equivocal flow measurements even though full erection and normal flow measurements can subsequently be obtained by retesting with the addition of 1 mg phentolamine.

The establishment of a simple reliable radionuclide technique of estimating penile arterial perfusion will have major consequences on the investigation and management of impotence. Such a test would enable investigation into the natural history of the disease, especially in ageing and diabetes where it appears to be multifactorial. Patients with occult arterial disease as the cause of their impotence would be detected early and no longer be subjected to inappropriate investigation and surgery to the venous system. Better patient selection would identify those patients who would benefit from arteriography and revascularization procedures. Finally, a reliable radionuclide technique would, for the first time, offer a means of objectively assessing the results of these revascularization procedures and enable comparison between the various techniques available. There can be little doubt that such a goal is worth pursuing, however evasive it may seem at times.

## References


Aboseif, S. R. and Lue, T. F. (1988) Hemodynamics of penile erection. *Urologic Clinics of North America*, **15**, 1–7

Bell, D., Lewis, R. and Kerstein, M. D. (1983) Hyperemic stress test in diagnosis of vasculogenic impotence. *Urology*, **22**, 611–613

Buvat, J., Buvat-Herbaut, M., Dehaene, J. L. and Lemaire, A. (1986) Is intracavernous injection of papaverine a reliable screening test for vascular impotence? *Journal of Urology*, **135**, 476–478

Casey, W. C. and Zucker, M. I. (1979) Technetium-99 pelvic scan: use in follow-up of penile revascularization bypass operations. *Urology*, **14**, 465–466

Daly, M. J. and Henry, R. E. (1980) Quantitative measurement of skin perfusion with xenon-133. *Journal of Nuclear Medicine*, **21**, 156–160

Fanous, H. N., Jevtich, M. J., Chen, D. C. P. and Edson, M. (1982) Radioisotope penogram in diagnosis of vasculogenic impotence. *Urology*, **20**, 499–502

Grech, P., Nave, S., Cunningham, D. A. and Witherow, R. O'N (1991) Combined papverine text and radionuclide penile blood flow in impotence: method and preliminary results. *British Journal of Urology* (in press)

Haden, H. T., Katz, P. G., Mulligan, T. and Zasler, N. D. (1989) Penile blood flow by xenon-133 washout. *Journal of Nuclear Medicine*, **30**, 1032–1035

Hashmat, A. I., Raju, S., Singh, I. and Macchia, R. J. (1989) $^{99m}$Tc penile scan: an investigative modality in priapism. *Urologic Radiology*, **11**, 58–60

Juenemann, K. P., Lue, T. F., Hellstrom, W. J. G. *et al.* (1985) Hemodynamics of papaverine and phentolamine-induced erection in monkeys and dogs (Abstract) *Journal of Urology*, **133**, 218

Lassen, N. A., Lindbjerg, J. and Munck, O. (1964) Measurement of blood flow through skeletal muscle by intramuscular injection of xenon-133. *Lancet* **i**, 686–688

Lin, S. N., Liu, R. S., Yu, P. C. *et al.* (1989) Diagnosis of vasculogenic impotence: combination of penile xenon-133 washout and papaverine tests. *Urology*, **34**, 28–32

Lue, T. F., Hricak, H., Schmidt, R. A. and Tanagho, E. A. (1986) Functional evaluation of penile veins by cavernosography in papaverine-induced erection. *Journal of Urology*, **135**, 479–482

Lue, T. F., Takamura, T., Schmidt, R. A. *et al.* (1983) Haemodynamics of erection in the monkey. *Journal of Urology*, **130**, 1237–1241

Masters, W. H. and Johnson, V. E. (1970) *Human Sexual Inadequacy*, Little Brown, Boston

Melman, A. (1988) The evaluation of erectile dysfunction. *Urologic Radiology*, **10**, 119–128

Morales, A., Condra, M. S., Owen, J. E. *et al.* (1988) Oral and transcutaneous pharmacologic agents in the treatment of impotence. *Urologic Clinics of North America*, **15**, 87–93

Mueller, S. C. and Lue, T. F. (1988) Evaluation of vasculogenic impotence. *Urologic Clinics of North America*, **15**, 65–76

Newman, H. F. and Northup, J. D. (1981) Mechanism of human penile erection: an overview. *Urology*, **17**, 399–408

Nseyo, U. O., Wilbur, H. J., Kang, S. A. *et al.* (1984) Penile xenon ($^{133}Xe$) washout: a rapid method of screening for vasculogenic impotence. *Urology*, **23**, 31–34

Oshima, M., Ijima, H., Kohda, Y. *et al.* (1984) Peripheral arterial disease diagnosed with high-count-rate radionuclide arteriography. *Radiology*, **152**, 161–166

Parkin, A., Robinson, P. J., Wiggins, P. A. *et al.* (1986) The measurement of limb blood flow using technetium-labelled red blood cells. *British Journal of Radiology*, **59**, 493–497

Schwartz, A. N., Graham, M. M., Ferency, G. F. and Randal, S. M. (1989) Radioisotope penile plethysmography: a technique for evaluation corpora cavernosal blood flow during early tumescence. *Journal of Nuclear Medicine*, **30**, 466–473

Shirai, M. and Nakamura, M. (1970) Differential diagnosis of organic and functional impotence by the use of $^{131}I$-human serum albumin. *Tohoku Journal of Experimental Medicine*, **101**, 317–324

Shirai, M. and Nakamura, M. (1975) Diagnostic discrimination between organic and functional impotence by radioisotope penogram with $^{99m}TcO_4^-$. *Tohoku Journal of Experimental Medicine*, **116**, 9–15

Shirai, M., Nakamura, M., Ishii, N. *et al.* (1976) Determination of intrapenal blood volume using $^{99m}Tc$-labeled autologous red blood cells. *Tohoku Journal of Experimental Medicine*, **120**, 377–383

Siegel, M. E. and Stewart, C. A. (1984) Peripheral vascular diseases. In *Textbook of Nuclear Medicine, Volume 2: Clinical Applications*, 2nd edn (eds J. Harbert and A. F. G. da Rocha), Lea and Febiger, Philadelphia, pp. 460–478

Siraj, Q. H., Hilson, A. J. W., Townell, N. H. *et al.* (1986) The role of the isotope phallogram in the investigation of vasculogenic impotence. *Nuclear Medicine Communications*, **7**, 173–182

Virag, R. (1982) Intracavernous injection of papaverine for erectile failure (Letter). *Lancet*, **ii**, 938

Wagner, G. and Uhrenholdt, A. (1980) Blood flow measurement by the clearance method in the human corpus cavernosum in the flaccid and erect states. In *Vasculogenic Impotence* (Proceedings of the 1st International Conference on Corpus Cavernosum Revascularization) (eds A. W. Zorgniotti and G. Rossi), Charles C. Thomas, Springfield, Illinois, pp. 41–46

Yeh, S. H., Liu, R. S., Lin, S. N. *et al.* (1987) Corporeal Xe-133 washout for detecting venous leakage (Abstract). *Journal of Nuclear Medicine*, **28**, 650

# 11

# Arteriography


## I. Nockler


## Introduction

During the past decade a better understanding of impotence has evolved, with an increased awareness of organic causes that may be amenable to treatment. Haemodynamic causes account for many of the organic cases, either in the flow of arterial blood to the corpus cavernosus or to the failure of venous occlusion.

Ginestie and Romieu (1977) recognized the value of demonstrating the internal iliac arterial tree and first performed selective pudendal arteriography puncturing the femoral arteries bilaterally to gain access to the internal iliac arteries. High osmolar contrast medium was used to delineate the pudendal and penile arteries. General anaesthesia was used as considerable pain is felt on injecting the pudenal arteries and no vasodilators were used.

Since then the technique has been refined and its quality improved by using vasodilators and the use of an artificial erection as well as other technical advances.

Increased flow in the penile arteries was first attempted by Michal and Pospichal (1978). Heparinized saline was infused into the corpora cavernosa and an artificial erection induced, and this produced dilated pudendal and penile arteries prior to arteriography. This method was named phalloarteriography and enabled improved visualization of the penile artery and distal branches.

## Pharmacoarteriography

The introduction of intracavernosal papaverine to produce an erection (Virag, 1982) led to a dramatic change in our perception of the physiology of erection. This is not only established the existence and mechanisms of veno-occlusion, but also provided a pharmacotherapeutic method for producing an erection. Intracavernosal papaverine with or without phentolamine is now widely used and enables excellent visualization of the distal internal pudendal arterial tree (Bahren *et al.*, 1988; Bookstein *et al.*, 1988b). Doses of 15–60 mg papaverine and 0.25–1.0 mg phentolamine mesylate are injected into the corpus cavernosus and dispersed throughout the corpora. Tumescence occurs within about 10–20 min in the normal male. This is an essential part of the examination as it stretches the penile arteries which are tortuous in the flaccid state, allows a good morphological study and avoids overlooking a possible stenosis (Delcour *et al.*, 1988). Comparative studies with and without papaverine have shown that it induces substantial dilatation especially of small calibre arteries of the penis (Virag, 1982; Zorgniotti and Lefleur, 1985; Delcour *et al.*, 1988). However, if a full erection is induced with an intracavernosal papaverine injection, the arterial flow in the cavernosal artery decreases (Lue *et al.*, 1985; Bahren *et al.*, 1988). These authors maintain that a graded dose of papaverine should be injected to induce an erection in any individual. Most authors inject 60 mg intracavernosally for all patients to induce tumescence and not a full erection, and we are now using the same regime.

## Anaesthesia

Controversy surrounds the use of anaesthesia. Proponents of the use of local anaesthesia to the groin also administer intra-arterial morphine and xylocaine to provide adequate analgesia and sedation (Gray *et al.*, 1982). Digital subtraction angiography (DSA), particularly using the less painful non-ionic or low osmolar contrast medium at half strength, allows the use of local anaesthesia.

Although general anaesthesia has the advanatge of a relaxed patient and a dilated vascular system, the action of intracavernosal vasoactive drugs and the availability of spinal anaesthesia renders it unnecessary. The quality obtained after intracavernosal injection of vasoactive substances under spinal anaesthesia is markedly superior to that seen under local anaesthesia (Bahren *et al.*, 1988).

We therefore perform pudendal arteriography under spinal anaesthesia using intracavernosal vasoactive drugs and have obtained excellent results.

## Selection of patients

Some centres first use non-invasive studies to assess the internal iliac artery and pudendal arterial bed. These include penile colour Doppler ultrasound, the penile brachial index and isotope phallograms.

All patients undergo pharmacological assessment by the clinician using intracavernosal injection of vasoactive agents such as papaverine. This is a simple test to perform and an excellent screening test to differentiate organic erectile failure from other causes (Lue and Tanagho, 1987). If the response to papaverine is normal, vasculogenic impotence may effectively be excluded (Sidi and Lange, 1986; Lue and Tanagho, 1987; Orvis and Lue, 1987). However, if the response is abnormal, vasculogenic impotence is implied. Our patients then undergo examination of the penile venous system by dynamic infusion pharmacocavernosometry and cavernosography.

If pudendal and penile vessel disease is suggested on the non-invasive studies, these have to be precisely documented arteriographically. Patients may have cavernosograms and cavernosometry performed at the time of doing the arteriogram but we usually perform the latter study on a separate date.

### Criteria for selection of patients

Internal pudendal arteriography should be performed on patients with organic impotence in whom endocrinological or neurological causes have been excluded. Performing selective pudendal arteriography is an expensive study and an invasive technique, and should only be performed where a good long-term result can be expected following vascular reconstructive surgery. The patients who benefit most from this surgery are those with congenital abnormalities such as arteriovenous malformations or fistulae, or post-traumatic impotence, (Lurie, Bookstein and Kessler, 1988). Satisfactory results may be expected in up to 70% of these patients, but in less than 50% of patients with arteriosclerosis (Nelson, 1988; Krysiewicz and Mellinger, 1989).

The study is thus reserved for those who wish to consider a vascular reconstructive procedure.

## Method

As always, informed consent is obtained. Spinal anaesthesia is performed by an anaesthetist and an intracavernosal injection of 60 mg papaverine and 0.5–1 mg phentolamine administered. The use of a gonadal shield to protect the scrotum from the X-rays is routine.

Single femoral artery puncture is performed (conveniently from the right side) and the distal aorta catheterized. About 40 ml of contrast medium is injected and images obtained of the distal aorta and major pelvic vessels (see Figure 11.3) either by conventional arteriography or by digital subtraction angiography. The inferior epigastric artery must be identified, especially where this vessel may be used for vascular bypass procedures. The catheter is then exchanged for a curved selecting catheter such as a small curve hook catheter or inferior mesenteric catheter. A long curve hook catheter may be useful especially on catheterizing the ipsilateral internal pudendal artery.

The contralateral internal iliac artery is then catheterized and the guide wire and catheter passed into the internal pudendal artery. Some authors state that the tip of the catheter should not pass beyond the branching of the internal iliac artery so as not to miss an accessory artery that may originate from the gluteal or obturator artery (Bahren *et al.*, 1988; Breza *et al.*, 1989). However we have found that the pudendal artery is always over-injected and contrast refluxes into other branches of the internal iliac artery.

The penis is positioned to overlie the contralateral greater trochanter and the patient rotated 30° in the posterior oblique projection. Contrast medium in a dose of 40 ml is injected at a rate of not more than 3–4 ml $s^{-1}$. This flow rate is chosen as a greater rate causes reflux into the iliac arteries which may detract from the quality of the examination by reducing the amout of contrast medium in the penile arteries in the late phase, and by superimposition over the pudendal artery. The exposure should last for 25–30 s as the pudendal arteries opacify about 5 s after commencing the injection and the distal pudendal arteries will not be demonstrated for about 10 s. They may only be seen at about 25 s, especially in the case of pathological vessels. The catheter is then withdrawn and the ipsilateral internal iliac artery and pudendal artery catheterized. The penis is repositioned over the contralateral greater trochanter, the patient rotated into the right posterior oblique position and images of the right arterial system obtained in the same way. Bilateral femoral puncture is thus avoided.

We do not catheterize the bladder as the arteries of interest are projected free of the bladder in the oblique position. Goldstein *et al.* (1990) and Bahren *et al.* (1988) make use of bladder catheterization to outline the urethra and course of the spongiosal artery, as well as to provide bladder drainage during the procedure.

### Contrast medium

Non-ionic contrast medium is generally used as it improves patient safety and comfort, especially where local anaesthesia is being used. Low osmolar contrast medium such as Hexabrix (ioxaglate meglumine and ioxolate sodium) may also be used, but a cautionary note should be sounded on the incompatibility of Hexabrix and papaverine hydrochloride as precipitates may be formed if accidentally mixed in the same syringe (Pilla *et al.*, 1986; McGill *et al.*, 1988).

## Normal arteriographic anatomy

Arteriogenic impotence requires precise demonstration of the penile arterial supply from the aortic bifurcation to the tip of the penis (Figures 11.1 and 11.2). The arterial supply to the penis is derived mainly from the anterior division of the internal iliac artery via the internal pudendal artery. The inferior

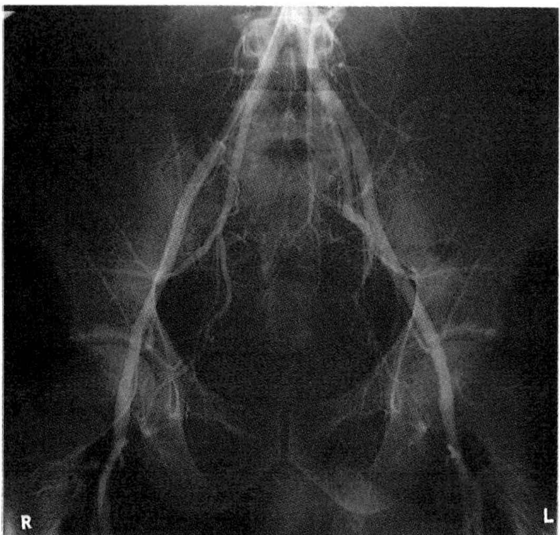


**Figure 11.1** Flush aortogram. Catheter tip in the distal aorta. The major branches of the aorta opacified and potential proximal vessel disease assessed

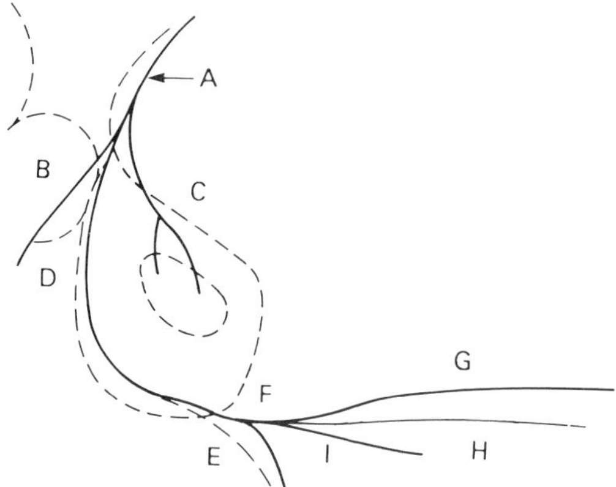


**Figure 11.3** Pudendal artery anatomy (present in about 50% of cases): A, internal iliac artery (anterior division); B, inferior gluteal artery; C, obturator artery; D. internal pudendal artery; E, scrotal branches; F, penile artery; G, dorsal artery of penis; H, cavernosal artery; I, bulbourethral artery

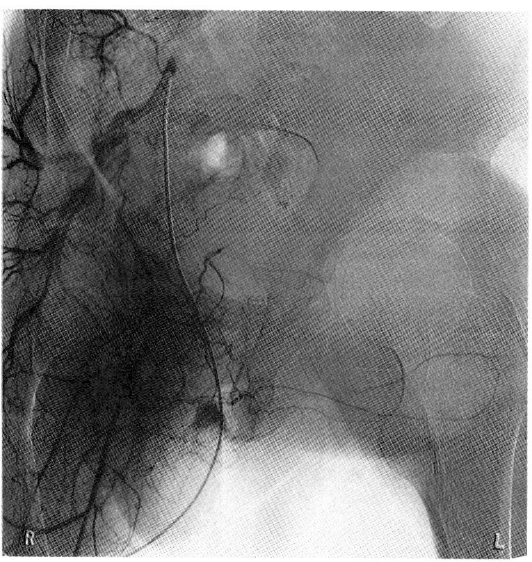


**Figure 11.2** Selective right internal iliac arteriogram showing normal pudendal artery and branches. There is retrograde filling of the contralateral dorsal penile artery

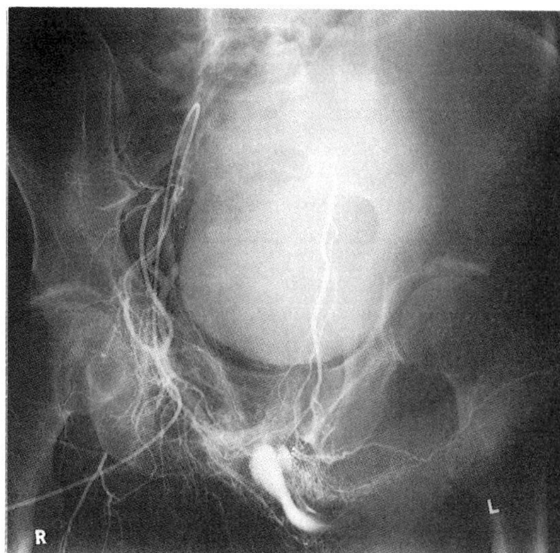


**Figure 11.4** Selective right pudendal artery study shows deep staining of the bulbourethral artery and both cavernosal and dorsal penile arteries filling. There is also filling of the contralateral pudendal artery

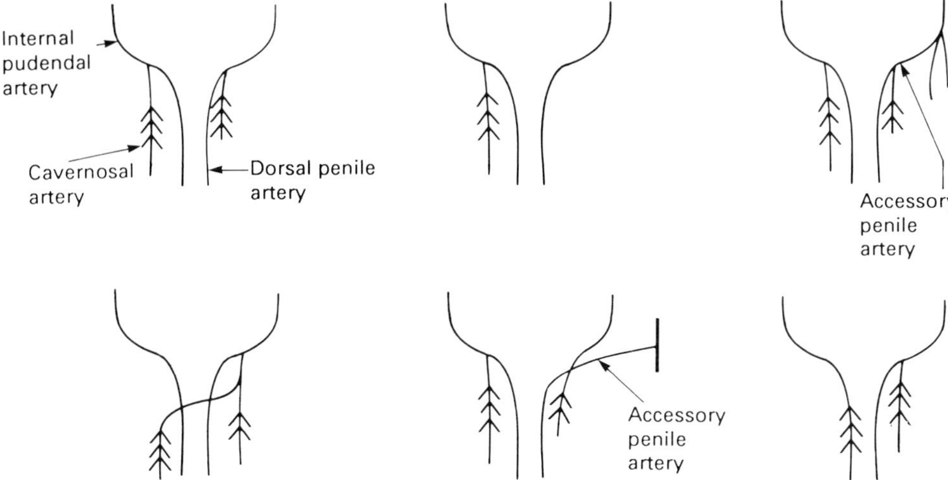


**Figure 11.5** Schematic representation of common anatomical variants of penile vasculature

gluteal artery and the obturator artery usually also arise as terminal branches of the anterior division of the internal iliac artery (Figure 11.3).

The internal pudendal artery (Figure 11.4) runs in a curve in the dorsolateral pelvic wall remote from the viscera. It enters the lesser pelvis, accompanied by the nerve, through the lesser sciatic notch. It enters the ischiorectal fossa where it courses along in Alcock's canal along the inferior insertion of the obturator internus muscle (Gray, 1973). In the dorsal aspect of the urogenital triangle it gives rise to the superficial perineal artery which supplies the scrotum, and thereafter it is known as the penile artery. The latter pierces the urogenital diaphragm and continues along the medial margin of the inferior ramus of the pubis. In the anterior perineum the penile artery divides into its terminal branches, the bulbourethral, cavernous or artery to the corpus cavernosus, and the dorsal or superficial artery of the penis.

The bulbourethral artery is short and of large calibre and passes medially to enter the bulb of the penis. It has a characteristic cone-shaped blush on the arteriogram.

The dorsal artery passes anterior to the crus and courses distally along the dorsum of the penis to the glans penis. It gives off several circumflex branches to the mid-dorsal corpora cavernosa (Flanigan *et al.*, 1985; Bookstein, 1988a) and, for this reason bypass into a proximally occluded dorsal penile artery can improve flow into the corpora cavernosa (Flanigan *et al.*, 1985; Bookstein, 1988a).

The cavernous or deep artery varies considerably in its origin, number and communication with other arteries (Valji and Bookstein, 1988; Bahren *et al.*, 1988). It gives off a short branch to the crus and then courses through the centre of the cavernous body almost to the tip. Along its course it characteristically gives off multiple terminal helicine branches to the cavernous spaces.

Anatomical variants are the rule (Figure 11.5) and include both cavernous arteries originating from the same side, hypoplasia or absence of one dorsal penile artery and accessory penile arteries (Figure 11.6) (Bookstein, 1988a; Breza *et al.*, 1989). The latter may occur in 6–9% (Flanigan *et al.*, 1985; Ginestie and Romieu, 1976). In a small series it was found in seven out of ten cases (Huguet, Cliressi and Juhan 1981). Because of the frequency of variants, non-visualization of a cavernosal artery on one side

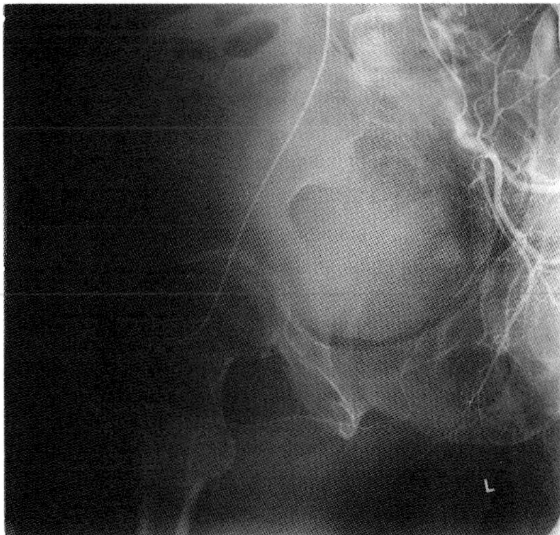


**Figure 11.6** An accessory penile artery arising from the proximal internal pudendal artery and supplying the dorsal and cavernosal artery. The internal pudendal artery supplies the scrotum

does not necessarily indicate obstruction as it could arise from the contralateral side or an accessory artery (Bookstein, 1988a). Collateral vessels may open up in the presence of obstruction in vessels of the penis (Flanigan *et al.*, 1985).

## The abnormal arteriogram

Arterial disease may be observed at any level, but the distal pudendal artery or proximal penile branches are more frequently involved (Figures 11.7 and 11.9) (Bookstein, 1988). It needs to be emphasized that significant bilateral arterial obstruction needs to be present for arteriogenic impotence and thus unilateral revascularization may restore potency (Flanigan *et al.*, 1985; Bookstein 1988). The selective arteriogram may be limited to the initial side if a normal ipsilateral cavernosal and dorsal artery is demonstrated and no collateral flow is shown to suggest contralateral disease.

Impotence associated with pudendal arteriovenous malformation (Figure 11.10) has also been described in a few cases with the early passage of contrast medium from the bulbar artery to a large tortuous vein or veins in the pelvis (Zorgniotti *et al.*, 1984). Although a malformation, it may not manifest itself until significant trauma or disease. In cases of non-iatrogenic trauma, arterial obstruction may be at variable and multiple levels (Lurie, Bookstein and Kessler, 1988). These may be from the internal iliac artery in pelvic fractures to the internal pudendal artery and the penile artery and its terminal branches. Venous leak may accompany the arterial abnormalities and should also be investigated. This group of patients is often successfully revascularized as the impotence is frequently vasculogenic and the patients are often young and in good health.

The presence of isolated stenoses in the common or internal iliac arteries makes percutaneous transluminal angioplasty (PTA) a feasible means of

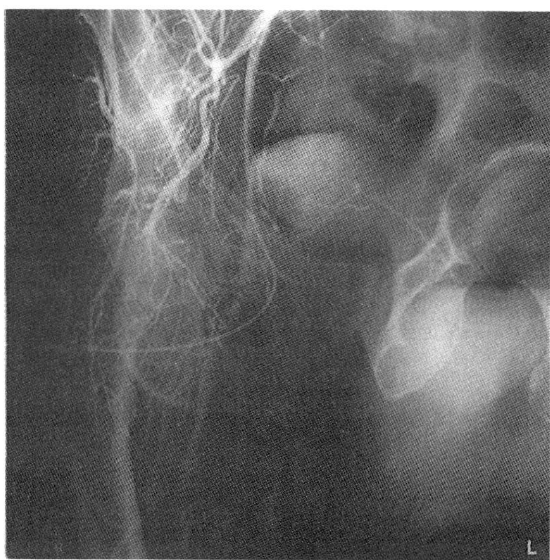


**Figure 11.8** Selective right internal iliac artery injection. Shows multiple strictures of the internal pudendal artery and no filling of the penile artery branches. Collateral vessels fill the opposite pelvic vessels. The contralateral internal pudendal artery was severely diseased

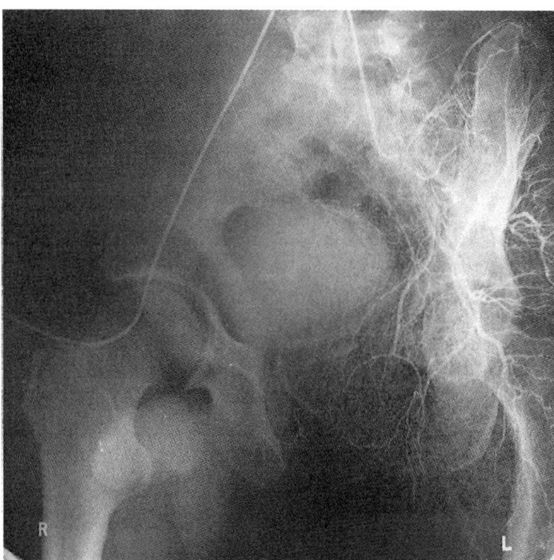


**Figure 11.7** Selective left internal iliac artery injection. The distal pudendal artery is occluded in Alcock's canal. Collateral arteries fill the cavernosal and dorsal arteries but both fail to opacify distally

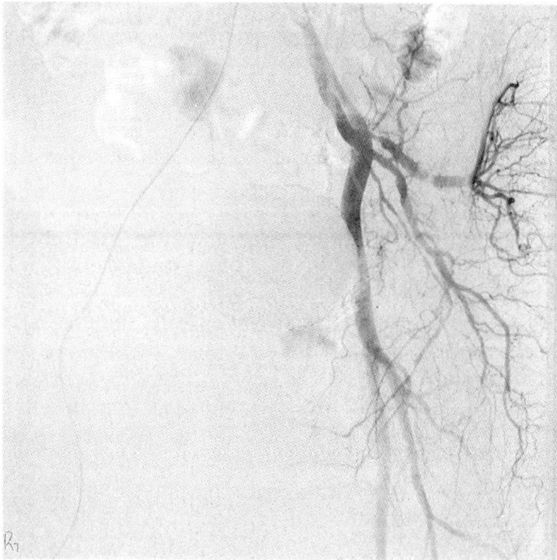

**Figure 11.9** Selective left internal iliac artery opacification shows multiple strictures of the pudendal artery and no distal filling of the penile artery branches

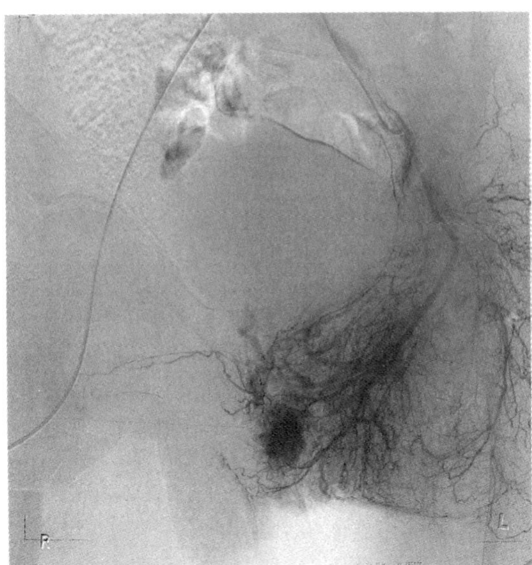


**Figure 11.10** Selective left internal iliac artery injection: early phase. Pelvic venous filling occurs due to an arteriovenous malformation. Normal arterial anatomy and the contralateral side was normal in this 26-year-old man with a 2-year history of impotence

treating vasculogenic impotence. However, before attempting PTA the distal arterial tree must be shown to be intact as the success of the procedure depends to a large degree on a normal distal internal pudendal artery and penile artery and branches, and a normal veno-occlusive mechanism. The results following PTA are mixed and only small series have been published (Valji and Bookstein, 1988).

## Complications

The complications found are those seen in any other diagnostic or therapeutic angiography. Bleeding, ecchymosis and haematomata overlying the femoral artery, intimal and arterial extravasation and lower limb claudication may occur. Contrast allergies and conditions associated with contrast allergies should be excluded before the procedure.

## Conclusion

The role of radiology is best understood in the light of currently available therapeutic options. These will be dealt with elsewhere in this book but a variety of revascularization procedures for arteriogenic impotence may be employed and precise demonstration of the arterial anatomy must be of utmost importance to the radiologist. The results following penile artery revascularization are mixed and many failures may reflect missed diagnosis of associated venous leak or distal arterial disease (Bookstein, 1988a).

Although serious complications are rare, use of arteriography should be restricted to those selected individuals with non-endocrinological, non-neurological organic impotence who are potential candidates for arterial revascularization surgery.

## References


Bahren, W., Gall, H., Scherb, W. *et al.* (1988) Arterial anatomy and arteriographic diagnosis of arteriogenic impotence. *Cardiovascular and Interventional Radiology,* **11**, 195–210

Bookstein, J. J. (1988a) Penile angiography: the last angiographic frontier. *American Journal of Radiology,* **150**, 47–54

Bookstein, J. J. (1988b) Penile vascular catheterisation in the diagnosis and treatment of impotence. *Cardiovascular and Interventional Radiology,* **11**, 183–184

Bookstein, J. J., Fellmeth, B., Moreland, S. and Lurie, A. L. (1988) Pharmacoangiographic assessment of the corpora cavernosa. *Cardiovascular and Interventional Radiology,* **11**, 218–224

Breza, J., Aboseif, S. R., Orvis, B. R. *et al.* (1989) Detailed anatomy of penile neurovascular structures: surgical significance. *Journal of Urology,* **141**, 437–443

Delcour, C., Vandenbosch, G., Delatte, P. *et al.* (1988) Techanical advances in penile arteriography. *American Journal of Radiology,* **150**, 803–804

Flanigan, D. P., Sobinsky, K. R., Schuler, J. J. *et al.* (1985) Internal iliac artery revascularisation in the treatment of vasculogenic impotence. *Archives of Surgery,* **120**, 271–274

Ginestie, J. F. and Romieu, A. (1977) *Radiological Exploration of Impotence.* (1978) Nijhoff, Boston

Goldstein, I., Krane, R. J., Greenfield, A. J. and Padma-Nathan, H. (1990) Vascular diseases of the penis: impotence and priapism. In *Clinical Urology* (ed. H. M. Pollack), pp. 2231–2252

Gray, H. (1973) Grays 'Anatomy of the Human Body (ed. C. M. Gross), Lea and Febinger, Philadelphia, p. 648

Gray, R. R., Keresteci, A. G., St. Louis, E. L. *et al.* (1982) Investigation for impotence by pudendal angiography: experience with 73 cases. *Radiology,* **144**, 773

Huguet, J. F., Clerissi, J. and Juhan, C. (1981) Radiological anatomy of the pudendal artery. *European Journal of Radiology,* **1**, 278–284

Krysiewicz, S. and Mellinger, B. C. (1989) The role of imaging in the diagnostic evaluation of impotence. *American Journal of Radiology,* **153**, 1133–1139

Lue, T. F., Hticak, H., Marich, K. W. and Tanagho, E. A. (1985) Vasculogenic impotence evaluated by high resolution ultrasonography and pelvic Doppler spectrum analysis. *Radiology,* **155**, 777–781

Lue, T. F. and Tanagho, E. A. (1987) Physiology of

erection and pharmacological management of impotence. *Journal of Urology,* **137**, 8279

Lurie, A. L., Bookstein, J. J. and Kessler, W. O. (1988) Angiography in post-traumatic impotence. *Cardiovascular and Interventional Radiology,* **11**, 232–236

Orvis, B. R. and Lue, T. F. (1987) New therapy for impotence. *Urologic Clinics of North America,* **14**, 569–581

McGill, J. E., Rysavy, J. A. and Frick, M. P. (1987) Experimental investigations of Hexabrix–papaverine interaction. *Radiology,* **166**, 577

Michal, V. and Pospichal, C. (1978) Phalloarteriography in the diagnosis of erectile impotence. *World Journal of Surgery,* **2**, 239–247

Nelson, R. P. (1988) Non-operative management of impotence. *Journal of Urology,* **139**, 2–5

Sidi, H. H. and Lange, P. H. (1986) Recent advances in the diagnosis and management of impotence. *Urologic Clinics of North America,* **13**, 489–500

Valji, K. and Bookstein, J. J. (1988) Transluminal angioplasty in the treatment of arteriogenic impotence. *Cardiovascular and Interventional Radiology,* **11**, 245–252

Virag, R. (1982) Intracavernous injection of papaverine for erectile failure. *Lancet,* **ii**, 938

Zorgniotti, A. W. and Lefleur, R. S. .1985) Autoinjection of the corpora cavernosa with a vasoactive drug combination for vasculogenic impotence. *Journal of Urology,* **133**, 39–41

Zorgniotti, A. W., Shaw, W. W., Padula, G. and Ross, G. (1984) Impotence associated with pudendal arteriovenous malformation. *Journal of Urology,* **132**, 128–131

# 12

# Neurophysiological testing

**I. Eardley, R. S. Kirby and C. J. Fowler**

## Introduction

Sacral autonomic innervation and higher centres which modulate basic sexual reflexes are essential for penile erection during sexual intercourse, and damage to these pathways may result in impotence. Damage can be focal or may occur as part of a generalized neurological disorder, so that erectile impotence may either be an isolated symptom or part of a widespread symptom complex. Although the history and examination may provide some information, neurophysiological testing offers the means of demonstrating the level and extent of the neurological lesion. The techniques which are currently available mostly test pathways of the somatic nervous system, although in recent years there have been increasing attempts to study the autonomic nervous system, upon which normal penile erection depends.

The neurophysiology of erection is outlined below and this is followed by a description of the clinical neurophysiological techniques available for studying pudendal innervation.

## Neuroanatomy and neurophysiology of penile erection

### Afferent pathways

Sensory information is carried in afferent fibres within the dorsal nerve of the penis which, after piercing the pelvic diaphragm, continues as the pudendal nerve and then enters the sacral cord through the dorsal roots of the second to fourth segments. Information concerning light touch is carried in large diameter, fast conducting, myelinated fibres, which is then transmitted within the dorsal columns to the cuneate and gracile nuclei, and from there to the thalamus and cerebral cortex. Temperature and pain sensation are carried to the spinal cord via small myelinated and unmyelinated fibres, and from there via the spinothalamic tracts to the thalamus.

### Efferent pathways

Somatic efferent pathways to the bulbocavernosus and ischiocavernosus muscles originate within the motor strip on the medial aspect of the cerebral hemispheres, from where the corticospinal tracts convey fibres to the ventral horn of the sacral spinal cord. After synapsing within the ventral horn, large myelinated fibres travel via the anterior sacral roots (S2–4) to joint the pudendal nerve which innervates the muscles of the pelvic floor. After the corpora have been filled with blood, contraction of the ischiocavernosus and bulbocavernosus muscles produces rigidity of the penis.

Autonomic pathways involved in sexual function originate in the hippocampus, the anterior cingulate gyrus and the thalamus. Via a variety of descending tracts, fibres pass to two spinal centres. The most important of these is the sacral erection centre which lies in the second to fourth segments of the sacral spinal cord (Lue *et al.*, 1984). The thoracolumbar centre lies in the intermediolateral grey matter of the spinal cord (segments T12–L3). From both these centres, fibres pass to the hypogastric and pelvic plexi, before fusing to form the cavernous nerves. These nerves travel along the posterolateral surface of the prostate (Walsh and Donker, 1982), then curve anteriorly to join the membranous urethra, and pierce the urogenital diaphragm to pass through the tunica albuginea to supply the corpora.

Penile erection depends upon the interaction of both sympathetic and parasympathetic nerves (see Chapter 3), although it seems that the sacral parasympathetic outflow is the more important. The parasympathetic cholinergic nerves appear to act synergistically with other vasodilator neurotransmitters (including VIP) to cause penile erection, while adrenergic impulses act mainly by maintaining flaccidity and causing detumescence.

## Methods of neurophysiological assessment

### Urethral sphincter electromyography

In striated muscle, the axon of each anterior horn cell innervates a number of muscle fibres, the whole being called a 'motor unit'. Using a concentric needle electrode to record the electromyographic (EMG) activity, the amplitude and duration of the potential produced by a motor unit is related to both the number and spatial distribution of muscle fibres within it. In a complete lower motor neurone lesion there is loss of all EMG activity, while following a partial lesion reinnervation ensues, either by regrowth of damaged axons or by collateral sprouting of surviving motor nerve fibres. EMG potentials recorded under these conditions show abnormalities of amplitude and duration which reflect the changes in architecture of the motor unit.

EMG of the urethral sphincter was first described by Petersen and Franksson in 1955. They found that unlike most other skeletal muscles, the sphincter motor units are tonically active. Analysis of motor units within the urethral sphincter (Chantraine, 1966; Fowler *et al.*, 1984), show that in control subjects the majority of motor units have a duration of less than 6 ms and an amplitude less than 2 mV. Following lower motor neurone damage with denervation and reinnervation, the motor units show an increased duration and amplitude and become polyphasic (Figure 12.1).

Urethral sphincter EMG with motor unit analysis can thus be used to demonstrate lower motor neurone damage to the innervation of the urethral sphincter, which arises from the same sacral cord segments as the pelvic parasympathetic outflow.

### Sacral reflex testing

The bulbocavernosus reflex (BCR) is the reflex contraction of the bulbocavernosus muscle produced by squeezing the glans penis. It is likely that both the afferent and efferent impulses for this reflex are carried by myelinated fibres within the pudendal nerve. This reflex response may be

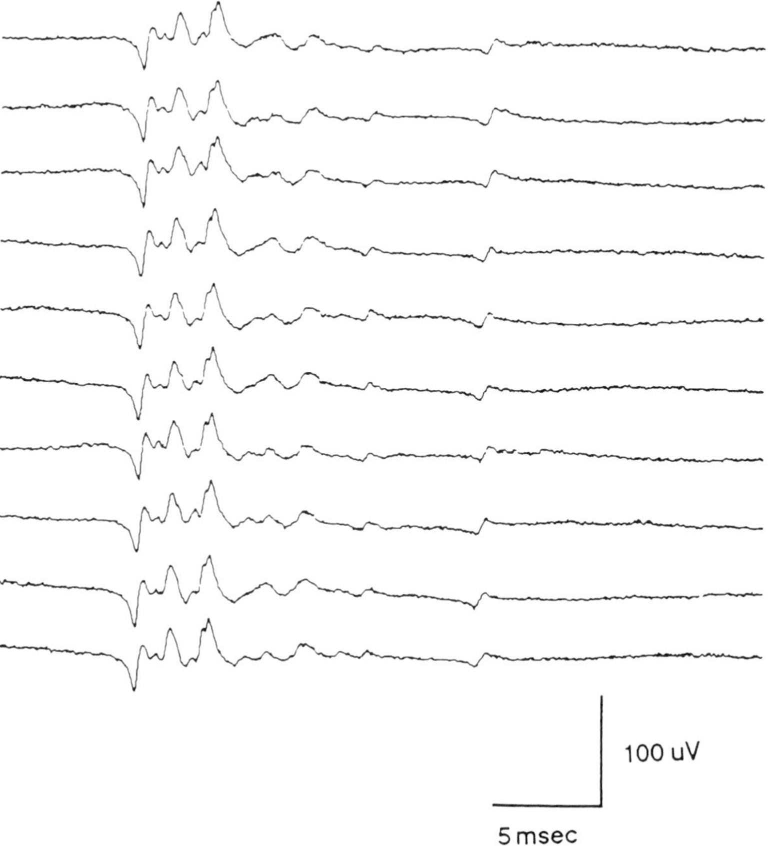


**Figure 12.1** A repetitively firing motor unit from a patient with a lower motor neurone lesion. Note the prolonged duration and polyphasic nature of the waveform

recorded with a needle electrode within the striated sphincter and single fibre EMG studies have demonstrated that it is an oligosynaptic reflex (Vodusek and Janko, 1990) (Figure 12.2).

In addition to the response in the bulbocavernosus muscle, other muscles of the pelvic floor contract in response to electrical stimulation of the glans penis. These sacral reflexes may be used to assess the integrity of both the afferent and efferent neurones and also the central connections within the sacral cord. In complete lesions the reflex is absent both clinically and electrically, while with incomplete lesions the reflex may or may not be present clinically (Blaivas, Zayed and Labib, 1981) and, in these circumstances, neurophysiological recordings may demonstrate either an increased latency or an absent response (Krane and Siroky, 1980).

## Pudendal nerve somatosensory evoked potentials

Electrical stimulation of a peripheral nerve will produce a recordable potential change over the contralateral sensory cortex and this response may be identified from the background activity by use of an averaging technique (Dawson, 1947). It has been shown that the impulses which produce this potential (called a somatosensory evoked potential or SSEP) are carried from the peripheral nerves via the posterior columns (Jones and Small, 1978) and represent activity in thalamocortical axons (Cracco, 1972).

The application of this technique to the pudendal nerve was first reported by Kaplan (1981), but since then several other groups have also reported results of studies of pudendal SSEPs (Haldeman, Bradley and Bhatia, 1982; Opsomer *et al.*, 1986). The most readily identifiable response is the first negative deflection of the potential (the P1 potential) and typically the latency of this response is between 37 and 45 ms (Figure 12.3).

The latency of the recorded response depends upon the integrity of the afferent pathways, so that neurological disease affecting the sensory innervation of the sacral segments may result in a prolonged latency or even in an absent response

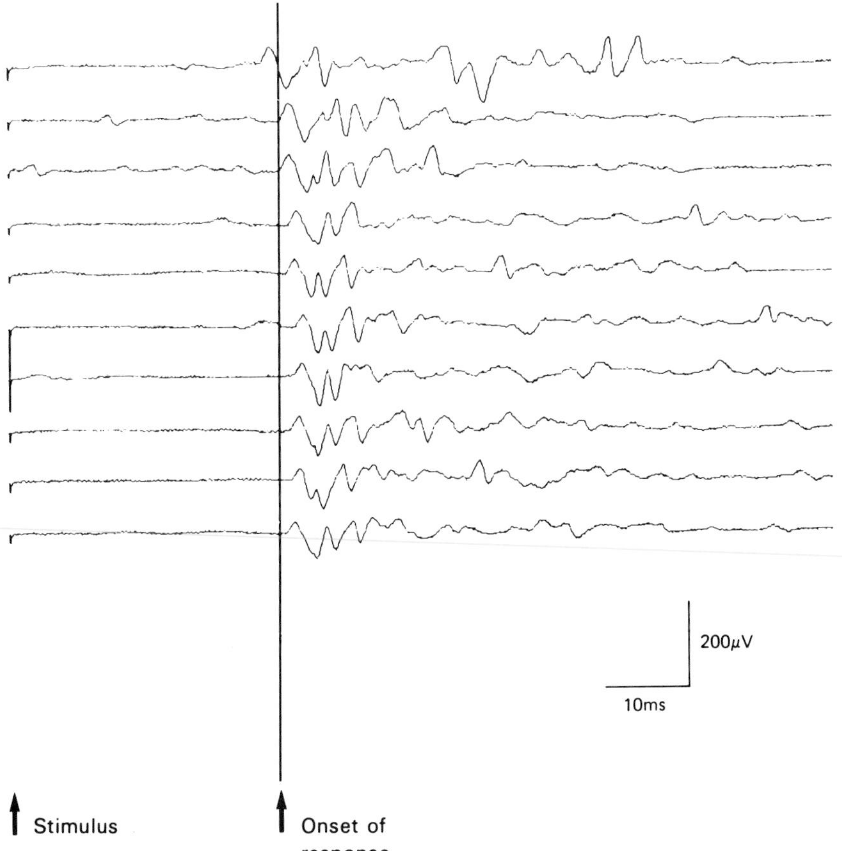


**Figure 12.2** A normal sacral reflex response to repetitive stimulation of the dorsal nerve of the penis

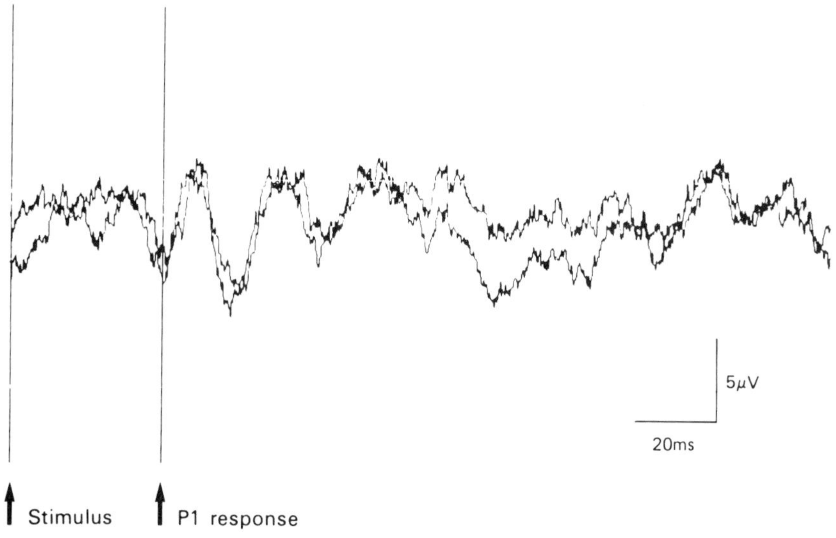


**Figure 12.3** A normal pudendal somatosensory evoked potential (two traces superimposed)

(Haldeman, Bradley and Bhatia, 1982). Little useful information can be gained from recording the sensory threshold to electrical stimulation, since unless specific precautions are taken, variation in the resistance of the stimulator–skin junction between subjects makes values obtained in this way unreliable (Fowler and Fowler, 1987).

## Nerve conduction studies

It is possible to measure the conduction velocity of large diameter myelinated sensory fibres of the pudendal nerve by electrically stimulating the dorsal nerve at the base of the glans penis and recording near the pubis (Bradley, Lin and Johnson, 1984). Neuropathies which primarily affect the large diameter myelinated fibres will slow conduction velocity, but such pathology is of little relevance to the complaint of impotence which is likely to result from small fibre or unmyelinated fibre dysfunction.

## Motor evoked potentials

In recent years, techniques to assess somatic motor conduction have been developed, using either electrical stimulation (Merton and Morton, 1980) or magnetic stimulation of the brain (Barker *et al.*, 1985). The application of these techniques to the study of the genitourinary system has thus far been confined to the study of urethral innervation (Snooks and Swash, 1984; Eardley *et al.*, 1990) and the bulbocavernosus muscle (Opsomer *et al.*, 1989). If there is damage to the descending motor tracts, then the EMG response to cortical stimulation will either be delayed or absent.

## Testing for small fibre neuropathy

The techniques described above test conduction in large myelinated fibres of the somatic nervous system. However most of the sensory fibres within the pudendal nerve are small myelinated and unmyelinated fibres which conduct nervous action potentials related to thermal and pain sensation (Halata and Munger, 1986).

Several methods of testing thermal thresholds are available (Fruhstorfer, Lindbloom and Schmidt, 1976; Fowler *et al.*, 1988), but in principle the smallest temperature change to cutaneous warming or cooling which a subject can detect is assessed for each subject. In patients with a small myelinated neuropathy (which is commonly seen in diabetes mellitus), larger temperature changes are necessary before the subject is able to notice a difference. Thus far these techniques have largely been confined to studies of the sensory nerves of the feet (which are commonly affected early in the course of the diabetic neuropathy), but with modification of the thermodes, examination of the genitalia can also be performed (Robinson, Woodcock and Stephenson, 1987).

## Electromyography of the corpus cavernosum

Wagner and his colleagues (1989) have recently reported that direct EMG recordings can be obtained from the smooth muscle of the corpus cavernosum. Following insertion of a concentric needle electrode into the flaccid penis, electrical activity was recorded which decreased with penile erection and then increased again with detumescence. However, in view of the extreme difficulties encountered in attempts to record the electromyographic activity of the detrusor muscle (Craggs and Stephenson, 1976), the results should be interpreted with caution. The study was a kinesiological investigation rather than an attempt to make out details of EMG activity and it may be that this technique will, in the future, provide further information regarding the timing of smooth muscle activity during erection.

## Applications of clinical neurophysiology

### Diagnosis of neurological disease

Clinical neurophysiology may, in selected patients, be useful to confirm a suspected neurological diagnosis. For example, in a pateint with parkinsonism associated with impotence and autonomic dysfunction, the presence of an abnormal urethral sphincter EMG suggests a diagnosis of multiple system atrophy (Eardley *et al.*, 1989). Similarly, abnormal pudendal SSEPs are associated with multiple sclerosis (Haldeman, Bradley and Bhatia, 1982), as are abnormalities of motor evoked responses. In all cases the appropraite neurophysiological study will be suggested by the clinical features, and the results must be interpreted in the light of these same clinical features.

A brief summary of the appropriate tests which will confirm a provisional clinical diagnosis is given in Table 12.1.

Several groups have attempted to use clinical neurophysiology either as a means of confirming a neurogenic aetiology for the impotence, or as a means of identifying subclinical neurological disease in patients with erectile dysfunction.

In one such study, to assess the value of the sacral reflex latency under these circumstances, Ertekin and Reel (1976) found that out of 16 cases of 'functional' impotence only one patient had a delayed sacral response. In contrast, Porst, Tackmann and Van Ahlen (1988) found that 35/83 (42%) of impotent patients with no history of neurological disease had an abnormality of the sacral reflex. Finally Lavoisier *et al.* (1989) found that of 90 impotent men, 19 (21%) had either an absent or a delayed bulbocavernosus response. They attempted to define the cause of the impotence in these patients on clinical grounds and concluded that 8/19 actually had psychogenic impotence.

Similar studies have been carried out using the pudendal nerve SSEP, again without any clear conclusion. Ertekin *et al.* (1985) found that of 24 impotent men with no evidence of neurological disease, only two (8%) had an abnormal somatosensory evoked potential. In contrast, Tackmann, Porst and Van Ahlen (1988) found that 30/167 (17.9%) similar patients had abnormalities of their pudendal nerve SSEP. In studies of patients with known neurological disease, Kirkeby, Poulsen and Dorup (1988) found that patients with impotence related to multiple sclerosis almost invariably had abnormalities of the pudendal nerve SSEP, while Ertekin *et al.* (1985) found that only six of 11 (55%) of a similar group of patients had abnormal responses.

Since the sacral reflex response assesses the sacral segments and the pudendal nerve SSEP assesses disease within the spinal cord, it would seem that a combination of these neurophysiological tests might provide a more sensitive and specific indicator of neurogenic impotence. Ertekin *et al.* (1985) used both the bulbocavernosus reflex and the pudendal nerve SSEP to study 90 patients with impotence. They concluded that the two tests were complementary, although there were many patients with known neurological disease, such as Parkinson's disease, multiple sclerosis or temporal lobe epilepsy, who had no neurophysiological abnormalities. Tackmann, Porst and Van Ahlen (1988) came to similar conclusions in a study of a large number of impotent men. Although abnormalities were common, there were many patients with known neurological disease and presumed neurogenic impotence who had normal studies, while conversely there were many patients with no clinically apparent neurological disease who had abnormalities of one or more neurophysiological parameters.

The main drawback of all these tests is that they assess somatic nervous pathways, while erection is

**Table 12.1 Tests used to confirm a provisional clinical diagnosis**

| *Provisional diagnosis* | *Test* | *Findings* |
|---|---|---|
| Pelvic nerve injury or cauda equina lesion | Urethral sphincter EMG<br>Sacral reflex latency | Abnormally prolonged polyphasic motor units<br>Delayed or absent response |
| Multiple system atrophy | Urethral sphincter EMG | Abnormally prolonged polyphasic motor units |
| Spinal cord disease, e.g. multiple sclerosis | Somatosensory evoked potential<br>Motor evoked potential | Delayed or absent response<br>Delayed or absent response |

largely under autonomic control. In practical terms, the main role of neurophsyiological testing is to confirm a clinical suspicion of neurological disease, and for that reason it should be used selectively, according to the clinical indications.

However, in several of the studies mentioned above, neurophysiological abnormalities were relatively common in patients with no clinically apparent neurological disease and these findings deserve further investigation. Firstly their validity must be confirmed, and then it is necessary to carefully follow the patients with abnormal results to see whether they then go on to develop overt neurological features.

### Investigation of diabetic impotence

In patients with diabetes mellitus, clinical neurophysiology has, in the past, been used to investigate the contribution of neuropathy to the pathogenesis of impotence. Most studies have concentrated upon the sacral reflex latency and the conclusions are often contradictory. In a study of 13 diabetic men, Karacan (1980) found abnormalities of the sacral reflex arc in 9 (69%) patients and concluded that neuropathy at sacral level played a major role in the impotence of most diabetics. However, Parys, Evans and Parsons (1988) in a study of 19 impotent diabetics found that only three (16%) had abnormal sacral reflex latencies, while Desai *et al.* (1988) found that five of 29 (17%) impotent diabetics had abnormal sacral reflex latencies. They further attempted to identify clinically those diabetics with neurogenic impotence, but even in this selected group, only five of 17 (29%) had abnormal sacral reflex latencies. Finally, Fowler *et al.* (1988) found that only four of nine (44%) patients with diabetic impotence had abnormal sacral reflex latencies.

Kaneko and Bradley (1987) compared the value of testing the bulbocavernosus reflex with assessing sensory conduction in the dorsal nerve of the penis, and found that the reflex latency in a group of impotent diabetics was similar to a group of non-diabetic impotent men. However, sensory conduction within the pudendal nerve was significantly delayed.

One of the problems with assessing the sacral reflex latency (and for that matter, sensory conduction within the dorsal nerve of the penis) is that in diabetes the small myelinated and unmyelinated fibres bear the brunt of the nerve damage (Said, Slama and Selva, 1983). Thus in some patients there may be selective nerve fibre damage, resulting in a defect in autonomic innervation while conduction in larger fibres is relatively preserved and this may explain the variable results of testing the sacral reflex arc in diabetes mellitus.

Small myelinated and unmyelinated fibres carry sensory information related to thermal sensation and, furthermore, it is the longest fibres carrying sensory information from the feet which are affected in the early stages of diabetic neuropathy. In an attempt to identify those patients with damage to these smaller nerve fibres, Fowler *et al.* (1988) investigated the value of thermal threshold testing in impotent diabetics. In this study, all patients with apparent neuropathic erectile dysfunction had abnormal thresholds to warming, which implied an unmyelinated peripheral neuropathy. Testing was applied only to the foot, but the findings were confirmed by Robinson, Woodcock and Stephenson (1987) who found that out of 27 impotent diabetics only two had normal penile thermal thresholds.

Another approach has been to use the recently described method of corpus cavernosum electromyography to identify those patients with neurogenic impotence. In a study of 10 insulin-dependent diabetics, Gerstenberg *et al.* (1989) found that four patients had no evidence of an arterial lesion but did have abnormalities indicative of an autonomic neuropathy, and they all responded to papaverine injections. The other patients all had Doppler studies suggestive of arterial problems, and although two of them also had EMG abnormalities, none responded to intracorporeal papaverine. This technique, however, is still at an early stage of development and further evaluation is required.

## Conclusion

Clinical neurophysiology is useful in assessing the somatic nervous pathways to the sacral segments. However, it is not yet possible to assess the autonomic pathways and it is these that are important in the nervous control of erectile function. Accordingly there is not yet a good neurophysiological test which is able to identify patients with neurogenic impotence.

Clinical neurophysiology does have a role, however, in confirming a diagnosis in patients in whom neurological disease is suspected. In some diseases, such as multiple system atrophy, impotence is one of the earliest clinical features of the disease and it is clearly of value to be able to make a firm diagnosis as early as possible. It is important for the urologist to be alert to the possibility of neurological disease in patients presenting with erectile impotence, and in these cases referral for a neurological opinion and specific neurophysiological investigations is often of value.

### References

Barker, A. T., Freeston, I. L., Jalinous, R. *et al.* (1985) Magnetic stimulation of the human brain. *Journal of Physiology*, **369**, 3P

Blaivas, J. G., Zayed, A. A. H. and Labib, K. B. (1981) The bulbocavernosus reflex in urology: a prospective study of 299 patients. *Journal of Urology,* **126**, 197–199

Bradley, W. E., Lin, J. T. Y. and Johnson, B. (1984) Measurement of the conduction velocity of the dorsal nerve of the penis. *Journal of Urology,* **131**, 1127–1129

Chantraine, A. M. (1966) Electromyographie des sphincters stries uretral et anal humains. Etude descriptive et analytique. *Renal Neurologie (Paris),* **115**, 393–403

Cracco, R. Q. (1972) The initial positive potential of the human scalp-recorded somatosensory evoked response. *Electroencephalography and Clinical Neurophysiology,* **32**, 623–629

Craggs, M. D. and Stephenson, J. D. (1976) The real bladder electromyogram. *British Journal of Urology,* **48**, 443–451

Dawson, G. D. (1947) Cerebral responses to electrical stimulation of peripheral nerves in man. *Journal of Neurology, Neurosurgery and Psychiatry,* **10**, 134–140

Desai, K. M., Dembny, K., Morgan, H. and Gingell, J. C. (1988) Neurophysiological investigation of diabetic impotence. Are sacral response studies of value? *British Journal of Urology,* **61**, 68–73

Eardley, I., Nagendran, K., Kirby, R. S. and Fowler, C. J. (1990) Magnetic stimulation of the human brain. A new technique of assessing efferent pathways to the striated urethral sphincter. *Journal of Urology,* **144**, 948–951

Eardley, I. Quinn, N. P., Fowler, C. J. *et al.* (1989) The role of urethral sphincter electromyography in the differential diagnosis of parkinsonism. *British Journal of Urology,* **64**, 360–362

Ertekin, C., Akyurekli, O., Gurses, A. N. and Turgot, H. (1985) The value of somatosensory evoked potentials and the bulbocavernosus reflex in patients with impotence. *Acta Neurologica Scandinivica,* **71**, 48–53

Ertekin, C. and Reel, F. (1976) Bulbocavernosus reflex in normal men and in patients with neurogenic bladder and/or impotence. *Journal of the Neurological Sciences,* **28**, 1–15

Fowler, C. J., Ali, Z., Kirby, R. S. and Pryor, J. P. (1988) The value of testing for unmyelinated fibre, sensory neuropathy in diabetic impotence. *British Journal of Urology,* **61**, 63–67

Fowler, C. J. and Fowler, C. G. (1987) In *The Physiology of the Lower Urinary Tract* (eds M. Torrens and J. F. B. Morrison), Springer Verlag, Chapter 10

Fowler, C. J., Kirby, R. S. Harrison, M. J. G. *et al.* (1984) Individual motor unit analysis in the diagnosis of disorders of urethral sphincter innervation. *Journal of Neurology, Neurosurgery and Psychiatry,* **47**, 637–641

Fruhstorfer, H. Lindbloom, U. and Schmidt, W. G. (1976) Method for quantitative estimation of thermal thresholds in patients. *Journal of Neurology, Neurosurgery and Psychiatry,* **39**, 1071–1075

Gerstenberg, T. C., Nordling, T., Hald, T. and Wagner, G. (1989) Standardised evaluation of erectile dysfunction in 95 consecutive patients. *Journal of Urology,* **141**, 857–862

Halata, Z. and Munger, B. (1986) The neuroanatomical basis for the protopathic sensibility of the human penis. *Brain Research,* **371**, 205–230

Haldeman, S., Bradley, W. E. and Bhatia, N. (1982) Evoked responses from the pudendal nerve. *Journal of Urology,* **128**, 974–980

Jones, S. J. and Small, D. G. (1978) Spinal and subcortical evoked potentials following stimulation of the posterior tibial nerve in man. *Electroencephalography and Clinical Neurophysiology,* **44**, 299–306

Kaneko, S. and Bradley, W. E. (1987) Penile electrodiagnosis. Value of bulbocavernosus reflex latency versus nerve conduction velocity of the dorsal nerve of the penis in the diagnosis of diabetic impotence. *Journal of Urology,* **137**, 933–935

Kaplan, P. E. (1981) A somatosensory evoked response obtained after stimulation of the contralateral pudendal nerve. *Electromyography and Clinical Neurophysiology,* **21**, 585–587

Karacan, I. (1980) Diagnosis of erectile impotence in diabetes mellitus. *Annals of Internal Medicine,* **92**, 334–337

Kirkeby, H. J., Poulsen, E. U. and Dorup, J. (1988) Erectile dysfunction in multiple sclerosis. *Neurology,* **38**, 1366–1370

Krane, R. J. and Siroky, M. B. (1980) Studies on sacral evoked potentials. *Journal of Urology,* **124**, 872–876

Lavoisier, P., Proulx, J., Courtois, F. and de Carufel, F. (1989) Bulbocavernosus reflex: its validity as a diagnostic test of neurogenic impotence. *Journal of Urology,* **141**, 311–314

Lue, T. F., Zeineh, S. J., Schmidt, R. A. and Tanagho, E. A. (1984) Neuroanatomy of penile erection: its relevance to iatrogenic impotence. *Journal of Urology,* **131**, 273–280

Merton, P. A. and Morton, H. B. (1980) Stimulation of the cerebral cortex in the intact human subject. *Nature,* **285**, 277

Opsomer, R. J., Caramia, M. D., Zarola, F. *et al.* (1989) Neurophysiological evaluation of central–peripheral sensory and motor pudendal fibres. *Electroencephalography and Clinical Neurophysiology,* **74**, 260–270

Opsomer, R. J., Guerit, J. M., Wese, F. X. and Van Cangh, P. J. (1986) Pudendal cortical somatosensory evoked potentials. *Journal of Urology,* **135**, 1216–1218

Parys, B. T., Evans, C. M. and Parsons, K. F. (1988) Bulbocavernosus reflex latency in the investigation of diabetic impotence. *British Journal of Urology,* **61**, 59–62

Petersen, I. and Franksson, C. (1955) Electromyographic study of the striated muscles of the male urethra. *British Journal of Urology,* **27**, 148–153

Porst, H., Tackmann, W. and Van Ahlen, H. (1988) Neurophysiological investigations in potent and impotent men. *British Journal of Urology,* **61**, 445–450

Robinson, L. Q., Woodcock, J. P. and Stephenson, T. P. (1987) Results of investigation of impotence in patients with overt or probable neuropathy. *British Journal of Urology,* **60**, 583–587

Said, G., Slama, G. and Selva, J. (1983) Progressive

centripetal degeneration of axons in small fibre diabetic polyneuropathy. *Brain,* **106**, 791–807

Snooks, S. J. and Swash, M. (1984) Perineal nerve and transcutaneous spinal stimulation: new methods for investigation of the urethral striated sphincter musculature. *British Journal of Urology,* **56**, 406–409

Tackmann, W., Porst, H. and Van Ahlen, H. (1988) Bulbocavernosus reflex latencies and somatosensory evoked potentials after pudendal nerve stimulation in the diagnosis of impotence. *Journal of Neurology,* **235**, 219–255

Vodusek, D. B. and Janko, M. (1990) The bulbocavernosus reflex. *Brain,* **113**, 813–820

Wagner, G., Gerstenberg, T. and Levin, R. J. (1989) Electrical activity of corpus cavernosum during flaccidity and erection of the human penis: a new diagnostic method? *Journal of Urology,* **142**, 723–725

Walsh, P. C. and Donker, P. J. (1982) Impotence following radical prostatectomy: insight into etiology and prevention. *Journal of Urology,* **130**, 1237–1241

# 13

# Psychological evaluation of erectile failure

J. LoPiccolo

This chapter discusses current approaches to psychological evaluation of erectile failure. Interviewing procedures and psychometric testing are reviewed. First, however, the purpose of psychological assessment is discussed, with a focus on the use of psychological evaluation in making differential treatment decisions.

## Purpose of psychological assessment: differential diagnosis or treatment planning?

In 1970, Masters and Johnson stated that 95% of all cases of erectile failure were purely psychogenic. New diagnostic procedures have revealed that neurological, vascular and hormonal abnormalities are involved in a considerable percentage of cases of erectile failure (Tanagho, Lue and McClure, 1988; Mohr and Beutler, 1990). While some studies (e.g. Spark, White and Connolly, 1980) have reported very high rates of physiological pathology in cases of erectile failure, selective referral seems to account for these extremely high rates; for example, Spark, White, Connolly (1980) found that almost one-half of erectile failure cases had hormonal abnormalities. More typical hormonal abnormality rates for unselected patients in various studies are 5–10% (Seagraves *et al.*, 1981; Bancroft, 1984).

In regard to differential diagnosis, serious conceptual and methodological flaws are evident in virtually all of the currently published research. Conceptually, most of the research suffers from the flaw of attempting to categorize patients into discrete, non-overlapping categories of organic *or* psychogenic erectile failure. Yet in many cases, *both* organic *and* psychogenic factors are involved. Recognizing this combined causality, Melman, Tiefer and Pedersen (1988) diagnosed patients with erectile failure along a bipolar scale, from exclusively psychogenic, through mixed aetiology, to exclusively organic in origin. Melman, Tiefer and Pedersen (1988) reported that of 406 patients evaluated, 39.7% were purely psychogenic, 25.1% had both organic and psychological problems, and 28.9% were characterized as purely organic in origin. While this bipolar scale is an advance over a simplistic two-category typology, there is a logical problem. As Bem (1974) has pointed out with the issues of masculinity and femininity, the dimensions of organic and psychogenic logically are not the opposite ends of a unidimensional biopolar scale, but rather represent two separate and independently varying dimensions. That is, a man may have a high degree of *both* organic and psychogenic causes of erectile failure, or a low degree of both factors, or any combination of high and low degrees of impairment on each separate dimension. While this fact may seem obvious, there are statements in the clinical literature that if one finds a clear psychological cause of the erection problem, one need not conduct any physiological evaluation. This point of view suggests, for example, that having a serious problem in a marital relationship prevents one from developing atherosclerotic disease processes in the arteries leading to the penis.

Similarly, many physicians currently will perform surgery to implant a penile prosthesis if *any* degree of organic abnormality is found. In many such cases the patient has only a mild organic impairment which then makes his erection extremely vulnerable to being disrupted by psychological, behavioural and sexual technique factors. Many times, cases with such partial organic impairment can be treated successfully by sex therapy. If psychological and behavioural difficulties are eliminated, the patient's mildly impaired physiological capacity may be sufficient to easily produce good erection.

In the author's ongoing study of aetiology of erectile failure, 63 men have been independently rated for degree of psychological impairment (scored 0–4) and degree of organic impairment (also scored 0–4), following complete psychological, vascular, hormonal, neurological and nocturnal penile tumescence evaluations. The results of these evaluations, shown in Figure 13.1, indicate that there is only a moderate negative correlation (−0.58) between degrees of organic and psycho-

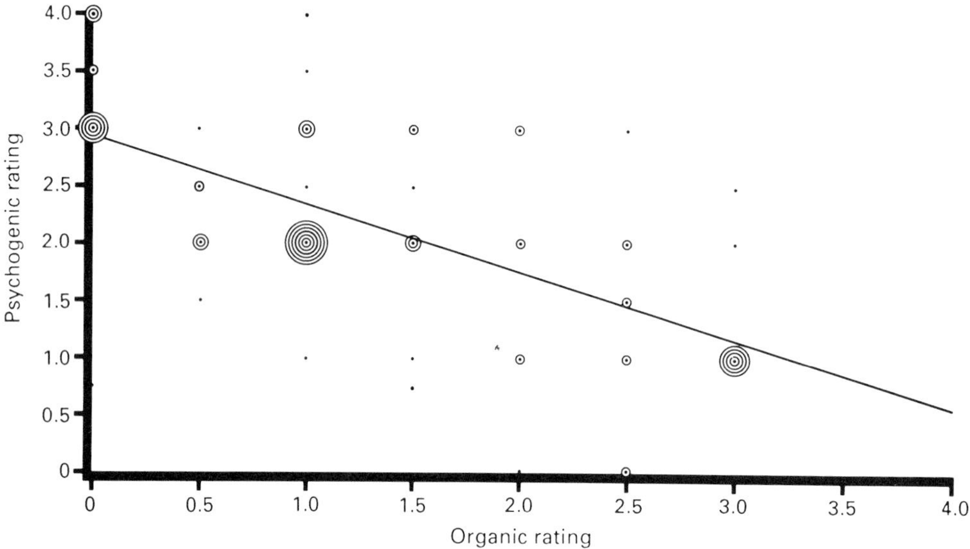


**Figure 13.1** Relationship between psychogenic and organic ratings (each circle represents one patient)

logical impairment, so a unidimensional biopolar scale is not an accurate representation of clinical reality. Furthermore, only ten men were found to be purely psychogenic, and only three to be purely organic in aetiology, so an 'either/or' two-category typology is even more inappropriate. Figure 13.1 also indicates that there are a considerable number of men (19/63 or 30%) with mild organic impairments (0.5–1.0 on our scale), but significant psychological problems (2.0 or greater on our scale). These men might, in a two-part typology, be considered to be 'organic' cases of erectile failure as there is some demonstrated physiological impairment. However, the greater degree of psychological aetiology seen in these cases argues against this categorization, and suggests that a physical intervention is probably not necessary to restore normal erectile functioning for these men.

Diagnosis into a two-dimensional schema also offers a comment on the long-term adjustment to implantation of a prosthesis. Consider, in Figure 13.1, the 16 men who scored at least 2.5 on the organic impairment scale, and for whom a prosthesis might therefore be an appropriate treatment. Of these 16 men, five (31%) received a rating of 2.0, 2.5 or 3.0 for presence of concurrent psychological problems. It might be anticipated that with this degree of psychological disturbance, long-term adjustment to the prosthesis would be poor. Although patients are typically very eager to have a prosthesis implanted, and report being very happy with it at short-term surgical follow-up, longer term follow-up indicates poor sexual adjustment in a significant percentage of cases (Tiefer, Pedersen and Melman, 1988). It seems reasonable that if a man has a number of psychological problems involved in his erectile failure, the implantation of the prosthetic device will only result in his now having these same difficulties, but with an artificially rigid penis. While erection is now present, one would not expect the frequency or quality of sexual activity to be high in such cases, and this result is what was found by Tiefer, Pedersen and Melman (1988). A thorough psychological evaluation is therefore indicated for all cases of erectile failure, even when an organic aetiology is clearly established and a surgical treatment is planned.

The focus in much of the clinical literature on making a differential diagnosis into mutually exclusive categories of organic or psychogenic aetiology is often at the expense of formulating the best treatment plan, which is ultimately the purpose of diagnostic assessment. The focus of psychological assessment should not only be to quantify the degree of psychological causality of the erection problem, but to identify issues to be focused upon in treatment, and assess prognosis for response to physical interventions such as vasoactive injections, vacuum erection devices, or prostheses. As it seems to be true that most erectile failure cases involve major psychological aetiology (regardless of degree of organic impairment present), assessment should focus on which psychological and/or somatic interventions are most likely to help each particular patient. As Mohr and Beutler (1990) have noted, prognosis, not diagnosis, must be the deciding factor in choice of treatment, and psychological evaluation is critical in making prognostic evaluations.

## Interviewing techniques

The clinician approaching a sexual assessment interview may be anxious about raising this topic with the patient. Sex is obviously a highly emotional, private subject for most people, and the clinician may find him or herself feeling uncomfortable in response to the patient's embarrassment, hesitancy and reticence in discussing sexual behaviour.

The therapist should acknowledge that sex is a sensitive and difficult area to discuss. A good therapeutic statement is: 'I know it's a little uncomfortable to talk about something as personal as your sexual relationship. I'll try to make this as easy for you as I can, and please let me know if there is anything I can do that will make you more comfortable'. We also tell our patients that we have seen literally hundreds of cases of erectile failure, so there is nothing new the patient can tell us that will shock or surprise us. Our interest is in gaining a complete picture of the problem so that we can choose the best treatment for the patient.

Before beginning the interview, the patient should be informed about therapeutic confidentiality and privilege. We tell our patients that in certain circumstances we are required, under law, to divulge information about them to relevant authorities. These circumstances involve threatened harm to others, child sexual abuse and disputed child custody. In most states, privilege and confidentiality do not apply in cases in which the therapist feels the patient is an imminent danger to another person or to himself. All states in the USA now have mandatory reporting laws on child sexual abuse which oblige the therapist to report sexual activity with children. Similarly, in most states, privilege and confidentiality are automatically waived by the patient in regard to child custody disputes before the court. The clinician should understand the privilege and confidentiality statutes in his or her state and explain that all information revealed is confidential, with these few specific exceptions.

Procedurally, to do sexual assessment requires asking some very specific questions. Clinicians are typically trained to ask broad, open-ended questions, but some stylistic change may be necessary in regard to the sexual area. A good strategy is to begin with a general question, and then move to a more specific question. For example, in assessing sexual arousal difficulties, the general question would be: 'Are you becoming physically aroused when you engage in sex?' More specific questions would then be asked about arousal response to different specific sexual activities, subjective experiences of arousal as opposed to physiological changes, factors that determine variability of arousal response, and so forth. A detailed, structured interview guide for assessment of erectile failure is included as Appendix 1 to this chapter.

In interviewing patients with erectile failure, it is crucial to conduct a conjoint interview with the wife present. Often her view of the cause of the problem will differ, and her reactions to the patient's erectile problem must be assessed directly. However, it is important to also see each member of the patient couple alone.

When assessing erectile failure, we routinely schedule patients for a 2-hour initial evaluation appointment. In doing our assessments, we will see the couple together for the first 45 min to 1 h. At this point, we explain to them that we always see each member of a couple individually as well.

Exactly what is discussed in the individual sessions depends, to a certain degree, on what has happened in the couple session. In the couple session we will ask open-ended questions that the patients can respond to in a number of ways. For example, we routinely ask: 'Are there other situations in which you get a better erection?' If the husband says that his erection does not work any better in masturbation or during sexual fantasies, and that he did have an affair recently in which his erection was no better, we may not need to pursue these topics very much in the solo interview. However, if in response to that same question the husband avoids meeting the therapist's eyes, shift uncomfortably in the chair and says 'not really', the therapist makes a mental note to inquire in great detail about these topics during the solo session.

The topic areas that are dealt with in the solo sessions are the fairly obvious ones. We inquire about the content of sexual fantasies; masturbation; extramarital sexual contacts; sexual functioning in contacts prior to the marriage; any non-typical or deviant sexual practices; homosexual thoughts, fantasies, or experiences; and unpleasant or traumatic sexual experiences. Similarly, we will explore the taboo areas in the general marital relationship. We will ask if they find their spouse physically attractive. Do they find their spouse to be sexually skilled and a good lover? Does their spouse have adequate personal hygiene habits? Finally, we will simply ask each person if they love their spouse. We explain to patients that information revealed in these sessions will not be reported to their spouse without their permission. We explain that only if information is revealed that we feel is crucial for the spouse to know for therapy to proceed, will we ask for this permission. Examples of such situations include active ongoing affairs, hidden homosexual orientation, and sexual deviations such as transvestism. In such cases we offer the patient the alternative of making the previously secret information available to the spouse for therapeutic discussion, or referral to another therapist for individual therapy. This strategy avoids placing the therapist in the position of colluding with the patient in a deception of the spouse that would prevent therapeutic progress.

Our psychological assessment interview is brief compared with traditional sex therapy programmes which often involve very long (up to 8 h) sex history interviews. While such detailed histories may be useful in building rapport in therapy, they are of limited value (to say nothing of being impractical) in assessing erectile failure with a goal of choosing the best treatment modality. The focused interview outline presented in Appendix 1 is more useful in making treatment recommendations than historical information regarding childhood and adolescent sexual development. If the treatment decision is for psychotherapy, a brief (1–2 h) sex history interview is then appropriate, and good outlines for sex history interviews are provided in LoPiccolo and Heiman (1978) and Lobitz and Lobitz (1978).

## Psychometric assessment

To be useful to the practising clinician, a psychometric assessment device must be specifically relevant; the connection between the test content, diagnostic schemes and treatment strategy must be direct and easily seen. To do sex therapy with a couple, information is needed on the relationship of the couple and, more specifically, the sexual aspect of that relationship. If proper instruments are selected and data collected at initial contact, information from standardized tests may be very valuable to the therapist in correctly diagnosing the problem, selecting a treatment plan, and discussing treatment prognosis with the couple.

In our work with erectile failure cases, the patient couple, after initial phone contact, are mailed an assessment packet. They are instructed to fill out the questionnaires in this packet and mail them back before their evaluation. We explain that therapeutic time is expensive, and that we can do a much more efficient initial interview if we have this information.

Our initial assessment packet contains a 28-item Sex History Questionnaire in a multiple-choice response format, which is included as Appendix 2 of this chapter. This questionnaire asks about frequency of a variety of sexual activities, sexual desire, feelings about sex, feelings towards the mate, etc. Norms from a sample of 200 non-clinical control couples have been developed for this questionnaire, so the patient's responses may be evaluated in the context of sexually functional relationships. Discrepancies in answers between the patient and his wife are often a rich source of insight into the genesis of the erectile problem.

Our initial packet also includes the Locke–Wallace Marriage Inventory (Kimmel and VanderVeen, 1974) to give us some measure of marital distress. A standardized, brief health history form is also included to give us information about diseases and medications. We also use a number of other questionnaires, but these are administered to the patient after the initial intake interview. These other questionnaires take longer for the patient to complete, or contain more threatening material, and so are best administered after a therapeutic relationship has been established in the initial interview. The other measures that we use include the Symptom Check List-90 (Derogatis, Lipman and Covi, 1973), the Zung Depression Scale (Zung, 1973) and goal sheets that ask the clients to write down, for both themselves and their partner, three specific changes they want in each of the areas of sex, marriage and general life adjustment. These questionnaires give an extremely thorough assessment of general psychiatric status and marital adjustment.

In seeking the most complete assessment of the couple's problems, clinicians working with erectile failure are operating at a disadvantage compared with the assessment of other behavioural problems. If a patient complains of social anxiety, for example, a standard behavioural assessment would be for the clinician to observe the patient in a structured analogue social interaction in the clinician's office. Obviously, for both ethical and practical reasons we cannot ask our patients to engage in sexual activity while we observe to identify behaviour patterns that contribute to erectile failure. While the Sex History Questionnaire provides an overview, it does not tell the clinician exactly what occurs when the patient engages in sex with the spouse.

The Sexual Interaction Inventory (LoPiccolo and Steger, 1974) was developed to provide, via questionnaire, just such a detailed assessment of the patient's sexual activity. The Sexual Interaction Inventory (SII) consists of a list of 17 heterosexual behaviours adopted from Bentler's (1968a,b) Guttman scaling of sexual behaviours. Husband and wife separately answer six questions for each behaviour using a response format of a six-point rating scale. The responses from each member of the couple are summed across all 17 behaviours. The totals are used to derive an 11-scale profile. Each SII scale has a mean of 50 and a standard deviation of 10, based on scores from two samples totalling 124 volunteer couples who reported a satisfactory sexual relationship. The 11 scales were chosen on the basis of clinical experience in treating dysfunctional couples. Factors found be be crucial in determining sexual satisfaction included dissatisfaction with frequency and range of sexual behaviours engaged in, self-acceptance, pleasure obtained from sexual activity, accurate knowledge of partner's preferred sexual activities, and acceptance of partner. Scoring is arranged so that higher scores indicate greater pathology (e.g. dissatisfaction, conflict) with scores above 70 indicative of a large degree of pathology. A Sexual Interaction Inventory Profile for a typical case of erectile failure is shown in Figure 13.2.

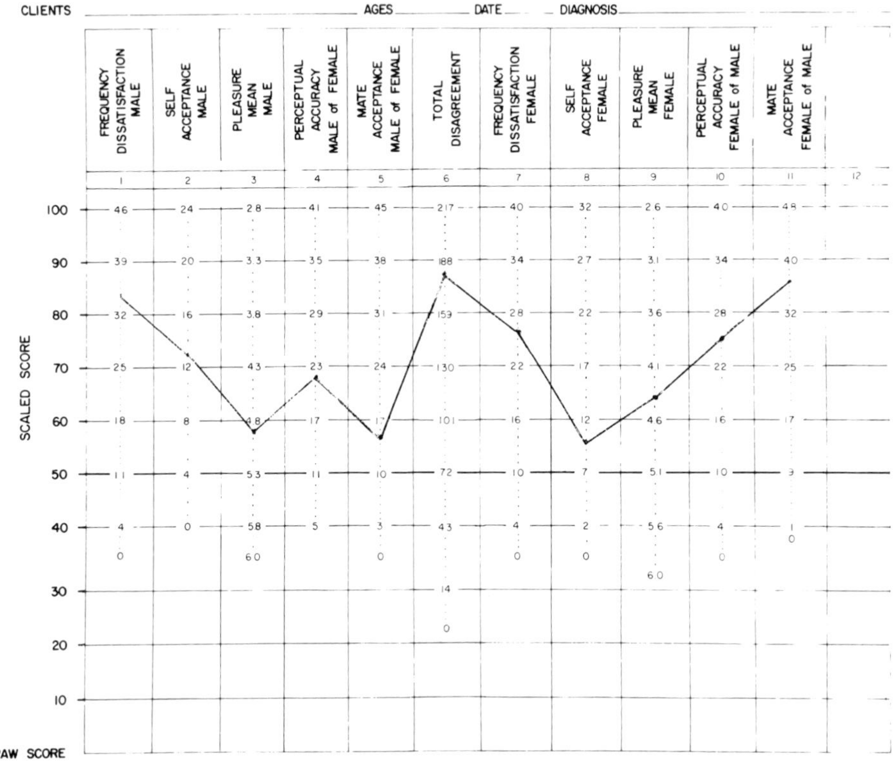


**Figure 13.2** Sexual interaction inventory (from LoPiccolo and Steger, 1974)

The SII has considerable diagnostic utility as well as serving as a means of assessing treatment outcome. Because the patterns of scale elevations indicate which aspects of the couple's sexual relationship are most distressed, the SII is very useful as an aid in planning treatment strategies.

## Prognostic indicators and choice of treatment

Based on the information gathered from the interview and questionnaire materials discussed above, the clinician can now make a prognostic decision about which type of treatment will best suit the individual patient couple. What follows is a brief review of prognostic indicators for psychotherapeutic tratment, and for medical interventions such as an implantation of a prosthesis, use of a vacuum erection device or vasoactive injections.

### Prognostic indicators for psychotherapy

The best prognosis for successful psychotherapy occurs in cases in which clear behavioural deficits or maladaptive thinking patterns which contribute to lack of erection can be identified. The most common behavioural and cognitive problems which respond well to psychotherapy are listed below.

1. Lack of adequate sexual stimulation. If the wife does not engage in any manual or oral stimulation of her husband's penis, but expects him to have an erection because he is kissing and caressing her, relatively simple behavioural directions for increasing physical stimulation have a good chance of success. These behavioural deficits can be identified clearly with the Sexual Interaction Inventory (LoPiccolo and Steger, 1974). This intervention is indicated in cases of partial organic impairment or ageing males, where the erection response requires a high intensity of physical stimulation of the penis.
2. The wife's sexual gratification is currently dependent upon the male obtaining an erection. If the wife only has orgasm during coitus, and does not consider an orgasm produced by her husband's manual, oral or electric vibrator stimulation to be normal, there is a good prognosis for sex therapy. If the husband can be reassured that he is providing full sexual satisfaction for his wife through manual, oral or electric vibrator stimu-

lation of her genitals, the pressure on him to perform for her by getting an erection will be greatley reduced.

3. Lack of knowledge about age-related changes in sexual functioning. Erectile failure is most commonly seen in men aged 50 or older. In these men, the slowing down of the erection response, the greater dependence upon physical as opposed to psychological stimulation to produce an erection, the longer duration of the refractory period, and the inability to ejaculate on every occasion of intercourse are normal ageing changes (Schover, 1984). However, many couples overreact to these changes with anxiety and distress, and produce erectile failure in the male. Simple education about normal ageing changes in sexuality, and behavioural techniques for dealing with these changes, can resolve the erectile failure.
4. Cognitive distortions regarding the male sex role stereotype, leading to unrealistic demands upon the male for sexual performance. Many men and women labour under a 'macho' set of unrealistic role demands for male sexual performance (Zilbergeld, 1978). Education to promote a realistic view of male sex roles and sexual performance can be very helpful.
5. Severe marital relationship problems. Hostility, resentment, anger and other negative emotions interfere with the man's ability to be aroused despite adequate physical stimulation. These problems can respond to psychotherapy, although these issues are not always easily resolved.
6. Specific relationship difficulties that make it functionally adaptive for the male to have an erection problem. Systemic approaches to erectile failure stress the functional or adaptive value of an erectile problem in dealing with interpersonal conflict (LoPiccolo, 1988). One common example would be a man who feels at a power disadvantage with his wife and has no good strategies for conflict resolution. His erectile failure may indeed give him a sense of power and a way to express his anger and his feelings of powerlessness in regard to his wife. While therapy in such cases is often more long-term, the prognosis is good if such systemic issues can be identified.

Having mentioned some good prognostic indicators for successful psychotherapy, a comment will now be offered on poor prognostic indicators.

1. An unwillingness on either the patient or the wife's part to reconsider male sex role demands, the role of the female in providing adequate stimulation for the male, or the means of stimulation by which the female reaches her orgasm.
2. Presence of a sexual deviation. Obviously if the male is aroused by an inappropriate sexual object (such as children), or has a paraphilia such as transvestism, therapy becomes much more difficult.
3. Extreme religiosity, with religious beliefs about sex interfering with sexual performance. These cases are best referred to a pastoral counsellor who may have some credibility in changing or at least helping the patient to re-examine these beliefs.
4. Moderate to severe clinical depression. Sex therapy is routinely unsuccessful in cases of clinical depression.

## Prognostic indicators for medical treatments

Good prognostic indicators for a prosthesis, use of a vacuum aided device or vasoactive injections include:

1. A presently adequate repertoire of sexual stimulation is being provided to the male by the female in terms of manual and oral stimulation of the penis during foreplay, but this is ineffective in producing an erection.
2. A clear understanding of exactly what sexual behaviour can be expected following the medical treatment and a willingness to adapt to the marked changes in sexual behaviour patterns that are caused by any of these medical procedures.
3. The female does enjoy penile–vaginal intercourse, but reports that size of the penis is not important to her. Since a prosthesis does not increase the size of the penis as occurs when a man gets a physiological erection, some women do report dissatisfaction with the prosthesis if they previously enjoyed the sensation of containment of the larger normally erect penis. These cases are routinely dissatisfied with the prosthetic implant (Melman, Tiefer and Pedersen, 1988).

There are also some indicators of poor prognosis for long-term adjustment to a medical intervention. The more commonly seen factors include:

1. Strong systemic gains for either the wife or husband in terms of the effects the erectile failure is currently having on the marriage. If either a husband or the wife is invested in maintenance of the erectile failure because it helps them deal with some issues of power, intimacy, closeness, trust or control in the relationship, adjustment to a prosthesis or medical procedure will be poor unless psychotherapy is also provided, preferably prior to surgery.
2. The wife is essentially uninterested in resuming active intercourse. In a recent case the wife stated: 'I've always done my wifely duty, but it's been a great relief not to have to do it these last

five years since he's been impotent'. This case was given a penile prosthesis. As might be expected, the results were psychologically disastrous with severe marital distress and an ultimate divorce occurring.

3. Unrealistic expectations that an artificial erection will deal with problems of differences in desired frequency of intercourse, willingness to engage in other forms of sexual activity, such as manual or oral stimulation, and general dissatisfaction with the partner's sexual techniques.
4. Significant psychopathology indicated on the psychometric devices discussed previously.

## Conclusion

This chapter has reviewed strategies and techniques for assessment of psychological factors involved in erectile functioning. The evaluation of a complex interpersonal problem, such as erectile failure, is difficult and time-consuming. It is hoped that clinicians will be thorough and careful before making treatment recommendations which have power to increase, as well as reduce, patient distress about erectile failure.

### References

Bancroft, J. (1984) Testosterone therapy for low sexual interest and erectile dysfunctions in man: a controlled study. *British Journal of Psychiatry,* **14**, 146–151

Bem, S. (1974) The measurement of psychological androgyny. *Journal of Consulting Clinical Psychology,* **42**, 155–162

Bentler, P. (1968a) Heterosexual behaviour assessment. I. Males. *Behavioural Research Therapy,* **6**, 21–25

Bentler, P. (1968b) Heterosexual behaviour assessment. II. Females. *Behavioural Research Therapy,* **6**, 27–30

Derogatis, L., Lipman, R. and Covi, L. (1973) SCL-90: an out-patient psychiatric rating scale. *Psychopharmacological Bulletin,* **9**, 13–28

Kimmel, D. and VanderVeen, F. (1974) Factors of marital adjustment in Locke's Marital Adjustment Test. *Journal of Marriage and Family,* **29**, 57–63

Lobitz, W. and Lobitz, G. (1978) Clinical assessment in the treatment of sexual dysfunctions. In *Handbook of Sex Therapy* (eds L. LoPiccolo and J. LoPiccolo), Plenum, New York, pp. 85–102

LoPiccolo, J. (1988) Management of psychogenic erectile failure. In *Contemporary Management of Impotence* (eds E. Tanagho, T. Lue and R. McClure), Williams and Wilkins, Baltimore, pp. 133–146

LoPiccolo, L. and Heiman, J. (1978) Sexual assessment and history interview. In *Handbook of Sex Therapy* (eds L. LoPiccolo and J. LoPiccolo), Plenum, New York, pp. 103–112

LoPiccolo, J. and Steger, J. (1974) The sexual interaction inventory: a new instrument for assessment of sexual dysfunction. *Archives of Sexual Behavior,* **3**, 585–595

Masters, W. H. and Johnson, V. E. (1970) *Human Sexual Inadequacy*. Little Brown, Boston

Melman, A., Tiefer, L. and Pedersen, R. (1988) Evaluation of the first 406 patients in urology department based center for male sexual deviation. *Urology,* **32**, 6–10

Mohr, D. C. and Beutler, L. E. (1990) Erectile dysfunction: a review of diagnostic and treatment procedures. *Clinical Psychology Review,* **10**, 123–150

Schover, L. (1984) *Prime Time: Sexual Health for Men over Fifty*. Holt, New York (for aging couples).

Seagraves, R. T., Schoenberg, H. W., Zarins, C. K. *et al.* (1981) Discrimination of organic versus psychological impotence with the DSFI: a failure to replicate. *Journal of Sexual Marital Therapy,* **7**, 230–238

Spark, R. F., White, R. A. and Connolly, P. B. (1980) Impotence is not always psychogenic. Newer insights into hypothalamic-pituitary-gonadal dysfunction. *Journal of the American Medical Association,* **243**, 750–755

Tanagho, E. A., Lue, T. F. and McClure, R. D. (1988) *Contemporary Management of Impotence and Infertility,* Williams and Wilkins, Baltimore

Zilbergeld, B. (1978) *Male Sexuality*. Bantam Books (for men), New York

Zung, W. (1973) From art to science. The diagnosis and treatment of depression. *Archives of General Psychiatry,* **29**, 328–337

## Appendix 1: Sexual Functioning Questionnaire



Questions 49–60 should *not* be asked in the presence of the partner.

The following set of questions should be administered during the initial intake. If the patient has a sexual partner who accompanies him to the interview, ask the man questions 1–48 in the presence of his partner. Record the male's response as the main response; note the partner's response in the margin of the page.

1. Which best describes your situation in terms of a *full* erection?
   a) never get a full rigid erection
   b) get a full rigid erection in some situations
2. Which best describes your situation in terms of a *partial* erection?
   a) never get at least a partial erection
   b) get a partial erection in some situations
   c) can almost always get at least a partial erection
3. Is this partial erection sufficient for intercourse?
   1 Always 2 Usually 3 Sometimes 4 Rarely 5 Never
4. How would you rate the *best* of the erections you have gotten in the recent past?
   Soft 1 2 3 4 5 Full and rigid
5. How would you rate the *average*, or usual, erections you have gotten in the recent past?
   Soft 1 2 3 4 5 Full and rigid
6. How would you rate the *worst* of the erections you have gotten in the recent past?
   Soft 1 2 3 4 5 Full and rigid
7. Are you ever aware of night-time or early morning erections?
   ____ yes ____ no
   If yes, then ask question 8.
8. How would you rate most of these erections?
   Soft 1 2 3 4 5 Full and rigid
9. Have you noticed a change in the frequency of these night-time or early morning erections?
   ____ yes ____ no
   If yes, then ask question 10.
10. Have they been occurring more often ____ or less often ____? (check one)
    Patient explanation (time course, onset, possible precipitating events, etc.)
11. Have you noticed a change in the firmness of these night-time or early morning erections?
    ____ yes ____ no
    If yes, then ask:
12. Have they become firmer ____ or softer ____? (check one)
    Patient explanation (time course, onset, possible precipitating events, etc.)
13. During sexual intercourse, does the position of your body in any way influence your ability to get an erection? (e.g. man on top, woman on top, standing, etc.)
    1 Always 2 Usually 3 Sometimes 4 Rarely 5 Never
14. Do you engage in female to male oral sex (fellatio)?
    ____ yes ____ no
    If yes, then ask 15–17:
15. During female to male oral sex, how would you rate the *best* of your erections?
    Soft 1 2 3 4 5 Full and rigid
16. During female to male oral sex, how would you rate your *average* erections?
    Soft 1 2 3 4 5 Full and rigid
17. During female to male oral sex, how would you rate the *worst* of your erections?
    Soft 1 2 3 4 5 Full and rigid
18. Do you engage in foreplay other than oral sex?
    ____ yes ____ no
    If yes, then ask 19–21:
19. During foreplay, other than oral sex, how would you rate your *best* erections?
    Soft 1 2 3 4 5 Full and rigid
20. During foreplay, other than oral sex, how would you rate your *average* erections?
    Soft 1 2 3 4 5 Full and rigid
21. During foreplay, other than oral sex, how would you rate your *worst* erections?
    Soft 1 2 3 4 5 Full and rigid
22. Which best describes your current situation?
    a) have never been able to have a full firm erection

b) this is the first episode of having difficulties with erection
c) have had difficulty with erection intermittently over the years

23. Did the start of your current erection problems happen . . .
a) suddenly, with a total loss of erection
b) suddenly, followed by periods of good erections and then becoming a problem again
c) slowly, with a gradual decrease in the firmness of your erection
d) the problem is currently happening intermittently

24. How would you rate your sexual interest; that is, how often do you *feel* an *urge* to have sex? This is different from *thinking* it would be nice to want sex, or that you *should* want sex.
a) never feel an urge
b) rarely feel an urge
c) sometimes feel an urge
d) very often feel an urge

25. In a sexual experience (e.g. oral sex, intercourse, etc.), do you currently ejaculate (climax)?
____ never
____ rarely
____ most of the time
____ always
If yes, then ask 26–28

26. When ejaculation (climax) occurs, how would you rate the *best* of your erections? In other words, during most of your ejaculation, how would you rate your best erections?
1 2 3 4 5
Soft Full and rigid

27. When ejaculation (climax) occurs, how would you rate the *average* of your erections? In other words, during most of your ejaculation, how would you rate your average erections?
1 2 3 4 5
Soft Full and rigid

28. When ejaculation (climax) occurs, how would you rate the *worst* of your erections? In other words, during most of your ejaculation, how would you rate your worst erections?
1 2 3 4 5
Soft Full and rigid

29. Compared to the time before you had problems with erection, the amount of time it takes you to reach orgasm now could best be described as . . .
a) taking much longer than it used to
b) taking slightly longer than it used to
c) same as always
d) slightly faster than it used to
e) much faster than it used to
f) not applicable

30. Compared to the time before you had problems with erection, which best describes the *amount* you *now* ejaculate?
a) much less than it used to be
b) less than it used to be
c) same as always
d) slightly more than it used to be
e) much more than it used to be
f) don't know
g) not applicable

31. During sexual activity, how concerned are you about getting and maintaining an erection? In other words, during the moments of your sexual activity, how much are you thinking about getting and maintaining an erection?
1 2 3 4 5
Very concerned No concern

32. Around the time your erection problems began, did you experience an extremely stressful event? That is, a single event rather than an ongoing stressful situation?
____ yes ____ no
Patient explanation.

33. Around the time your erection problems began, were you under any chronic, long-term stress?
____ yes ____ no
Patient explanation.

## Head injury

34. Have you ever been rendered unconscious by a head injury?
____ yes ____ no
If yes, explain circumstances

35. Have you ever received a concussion from a head injury?
____ yes ____ no
If yes, explain circumstances

36. Have you ever severely injured your head without losing consciousness or receiving a concussion?
____ yes ____ no
If yes, explain circumstances

37. Have you ever lost consciousness without suffering from any type of head injury?
____ yes ____ no
If yes, explain circumstances

38. How many cups of coffee/tea do you drink per day?
____ caffeinated coffee
____ decaffeinated coffee ____ tea

39. At what age did you start to drink coffee/tea?
____.

40. Do you drink or eat any other caffeinated products (e.g. soda, chocolate)?
____ yes ____ no
If yes, number per day ____

41. Do you use any tobacco products?
____ yes ____ no
If yes, cigarrettes ____ packs per day
cigars ____ per day
pipe ____ often
____ occasionally
____ rarely
chew tobacco ____ yes ____ no

42. How often do you drink alcoholic beverages?
a) never
b) once or twice a year
c) once or twice a month
d) every weekend
e) several times a week
f) every day

43. How much do you drink when you drink alcoholic beverages?
a) don't drink
b) 1 drink
c) 2–3 drinks
d) 4–7 drinks
e) 8 or more drinks
f) until 'high' or drunk

44. What is your usual drink?

45. What drugs are you taking, or have taken within the past 12 months? (This includes both prescription *and* over-the-counter drugs)

| *Dates of start/end of regimen* | **drug* | *dosage/ per day* | *reason* |
|---|---|---|---|
| ____ | ____ | ____ | ____ |
| ____ | ____ | ____ | ____ |
| ____ | ____ | ____ | ____ |
| ____ | ____ | ____ | ____ |
| ____ | ____ | ____ | ____ |

46. What drugs were you taking within one year of onset of your problem?

| *Dates of start/end of regimen* | **drug* | *dosage/ per day* | *reason* |
|---|---|---|---|
| ____ | ____ | ____ | ____ |
| ____ | ____ | ____ | ____ |
| ____ | ____ | ____ | ____ |
| ____ | ____ | ____ | ____ |
| ____ | ____ | ____ | ____ |

*If a patient does not know the name of drug, get a description of drug and name of physician, and get a signed release

47. Do you use any street drugs (e.g. heroin, quaaludes, etc.)?
____ yes ____ no
If yes, name of drug and amount

48. Have you, in the past, used any street drugs (e.g. heroin, quaaludes, etc.)?
____ yes ____ no
If yes, name of drug and amount

## The following questions should not be asked in the presence of the partner

49. During sexual activity, how does your partner react to you not getting or maintaining an erection?
1 2 3 4 5
Cold and rejecting — Warm and understanding

50. Since your erection problem began, have you had any sexual activity with somebody other than your usual partner?
Patient explanation
____ yes ____ no
If yes, then ask:

51. Did you have any problems achieving and/or maintaining erections with this partner?

| 1 | 2 | 3 | 4 | 5 |
|---|---|---|---|---|
| Always | Usually | Sometimes | Rarely | Never |

52. On the scale line below, select the number which best describes the degree of happiness, everything considered, of your marriage. The middle point, 'happy', represents the degree of happiness which most people get from marriage, and the scale gradually ranges on one side to those few who experience extreme joy in marriage and on the other side to those few who are very unhappy in marriage.
1 2 3 4 5
Very unhappy — Perfectly happy

53. How aroused are you by looking at your partner in a sexual situation, regardless of the degree of erection?
1 2 3 4 5
Not at all aroused — Very aroused

54. How physically attractive is your partner?
1 2 3 4 5
Not at all attractive — Very attractive

55. How skilled is your partner as a lover?
1 2 3 4 5
Unskilled — Very skilled

56. When you masturbate yourself, how would you rate your erection?

    1 2 3 4 5

    Soft Full and rigid

57. Patient does not masturbate ____ Patient does masturbate ____

58. Have you ever had a sexual experience with another man?

    ____ yes ____ no

59. If yes, is this current? ____ In the past? ____ Does not apply ____

60. Have you ever been aware of being attracted to or aroused by other men?

    ____ yes ____ no

    If yes, current ____, past ____

    Does not apply ____

61. Are there any *fantasies* for which you get better erections than those described above?

    ____ yes ____ no

    If yes, check (√)

    ____ Cross-dressing
    ____ Exhibiting
    ____ Watching other people have sexual activity
    ____ Forcibly having sexual activity with someone
    ____ Displaying some kind of violent behaviour
    ____ Being humiliated sexually
    ____ Humiliating someone else sexually
    ____ Sex with a child
    ____ Sex associated with some particular item of clothing or object
    ____ Sex with a member of your family
    ____ Other (explain)

62. Are there any *activities* for which you get better erection than those described above?

    If yes, check (√)

    ____ Cross-dressing
    ____ Exhibiting
    ____ Watching other people have sexual activity
    ____ Forcibly having sexual activity with someone
    ____ Displaying some kind of violent behaviour
    ____ Being humiliated sexually
    ____ Humiliating someone else sexually
    ____ Sex with a child
    ____ Sex associated with some particular item of clothing or object
    ____ Sex with a member of your family
    ____ Other (explain)

# Appendix 2: Sexual History Form



(Please find the most appropriate response for each question).

1. How frequently do you and your mate have sexual intercourse or activity?
   1) more than once a day
   2) once a day
   3) 3 or 4 times a week
   4) twice a week
   5) once a week
   6) once every two weeks
   7) once a month
   8) less than once a month
   9) not at all
2. How frequently would you like to have sexual intercourse or activity?
   1) more than once a day
   2) once a day
   3) 3 or 4 times a week
   4) twice a week
   5) once a week
   6) once every two weeks
   7) once a month
   8) less than once a month
   9) not at all
3. Who usually initiates having sexual intercourse or activity?
   1) I always do
   2) I usually do
   3) my mate and I each initiate about equally often
   4) my mate usually does
   5) my mate always does
4. Who would you like to have initiate sexual intercourse or activity?
   1) myself, always
   2) myself, usually
   3) my mate and I equally often
   4) my mate, usually
   5) my mate, always
5. How often do you masturbate?
   1) more than once a day
   2) once a day
   3) 3 or 4 times a week
   4) twice a week
   5) once a week
   6) once very two weeks
   7) once a month
   8) less than once a month
   9) not at all
6. For how many years have you and your mate been having sexual intercourse?
   1) less than 6 months
   2) less than 1 year
   3) 1 to 3 years
   4) 4 to 6 years
   5) 7 to 10 years
   6) more than 10 years
7. For how long do you and your mate usually engage in sexual foreplay (kissing, petting, etc.) before having intercourse?
   1) less than 1 minute
   2) 1 to 3 minutes
   3) 4 to 6 minutes
   4) 7 to 10 minutes
   5) 11 to 15 minutes
   6) 16 to 30 minutes
   7) 30 minutes to 1 hour
8. How long does intercourse usually last, from entry of the penis until the male reaches orgasm (climax)?
   1) less than 1 minute
   2) 1 to 2 minutes
   3) 2 to 4 minutes
   4) 4 to 7 minutes
   5) 7 to 10 minutes
   6) 11 to 15 minutes
   7) 15 to 20 minutes
   8) 20 to 30 minutes
   9) more than 30 minutes
9. Overall, how satisfactory to you is your sexual relationship with your mate?
   1) extremely unsatisfactory
   2) moderately unsatisfactory
   3) slightly unsatisfactory
   4) slightly satisfactory
   5) moderately satisfactory
   6) extremely satisfactory
10. Overall, how satisfactory do you think your sexual relationship is to your mate?
    1) extremely unstatisfactory
    2) moderately unsatisfactory
    3) slightly unsatisfactory
    4) slightly satisfactory
    5) moderately satisfactory
    6) extremely satisfactory
11. When your mate makes sexual advances, how do you usually respond?
    1) usually accept with pleasure
    2) accept reluctantly
    3) often refuse
    4) usually refuse
12. If you try, is it possible for you to reach orgasm through masturbation?
    1) nearly always, over 90% of the time
    2) usually, about 75% of the time

3) sometimes, about 50% of the time
4) seldom, about 25% of the time
5) never
6) have never tried to

13. If you try, is it possible for you to reach orgasm through having your genitals caressed by your mate?
    1) nearly always, over 90% of the time
    2) usually, about 75% of the time
    3) sometimes, about 50% of the time
    4) seldom, about 25% of the time
    5) never
    6) have never tried to

14. If you try, is it possible for you to reach orgasm through sexual intercourse?
    1) nearly always, over 90% of the time
    2) usually, about 75% of the time
    3) sometimes, about 50% of the time
    4) seldom, about 25% of the time
    5) never
    6) have never tried to

15. What is your usual reaction to erotic or pornographic materials (pictures, movies, books)?
    1) greatly aroused
    2) somewhat aroused
    3) not aroused
    4) negative – disgusted, repulsed, etc.

16. Does the male have any trouble in getting an erection, before intercourse begins?
    1) never
    2) rarely, less than 10% of the time
    3) seldom, less than 25% of the time
    4) sometimes, 50% of the time
    5) usually, 75% of the time
    6) nearly always, over 90% of the time

17. Does the male have any trouble keeping an erection, once intercourse has begun?
    1) never
    2) rarely, less than 10% of the time
    3) seldom, less than 25% of the time
    4) sometimes, 50% of the time
    5) usually, 75% of the time
    6) nearly always, over 90% of the time

## Women only

18. Can you reach orgasm through stimulation of your genitals by an electric vibrator or any other means such as running water, rubbing with some object, etc.?
    1) nearly always, over 90% of the time
    2) usually, about 75% of the time
    3) sometimes, about 50% of the time
    4) seldom, about 25% of the time
    5) never
    6) have never tried to

19. Can you reach orgasm during sexual intercourse if at the same time your genitals are being caressed (by yourself or your mate or with a vibrator, etc.).
    1) nearly always, over 90% of the time
    2) usually, about 75% of the time
    3) sometimes, about 50% of the time
    4) seldom, about 25% of the time
    5) never
    6) have never tried to

20. When you have sex with your partner, including foreplay and intercourse, do you notice some of these things happening: your breathing and pulse speeding up, wetness in your vagina, pleasurable sensations in your breasts and genitals?
    1) nearly always, over 90% of the time
    2) usually, about 75% of the time
    3) sometimes, about 50% of the time
    4) seldom, about 25% of the time
    5) never

## Men only

21. Do you ever ejaculate (climax) without any pleasurable sensation in your penis?
    1) never
    2) rarely, less than 10% of the time
    3) seldom, less than 25% of the time
    4) sometimes, 50% of the time
    5) usually, 75% of the time
    6) nearly always, over 90% of the time

## All the remaining questions are to be answered by both men and women

22. Does the male ejaculate (climax) without having a full, hard erection?
    1) never
    2) rarely, less than 10% of the time
    3) seldom, less than 25% of the time
    4) sometimes, 50% of the time
    5) usually, 75% of the time
    6) nearly always, over 90% of the time

23. Does the male ever reach orgasm (climax) while he is trying to enter the woman's vagina with his penis?
    1) never
    2) rarely, less than 10% of the time
    3) seldom, less than 25% of the time
    4) sometimes, 50% of the time
    5) usually, 75% of the time
    6) nearly always, over 90% of the time

24. Is the female's vagina so 'dry' or 'tight' that intercourse cannot occur?
    1) never
    2) rarely, less than 10% of the time

3) seldom, less than 25% of the time
4) sometimes, 50% of the time
5) usually, 75% of the time
6) nearly always, over 90% of the time

25. Do you feel pain in your genitals during sexual intercourse?
1) never
2) rarely, less than 10% of the time
3) seldom, less than 25% of the time
4) sometimes, 50% of the time
5) usually, 75% of the time
6) nearly always, over 90% of the time

26. How frequently do you feel sexual *desire*? This feeling may include wanting to have sex, planning to have sex, feeling frustrated due to a lack of sex, etc.
1) more than once a day
2) once a day
3) 3 or 4 times a week
4) twice a week
5) once a week
6) once every two weeks
7) once a month
8) less than once a month
9) not at all

27. When you have sex with your mate, do you feel sexually aroused (i.e. feeling 'turned on', pleasure, excitement)?
1) nearly always, over 90% of the time
2) usually, about 75% of the time
3) sometimes, about 50% of the time
4) seldom, about 25% of the time
5) never

28. When you have sex with your mate, do you have negative emotional reactions, such as fear, disgust, shame or guilt?
1) never
2) rarely, less than 10% of the time
3) seldom, less than 25% of the time
4) sometimes, 50% of the time
5) usually, 75% of the time
6) nearly always, over 90% of the time

# Section Three

# Management of erectile dysfunction

# 14

# Role of sex therapy in the management of erectile dysfunction

**P. Barnes**

This chapter aims to describe one method of behavioural sex therapy used in the management of erectile dysfunction. Other chapters deal with the types of intervention more commonly used by medical practitioners. It should be noted that although this chapter discusses the type of treatment suitable for psychogenic impotence, this method should not be considered as entirely separate or indeed an alternative. These methods can certainly cure the patient with psychologically-induced secondary erectile dysfunction and they can also be used in conjunction with surgical or drug-related intervention.

## Relate

The behavioural modification programme represented below is that used by sex therapists working for Relate, formerly the National Marriage Guidance Council. This is a national organization that operates throughout the UK helping couples and individuals with relationship problems. The sex therapists have all worked as marital counsellors prior to taking the training course in sex therapy. The training and the work are highly regarded and professionally recognized but many therapists work as volunteers. Relate is a charity and its services are offered to the public irrespective of their ability to pay. Most clients, however, make financial contributions to the organization and some will even pay the full market rate for the services received. Approximately 180 therapists work in the UK in 110 Relate centres. The method of treatment used is based loosely on the work of Masters and Johnson (1970) and is most appropriate for couples.

## Brief history of sex therapy

Doctors have been devising methods of treating erectile dysfunction since the 18th century. At the turn of the 20th century Moll and Chanot (Bancroft, 1974) advocated direct behavioural intervention. Although we would see this as very crude by present-day standards, it actually contained the essence of modern behavioural methods. The first half of the 20th century saw psychoanalysis as the most dominating influence. Sexual problems were perceived as a disorder of the personality and so the most suitable form of treatment was Freudian-style psychoanalysis. In the late 1950s and 1960s modern behavioural treatment became established when treatments evolved for specific dysfunctions. 1970 was a crucial year in the development of behavioural therapy when Masters and Johnson published their book *Human Sexual Inadequacy*. Not only did this describe a treatment programme which was a unique combination of behavioural, psychotherapeutic and educational elements, but it also presented follow-up data for at least 5 years. The book was not without its critics but, on the whole, it was accepted and is now the basis of modern sex therapy. Modern therapists mainly adopt a more eclectic approach and Kaplan (1974) in particular emphasized the importance of incorporating behavioural with psychoanalytical principles.

The programme followed by Relate therapists is an eclectic approach but would probably fall between the Masters and Johnson method and the very flexible approach of Kaplan. A lengthy assessment gives the therapist a detailed analysis of the problem and he or she will not offer behavioural modification if a more psychoanalytical mode is indicated. There are many ways of resolving sexual difficulties and for some clients, especially those who are single, counselling, psychotherapy, group therapy or psychoanalysis might be more appropriate.

## Basic principles of behavioural sex therapy

Before discussing the precise details of the programme that a client with sexual difficulties can expect to participate in, it is necessary to look at the basic principles, goals and objectives of the sex therapist. These are as follows:

1. Understanding the nature of the problem.
2. A carefully programmed relearning of sexual behaviour.
3. Removal of anxiety.
4. Teaching communication skills.
5. Redefining success.
6. Permission giving.

## Understanding the nature of the problem

Every patient suffering from erectile dysfunction is different. It is often difficult to dichotomize patients into those with psychogenic impotence and those with organic problems. One can safely say though that, whatever the diagnosis, there will always be *psychological factors* contributing to the problem. In some clients these may be predominant and the dysfunction may date from an early trauma, a period of stress or an early relationship problem. Even where the problem is organic in origin it will have been maintained by psychological factors, for example, performance anxiety, discord in the relationship, self-image and guilt.

> An example of a client whose erectile dysfunction was caused by a psychological trauma was Mr W. He was 40 when he came to the clinic with his partner. He had been impotent since the age of 22. He had had sexual experiences as an adolescent and had had intercourse many times. The trauma occurred when he had intercourse with his girlfriend in the house where he lived with his mother. He didn't realise that his girlfriend was menstruating and the following day his mother presented him with the bloody sheets when he arrived home from work. His mother was obsessed by personal hygiene and it was a relationship ridden with guilt. Mr W's guilty feelings were so intensified from that moment on that he was never able to have a satisfactory sexual relationship.

In addition to assessing the psychological well-being of the client the *behavioural conditions* must be clearly understood. It is essential to gather very specific information about the dysfunction. Each client is unique and will present a different pattern of sexual difficulties as the following examples clearly show.

> Mr A. had intercourse with his wife for 10 years, was celibate for 30 years and was then unable to achieve an erection. Mr B., a 50-year-old virgin, was able to have a firm erection during foreplay but lost it immediately prior to penetration. Mr C. had an erection firm enough for penetration but lost it within a minute of vaginal containment. Mr D. was able to have a firm erection and climax with his girlfriend but not his wife. Mr E. had successful intercourse approximately three times a year when on holiday but did not achieve an erection at other times.

These examples clearly indicate that erectile dysfunction can mean many different things. It is not only sexual behaviour that has to be fully understood, but the therapist needs an understanding of the client's *lifestyle* and the behaviours associated with it. Drugs and alcohol dependency may drastically change a person's sexual behaviour and even sporting activities can affect a person's sexuality. Desai and Gingell (1989) recently reported the case of a man who suffered short term erectile impotence after a 32 km cycle race. It was speculated that dysfunction might be more common in long distance cyclists than is recognized. The possibilities are endless and emphasize the importance of fully understanding the nature of the problem. Some of the above examples also suggest that the sexual dysfunction may be linked to the kind of relationships a man may have.

The nature of the *relationship* plays a key role in the assessment *and* treatment of the client. Not only is it possible that the relationship may be causing the dysfunction, but it may also be the key to successful treatment. Sometimes the problem is created when a man enters into a new relationship or by changes in an existing one.

> Mr A.'s wife had been seriously ill and they had not had intercourse for 30 years. Two years after she died he met another woman who was sexually demanding. However, because he was so conditioned to an absence of sexuality in a relationship he couldn't have an erection. Mr F.'s occasional inability to have an erection caused his wife to become extremely critical and prompted castrating remarks. Eventually he failed to have an erection on all occasions when they tried to make love.

A loving supportive partner is essential to successful treatment. The treatment programme discussed below is for a couple and the female partner has a very active role to play. In addition to being understanding and encouraging she may also be required to play a role that may or may not be natural to her, i.e. the 'femme fatale'. To enable her partner to become aroused she could decide to wear 'sexy' underwear or experiment with sexual practices not tried before, for example, oral sex. Although the sex therapist will give her permission to try out new things and will encourage where appropriate, she will never be forced to do anything she is uncomfortable with. Generally she will be willing to do anything to solve the problem and will undoubtedly enjoy the benefits of an enriched sex life herself. Familiarity with different types of sexual technique will depend on the experiences and sexual education of the couple.

In her efforts to gain a complete understanding of the nature of the problem, its causes and its maintaining factors, the therapist will make a full assessment of the client. This will include the type of *sexual education* he has had. A lack of this could certainly mean that he is ignorant about the actual mechanics of intercourse and could also mean that he is quite fearful of the process. Many boys will learn about reproduction (usually in animals) at school, but it is very unlikely that they will ever have seen a close-up photograph of the vulval area of a woman. Sometimes clients who present with erectile dysfunction have developed fantasies about the vulval area and the vagina. One client imagined the vagina as a huge chasm that would engulf his penis. Another saw it as a wound and associated it with surgery and blood. A third imagined that it was linked with the intestines. In addition to a poor knowledge of anatomy and its consequent fears and fantasies, an inadequate knowledge of techniques can be equally debilitating. Lack of experience and exposure to sexual material may mean that the client's view of sex is confined to intercourse in the missionary position. When problems occur the person with a limited repertoire will have little or no resources to call upon in an attempt to find a solution. The client's knowledge will also influence his expectations.

A client's *expectations* will complete the picture that the therapist has built up about the individual. In our society potency is linked with masculinity and when a man fails to have an erection he begins to feel worthless and helpless. Men have securely tied their self-respect to the upward mobility of their penises and when their penises do not rise to the occasion they no longer feel like men (Zilbergeld, 1978). The men who seek out the help of a sex therapist generally have very high expectations and want nothing less than a very firm erection every time they make love. Anything less will undermine their feelings about their own masculinity. Often they view sexual intercourse as the only way of making love and this ties them into a sexual tyranny. It has been suggested that a belief in sexual intercourse as true sex invites women into sexual submission and men into sexual dominance (Sanders, 1988). If men expect to play a dominant role, failure in bed is perceived as a failure in their relationship and maybe in society as a whole. The female partner who accepts the submissive role will also see her partner as a failure and this will heighten her feelings of discontent and put added pressure on him.

Underlying any treatment programme is the therapist's need to fully understand the problem. If any of the above issues – psychological factors, behavioural conditions, relationship, sexual education and expectations – are omitted from the assessment procedure, diagnosis will be incomplete. Accurate assessment is one of the main goals of any therapist and it will be seen later in the chapter that the Relate therapist adopts a lengthy systematic approach to this task.

## A carefully programmed relearning of sexual behaviour

A couple experiencing sexual difficulties will probably be entrenched in a pattern of sexual activity that ends in failure. Without help it is unlikely that the couple will be able to alter this pattern. Inadequate or inaccurate information will prevent them from establishing an alternative pattern. Behavioural sex therapy aims to provide a structured approach which allows the couple to rebuild their programme of sexual action gradually with the constant guidance and support of the therapist. Although every couple is different and may need to be treated differently, the programme is basically the same for all clients. When they are babies people enjoy the pleasure of touch in an uninhibited way, but as children get older this is often discouraged and by the time they are adults they might be unaware of their own bodies and their sensuality. The programme of sex therapy aims to give adults the opportunity to experience these sensuous feelings again before moving on to more sexual sensations. The process of lovemaking is broken down into many small steps and the couple will master each of these before being directed to move on by the therapist.

## Removal of anxiety

Although some progress has been made in our society towards more free discussion of sexual matters, many myths still abound. Many men and, indeed, women still feel it is the man's responsibility to assume a dominant role and lead the lovemaking. This link between sexual competence and self-image is so powerful that when a man fails to achieve intercourse his feelings of failure are intense and his anxiety level so high that he is likely to abandon sexual activity completely. Sex therapy aims to reduce this anxiety in two ways. The first way is to ban intercourse. The act of lovemaking is broken down into so many small steps that the client knows that he is not going to have to 'go all the way'; indeed it is forbidden. Secondly, because the exercises are shared and the woman plays an equal role in the initiation of their physical relationship, the man does not have to dominate.

### Teaching communication skills

Enhanced communication permeates the entire therapeutic process. The moment the clients enter into a discussion with the therapist they are requested to talk about sexual issues. This normally is a new experience for the clients who will be encouraged to use the correct terminology for their genitals and asked to describe in some detail the nature of their lovemaking. During the exercises the couple will express their dislikes and preferences using body language in addition to verbal signals. The sessions with the therapist also provide an opportunity to improve communication skills: the couple give feedback and share with each other their feelings about the exercises.

### Redefining success

Some men who enter the clinic have unrealistic expectations of treatment. They aspire to the very firm, obtuse angled erections of their youth or they want to have intercourse very frequently. Their expectations may be based on previous experience or on fantasy and myth. Zilbergeld (1978) and Ellis (1958) have written at length to debunk the myth that 'sex equals intercourse'. More recently Bass (1986) discusses the difficulty he has working with the sort of man who pleads with him that he wants 'his penis to work'. Through a form of treatment known as Rational Emotive Therapy, Bass approaches the problem of erectile dysfunction from a more elegant philosophical perspective. His treatment programme is aimed at reducing the amount of client disturbance as well as increasing sexual satisfaction rather than simply helping the client to regain his potency.

Whatever the expectations of the couple, the Relate therapist will work with realistic goals. Bearing in mind their current lifestyle, their commitments and responsibilities, the couple will establish, with the help of the therapist, an appropriate physical relationship to aim for. Therapists must be wary of their own values and there may have to be some compromise. We may judge that a man's aims are unachievable but it may not always be straightforward to convince him of this. Daines (1988) gives examples of the 'unrealistic' expectations of two of his clients. One was a man who complained that he could only have intercourse once in an evening! The other was a man who sought treatment because, after working 14 hours a day, 6 days a week, he sometimes couldn't get an erection!

Through therapy the couple will be able to see that they can have a very pleasurable physical relationship without necessarily having intercourse. An older man may need some counselling to help him come to terms with the fact that his erection will not be the same as it was when he was 19. It will help him when he realizes that other parts of his body have also changed. When a couple is accepted into the treatment and accept the programme, their goals must be realistic so that successful treatment is achievable.

### Permission giving

One of the most valuable roles of the therapist is creating the atmosphere where a couple can talk freely about sex. It is still regarded by many as a taboo subject. The author was reminded of this recently when she visited the library of the British Museum in London to read some journal articles about erectile dysfunction. Because of the nature of the material she was ushered into a special room where the journals had to be read at a special table, closely supervised by a librarian! Although a therapist can give information and permission he or she must be wary of imposing his or her own values on the clients. There will be exceptions but the majority of therapists tend to be white and middle class. Daines observes that marital and sexual therapists often hold the following values:

(a) Sex is a good thing.
(b) Communicating is better than not communicating.
(c) Time should be taken over lovemaking.
(d) Lovemaking can be satisfactory without penetration.

His research has shown that these values are not always shared by working class men and women and by men in general. However, the therapist can encourage the clients to be more open about their sexuality without necessarily sharing their views.

There may be some aspects of their sexuality that the client has felt unable to share with his or her partner. Also the couple may have felt inhibited in their lovemaking because in their sexual development they were told that certain activities were unhygienic or dangerous or distasteful. The therapist will allow the couple to discuss their inhibitions and desires openly and provided the couple are equally motivated they will be encouraged to try out new things. The value of the woman being less inhibited during the treatment programme for erectile dysfunction has already been discussed.

The above represent the principles on which the work of the sex therapists at Relate is based. The following describes the actual procedure by which these are put into effect and gives an indication of what a client approaching Relate could expect.

## Assessment

Careful assessment is one of the main tasks of the therapists working for Relate. Six or seven hours in total are spent on this part of the therapy. Although at this stage the therapist will form an initial hypothesis about the cause of the sexual difficulties, the precise origins of the problem are often unclear and can only be clarified during treatment (Hawton, 1985). The therapist will not know with certainty whether the couple will benefit from sex therapy, but by following a very careful procedure it can be ascertained whether or not the couple is *likely* to benefit.

When a client first contacts Relate it will be emphasized to him that he needs to attend the clinic with a partner. The behavioural sex therapy methods used by Relate are not appropriate for single people and if there is no partner available the client will be referred to a counsellor in Relate or given a modified programme. If the man presenting with erectile dysfunction has a partner, the assessment procedure comprises an initial assessment, a history taking with each partner and a roundtable or feedback session.

## Initial assessment

This normally lasts for an hour during which time the therapist will ask the couple about the sexual difficulty, the length of time it has been present, their relationship (the couple will not always be married), their general health (including the use of alcohol and drugs) and their motivation for wanting to solve the problem. Some couples will only feel motivated to seek out help for a long-standing sexual difficulty when they wish to have children. In the case of erectile dysfunction if the client has not had a full medical examination this will be recommended. Some therapists would refer the client to his general practitioner to be referred on to a specialist whereas others might refer him directly to a urologist. During this initial assessment the therapist will give information about the therapy with the purpose of indicating the commitment the couple will have to make. They will be told that they must carry out their exercises at home on three separate days for at least an hour each time and that they must visit the clinic once a week for a 30–60 minute session. They should expect the programme to continue for an average of 20 weeks or longer if treatment does not go according to plan. The therapist needs to be sure that the couple have the space, the privacy and the time available to embark on the programme.

At this stage the two main contraindications to treatment would be obvious physical reasons for the dysfunction and very serious marital conflict. One would expect a certain amount of disharmony or conflict, especially if the problem has been present for some time, but if the tension in the relationship appears to be the cause rather than the effect of the dysfunction the couple will be advised to have relationship counselling. This can be a very straightforward referral to one of the counsellors in Relate and need not arouse too much anxiety. There is still much information to ascertain before the couple is finally accepted into treatment. If, during this initial assessment the therapist feels they might benefit, she invites them back individually for history taking.

## History taking

The therapist sees each partner for 1.5–2 h and completes a questionnaire as the questions are answered. The couple are seen as individuals in order to create a more confidential atmosphere where the clients can be honest and unembarrassed and to help them accept their own responsibility in the situation. The information that the couple give the therapist about themselves and their perceptions of their partners is very important in terms of evaluating the relationship. How much or how little the couple blame each other for the problem is a measure of how stable the relationship is. Research has shown that happily married men will blame themselves for the dysfunction and their partners will tend to agree (Fichten, Spector and Libman, 1988).

The areas of a client's life that are closely examined are as follows:

1. Early childhood.
2. Family relationships.
3. Sexual development, in particular, traumas.
4. Family attitudes to sex.
5. Adolescent sexual relationships.
6. Adult sexual relationships.
7. General relationship with current partner.
8. Specific details of current sexual behaviour.
9. Sexual fantasies.
10. Perceptions of own and partner's personalities.
11. Goals for treatment.

Discussion of the above can be therapeutic in itself and occasionally will be an end in itself.

> After looking more closely at her marriage one client realised that the sexual problem was only a screen behind which the marriage had broken down and was beyond repair. Mr A. who has been referred to previously, didn't proceed into treatment because the history taking gave him the opportunity to talk about his feelings and release some of the tension that was preventing him from having a satisfactory sex life. His wife had been seriously ill for many years and this had prevented him from having a sexual relationship. She had been dead for 2 years when he came to the clinic but he had never expressed or resolved some of the negative feelings he had towards her. During the history taking he was able to express not only the anger he felt towards her but also that which

he felt towards himself for accepting such an intolerable situation for all those years. Previously his anger had been directed towards his new girlfriend and his penis. He was able to see that his anger belonged elsewhere and his ensuing calmness improved his sexual situation.

The information revealed at these sessions will usually enable the therapist to decide whether or not to offer the couple treatment. The information obviously needs to be formulated into a structure to clarify it for the therapist and for the clients when it is fed back to them. Many therapists use Hawton's method of categorizing the information. He divides the factors creating the problem into three groups.

*Predisposing factors* will relate to childhood. Obviously certain types of family background, for example, repressive, strongly religious and incestuous, will make a person more vulnerable to developing sexual difficulties in later life.

Mr W., mentioned earlier, was the only child of a single parent. The mother was obsessive about hygiene, repressive sexually and produced a very guilty relationship between mother and son. Mr B. was himself a cleric, had been an only child in a family where sex was a taboo subject and had been sent to a boys' boarding school where the headmaster's sexual preferences were of a dubious nature.

*Precipitants* are the events or experiences associated with the initial appearance of the dysfunction. This could be a sexual trauma, or a change of circumstances, for example unemployment, a new partner, infidelity or childbirth.

One client lost interest in sex after bursting a blood vessel in his penis during intercourse. Mr A.'s precipitant was the development of a relationship with a younger, more sexually active woman.

Finally the *maintaining factors* explain why the dysfunction persists. The strongest force which prevents improvement and often causes deterioration is performance anxiety. Whereas a man can accept that his arm may feel weak one particular day and unable to lift something, he cannot accept that his penis might be too weak to perform once in a while. The performance of his penis is very much linked to his emotional wellbeing. In addition, the amount of conflict in the relationship will certainly affect whether or not the problem is maintained. A sympathetic wife who warmly supports her husband and accepts his problem is more likely to encourage improvement than a wife who criticizes him for his inability to have erections and has tantrums claiming that she is being rejected. Restricted foreplay is another reason why erectile functioning cannot be improved without the help of a therapist. Often a man will feel that he should be able to have an erection the minute he decides he is going to have sex and cannot accept that sensuous and arousing caresses might be a necessary prerequisite. Lastly, in this group are strong emotions that impair communication.

Mr W., for example, still, at the age of 40, felt guilty about his mother and his feelings of responsibility weighed heavily on his shoulders. Mr A. was still incredibly angry with his first wife.

If the information acquired in the history takings reveals serious disharmony in the relationship or if it is discovered that one of the partners is having an affair, the couple will be referred for counselling. If it becomes apparent that one of the partners is seriously psychologically disturbed and unlikely to benefit from a programme of behaviour modification, then the person will be referred to a counsellor or a psychotherapist or possibly a psychiatrist. Sometimes the therapist must keep the secret of one of the partners but, despite this, she will give the couple as much information as possible about their problem in the final assessment session – the roundtable session.

### Roundtable session

This session lasts approximately 1 h during which the therapist will tell the couple all that has been learned about them, the families they come from, their problem and its causes. The couple will be encouraged to comment on the therapist's observations. If the couple fulfil the criteria they will be told that behavioural sex therapy could be a helpful form of treatment. The criteria that the therapist will have been looking for are relative stability of the relationship and absence of serious conflict, a clearly defined sexual dysfunction, no deep psychological disturbance, sharing of goals and commitment. The therapist will explain the general principles of sex therapy and will clarify the goals. The couple must accept that they are embarking on a relearning programme and that all instructions must be taken from the therapist and they are not to attempt intercourse until told to do so. If the couple do set unrealistic goals or do not fully understand the time commitment necessary, they will certainly be disappointed.

## Treatment programme

When the couple have all the information, have agreed on objectives and confirmed that they are keen to try the treatment, the therapist will set the first exercises. The treatment programme can be broken down into four stages:

1. Sensate Focus 1.
2. Sensate Focus 2.
3. Sensate Focus (sexual).
4. Specific treatment.

## Sensate Focus 1

Masters and Johnson gave this part of the treatment its name. Kaplan (1976) prefers to call it 'pleasuring' as this is perhaps more decriptive of the activity of the exercises. Whereas Masters and Johnson, Relate therapists and Hawton would prescribe these exercises for all clients with sexual dysfunction, Kaplan uses it only with certain problems. She would, however, employ it with men with erectile dysfunction.

This part of the treatment is intended to give the couple permission to experience pleasure. They are asked to caress, stroke and touch one another in a sensual and not sexual way. Clinical evidence suggests that mutual, gentle, tactile stimulation can enhance the affectionate bond between people. This will create conditions ideal for the elimination of sexual anxiety.

Practically speaking the couple are asked to decide in the clinic when they are going to do the exercises. Some people feel more relaxed in the morning whereas some prefer the evening when all their other responsibilities and chores are out of the way. They also decide which days will be best and they make a mutual commitment. It is very easy for a couple to find distractions in the early days of the programme. This is not necessarily because they lack motivation but because they are generally anxious at the beginning. They also need to decide which room in the house they are going to use. It needs to be warm, comfortable and softly lit. It doesn't have to be in the bedroom where sometimes the bed can be uncomfortable in the physical or emotional sense. If the bedroom has been the scene of many sexual failures it is best to avoid it in the early days of the programme.

The instructions for the first set of exercises are as follows. The couple are told to have a bath or a shower to help them relax and then go to the prepared room where they will carry out their exercises. They will be naked. In the case of erectile dysfunction the man will be told to adopt the passive role first of all. The woman uses his body to get in touch with her own feelings. She can use touch, taste, smell, and she must look at and even listen to his body but she must avoid his genitals. The aim is not to give him pleasure but to explore and become aware of the different sensations, for example, the contrast between hairy and smooth skin. He is instructed to concentrate on his feelings too. They are both advised not to say much to one another in these early stages. After 15 min on his back he turns over on to his stomach for a further 15 min. Then the woman takes on the passive role for 30 min and again the man must not touch her breasts or genitals. The couple are encouraged to experiment and try behaviours that may be unusual for them. Perhaps they will have an urge to tickle their partner or gently slap their more fleshy parts. This exercise takes at least an hour and is repeated twice more on the days agreed at the previous meeting with the therapist. If the couple seem comfortable with this stage they will be encouraged to make some minor variations. The woman may take the passive role first or they might use massage oil or talcum powder to further increase their awareness of their bodies. At the end of each session they must lie quietly in one another's arms.

During the therapy sessions the couple will give feedback to the therapist and to each other. They will be encouraged to give positive reinforcement and to avoid making critical negative comments. Obviously if there is so much negativism as to impede progress the therapist will examine more closely the feelings of the couple. Sensate Focus can often be the catalyst for unspoken conflicts that have not surfaced during history taking.

> Mr W. found this part of the treatment extremely anxiety provoking. The intimacy was so threatening to him that he began to sabotage the programme. He insisted on only doing the exercises twice weekly. Eventually he withdrew from treatment.

When good communication has been established in the therapy room the couple will be permitted to talk to one another during the exercises at home. It should not, however, become a running commentary and the couple should also practise using non-verbal techniques to express their likes and dislikes.

## Sensate Focus 2

Throughout the entire programme the couple must always start with the Sensate Focus, although as they progress into more specific exercises the time spent on this will be less. In this second stage they are allowed to look at each others' genitals but not to stimulate. The goal is one of exploration. In conjunction with this the therapist, with the aid of diagrams and photographs, teaches the couple about the sexual anatomy and the process of arousal and sexual climax. At the end of this stage the couple will have built up a mental picture of their partner's genitals. Sometimes it is appropriate to discuss the effects of ageing; the change in the angle of the erection and the lengthening of the refractory period.

## Sensate Focus (sexual)

Following the preliminaries of the non-genital touching, the couple will begin to include them.

They will be asked not to concentrate on them but to touch them in a gentle, teasing way. The woman, for example, should caress the penis gently and then go back to the thighs or the chest. By this time the couple will be beginning to feel aroused but they should also use this time to make discoveries or confirm knowledge about their own and each others' bodies. In the role of 'femme fatale' this will be the time for the wife to experiment with 'sexy' underwear or new techniques. From the feedback the therapist will learn whether the man is beginning to experience erections or not. When there are indications that the man is relaxed and having erections the couple can move on to the more specific exercise programme.

### Specific treatment

The couple will reach the part of the exercise described in the section above and then they will adopt a new position called the Male Training Position. In this posture the woman stimulates the man to an erection and when this is achieved she ceases the stimulation, lets the erection subside and then repeats the process twice again. The man is encouraged to concentrate on the pleasurable sensations and to use fantasy if this helps. Occasionally clients have had little or no experience of fantasy and if they are interested they will be directed to two books by Nancy Friday: *Men in Love* and *My Secret Garden*. The contrast of erection with flaccidness will enable a man to build up confidence in his sexual performance and at this stage he can relax in the knowledge that he doesn't have to do anything with it. This part of the programme might last 2 or 3 weeks so that the client can feel confident that he is able to have an erection and sustain it.

Following this the next addition to the exercise programme is for the woman to move into the Female Superior Position; kneeling astride, she stimulates her partner's penis. In this position she can put the erect penis into her vagina. She must not move and when the penis becomes flaccid she lifts herself off and restimulates it and repeats it twice more. In the earlier part of the exercise the man will have stimulated the woman in a sexual way so that she will be aroused or may have had an orgasm and will be lubricated when she is in the superior position. For many clients this is a fairly crucial stage of the treatment because this has often been the point at which failure occurred in the past.

> For Mr B. the experience of vaginal containment was so traumatic that at first he couldn't continue. His wife had to make him a cup of tea to help him calm down. He needed to repeat this part of the exercise many times before he could feel relaxed and confident.

Once competence is reached at this stage the woman can begin to move around and stimulate the penis. Ejaculation should occur fairly soon and when this happens the goal has usually been achieved and the treatment programme is over. Most couples will continue to attend the clinic for a few weeks because they will almost certainly want to try out other positions for intercourse.

In addition to the basic programme described above the therapists might employ some additional techniques where indicated. There are three extra tasks and the man might benefit from any one of them and sometimes all three. Those most often used in the treatment of erectile dysfunction are relaxation, self-focus and Kegel exercises. Relaxation therapy will be particularly useful with a tense and anxious client. During the therapy sessions the client will be shown how to contract and relax muscles and how to breathe deeply. Usually information sheets are given or it might be suggested that the client buys a commercially produced relaxation programme on audiotape. Relaxation must be practised at home.

The self-focus programme might be indicated for one or both partners according to information gained at history taking. Awareness of self can be enhanced through a self-focus programme. These exercises are carried out in private and follow a very similar pattern to the Sensate Focus programme. After becoming more aware of their bodies the clients discover the sort of touches they like most. They can then pass on this information to their partners and have a much fuller and more enjoyable sex life. Each week they receive a handout with clear instructions on each exercise.

Thirdly, the man might find Kegel exercises helfpul. Traditionally this is an exercise for women but through flexing and relaxing the muscles in the pelvic area men can also increase awareness and control of their bodies. To stimulate further a man's awareness of himself and his needs Bernie Zilbergeld's book *Men and Sex* is often recommended.

At the end of treatment the couple fill in a questionnaire expressing their thoughts and feelings about the treatment programme. They are also asked to return to the clinic after 3 months when they have had a chance to incorporate their recently learned sexual behaviour into their relationship and lifestyle without the supervision of the therapist.

## Results

Anyone interested in ways of helping clients suffering from erectile dysfunction will be anxious to find a method that is successful. The findings of Relate are very positive. Between 1985 and 1989, Relate therapists saw 4926 clients; 422 (23.1%) presented with secondary erectile failure. As with other sexual dysfunction clinics, Relate reports a high dropout rate. Of the 422 who applied, 252 attended for initial assessment and 156 completed treatment; of those who did so, the majority reported erections sufficient for intercourse on more than 50% of occasions. Most clients who complete the treatment programme achieved their goals and emerged with an enhanced sexual relationship. Most clients also report that their general and sexual communication have improved. Both the exercises and the feedback sessions have given them opportunities and practice in talking to one another.

Relate clinics have a lower percentage of clients presenting with erectile dysfunction than clinics that are attached to hospitals. Relate reports that 23.1% of their clients had secondary impotence whereas Bhugra (1987) reports that 67% of male clients presented with erectile dysfunction at a well known sexual dysfunction clinic linked with a hospital. These were mainly referrals from general practitioners, surgeons and psychiatrists unlike Relate where 30% of the clients are self-referred. Bhugra reports a high drop-out rate: one-third did not attend for the assessment and one-quarter did not continue after assessment. This may reflect poor engagement in the therapeutic process or improvement in some clients after initial contact counselling and recommendation of reading material. Of the 32 who completed treatment, however, only 3 did not improve. Warner, Bancroft *et al.* (1987) report satisfactory results in their clinic in Edinburgh; 87% of their clients showed moderate to good improvement.

## The future

There is increasing evidence that there is a need for medical practitioners and therapists to work together in this field. There is a considerable amount of overlap between psychogenic and biogenic impotence. Kosch, Curry and Kuritzky (1988) report that in a small sample of patients with erectile dysfunction the majority had marital problems, anxiety or depression and the majority showed positive signs of biogenic impotence. The reader must certainly conclude that the behavioural methods described above, with their relearning and educational elements, would complement the medical treatment of sexual dysfunction.

Obviously it is a type of treatment that takes considerable amounts of the professional's time. This works very well at Relate and the waiting lists are not excessively long. Busy medical clinics will not have the time and resources to provide this type of behavioural therapy. Some have therefore devised abbreviated forms of treatment that incorporate some of the principles discussed earlier in this chapter. An example of this is described in a letter to the *British Medical Journal* in 1986 by Deacon and Snaith of the Department of Psychiatry, St James University Hospital, Leeds, where patients are given six or seven 10 min weekly sessions in which they are taught to control their anxiety. They can practise this at home and it can be useful when a cooperative partner is unavailable.

One aspect of the behavioural approach that can never be shortened is the assessment process. Few doctors have time to really explore the nature of the problem. Patients whose relationships have not been assessed are sometimes given papaverine-induced erections. Research has shown that this does not necessarily improve their sex lives and follow-up studies reveal that many of these have intercourse infrequently. General practitioners and urologists could be helped by completing personality and relationship inventories for their patients. Collier, in a study of the use of GRIMS and GRISS inventories, stresses the need for careful psychological assessment and suggests more research could be carried out into referral practices. He also says that penile implant surgery should only be offered after suitable preoperative assessment and counselling. It is important to detect and help those couples where there is a high degree of marital dysfunction and who may in fact *not* benefit from surgical intervention. He quotes the following case:

> Mr X., a 50-year-old Asian banker, attended with his wife, the referral stating that he was impotent and in need of injections. In fact, increasing work was taking him away from home more often and his wife was dissatisfied with the frequency of lovemaking which was now only twice a month. During this he had normal erections and normal sexual function. They were offered marital counselling and happily accepted, stating they wanted no injections. It was concluded that the general practitioner must have misunderstood his request for help.

Medical practitioners cannot be blamed for using physical intervention where it is unnecessary because so often it is the patients who demand certain forms of treatment. Following the publicity about papaverine there was an enormous demand for injections. Naturally, the urologists administering the injections didn't have the time to ascertain whether there were relationship difficulties or emotional problems which might have been treated in some other way. Renshaw (1988) advises doctors not always to accept what the patient desires. The patient might not always be aware of the alternatives. This applies particularly to the older patient who thinks that he wants an implant but could be persuaded that there are more appropriate methods of sexual expression than coitus.

It appears that erectile dysfunction is a problem that is not as clearly defined as once believed. Behavioural therapy as offered by Relate sex therapists is an ideal method of treatment for a couple whose relationship is relatively stable, who are sufficiently motivated, whose medical problems have been treated and who are willing to make available the time necessary for successful treatment. Every day, in all types of agency, professionals are presented with clients and patients who do not completely fit into this category. We all need to develop the types of treatment that we have on offer so that the problem can be addressed as a whole and where possible resources can be pooled. Those with unquestionable physical problems should have the necessary medical intervention with some counselling and re-education, but for others a compromise needs to be found somewhere along the continuum of surgery to psychoanalysis.

## References


Bancroft, J. (1974) Deviant sexual behaviour: modification and assessment. Clarendon Press, Oxford

Bancroft, J. (1983) *Human Sexuality and Its Problems,* Churchill Livingstone, Edinburgh

Bass, B. A. (1986) The elegant solution to the problem of impotence. *Journal of Rational Emotive Therapy,* **4**, 113–118

Belliveau, F. and Richter, L. (1970) *Understanding Human Sexual Inadequacy,* Coronet, London

Bhugra, D. (1987) A retrospective view of a sexual dysfunction clinic. *Sexual and Marital Therapy,* **2**, 73–82

Desai, K. and Gingell, J. C. (1986) Hazards of long distance cycling. *British Medical Journal,* **298**, 1072

Collier, J. L. (1989) Surgical impotence clinics: a preliminary study of the use of GRIMS and GRISS in initial assessment and efficacy of treatment. *Sexual and Marital Therapy,* **4**

Daines, B. (1988) Assumptions and values in sexual and marital therapy. *Sexual and Marital Therapy,* **3**, 149–164

Deacon, V. and Snaith, P. (1986) *British Medical Journal,* **292**

Ellis, A. (1986) Sex without guilt. Kyle Stuart, New York

Fichten, C. S., Spector, I. and Libman, E. (1988) Client attributions for sexual dysfunction. *Journal of Sex and Marital Therapy,* **14**, 208–224

Hawton, K. (1985) *Sex Therapy: A Practical Guide,* Oxford University Press, New York

Kaplan, H. S. (1974) The new sex therapy. Baillière Tindall, London

Kaplan, H. S. (1976) *The Illustrated Manual of Sex Therapy,* Souvenir Press, London

Kosch, S. G., Curry, R. W. and Kuritzky, L. (1988) Evaluation and treatment of impotence: a pragmatic approach addressing organic and psychogenic components. *Family Practice Research Journal,* **7**, 162–174

Masters, W. H. and Johnson, V. E. (1970) *Human Sexual Inadequacy,* Churchill, London

Renshaw, D. C. (1988) Sexual problems in later life: a case of impotence. *Clinical Gerontologist,* **8**, 73–76

Sanders, G. (1988) An invitation to escape sexual tyranny. *Journal of Strategic and Systemic Therapies,* **7**, 23–44

Warner, P., Bancroft, J. and Edinburgh Human Sexuality Group A (1987) A regional clinical service for sexual problems. *Sexual and Marital Therapy,* **14**, 208–244

Zilbergeld, B. (1978) *Men and Sex*, Little Brown, Boston and Fontana, London (1980)


## Recommended reading for clients


Delvin, D. *The Book of Love,* New English Library. An illustrated book on sexual techniques for the inexperienced

Friday, N. *My Secret Garden,* Quartet. The sexual fantasies of women graphically described

Friday, N. *Men in Love,* Arrow. The fantasies and fears of hundreds of men

Inkeles, G. and Todris, M. *The Art of Sensual Massage,* Allen and Unwin

Ward, B. *Sex and Life,* Macdonald. Illustrated and factual book about sex, birth, contraception, etc.

Zilbergeld, B. *Men and Sex,* Fontana. A guide to sexual fulfilment. Fontana

# 15

# Setting up and running a male erectile dysfunction clinic

J. C. Gingell and H. W. Gilbert

## Introduction

It is now within the capability of every urologist to provide a service for men with erectile dysfunction. This was certainly not the case before the discovery of the use of intracorporeal vasoactive agents. However, since the early pioneering work of Virag (1982) and Brindley (1983) the use of intracorporeal papaverine (ICP), papaverine/phentolamine mixtures and, more recently, prostaglandin $E_1$ ($PGE_1$) have been widely reported for both the diagnosis and therapy of impotence. At the present time reports on more than 3000 patients given ICP have been published, almost 4000 patients with the drug combination papaverine/phentolamine and 1284 patients with $PGE_1$ (Juenemann and Alken, 1989). As almost all patients with psychogenic impotence or erectile failure due to neurological causes will respond to ICP; it is a valuable outpatient or office procedure. Those patients with impotence due to a significant vascular aetiology are unlikely to respond and may from a practical point of view be offered the choice between penile prostheses or external suction devices. There is, however, increasing interest in penile revascularization and 'venous leak' surgery which demands more sophisticated investigative modalities for diagnosis. Penile duplex sonography, first described by Lue *et al.* (1985), has been used by Collins and Lewandowski (1987), Desai *et al.* (1987), Mellinger *et al.* (1987) and Benson and Vickers (1989) to evaluate cavernosal arterial blood flow. More recently colour flow Doppler sonography has become available and has significant advantages including superior visualization of the cavernosal arteries in the flaccid state and improved determination of the Doppler angle (Quam *et al.*, 1989; Schwartz *et al.*, 1989; Gilbert and Gingell, 1990). Penile arteriography (Ginestie and Romien, 1978; Gray *et al.*, 1982; Bookstein *et al.*, 1987) is invasive and together with digital subtraction angiography (Nessi *et al.*, 1987) should be confined to those patients likely to be candidates for correctable vascular surgery, e.g. congenital or traumatic arteriovenous fistulae or post-traumatic local vascular injury in younger patients rather than vasculopaths (Bennett *et al.*, 1986; Nelson, 1988).

If a patient has not responded to ICP and has a normal penile arterial inflow, then dynamic cavernosometry/cavernosography needs to be performed in order to detect and assess 'venous leak' (Puyau and Lewis, 1983; Delcour *et al.*, 1986; Lue *et al.*, 1986; Malhotra *et al.*, 1986; Bookstein, 1987; Lewis, 1988). Although the current results of venous leak surgery are not outstanding, there is room for improvement by better patient selection.

The mainstay of initial diagnosis and treatment rests with a detailed medical and sexual history and the response to ICP.

## The clinic

There are, of course, significant and well known differences in urological practice in the USA, the UK and Europe. In the UK almost all practising urologists have a major commitment to the National Health Service (NHS). This entails an enormous clinical workload. How can one justify attracting more work by setting up special clinics within the NHS to investigate and treat male erectile dysfunction? It is not surprising that at the present time in the UK very few urologists are interested in setting up a male erectile dysfunction clinic within the NHS. The general feeling is that the 'floodgates' will open and they will not be able to cope with the demands made upon their services. Certainly patients with erectile dysfunction cannot be integrated into a busy general urological outpatient clinic. Many urologists, however, are able to organize special clinics for stone disease, haematuria, incontinence, prostate cancer, etc. The patient demand is certainly there to establish special clinics for erectile dysfunction. Such clinics are necessary for the education of urological trainees. The opportunity exists for integration with psychosexual counsellors and for interested general practitioners to become involved as clinical assistants. There is also the opportunity of acquiring research monies so that the large clinical database provided by the clinic can be utilized to further our knowledge of the investigation and treatment of erectile dysfunction.

In the UK the opportunity exists for urologists to practise their specialty outside the NHS and hence to undertake 'office urology'. In a postal questionnaire of 1000 German urologists, practising on an outpatient basis, regarding their use of ICP 219, 43.8% used pharmacotherapy for erectile failure on a constant basis (Porst *et al.*, 1988). It is, of course, possible to integrate the investigation and treatment of erectile dysfunction into a general urological practice provided sufficient time is allowed per consultation for a thorough unhurried medical and sexual history to be taken. One must have access to a supply of vasoactive agents and the necessary syringes and needles to inject, to teach self-injection and supply for domestic use. For any one initiating and supervising a self-injection programme it is vital that facilities are available 24 h a day to deal with the potential hazard of prolonged erections.

## The history

Whether one establishes a clinic for the specific evaluation of patients with erectile dysfunction or integrates such patients into a general urological practice, sufficient time must be apportioned to allow the extraction of a comprehensive history. According to Benson (1988), most urologists have a 'gut' feeling as to the direction of future therapy following an initial office visit and although time-consuming, a detailed sexual and medical history directs further investigation. It is therefore important to consider the direction of questioning to establish the likely contributing factors to the patient's problem of erectile dysfunction.

### Medical history

The possible aetiological factors contributing to or directly causing erectile failure are usually obtained from the history. The commonest causes of organic impotence are as follows:

1. Diabetes mellitus.
2. Arterial occlusive disease.
3. Neurological disorders.
4. Disease of the erectile tissue of the penis, e.g. Peyronie's, post-priapism fibrosis.
5. Radical pelvic surgery and trauma.
6. Side effects from certain medications.
7. Chronic disease such as kidney or liver failure.
8. Hormonal abnormalities.
9. Alcoholism and drug abuse.

The cause of impotence in diabetes may be neurogenic, vasculogenic or a combination of these factors. The problem may be contributed to or caused by antihypertensive and diuretic medication. There may be a penile abnormality such as Peyronie's disease or the erectile failure may be entirely psychogenic. The arterial inflow to the penis may be reduced as a result of atheroma affecting the common and internal iliac arteries or occlusion of the pudendal artery itself in Alcock's canal or its small cavernosal and dorsal branches supplying the penis. It is important to ascertain from the history any vascular risk factors including smoking.

A large number of drugs are associated with the side effect of erectile failure. Any drug which has a marked effect on the autonomic nervous system may interfere with erectile function. Antidepressants with anticholinergic actions such as the phenothiazines and tricyclics, and antihypertensives such as beta-blockers, methyldopa and the thiazide diuretics, are perhaps the most common. Drugs with endocrine effects include spironolactone and cimetidine (anti-androgen) and metoclopramide (hyperprolactinaemia). The potential exists for changing medication and favourably influencing the erectile dysfunction.

### Sexual history

The single most important piece of information forthcoming from direct questioning is whether the patient ever perceives the presence of good quality spontaneous nocturnal or morning erections. If they do, no matter how infrequently, then they should respond to ICP. Questioning should be directed to finding out the exact nature of the patient's problem and its duration. Was the onset sudden or gradual? Has there been a significant passage of time without the opportunity of intercourse (widowers)? Are erections obtained but of poor quality and not maintained? Is penetration possible but the erection rapidly lost? Is the problem partner-related? What is the attitude of the partner to the patient's problem? Some urologists consider it important to interview the couple. Most do not consider this necessary but the invitation should be extended to the sexual partner to attend for consultation if the patient thinks that it might help.

## Clinical examination

A general routine physical examination must include an assessment of the cardiovascular system. A neurological examination is not necessary unless indicated by the history. Particular attention should be directed to the genitalia. Careful palpation of the penis may reveal unsuspected nodules of Peyronie's. Testicular size should be evaluated.

## ICP diagnostic test

After completion of the history and physical examination, the opportunity exists to test the patient's response to ICP. The very time-consuming explanation required by urologists in the USA for medicolegal reasons may well defer this to the next office visit as the patient can be given a written comprehensive explanation of the possible complications. My own preference is to test the response to ICP at the first consultation. The dose of vasoactive agent is determined from the likely cause of the erectile dysfunction obtained by the history. Papaverine is generally used in the author's clinic, but the same remarks are appropriate for urologists wishing to use papaverine/phentolamine mixture or $PGE_1$. If the problem is obviously neurogenic or probably psychogenic, a low test dose should be used to minimize the possible complication of a prolonged erection. It should be explained to the patient that the purpose of the injection is to test if the blood flow to the penis can be improved sufficiently to induce an erection, and to emphasize to the patient that only a test dose is being given and that they should not be disappointed if a full erection is not achieved as the potential exists to increase the dose next time if necessary. The patient should be informed that it is not desirable to induce a prolonged erection and that the actual dose given is based on informed guesswork.

### Technique of injection

There is a skill in giving injections and this must not be underestimated, particularly when dealing with the penis. The finest possible needle should be used, i.e. 27SW gauge integral needle with insulin syringes, either 1 ml or 2 ml. The rapid insertion of the needle should be followed by a pause in which the patient can be asked to relax and perhaps expect to experience a transient burning or tingling feeling in the penis when the injection is given. The injection should be made rapidly and the base of the penis compressed between the thumb and finger of the free hand to minimize systemic loss of the vasoactive agent. Firm massage of the shaft of the penis should then be undertaken after withdrawal of the needle and compression over the injection site. It is important that the patient should then be asked to stand and, with the index and middle finger of one hand, digitally compress the dorsal veins of the penis and with the other hand massage the shaft of the penis. As tumescence ensues the patient should be encouraged to contract the perineal musculature so that blood from the crura is pumped into the penis to enhance the effect. Attention to the above details have enabled the successful treatment of patients referred as 'non-responders' when usually the patient has been injected and left horizontal on a couch and the response assessed by the clinician 0.5 h later.

If an erection or good tumescence is obtained, the patient must be given a note with a statement to the effect that if an erection is still present in 6 h time they must contact the urologist without fail. Any urologist undertaking a programme of self-injection therapy must provide fail-safe facilities for patients to contact them if a prolonged erection occurs. It is extremely important to have a ready made-up tray to deal with this eventuality (Table 15.1). The patient is at greatest risk from developing a prolonged erection following the first dose and it is fortunately a rare occurrence in patients established on a self-injection programme. When it does occur under these circumstances it is usually due to the patient not conforming with instructions and overdosing. Any patient living outside a 50 mile radius of the base hospital or clinic is given a typed sheet with detailed instructions of how to deal with a prolonged erection (Figure 15.1).

**Table 15.1 Priapism kit**

1. 60 ml syringe (luer fitting)
2. 1% plain lignocaine 2 ml
3. Normal saline ampoules 10 ml
4. 1 ampoule metaraminol (Aramine) 10 mg/ml
   Use only 0.1 ml = 1 mg diluted to 10 ml with normal saline
5. 19 SW gauge butterfly needle
6. Sterile foil bowl
7. 10 ml and 2 ml syringes
8. 25 gauge needles (orange)
9. Medi-swabs
10. Rubber band or soft catheter and artery forceps

## The second visit

The follow-up visit is just as time-consuming as the first consultation. If the patient responded by producing an erection to ICP at the first visit, it is important to determine for how long the erection persisted. If this was less than 4 h then the dose of vasoactive agent has been established and the patient can be taught to self-inject. Instruction must include how to open the ampoule of vasoactive agent and aspirate the required amount from the ampoule. The patient must be instructed how to hold the penis in such a way that risk of injecting other than into the corpus cavernosum is minimized. Care must be taken to prevent the penis from being twisted with the possibility of injecting into the urethra via the corpus spongiosum or of allowing the glans to retreat inside the foreskin and risk being injected. Before the patient is given a supply of papaverine, needles and syringes and Sterets™ for self-injection, it is important that he signs a consent form for treatment (Figure 15.2). The consent should include a statement to the effect that he understands the risk of prolonged erection, bruising, fibrous nodules, possible loss of effect and infection. They should also be given a chart (Table 15.2) to fill in which details the results of each injection and this has to be returned before a further supply of papaverine is issued. Instructions are given to limit the frequency of injections to once per week for the first month but then twice weekly subsequently if desired. If the patient responded to the first

**If a prolonged erection occurs:**

In the event of an erection persisting beyond 6 h, you should take this form to your local hospital without delay.

*Practical procedure for management*

Insert a 19 SW gauge butterfly needle into one corpus cavernosum using the usual aseptic technique. Preliminary infiltration with a local anaesthetic is not necessary. Take the cap off the luer fitting and let the dark blood gradually trickle out into a sterile foil receiver over a period of 5–10 min. In the meantime, take a 1 ml ampoule of Aramine which contains 10 mg of metaraminol, an alpha-adrenergic agent. Using a 1 ml syringe draw up 0.1 ml (= 1 mg of metaraminol) of the drug and dilute up to the 1 ml mark with sterile normal saline. Also have ready a further 10 ml of normal saline drawn up in another syringe. Once the penis feels easily compressible, place a rubber cuff around its base. Then inject the diluted 1 mg of metaraminol, and immediately follow this through slowly with 10 ml of normal saline, gently massaging the penis at the same time. Release the cuff. Now *aspirate* a further 40–60 ml of blood through the same butterfly using a 60 ml syringe. This should normally succeed in producing detumescence. If not, repeat the above procedure. Failure means priapism and urgent surgical referral for decompression or shunt procedure is required. Once the penis is flaccid, remove the butterfly and apply manual compression with a swab for 1–2 min. No dressing is required. Observe the patient for at least an hour afterwards and discharge if all is well.

**Figure 15.1** Instruction sheet giving details of how to deal with a prolonged erection

I ________________________________________

of ________________________________________

________________________________________

suffer from sexual dysfunction which is preventing me from having normal sexual intercourse. I hereby elect to undertake treatment to alleviate this problem by means of self-administered injection into the penis of papaverine either alone or in combination with phentolamine. I agree to fully comply with the specified instructions, particularly with regard to sterile injection technique, injecting only the designated sites on the penis, and to restrict the frequency and dose of injections as ordered. I understand that there is no long-term knowledge concerning this treatment or of possible side effects resulting from either repeated injection into the penis, or the use of the aforementioned drugs. Although no serious complications have been documented to date, I accept that the risks include (a) prolonged erections (possibly requiring medical or surgical remedy), (b) scarring or deformity of the penis, (c) eventual loss of effect, (d) bruising of the penis, (e) difficulty in ejaculating, (f) infection in the penis. I am aware of alternative methods of treatment for my impotence which have been explained to me by ______________.
I have been instructed in the method of injection and have also had a full opportunity to clarify matters pertaining to this treatment.
I confirm that I have read this consent form prior to signing.

________________________
(PATIENT)

________________________
(WITNESS)

________________________
(DOCTOR)

**Figure 15.2** Consent form for treatment by self-injection. Reproduced from *Controversies and Innovations in Urological Surgery* (1989), Springer Verlag with permission of the publishers

**Table 15.2 Chart to be completed by patient on self-injections of papaverine**

| Date | 1 | 2 | 3 | 4 | 5 | 6 | 7 | 8 | 9 | 10 |
|---|---|---|---|---|---|---|---|---|---|---|
| Duration of erection | | | | | | | | | | |
| Frequency of intercourse (per injection) | | | | | | | | | | |
| Ejaculation (Yes or No) | | | | | | | | | | |
| Frequency of ejaculation (per injection) | | | | | | | | | | |
| Any other comments | | | | | | | | | | |

injection by producing moderate to good tumescence, they can also be taught to self-inject but with a larger dose, i.e. 60 mg papaverine if 30 mg was first used. If the response is better but short of rigidity it is still worth trying self-injection therapy on the basis that the response may be enhanced in the domestic situation. If this is not the case and sufficient rigidity is not achieved for penetration, nothing is lost and the patient can return for further advice. If the patient did not respond to the first injection or produced only minimal tumescence they are extremely unlikely to respond to an increased dose. It is, however, worth trying a larger dose if only to convince the patient that it is not worth pursuing this line of therapy further.

### Papaverine failures

From a practical point of view these patients can be offered a choice between external suction devices and prostheses. It is useful to give them manufacturer's literature and simple review articles to read so that they are better informed regarding the options available to them on their next visit. It is possible to obtain samples of the different suction devices and various prostheses from the manufacturers so that at the next review the choice of treatments can be discussed in some detail. If penile prostheses are chosen, it is important that the sexual partner is also interviewed before proceeding and that they see examples of the range of prostheses available for implantation.

## Conclusion

If ICP can produce an erection then the patient can be taught to perform the injection at home with resumption of sexual intercourse. Almost all patients with psychogenic impotence and those with a neurological cause will respond. If the cause is likely to be vasculogenic, it is still worth trying and only in those failing to respond should it be necessary to proceed to further investigation. The development of successful self-injection programmes with a variety of vasoactive agents has revolutionized the management of impotence and greatly simplified the investigation of erectile failure.

## References

Bennett, A. H., Rivard, D. J., Blanc, R. P. and Moran, M. (1986) Reconstructive surgery for vasculogenic impotence. *Journal of Urology,* **136**, 599–601

Benson, C. B. and Vickers, M. A. (1989) Sexual impotence caused by vascular disease: diagnosis with duplex sonography. *American Journal of Roentgenology,* **153**, 1149–1153

Benson, G. S. (1988) *Office Evaluation of Impotence.* Boston University School of Medicine Department of Urology, Pre-congress clinical Teaching Session, pp. 17–19

Bookstein, J. J. (1987) Cavernosal veno-occlusive insufficiency in male impotence: evaluation of degree and location. *Radiology,* **164**, 175–178

Bookstein, J. J., Valji, K., Parsons, L. and Kessler, W. (1987) Pharmacoarteriography in the evaluation of impotence. *Journal of Urology,* **137**, 133–138

Brindley, G. S. (1983) Cavernosal alpha-blockage: a new technique for investigating and treating erectile impotence. *British Journal of Psychiatry,* **143**, 332–337

Collins, J. P. and Lewandowski, B. J (1987) Experience with intracorporeal injection of papaverine and duplex ultrasound scanning for assessment of arteriogenic impotence. *British Journal of Urology,* **59**, 84–88

Delcour, C., Wespes, E., Vandenbosch, G. *et al.* (1986) Impotence: evaluation with cavernosography. *Radiology,* **161**, 803–806

Desai, K. M., Gingell, J. C., Skidmore, R. and Follett, D. H. (1987) Application of computerised penile arterial waveform analysis in the diagnosis of arteriogenic impotence: an initial study in potent and impotent men. *British Journal of Urology,* **60**, 450–456

Gilbert, H. W. and Gingell, J. C. (1990) The role of colour

Doppler in vasculogenic impotence. *British Journal of Urology* (in press)

Ginestie, J. F. and Romien, A. (1978) *Radiologic Exploration of Impotence,* Nijhoff, Boston

Gray, R. R., Keresteci, A. G., St. Louis, E. L. *et al.* (1982) Investigation of impotence by internal pudendal angiography. *Radiology,* **144**, 773–780

Juenemann, K.-P. and Alken, P. (1989) Pharmacotherapy of erectile dysfunction: a review. *International Journal of Impotence Research,* **1**, 71–93

Lewis, R. W. (1988) Venous surgery for impotence. *Urologic Clinics of North America,* **15**, 115–121

Lue, T. F., Hricak H., Marich, K. W. and Tanagho, E. A. (1985) Evaluation of arteriogenic impotence with intracorporeal injection of papaverine and the duplex ultrasound scanner. *Seminars in Urology,* **3**, 43–48

Lue, T. F., Hricak H., Schmidt, R. A. and Tanagho, E. A. (1986) Functional evaluation of penile veins by cavernosography in papaverine-induced erection. *Journal of Urology,* **135**, 479–482

Malhotra, C. M., Balko, A., Wincze, J. P. *et al.* (1986) Cavernosography in conjunction with artificial erection for the evaluation of venous leak in impotent men. *Radiology,* **161**, 799–802

Mellinger, B. C., Vaughan, E. D. Jr., Thompson, S. L. and Goldstein, M. (1987) Correlation between intracavernous papaverine injection and Doppler analysis in impotent men. *Urology,* **30**, 416–419

Nelson, R. P. (1988). Non-operative management of impotence. *Journal of Urology,* **139**, 2–5

Nessi, R., de Flavus, L., Bellizoni, G. *et al.* (1987) Digital angiography of erectile failure. *British Journal of Urology,* **59**, 584–589

Porst, H., Weller, S., Hermanns, M. and Vahlensieck, W. (1988) Acceptance and side effects of vasoactive drugs in erectile dysfunction: results of an enquiry of over 1000 urologists. In *Proceedings of the Sixth Biennial International Symposium for Corpus Cavernosum Revascularization* (Third Biennial World Meeting on Impotence, Boston), International Society for Impotence Research (ISIR), p. 176

Puyau, F. A. and Lewis, R. W. (1983) Corpus cavernosography: pressure, flow and radiography. *Investigative Radiology,* **18**, 517–522

Quam, J. P., King, B. F., James, E. M. *et al.* (1989) Duplex and color Doppler sonographic evaluation of vasculogenic impotence. *American Journal of Roentgenology,* **153**, 1141–1147

Schwartz, A. N., Wang, K. Y., Mack, L. A. *et al.* (1989) Evaluation of normal erectile function with colour flow Doppler sonography. *American Journal of Roentgenology,* **153**, 1155–1160

Virag, R. (1982) Intracavernous injection of papaverine for erectile failure. *Lancet,* **ii**, 938

# 16

# Medical treatment of erectile dysfunction

R. S. Kirby and I. Eardley

One of the most common questions posed to clinicians by patients suffering from erectile dysfunction is whether there is an oral medication available that they can take to resolve their problem. Notwithstanding the success of intracavernosal pharmacotherapy and prosthetic implants, there is an understandable reluctance on behalf of the patient either to self-inject or to undergo surgery if simple recourse to oral or transcutaneous therapy will achieve the same result. Unfortunately, as yet, there is no universally efficacious oral or transcutaneous therapy with which to treat impotence. However, selected patients may respond to one or more of several agents, the use of which will be reviewed in this chapter.

## Endocrine therapy for impotence

Although in specialist endocrine clinics the incidence of endocrine-related impotence is high, in most general urological units the proportion of patients with remediable endocrine causes for their symptoms is rather less than 10%. Nonetheless these cases will be overlooked unless the relevant screening investigations are performed. Serum testosterone and prolactin levels are important, and in addition luteinizing hormone (LH) and follicle-stimulating hormone (FSH) measurements can be helpful. However, it must be borne in mind that a single LH determination will only have an accuracy of about 50% because of the episodic nature of LH secretion and its short serum half-life (Santen and Bardin, 1973). In addition, testosterone is transported in the serum bound to both albumin and a protein named sex hormone binding globulin (SHBG). Androgen radioimmunoassays measure total serum steroid concentration (i.e. the sum of the free biologically active hormone and the protein bound fraction). In most situations it is not necessary to determine the amount of free hormone, but it must be remembered that low concentrations of SHBG may occur in patients with obesity, hypothyroidism and acromegaly; conversely oestrogens and thyroid hormone both raise SHBG levels. Serum prolactin levels are not usually significantly raised without associated depression of serum testosterone, but the combination of impotence with reduced libido, gynaecomastia and hypogonadism should raise the important suspicion of a prolactin-secreting pituitary tumour (Carter *et al.*, 1978). In fact, many patients with hyperprolactinaemia (verified by thrice-repeated assay of prolactin) are found to be taking medications known to be associated with over-production of prolactin, e.g. oestrogens, phenothiazine, reserpine or methyldopa. The necessary action in these cases is obviously to simply adjust their medication. Only a small number of patients are actually confirmed as having adenomata or microadenomata or the pituitary on computed tomographic scanning and many of these respond to bromocriptine at doses of 5–10 mg per day (Perryman and Thorner, 1981). Referral of these patients to a specialized endocrinological unit is clearly indicated as larger tumours, unresponsive to bromocriptine or causing visual disturbances due to pressure on the optic chiasma, will require surgical ablation.

The most common endocrinological abnormality detected in patients with reduced potency is a reduction in serum testosterone levels. As discussed in Chapter 5 this may be the result of an abnormality of hypothalamic–pituitary function or primary gonadal abnormalities. In the absence of any specific abnormality free testosterone levels tend to decline progressively with age, although SHBG values rise (Vermeulen, Rubens and Verclonck, 1972). The aim of androgen replacement therapy for any of these causes is to maintain serum testosterone within the physiological range. Unmodified crystalline testosterone administered by mouth is rapidly absorbed but is metabolized by the liver; therefore, all orally active agents require chemical modification. Unfortunately these alkylated testosterone compounds still possess the disadvantage of erratic absorption and, moreover, they exhibit significant hepatotoxicity. As a consequence it is mandatory that patients prescribed either methyltestosterone or fluoxymesterone should undergo regular evaluation of hepatic enzyme levels. For this reason parenteral administration of the steroid esterified on the 17β hydroxyl group (i.e. testosterone cypionate or enanthate) is the treatment of choice for replacement therapy in male hypogonadism. Snyder and Lawrence (1980) reported that 200 mg of testosterone enanthate every 2 weeks or 300 mg every 3 weeks appears to be the most effective regime and we have found this satisfactory. If a response is seen with this treatment the effect is usually obvious within the first 4 weeks. If no effect is discernible by this time, there is probably little point in continuing this form of therapy beyond 2–3 months.

As mentioned above, severe hepatoxicity has been seen with oral 17α alkylated androgens, but not with the esterified compounds (Wilson and Griffin, 1982); with either form, however, occasionally hepatomas and bleeding into hepatic cysts have been reported (Shapiro *et al.*, 1977). Paradoxically, large doses of testosterone may exert a feminizing effect. This is the result of peripheral aromatization to oestradiol which may occasionally result in gynaecomastia; as would be expected this effect is more prominent in patients with pre-existing cirrhosis (Griffin and Wilson, 1986). Since prostatic growth is androgen-dependent, benign prostatic enlargement may be accelerated by androgen therapy and patients should be monitored by uroflowmetry and ultrasonic determination of residual urinary volume. In addition, there is at least a theoretical risk of promoting latent prostatic adenocarcinoma and it could be argued that patients should be informed of this and undergo both prostate-specific antigen (PSA) evaluation and transrectal prostatic ultrasound before therapy is commenced.

## Non-endocrine therapy

### Yohimbine

Yohimbine is an indole alkaloid derived from the bark of the yohimbine tree (*Pausinystalia yohimbe*). The drug has long enjoyed the reputation of being an aphrodisiac and has been used in the treatment of sexual difficulties in both sexes. Formerly it was sold as a combination product in association with a variety of compounds including strychnine and testosterone. In this form, known as Afrodex, it was reported to have produced improvement in 80% of 10 000 impotent males treated (Margolis *et al.*, 1971).

More recently several rather more scientific studies have been performed to objectively assess the effect of this medication in the treatment of impotence. Although Lordling (1978) detected no effect of yohimbine when used in combination with testosterone, Morales *et al.* (1987) reported the use of the drug in 100 patients with organic impotence. They noted an overall response rate of 43%, which included 20% patients with a complete response to medication. However, the placebo response rate was also high at 27%. The same group (Reid *et al.*, 1987) also reported the use of yohimbine in a 10-week placebo-controlled study of patients with psychogenic impotence where they observed a 56% overall response rate to the drug. A rather similar study, but using higher doses of yohimbine, was performed by Susset and colleagues (1989) who detected an overall response rate of 34%, including 14% complete responses. In 1989, Riley *et al.* reported the effects of yohimbine in 61 patients. After 8 weeks of treatment 36.7% of men treated with yohimbine at a dose of 5.4 mg t.d.s. reported an improvement compared with only 12.9% treated with placebo. Furthermore, when the treatment was changed to yohimbine for the men who received placebo in the first treatment period the proportion of men reporting good erections increased from 12.9% to 41.9%. Interestingly, no change in early morning erections or spontaneous erections was noted. This is in keeping with the data of Condra *et al.* (1986) who reported that men with organic impotence who respond subjectively to yohimbine may show little or no nocturnal tumescence. They suggested that the drug has a selective effect on sexually stimulated erections.

Side effects in all these studies were minor; however, yohimbine may induce hypertension so that blood pressure monitoring is essential in all patients treated. Panic attacks or, more commonly, a feeling of general unease, may also occur and require cessation of the medication. Rashes and other side effects may occur but are unusual.

The mechanism of action of yohimbine is still incompletely understood. The several different pharmacological effects of the drug have been reviewed by Goldberg and Robertson (1983). They include antagonist at dopamine receptors, inhibition of monoamine oxidase and cholinesterase as well as a local anaesthetic effect and both agonist and antagonist activity at 5-hydroxytryptamine receptors. These actions, however, are present only at high concentrations of the drug and the most important effect in man is undoubtedly antagonism at $\alpha_2$-adrenoceptors (Levin and Robertson, 1983). Human corpus cavernosal tissue has abundant $\alpha_2$-adrenoceptors (Levin and Wein, 1980). Although several α-adrenoceptor blocking agents have been shown to induce erection, the intracavernosal injection of idazoxan, an $\alpha_2$ selective adrenoceptor blocker, failed to induce erection. It follows that the erection-inducing action of adrenoceptor blockers peripherally is mainly an $\alpha_1$ mediated effect. It is unlikely, therefore, that yohimbine promotes erection through a peripheral mechanism.

It is much more probable that yohimbine exerts its beneficial effect on erections through central mechanisms. Through blockade of central $\alpha_2$-adrenoceptors, yohimbine probably produces increased sympathetic drive by increasing noradrenaline release and the firing rate of cells located in the brain noradrenergic nuclei (Cedarbaum and Aghajanian, 1976). Evidence for yohimbine-enhanced sympathetic drive is provided by the finding of increases in plasma free 3-methoxy-4-hydroxy phenylglycol and both anxiety (Charnley and Heninger, 1986) and pressor responses (Charnley, Heninger and Sternberg, 1982) following yohimbine administration in man.

### Isoxsuprine

Beta-adrenergic receptors are also present in corporeal tissue (Levin and Wein, 1980) as well as in the central nervous system and β-blockers are known to cause erectile dysfunction (Papadapoulos, 1980). Beta-receptor agonists, such as isoxsuprine, might therefore be expected to be mildly beneficial in impotent men. Isoxsuprine has been reported to be of value in men who are heavy smokers (Elist, Jarman and Edson, 1984) but there are few properly conducted double blind studies to confirm this. There is also anecdotal evidence that isoxsuprine is of value when used in combination with yohimbine, but again confirmation of the clinical value of this combination awaits rigorous scientific study.

### Nitroglycerine

The erection-inducing qualities of the smooth muscle relaxant papaverine are now well known, but this agent suffers the drawback of the need for intracorporeal injection each time it is used. Moreover, intracorporeal fibrosis may develop after multiple injections, probably because of the acidity of the compound. A transdermally acting smooth muscle relaxant would have obvious advantages and there have been one or two reports of the use of nitroglycerine in this context (Morales, 1986). Nitroglycerine paste was compared with placebo when applied to the shaft of the penis in 30 patients with erectile failure; 26 (85%) developed better quality erections with nitroglycerine than placebo in response to visual erotic stimulae (Morales *et al.*, 1988). Nitroglycerine may induce severe headaches in the user by causing relaxation of cerebral blood vessels; in addition, since it is readily absorbed across mucous membranes, it is perhaps not surprising that there is also a report of it causing reciprocal headaches in the spouse (Talley and Crawley, 1985).

## Conclusions

The bulk of patients with erectile impotence who respond to medical management will require intracorporeal pharmacotherapy with papaverine, phentolamine or prostaglandin $E_1$ and the use of these agents will be discused in detail in the next two chapters. At present we lack really rigorous evidence for the efficacy of any of the orally active agents. However, intramuscular depot testosterone preparations are undoubtedly effective in hypogonadal patients in whom pituitary dysfunction has been excluded. Yohimbine also seems effective in some patients, probably by a central mechanism, and it seems probable that more selective agents acting both centrally and peripherally will be developed in the future. With a potential market of ten million impotent males in the USA alone, there would seem to be ample incentive for the pharmaceutical companies to investigate this area.

## References


Carter, J. N., Tyson, J. E., Tolis, G. *et al.* (1978) Prolactin secreting tumours and hypogonadism in 22 men. *New England Journal of Medicine,* **299**, 847

Cedarbaum, J. M. and Aghajanian, G. K. (1976) Noradrenergic neurones of the locus coeruleus: inhibition of epinephrine and activation by the alpha agonist piperoxane. *Brain Research,* **112**, 413–419

Charnley, D. S. and Heninger, G. R. (1986) Alpha-2 adrenergic and opiate receptor blockage. *Archives of General Psychiatry,* **43**, 1037–1041

Charnley, D. S., Heninger, G. R. and Sternberg, D. E. (1982) Assessment of alpha-2 adrenergic autoregulator function in humans: effects of oral yohimbine. *Life Sciences,* **30**, 2033–2041

Condra, M., Morales, A., Surridge, D. H. *et al.* (1986) The unreliability of nocturnal penile tumescence recording as an outcome measurement in the treatment of organic impotence. *Journal of Urology,* **135**, 280–282

Elist, J., Jarman, W. D. and Edson, M. (1984) Evaluating medical treatment of impotence. *Urology,* **23**, 374

Goldberg, M. R. and Robertson, D. (1983) Yohimbine: a pharmacological probe for study of the alpha-2 receptor. *Pharmacological Reviews,* **35**, 143–180

Griffin, J. E. and Wilson, J. D. (1986) Disorders of the testes and male reproductive tract. In: *Textbook of Endocrinology,* 7th edn (eds J. D. Wilson and D. Foster), W. B. Saunders, Philadelphia, 259–311

Levin, R. M. and Robertson, D. (1983) Yohimbine: a pharmacological probe for study of the alpha-2 receptor. *Pharmacological Reviews,* **35**, 143–180

Levin, R. M. and Wein, A. J. (1980) Adrenergic alpha receptors outnumber beta receptors in human penile corpus cavernosum. *Investigative Urology,* **1**, 199–201

Lordling, D. W. (1978) Impotence: role of drug and hormonal treatment. *Drugs B,* 144

Margolis, R., Prieto, P. Stein, L. and Chinn, S. (1971) Statistical summary of 10 000 male cases using Afrodex in the treatment of impotence. *Current Therapeutic Research,* **13**, 616–622

Morales, A. (1986) Clinical use of systemic erectile agents. *Journal of Urology,* **136**, 233–236

Morales, A., Condra, M., Owen, J. A. *et al.* (1987) Is yohimbine effective in the treatment of organic impotence? Results of a controlled trial. *Journal of Urology,* **137**, 1168–1172

Morales, A., Condra, M., Owen, J. A. *et al.* (1988) Oral and transcutaneous pharmacologic agents for the treatment of impotence. In *Contemporary Management of Impotence and Infertility* (eds E. Tanagho, T. F. Lue and D. R. McClure), Williams and Wilkins, Baltimore, pp. 178–185

Papadopoulos, C. (1980) Cardiovascular drugs and sexuality. *Archives of Internal Medicine,* **140**, 1341

Perryman, R. L. and Thorner, M. U. (1981) The effects of hyperprolactinaemia on sexual and reproductive function in men. *Journal of Andrology,* **5**, 233

Reid, K., Surridge, D. H. C., Morales, A. *et al.* (1987) Double blind trial of yohimbine in the treatment of psychogenic impotence. *Lancet,* **i**, 421–423

Riley, A. J., Goodman, R. E., Kellett, J. M. and Orr, R. (1989) Double blind trial of yohimbine hydrochloride in the treatment of erection inadequacy. *Sexual and Marital Therapy,* **4**, 17–26

Santen, R. J. and Bardin, C. W. (1973) Episodic luteinizing hormone secretion in man: pulse analysis, clinical interpretation, physiological mechanisms. *Journal of Clinical Investigation,* **52**, 2617

Shapiro, P., Ikeda, R. M., Reubren, B. H. *et al.* (1977) Multiple hepatic tumours and petiosis hepatis in Fanconi's anaemia treated with androgens. *American Journal of Diseases of Children,* **131**, 1104

Snyder, D. J. and Lawrence, D. A. (1980) Treatment of male hypogonadism with testosterone enanthate. *Journal of Clinical Endocrinology and Metabolism,* **51**, 1335

Susset, J. G., Tessier, C. D., Winieze, J. *et al.* (1989) Effect of yohimbine hydrochloride on erectile impotence; a double blind study. *Journal of Urology,* **141**, 1360–1363

Talley, J. D. and Crawley, J. S. (1985) Transdermal nitrate, penile erection and spousal headache. *Annals of Internal Medicine,* **103**, 804

Vermeulen, A., Rubens, R. and Verclonck, L. (1972) Testosterone secretion and metabolism in male senescence. *Journal of Clinical Endocrinology and Metabolism,* **34**, 730

Wilson, J. D., Griffin, J. E. (1982) The use and misuse of androgens. *Metabolism*, **29**, 1278

# 17

# Cavernosal pharmacotherapy

C. M. Evans

## Introduction

Cavernosal pharmacotherapy is the treatment of erectile disorders by drugs injected into the corpora cavernosa.

The direct effect of pharmacological agents on the cavernous tissue was noted in 1977 when papaverine was accidentally injected into the cavernous tissue during a surgical shunt for vasculogenic impotence (Michal, Kramer and Pospichal, 1977). This led Virag to study the effect of papaverine on 25 patients with impotence, whilst measuring the intracavernous pressure (ICP) (Virag, 1982). Papaverine in a dose of 80 mg was injected into one corpus and a 21 G plastic cannula was inserted into the other to measure ICP. Under general anaesthesia there was a mean increase of 70 mmHg compared with 40 mmHg under local anaesthesia. The peak effect was obtained within 15–20 min and lasted 10–120 min. Seven of the patients reported improved erections after the procedure. This led to the use of papaverine for the management of impotence. Other workers discussed the value of differing agents, e.g. phenoxybenzamine (Brindley, 1983), phentolamine (Brindley, 1983) which he commenced using at the same time but prior to any publication by Virag, and prostaglandin $E_1$ (Stackl, Hasun and Marberger, 1988).

The mechanism of action of these drugs is not entirely known. Papaverine is a smooth muscle relaxant; phentolamine and phenoxybenzamine produce vasodilatation through α-adrenergic blockade. This produces an increased blood flow in the penis measured by Doppler ultrasound (Zorgniotti and Lefleur, 1985) and also results in a decrease in venous outflow.

There followed a confusion of names and abbreviations to describe the technique: pharmacologically-induced prolonged erection (PIPE) (Virag, 1985a); cavernosal alpha-blockade (CAB) (Brindley, 1983); cavernosal unstriated muscle relaxant injection (CUMRI) (Brindley, 1988); intracavernous pharmacotherapy (ICPT).

## Drugs available

### Phenoxybenzamine and phentolamine

A large oral dose (40–120 mg) of the long-acting α-sympathetic blocker, phenoxybenzamine, was used to prevent penile erection by Wagner and Brindley (1980), but it was noted to cause moderate penile tumescence in two of the three subjects studied. Brindley then injected himself intravenously with 20 mg phentolamine causing penile tumidity lasting 1 h. He then injected 1–40 mg phentolamine into one of his own corpora cavernosa, the latter dose causing a full erection lasting 8 min (Brindley, 1983). The technique was then also tried on a healthy colleague and on 13 patients with either impotence or anorgasmia. Six impotent patients were able to have sexual intercourse and one infertile patient with anorgasmia was made fertile. No short-term side effects were noted. The author considered intracavernosal phenoxybenzamine in the dose of 5 mg to be more useful as the erection caused by phentolamine was inconveniently brief, but he did note that phenoxybenzamine was painful on injection.

### Papaverine

This smooth muscle relaxant which acts as a vasodilator was initially used in a dose of 80 mg (Virag, 1982) but a considerable incidence of prolonged painful erections (15 out of 72 erections, 21%) lasting 6–18 h was noted (Virag, 1985a). A recommended dose of 10–30 mg was used in 11 diabetics (Zorgniotti, 1984) and nine of these, using 30 mg papaverine just prior to coitus, had a satisfactory performance. The tumescence persisted for up to 1 h. No complications were encountered.

### Prostaglandin $E_1$

This is a smooth muscle relaxant which produces vasodilatation and occurs naturally in high concentrations in the seminal fluids. This drug has been injected into the corpora in a dose of 20–40 μg in a series of 210 patients with impotence with a response rate of 68% (Stackl, Hasun and Marberger, 1988). The drug is more painful to inject and the pain persists throughout erection but does not appear to cause prolonged erections as it is rapidly metabolized, probably in the cavernous tissue.

## Drug dosage

Papaverine is still the most commonly used intracorporeal agent. In patients with organic impotence not associated with neuropathy, the recommended starting dose is 30 mg (Zorgniotti, 1984). For those patients with a neurological cause for impotence a very much smaller dose of 10–15 mg is advised as the corporeal tissues are highly sensitive to the drug. Those patients with psychological impotence should also be commenced on a small dose of 15–20 mg. The drug is available in vials of 30 or 60 mg in 2 ml.

Phentolamine is now usually used in conjunction with papaverine in those patients not fully rigid using papaverine in a dose of 60–90 mg. It has a longer action than papaverine and the adjunctive dose varies from 1–5 mg. Its preparation in a combined vial is available through a local hospital pharmacy. It has a shelf-life of 3 months at room temperature.

Prostaglandin $E_1$ is commenced at a starting dose of 20 μg. A dose of 10 μg is advised in patients with neurological impotence. The drug is available in ampoules of 500 μg at a cost of £65.50 per ampoule and preparation of this amount into smaller aliquots of 20 μg is possible (Chouhan, 1989). The vials are stored in a refrigerator and arbitrarily given an expiry date of 3 months, but this is currently under investigation. To administer, 1 ml of sodium chloride is injected into the vial.

It is important to note that none of these agents is licensed for use in impotence. The onus of using these agents is at present entirely on the clinician although this hopefully will be rectified shortly.

Other drugs available for use are ketanserin (Virag, 1985b), thymoxamine, imipramine, naftidrofuryl and verapamil (Brindley, 1986).

## Indications for use (Table 17.1)

### Impotence

Intracavernosal pharmacotherapy is useful in the diagnosis and treatment of impotence.

#### Diagnosis

Although treatment of impotence is sought by the patient, it is advisable to establish a cause. If the arterial blood supply to the penis is not adequate then the relaxation of the smooth muscle by agents causing vasodilatation within the corporeal tissue will not persuade enough arterial blood to get into the tissues to cause a rigid erection. Likewise, if the venous drainage of the corpora is too rapid, full rigidity does not take place. The incorporation of injection of papaverine with dynamic cavernosography is at present used for the diagnosis of venous leakage (Lue and Tanagho, 1987).

#### Treatment

*Neurological*

Those patients with impotence due to neurological problems, e.g. disseminated sclerosis, spinal cord

**Table 17.1 Uses and abuses of intracorporeal drugs**

| *Uses* | *Abuses* |
|---|---|
| Diagnosis:<br>Vascular insufficiency<br>Venous leakage<br>Treatment of impotence:<br>Confidence in single men without partners<br>Short-term therapy in psychogenic impotence, including premature ejaculation<br>Long-term self-injection for organic impotence<br>Treatment of infertility:<br>In anorgasmia<br>In conjunction with electro-ejaculation in paraplegics | Failure to instruct patients in the proper use and complications of the technique<br>Widespread use in men with no erectile problems (as an aphrodisiac)<br>Use by non-medical practitioners<br>Failure of review of patients |

injury, spina bifida, diabetic autonomic neuropathy and lower motor neuropathy following extensive pelvic surgery, are the most responsive to intracavernous papaverine.

*Vascular*
Patients with impotence thought to be mainly due to vascular insufficiency should initially be treated with intracorporeal drugs as surprisingly quite a few will respond, although the rationale for this is not entirely clear. Certainly, the use of prostaglandin $E_1$ in this group has been more than a little effective. The use of more invasive tests for vascular insufficiency is time-consuming and not always available and the patient often wants to get established on treatment. Also, especially in the older population, vascular problems may not be the sole cause and comcomitant psychological problems may compound the problem. Frequently it can be difficult to make an exact diagnosis of the cause of impotence or the problem may be multifactorial.

*Psychological*
Patients with purely psychological impotence, especially primary impotence, respond extremely well to intracorporeal drugs. In 50% of cases they re-establish their own adequate spontaneous erections even after one injection, and most will only need a short course of self-injections to re-establish confidence and thus normal sexual activity. Men with premature ejaculation can also be improved as the erection obtained after intracorporeal papaverine does not necessarily disappear after ejaculation (Zorgniotti and Lefleur, 1985). It is felt by some clinicans that patients with psychological impotence should not be treated by this technique but, again, since this treatment is so effective and psychotherapy so often protracted, the immediate needs of the patient are dealt with. The treatment, however, should not be prolonged and counselling should be provided in addition as problems of the relationship will still be present. If the patient has no partner then a permanent relationship will need to be established once confidence has been gained.

### Peyronie's disease

The presence of fibrosis in the tunica albuginea leads to penile angulation, often painful, which initially causes problems with vaginal penetration and may proceed to impotence. Injection of intracorporeal papaverine will establish with the patient the degree and site of angulation and also the rigidity of erection, especially distally. For those patients with adequate rigidity, spontaneously or at the time of injection, the treatment of severe curvature by penoplication is initially advised. For those with inadequate erections insertion of a penile prosthesis may be offered.

Although it is presumed that intracorporeal therapy would be of no value in patients following removal of a penile implant, it is worth considering as it has been reported to be successful (Zorgniotti and Lefleur, 1985).

## Technique of injection

The treatment of impotence is best undertaken in a clinic which ensures privacy and plenty of time for adequate consultation with the patient.

Before starting intracorporeal drug injection informed consent is essential, highlighting the slight complication risk. Many patients are now aware of the possibility of this technique when attending for the first visit and although apprehensive are willing to start treatment immediately.

The initial injection is given by the clinician. It is advisable to lay the patient supine and to warn him of a tingling sensation during injection. A site 2–4 cm distal to the base of the penis away from the midline anteriorly is selected and cleaned. Using the starting dose of the drug in a 2 ml syringe with a 25 or 26 G needle, the needle is inserted at right angles *into* the cavernosal tissue, avoiding going too far out the other side or into the urethra. The base of the penis is then held to prevent escape of the drug and the area massaged to allow the drug to penetrate the cavernosal tissue. Although recommended by some workers (Zorgniotti and Lefleur, 1985), standing up on this first occasion is not necessary. If standing the patient may feel light-headed if the drug gets into the general circulation. The response to the injection should be assessed 5–10 min later. If there is very little or no response the injection may be repeated after 0.5 h. It may be necessary to increase the dose of the drug stepwise to get an adequate response. A moderate or good response to initial therapy is seen in 70% of all patients. Patients on antihypertensives should be watched carefully after injection. Those patients on anticoagulants should have their prothrombin ratios checked; if it is within therapeutic range the patient can still be given intracorporeal drugs but local pressure should be applied for longer to prevent bruising.

### **Self-injection** (Figures 17.1–17.3)

Most patients who have a good response to intracorporeal drugs will be more than willing to undertake self-injection. It is advisable to have the partner present, especially in those patients with poor coordination (multiple sclerosis), poor eyesight or obesity, as the partner may well be able to inject the drug instead.

The patient is taught, either leaning against the couch or sitting on the edge of a chair, taking his penis in the left hand (if right-handed) firmly behind the glans penis and stretching slightly towards the

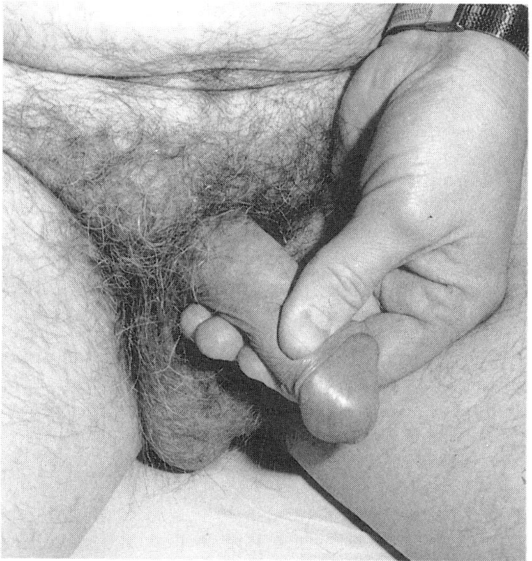

**Figure 17.1** Penis held in left hand, with fingers behind, stretching the penis towards the left leg

left leg (Figure 17.1). The needle is inserted at right angles into the corpus cavernosum anteriorly to the right of the midline about 2 cm from the root of the penis (Figure 17.2). The plunger is pushed in without aspiration, withdrawn smoothly and pressure applied to the area for 1 min (Figure 17.3).

All patients who have intracorporeal injections should be supplied with a typewritten paper advising them that if any full erection lasts more than 4 h following injection they should return to the clinician or local hospital where arrangements for decompression are available.

The frequency of self-injection is dependent on the advice of the clinician but most patients are satisfied with satisfactory sexual activity once every 2 weeks and, at the most, once a week. This will reduce complications. It is also important to advise that if the injection fails it should not be repeated immediately but a period of at least 24 h should intervene. Adjustment of dose should only be made in consultation with the clinician. All patients' techniques should be reviewed after 2–3 months. Routine liver function tests should be performed (Nelson, 1988).

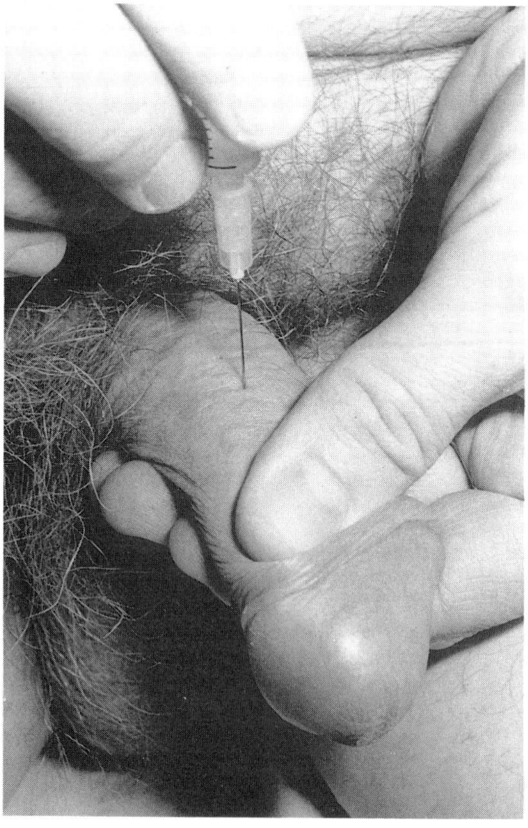

**Figure 17.2** The needle is inserted at right angles into the corpus cavernosum anteriorly to the right of the midline

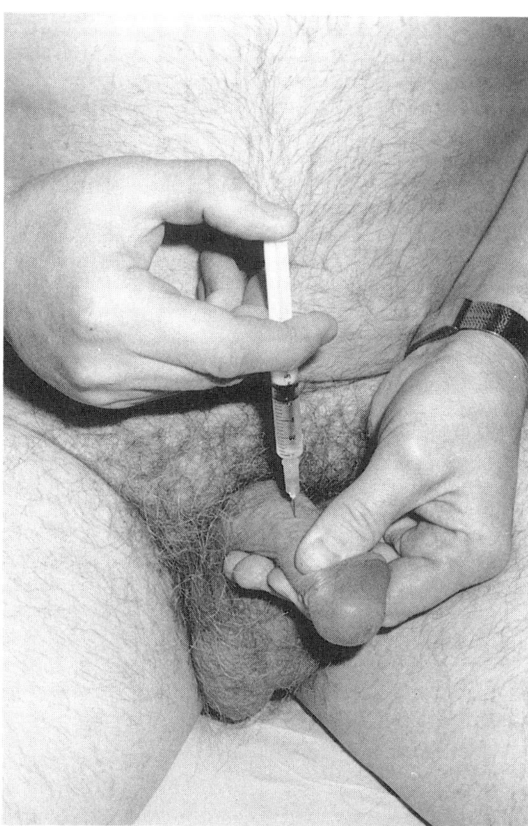

**Figure 17.3** The plunger is pushed in without aspiration

## Complications

### Local

Bruising at the site of injection denotes the needle has been inserted subcutaneously or withdrawn inadvertently during injection. The bruising settles spontaneously. Injection into the corpus spongiosum and urethral bleeding means the needle is incorrectly sited or in too far. In both these situations review of patient technique is required. Occasionally the patient injects into the glans which is painful.

The drug may not be effective; this occurs if compound mixtures which have exceeded their shelf-life are used or prostaglandin $E_1$ has not been adequately shaken with the diluent.

### Priapism/prolonged erection

Prolonged erection after intracorporeal pharmacotherapy was noted by the early workers and was related in part to the initial large doses. There is still a small incidence of prolonged erection of less than 1%. Delay in reporting this complication makes the treatment much more difficult.

The initial treatment if the erection is over 4 h is to insert a 19 G butterfly flushed with heparinized saline into one corpus cavernosum, aspirate and flush the corpora out using manual pressure; a second butterfly is sometimes needed into the other corpus. This will deflate the erection and usually nothing else is required. If, however, deflation fails to take place or if the penis becomes rigid again the procedure can be repeated and metaraminol (a sympathomimetic drug) in a dose of 1 mg inserted and massaged (Brindley, 1984). In order to prevent this drug entering the general circulation and causing potentially hazardous hypertension, a tourniquet can be placed around the base of the penis. Since this procedure can be most uncomfortable, some form of regional anaesthesia at least is advisable. Phenylephrine, noradrenaline or adrenaline can be used instead of metaraminol.

Failure to treat this complication properly will lead to thrombosis and fibrosis of the corpora and permanent impotence. Penile prostheses are not as easy to insert in patients with marked corporeal fibrosis.

### Fibrosis

Significant pathological changes were noted to occur in monkeys given 100 injections of papaverine over a year. Fibrosis at the injection site and hypertrophy of the smooth muscle occurred (Abozeid *et al.*, 1987). Since the fibrosis could occur even after one injection it was felt that this complication arose, not just from the needling itself, but from the irritant properties of papaverine, possibly the low pH. This led to the questioning of the use of these agents on a long-term basis, especially in those patients with impotence of a purely psychological nature. The incidence of this complication will be less if the patient self-injects less frequently. It also means that careful patient selection is necessary (Benson, 1987). However, if patients are aware of the problem and report early when it occurs, they can be considered for a penile prosthesis.

### General

Drugs injected into the corpora usually cause no general systemic effects. However, patients will complain occasionally of facial flushing and light-headedness associated with a drop in blood pressure, indicating the drug has entered the systemic circulation. This side effect responds to lying the patient supine and also to atropine. It may indicate that the patient has venous leakage.

Liver function problems have been recorded but are reversible when the drug is stopped (Nelson, 1987).

### Failure to respond

Some patients after many months may find that the drug in the recommended dose is less effective. It is possible that tolerance develops due to secondary depletion of neurotransmitters available in the corporeal tissue (Nelson, 1988). Increasing the dose, using combined agents such as papaverine and phentolamine, or even changing to another agent, e.g. prostaglandin $E_1$, may be efficacious.

Some patients can become disenchanted with long-term injection, finding the technique artificial, lacking in spontaneity and time-consuming.

## The future

There is no doubt that intracorporeal pharmacotherapy has revolutionized the management of impotence and made treatment of this desperately troublesome condition available on a widespread basis. There are still, however, many patients reluctant or embarrassed to present themselves. A good response to treatment is seen in 70% of patients, 50% of whom will embark successfully and remain on self-injection for months, even up to 4 years (Brindley, 1988). Of these a proportion may grow weary of injection, develop fibrosis or fail to respond. For these patients additional treatment in the form of either a penile prosthesis or an external appliance or even nothing further will be considered. The fact they have had intracorporeal drugs does not preclude them from further treatment and; in the meantime, has allowed them to enjoy a satisfactory sexual life using their own erectile mechanism for as long as possible. There is no reason why any impotent male should not be treated by intracorporeal drugs.

## References

Abozeid, M., Juenemann, K. P., Luo, J. A. *et al.* (1987) Chronic papaverine treatment. The effect of repeated injections on the simian erectile response and penile tissue. *Journal of Urology,* **138**, 1263–1266

Benson, G. S. (1987) Intracavernosal injection therapy for impotence. *Journal of Urology,* **138**, 1262

Brindley, G. S. (1983) Cavernosal alpha blockade. A new treatment for investigation and treating erectile impotence. *British Journal of Psychiatry,* **143**, 332–337

Brindley, G. S. (1984) New treatment for priapism. *Lancet,* **ii**, 220–221

Brindley, G. S. (1986) Pilot experiments on the actions of drugs injected into the human corpus cavernosum penis. *British Journal of Pharmacology,* **87**, 495–500

Brindley, G. S. (1988) Treatment of erectile impotence by intracorporeal injection. *British Journal of Sexual Medicine,* **15**, 20–24

Chouhan, M. (1989) Preparation of alprostadil for male impotence. *Pharmaceutical Journal,* **243**, 36

Lue, T. F. M. and Tanagho, E. A. (1987) Physiology of erection and pharmacological management of impotence. *Journal of Urology,* **137**, 829–836

Michal, V., Kramer, R. and Pospichal, J. (1977) Arterial epigastrico-cavernous anastomosis for the treatment of sexual impotence. *World Journal of Surgery,* **1**, 515–520

Nelson, R. P. (1987) Pathophysiology, diagnosis and management of erectile dysfunction. In *Urology Annual,* Vol. 1 (ed. S. Rous), Appleton and Lange, Norwalk, Conneticut, pp. 139–169

Nelson, R. P. (1988) Non-operative management of impotence. *Journal of Urology,* **139**, 2–5

Stackl, N., Hasun, R. and Marberger, M. (1988) Intracavernous injection of prostaglandin $E_1$ in impotent men. *Journal of Urology,* **140**, 66–68

Virag, R. (1982) Intracavernous injection of papaverine for erectile failure. *Lancet,* **ii**, 938

Virag, R. (1985a) About pharmacologically induced prolonged erection. *Lancet,* **ii**, 519–520

Virag, R. (1985b) Du bon usage de la papaverine intra-cavernous et d'autres drogues vasoactives dans la traitment de l'impuissance. *Gazette Medicale,* **92**, 19–24

Wagner, G. and Brindley, G. S. (1980) The effect of atropine, alpha and beta blockers on human penile erection; a controlled pilot study. In *Vasculogenic Impotence* (eds A. Zorgniotti and G. Rossi), Charles C. Thomas, Springfield, Illinois, pp. 77–82

Zorgniotti, A. W. (1984) Self-administered intracavernous injection of a vasoactive drug for impotence in diabetics. *Journal of Urology,* **131**

Zorgniotti, A. W. and Lefleur, R. S. (1985) Auto-injection of the corpus cavernosum with vasoactive drug. Combination for vasculogenic impotence. *Journal of Urology,* **133**, 39–41

# 18

# External appliances

R. Witherington

## Introduction

In recent years, high sexual expectations and an ageing world population have caused an immense upsurge of interest in the management of erectile impotence. Medications including hormones, yohimbine and intracavernosally injected vasoactive drugs are often quite effective and penile implants have generally met with remarkable success. Additionally, a variety of vascular surgical procedures are of benefit to a subset of the impotent population. However, a reversible non-invasive form of treatment for this troublesome affliction appears ideal. A quest for the latter has resulted in the development of some ingenious mechanical devices. Some have been quite effective but many have been cumbersome and less than satifactory.

Since the beginning of time man has tried to combat impotence with a variety of external mechanical aids. Prior to the development of satisfactory internally positioned penile prostheses and intracavernosal pharmacological therapy, external penile splints were frequently employed and one marketed by the now defunct Fre-San Company was quite popular. Placement of a constriction band around the base of the penis to help maintain or enhance an erection has been used by men for as many years as elastic materials have existed. The use of negative pressure devices to produce penile tumescence which could then be maintained by a compression band placed around the base of the penis is far from a new idea. Indeed, since 1917 the United States Patent Office has issued several patents to inventors of such negative pressure devices (Witherington, 1988). About 1960, Osbon developed a vacuum tumescence device which he personally used for more than 20 years. His prototype system utilized mouth suction to achieve vacuum and large rubber bands to accomplish tension. This device was made commercially available many years ago and has since been marketed under several names. Originally called the Youth Equivalent Device, the name was later changed to the Vita-Life System, then the Sta-Potent System and more recently the ErecAid System. The newer systems have incorporated a negative pressure pump to achieve vacuum. Additionally, more sophisticated and aesthetically pleasing tension bands have been made a part of the newer negative pressure systems. Osbon's system was patented in 1983 and, since then, at least nine other negative pressure plus tension band devices have been patented and made available commercially.

Use of external penile appliances has gained the acceptance of the medical community only in recent years and currently several are commercially available. Features incorporated into these devices include an external splinting effect, negative pressure (vacuum), and tension (constriction). Using these features, currently available external devices can be divided into three types. Each basic system will be described.

## External mechanical devices currently available (Table 18.1)

### The tension band

These simple systems utilize tension (constriction) only. Several devices, including the ERU-1, Restore, Revive and StayErec Systems consist of a loading cone, sleeve and tension band (Figure 18.1). The cone permits easy placement of the band onto the sleeve. Once the sleeve is loaded, it is placed around the penis where the tension band is then guided proximally to encircle and compress the base of the penis. Simple tension bands without the loading cone and sleeve, such as the Confidence Ring and Barretta Laso, are also available. Repeated manual compression of the perineum can be used to force blood into the erectile tissue distal to the point of constriction in order to enhance tumescence. After adequate penile rigidity is achieved, sexual intercourse can be accomplished. The re-useable tension band is then removed and it is important that it not be left on the penis for more than 30 min. When the tension band is on the penis,

**Table 18.1 External devices for management of impotence in USA (1990)**

| *Name* | *Distributor* | *Features* | | | | |
|---|---|---|---|---|---|---|
| | | *Negative pressure* | *Tension band* | *Splint effect* | *Loading cone* | *Pressure limiting valve* |
| Confidence Ring | Performance medical | – | + | – | – | – |
| ERU-1 System | Encore Medical Products Inc. | – | + | – | + | – |
| Barretta Laso | Barretta Products | – | + | – | – | – |
| Restore System | Mentor Corporation | – | + | – | + | – |
| Revive System | Revive System Corporation | – | + | – | + | – |
| StayErec System | Osbon Medical Systems Ltd | – | + | – | + | – |
| Synergist Erection System | Synergist Ltd | + | – | + | – | – |
| Better Erection System | Potency Inc. | + | + | – | + | + |
| Catalyst Vacuum System | Dacomed Corporation | + | + | – | – | – |
| VTU-1 System | Encore Medical Products Inc. | + | + | – | + | + |
| ErecAid System | Osbon Medical Systems Ltd | + | + | – | – | – |
| Erection Inducer Device | Performance Medical | + | + | – | – | – |
| Pos-T-Vac System | Pos-T-Vac Inc. | + | + | – | + | + |
| Response Piston System | Mentor Coporation | + | + | – | + | + |
| Response System | Mentor Corporation | + | + | – | + | + |
| Touch System | Mentor Corporation | + | + | – | + | + |
| Vacuum Erection Device | Mission Pharmaceutical Co. | + | + | – | – | + |
| ErecTek | Surgitek | + | + | – | + | + |

it compresses the urethra and usually prevents forward ejaculation. This trapping of ejaculate may produce distension of the bulbous urethra which can be painful. Use of a simple tension band appears to be of most benefit in the management of mild partial impotence where it can potentially upgrade an inadequate erection to one that may allow satisfactory intercourse. These devices are intended for use by men with inadequate erections who need or desire erectile augmentation.

## External splint plus negative pressure

Presently, only a single device of this sort is commercially available (Figure 18.2). This Synergist Erection System is available from Synergist Limited, Houston, Texas, USA. Many sizes are available and each patient must be measured to obtain a proper fit. Composed of soft silicone and shaped like a condom, this device is rigid enough to allow vaginal penetration. A small tube with an attached vacu-lock valve is connected to it that permits air to be evacuated from its interior. The undersurface of the distal end of the sheath is thinned out to improve sensitivity. To use it, water-soluble lubricant is placed inside the device and over the entire penis. The penis is placed at the base of the device and suction applied to the tube. Negative pressure pulls the flaccid penis into the device and simultaneously produces tumescence. After the penis has expanded to fill the sheath, the thin proximal collar is unfolded toward the base of the penis to improve seal and reduce the chance of losing vacuum. The suction tube is occluded to retain vacuum by closing the vacu-lock and then wrapped around the base of the device to get it out of the way. When properly positioned, the penis should feel stretched and be slightly tight, a state that resembles a normal erection. Tumescence is maintained as long as the device is worn. Intercourse is accomplished following application of water soluble lubricant to the exterior of the device. Following intercourse, the vacu-lock valve is opened to release the vacuum. The device can then be removed, cleaned and stored according to distributor's instructions. This system can be used by any impotent man and because of its external splinting feature, it may be of significant benefit in the management of total impotence. Osopa and Williams (1989), in a study on 20 unselected patients, concluded that the device was a useful, non-invasive alternative for the treatment of impotence in well selected, motivated patients and their partners.

Possible adverse effects from use of this device are vaginal discomfort, penile irritation and penile enlargement. Vaginal discomfort is usually avoidable by adequate lubrication of the outside of the device prior to intercourse. Penile irritation can appear as redness, swelling and occasionally small blisters at either the base or head of the penis and it usually subsides by giving the penis a rest. Associated penile enlargement can occur when the device is either worn for protracted periods of time or frequently used. Fortunately, cessation of repetitive use will usually resolve this problem.

Potential added benefits from use of the Synergist Erection System include a diminished likelihood of transmission of sexually transmitted diseases and a markedly reduced possibility of impregnation of the sexual partner.

## The negative pressure plus tension band devices

At least 11 devices of this sort are now commercially available in the USA and each incorporates both vacuum and tension. The basic components of each system include a vacuum chamber, negative pressure pump and tension band. A typical device is

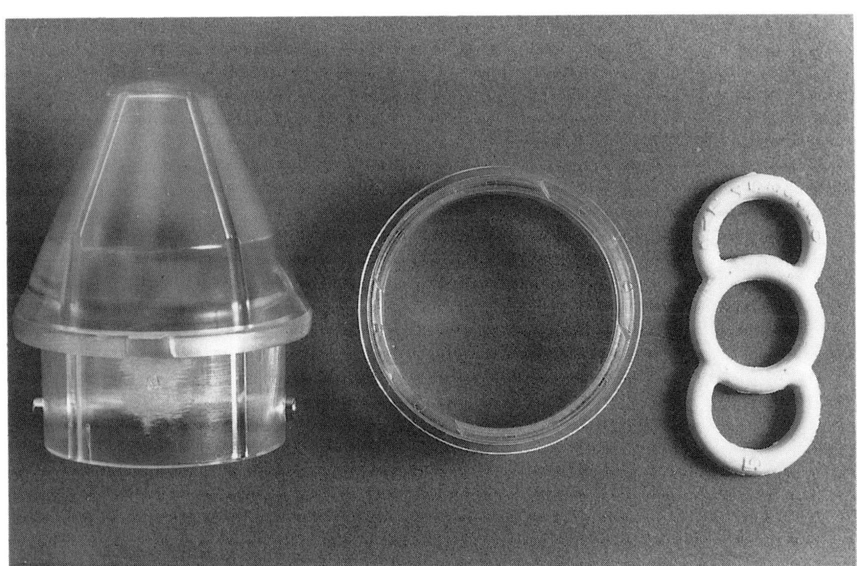

**Figure 18.1** Revive System. The cone (left) is used to load the tension band (right) onto the sleeve (centre). The loaded sleeve can then be placed around the base of the penis where the band can be easily transferred to produce compression

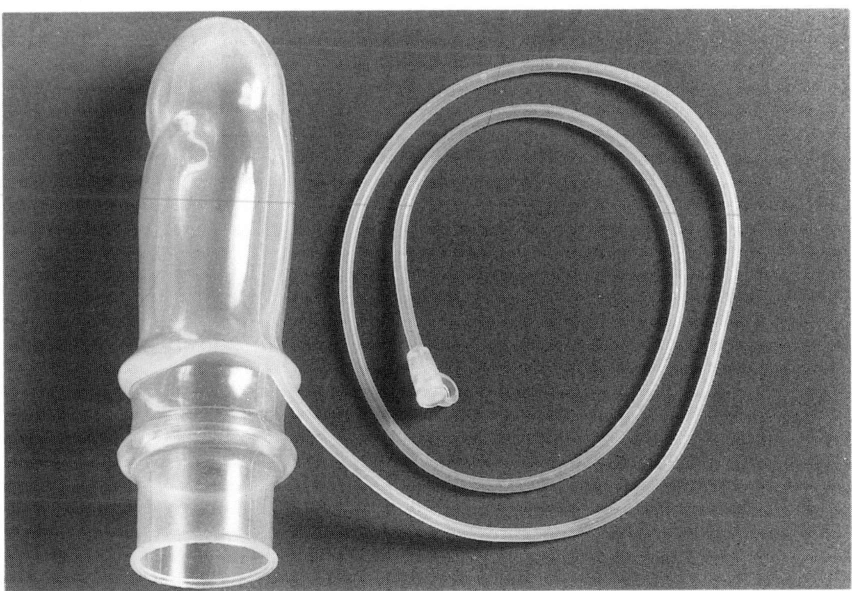

**Figure 18.2** Synergist Erection System. Note the tube used to evacuate air from the device interior during placement over the penis

shown in Figure 18.3. Prior to use, a correct fit of vacuum chamber to penis is obtained by placement of a proper size adapter sleeve or insert into the base of the chamber. A snug fit significantly lessens the chance of pulling scrotal tissue into the device when vacuum is applied. A proper tension band is then placed around the base of the chamber. In order to use the system, water-soluble lubricant is applied to the inside of the open end of the chamber and to the entire penis. The vaccum chamber is placed over the flaccid penis and an air-tight seal obtained (Figure 18.4a). By activating the pump, negative pressure is created within the vacuum chamber which draws blood into the penis to produce either erectile augmentation or an erection-like state (Figure 18.4b). When adequate tumescence is achieved, the tension band is guided from the chamber to the base of the penis where it produces penile compression and entrapment of blood. Vacuum is then released and the chamber removed (Figure 18.4c). If there is significant loss of tumescence during this step, the vaccum chamber can be repositioned over the penis and negative pressure again applied while the previously placed tension band encircles the base of the penis. Adequate sustained rigidity can nearly always be achieved by this simple manoeuvre. The erection-like state is maintained long enough to permit intercourse and it is recommended that the tension band be left on the penis no longer than 30 min. If a longer period of penile rigidity should be required, the band can be removed for a few mionutes to give the penis a rest and repeat tumescence achieved. Following use, the device should be cleaned and stored according to distributor's instructions.

The tension band usually prevents normal antegrade ejaculation which may allow sudden, painful distension of the bulbous urethra. However, painful ejaculation is seldom described. In men with complete impotence, tumescence is achieved only distal to the point of tension which may allow the penis to pivot at its base. This lack of proximal physioanatomical fixation may prevent some users from achieving vaginal intromission. However, despite this lack of proximal rigidity, the majority of men are able to use the devices successfully.

## Results achieved with external devices

Differences between a normal erection and the erection-like state obtained by use of these negative pressure plus tension band devices have been well described by Nadig, Ware and Blumoff (1986) in a study involving 35 men with organic impotence.

1. Blood flow into the penis decreases while the tension band is in place.
2. The penile skin temperature drops approximately 1°C as a result of decreased arterial blood flow.
3. Congestion of extracorporeal penile tissue occurs, resulting in distension of superficial veins and cyanosis of the penis. Additionally, these

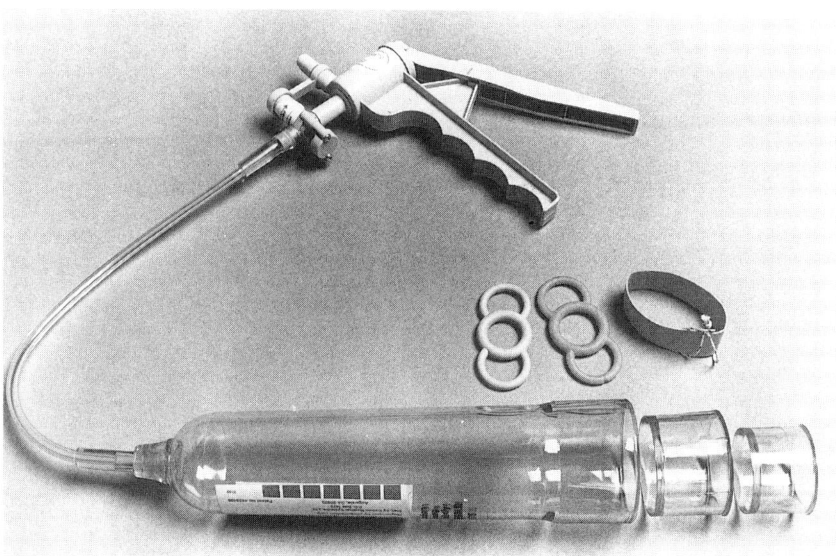

**Figure 18.3** Typical negative pressure/tension band system. The tube connects the vaccum chamber to the pump. Note the adapter sleeves or inserts at the base of the chamber and variety of tension bands

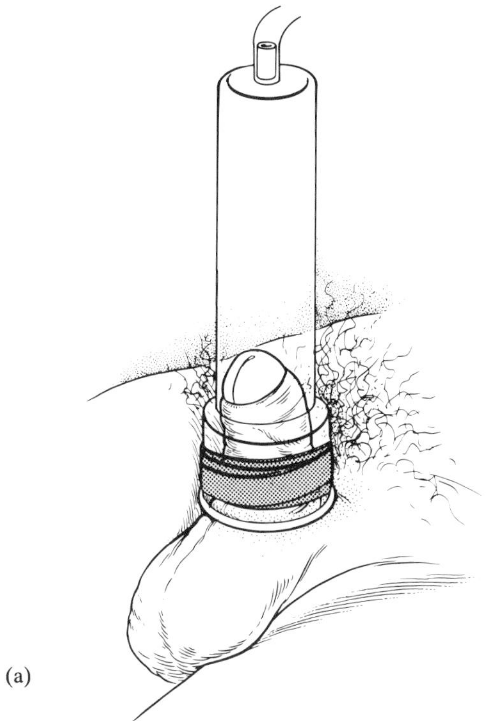
(a)

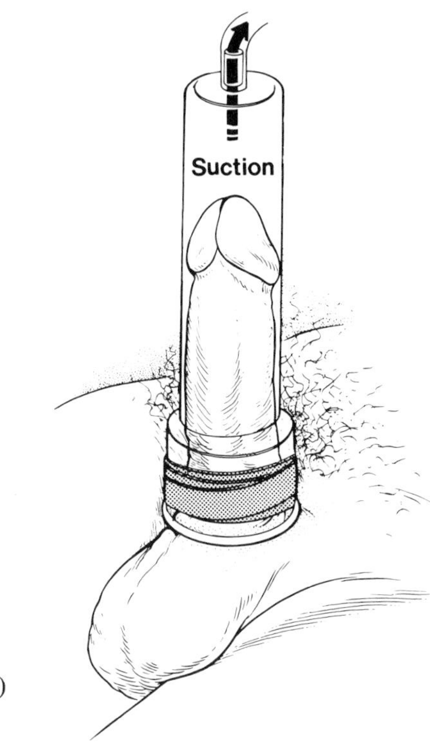

(b)

authors observed that penile circumference increased more when this device was used (mean = 4.3 cm) than during normal erections (mean = 2.8 cm).
4. The penis is rigid only distal to the tension band and thus the penis may pivot at its base.
5. Ejaculate is trapped in the proximal urethra until the tension band is removed.

Despite the aforementioned, these authors found that only a third of sexual partners noted coldness of the penis. Additionally, no user in their study complained of painful ejaculation and pivoting of the penis rarely interfered with intercourse. An erection-like state was achieved in 32 (91%) patients and 27 (77%) achieved a penile longitudinal rigidity of over 454 g buckling force, the minimum criterion for adequate rigidity used by many sleep laboratories. Five men with apparent full erections had penile longitudinal rigidity of less than 454 g buckling force. Despite this, four of these five subjects used the device successfully and regularly. The subjects required 3–7 min in the vacuum chamber for attainment of maximum rigidity with negative pressures ranging from 175 to 380 mmHg. Development of penile discomfort at the time of negative pressure application varied from subject to subject and was noted with pressures that ranged from a low

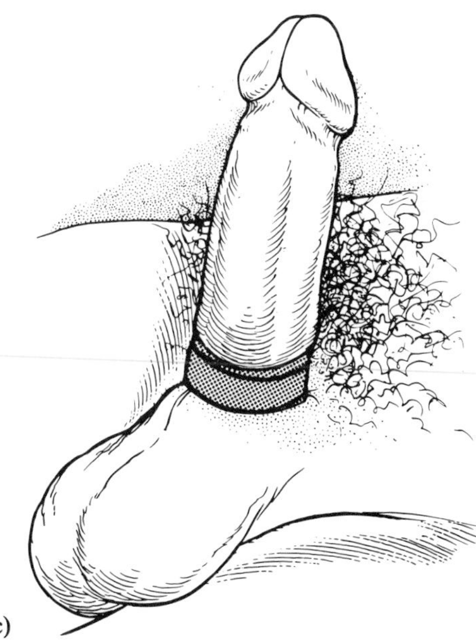
(c)

**Figure 18.4** (a) Negative pressure chamber placed over penis; (b) vacuum pulls blood into penis to produce tumescence; (c) tension band transferred from chamber to base of penis. Entrapment of blood occurs, which maintains erection-like state. Reproduced from Witherington (1987) with permission

of 150 mmHg to over 300 mmHg. Petechiae developed on the penile skin in eight of their subjects. These petechiae were painless, required no treatment, and resolved spontaneoulsy. No significant change in the penile brachial index was noted in a subgroup of nine individuals who were tested before and after use of the device. Twenty-four (69%) of their subjects were satisfied with the device and continued to use it regularly at the time of their report.

Impressive results from use of these devices have been reported by others also (Wiles, 1988; Witherington, 1987, 1988, 1989, 1990a). Osbon Medical Systems has surveyed well over 2000 users of their system and their most recent survey dealt with a subgroup of 439 users who had acquired the system since 1987. The average user was 64 years old and had used the device for less than a year. Prior to use, 83% either had no erection or one of such poor quality as to make vaginal penetration impossible. Achievement of an erection-like state that was adequate for satisfactory intercourse was reported in 92% of users and 78% had intercourse at least every 2 weeks; 27% were occasionally able to have satisfactory intercourse without using the device. The usual man required one week, or about five practice sessions, to learn to use the system satisfactorily. The seasoned user required an average of 2.5 min to achieve an erection-like state suitable for intercourse. Most indicated a solid relationship with their sexual partners and noted an improved self-image. Prior to using this system, participants had been sexually inactive for from 6 months to more than 10 years and 74% either had no erection or a feeble one that made vaginal intromission impossible. Pain or discomfort was reported by 40% when the device was initially used, but in the majority this nuisance disappeared with time. Orgasm was rated as pleasant by 57% of users; 12% were unable to ejaculate, a predicament that reflected the underlying cause for impotency in most cases; 14% described discomfort at the time of ejaculation and this had been present in a third of them prior to using the device. This discomfort may reflect painful distension of the bulbous urethra due to trapped ejaculate caused by the tension band.

Marmar, DeBenedictis and Praiss (1988) reported use of a negative pressure plus tension band device to augment erections in men with partial tumescence after an intracavernous injection of vasoactive drug. In a group of 22 men, the penis was not rigid and buckling pressures were low following intracavernosal injections; 21 (95%) responded to the use of negative pressure plus tension within 30–60 s and achieved a rigid erection that did not buckle under pressures ranging from 60–100 mmHg. Their findings showed that a negative pressure plus tension device could be used to augment a partial response to intracavernous injection. These authors suggested that the combination of vasoactive injections and a negative pressure device provided impotent men with a more complete non-operative treatment programme. Additionally, since some centres limit intracavernosal injections to two per week, the use of a negative pressure plus tension band device may represent a viable therapeutic alternative for men who desire intercourse more frequently.

Moul and McLeod (1989) reported use of a negative pressure plus tension band device in 11 explanted penile prothesis patients. The device was used at home for a minimum of a month after an acceptable office demonstration. Ten (91%) reported satisfactory erections and successful intercourse when using the device. Interestingly, five of six patients in whom explantation was due to infection were able to use the negative pressure device successfully. These authors concluded that the negative pressure device can be a useful therapy for erectile impotence even in the challenging explant population. Despite previous corporeal infection and presumed fibrosis, negative pressure devices can provide patients with a functional erection-like state. It is noteworthy that all patients in their study group commented that they wished the negative pressure device had been available and offered to them as a treatment alternative before they had received an implant.

Following implantation of penile prostheses, many men feel that they have inadequate erections. Cautious use of a negative pressure plus tension band device in this group can frequently result in satisfactory erectile augmentation. The added tumescence achieved by use of this device can often convert an unhappy implant patient into one with an acceptable outcome.

Additional potential uses for the negative pressure devices include the following:

1. In office attainment of an erection-like state to permit assessment of suspected penile chordee and curvature.
2. To stretch fibrotic areas and perhaps lessen penile curvature in patients with Peyronie's disease.
3. To stretch and perhaps enlarge the penis in carefully selected cases.

## Discussion

The spectrum of impotence ranges from a mild or partial form which may be transient to a more severe or total type where the penis is hopelessly flail. Most spontaneously acquired impotence is partial, at least initially. A safe non-invasive method for management of impotence appears ideal and an external mechanical aid may fulfil this criterion. The external devices herein described represent a reversible therapeutic modality that can augment an inadequate erection and they should prove useful in any man who needs erectile enhancement. These devices appear to be particularly effective in men with partial impotence in whom only erectile enhancement is needed. Consequently, it would appear that these devices could be used by a large segment of the impotent population since a very large proportion of afflicted men have only partial impotence. The marked improvement in self-image noted by over two-thirds of individuals using the negative pressure plus tension band devices indicates that these mechanical aids allow them to achieve sufficient penile rigidity to accomplish sexual intercourse. These devices have proven to be safe if used correctly and users must be carefully counselled and warned to use them properly. Users who have impaired penile sensation are particularly suseptible to injury. They are especially apt to suffer ischaemia and injury if tension bands are left on the penis longer than 30 min. The new user nearly always experiences some pain and bruising when learning to use the negative pressure plus tension band devices. However, by careful titration of tension and vacuum, these aggravations usually cease to be a problem.

A major drawback to use of these devices is the necessity for their precoital application. Initially most appear cumbersome and proper use requires learning time, practice, patience and persistence. The new user must be admonished to not get discouraged and give up easily. Time and persistence allow the majority of men to become proficient with the devices and then they can achieve an erection-like state in a very short period of time. Another possible negative feature to external appliance use is that sex is not spontaneous and natural. However, all options available to the impotent man suffer this same drawback. On the positive side, precoital application of these devices by an understanding couple potentially permits foreplay which can appreciably enhance the total sexual experience for both. With two good hands, or with an understanding cooperative sexual partner, any of these external devices can be used. Even if the man has only one good hand, several systems are available that can probably be used.

All of the devices herein described represent a potential non-surgical therapy for most types of venogenic impotence. Additionally, an external device can be used by the man who fails to adequately respond to surgical obliteration of abnormal venous shunts.

When managing impotence, there is occasionally reluctance by either the patient, the physician or both to proceed with either surgical therapy or intracavernosal injections. This reluctance can stem from either poor patient–physician interaction, patient distrust, or a history of patient unhappiness with things related to medicine generally. Under this circumstance, an external erection device may be quite useful to determine patient and partner ability to cope with a useable erection. Such use can be termed ‘preimplant conditioning’ and it often allows the patient to have an erection adequate for intercourse. If both the user and his partner are pleased with the result obtained by use of an external device, the chance of obtaining a satisfactory outcome from either appropriate intracavernosal injection or surgical therapy appears good. However, if device use allows the man to have a useable erection and either he or his partner should be displeased, more invasive therapy may terminate with an unhappy outcome even despite a potentially superior functional and anatomical result.

Frequently men are seen who are excellent candidates for a penile implant. However, surgery must be postponed for some reason. Such reasons may include recent removal of an implant because of infection or erosion, recent myocardial infarction, recent hepatitis or some other medical reason. Use of a negative pressure device in many of these men may allow them to enjoy an active sex life until more definitive therapy can be accomplished. Interval use of such a device may additionally prevent both penile scarring and atrophy.

Men on anticoagulants may safely utilize external penile appliances (Witherington, 1990b). However, they should be very careful to avoid excessive use of both negative pressure and penile compression. During the learning phase, men on anticoagulants should very cautiously apply both vacuum and tension and gradually increase each to an amount that can both produce and maintain an adequate erection-like state without excessive bruising.

There are no absolute contraindications to use of external penile devices and potential contraindications are few. Any man having a blood dyscrasia or who is on an anticoagulant should use them with caution. Additionally, any man who lacks good manual dexterity may not be able to easily use them without assistance.

Reported complications from use of these devices are few. Specifically, there has been no report of urethral stricture, skin necrosis, penile gangrene or spongy tissue fibrosis in a compliant user.

External penile appliances belong in the armamentarium of any physician who treats erectile impotence. All impotent patients should be counselled concerning their use as a potential means for management of their problem. These devices represent an attractive alternative to either sexual abstinence or invasive therapy such as insertion of penile prostheses, vascular surgery and intracavernosal injection of vasoactive drugs. If they fail to produce an adequate erection for any reason, an invasive method of therapy may still be chosen.

## References


Marmar, J. L., DeBenedictis, T. J. and Praiss, D. E. (1988) The use of a vacuum constrictor device to augment a partial erection following an intracavernous injection. *Journal of Urology,* **140**, 975–979

Moul, J. W. and McLeod, D. G. (1989) Negative pressure devices in explanted penile prosthesis population. *Journal of Urology,* **142**, 729–731

Nadig, P. W., Ware, J. G. and Blumoff, R. (1986) Non-invasive device to produce and maintain an erection-like state. *Urology,* **27**, 126–131

Osopa, R. and Williams, G. (1989) Use of the 'Correctaid' device in the management of impotence. *British Journal of Urology,* **63**, 546–547

Wiles, P. G. (1988) Successful non-invasive management of erectile impotence in diabetic men. *British Medical Journal,* **296**, 161–162

Witherington, R. (1987) External aids for treatment of impotence. *Journal of Urological Nursing,* **6**, 10–16

Witherington, R. (1988) Suction device therapy in the management of erectile impotence. *Urologic Clinics of North America,* **15**, 123–128

Witherington, R. (1988) Vacuum constriction device for management of erectile impotence. *Journal of Urology,* **141**, 320–322

Witherington, R. (1990a) External penile appliances for management of impotence. *Seminars in Urology,* **8**, 124–128

Witherington, R. (1990b) External devices for the treatment of impotence. In *Common Problems in Infertility and Impotence* (ed. J. Rajfer), Year Book Medical Publishers, Chicago, pp. 300–310

# 19

# Penile prostheses

C. C. Carson

The problem of male sexual dysfunction has been described since ancient times. Treatment for impotence, however, was not available until the beginning of the 20th century. At that time, a variety of surgical procedures including dorsal penile vein ligation, corpus cavernosum plication, and early attempts at replication of the os penis using segments of rib cartilage were tried (Wooten, 1902; Macht and Teagarden, 1923; Lowsley and Bray, 1936; Gee, 1975). In 1902, Wooten reported restoration of erectile activity through the ligation of the dorsal penile vein. Steinach in 1906, suggested bilateral vasectomy as a surgical cure for impotence and the 'Steinach procedure' remained popular until the objective study of Macht and Teagarden in 1923 proved bilateral vasectomy to be no more effective than placebo treatment. The first attempt to use prostheses in the management of erectile failure was reported in 1936 by Bogaras (Gee, 1975). Bogaras used a tailored section of rib cartilage to produce penile rigidity in a fashion similar to the os penis of walruses, squirrels and other animals. These cartilage grafts, however, suffered from reabsorption, extrusion, progressive curling and infection, and were abandoned. Bergman, Howard and Barnes in 1948 also reported the use of a rib graft for penile rigidity with similar complications and results.

The development of newer synthetic materials in the 1950s allowed further advancement of medical prosthetic devices. Goodwin and Scott, in 1952 were the first to report the use of a silicone implant for prosthetic treatment of impotence (Goodwin, Scardino and Scott, 1981). They reported success in two of five patients implanted with an acrylic rod which was placed beneath Buck's fascia. Similar acrylic and polyethylene devices were implanted by Loeffler and Sayegh as well as Behairi in the early 1960s (Loeffler and Sayegh, 1960; Gee, 1975). Behairi's implants were especially important since he demonstrated the ability to place prosthetic rods within the corpora cavernosa rather than beneath Buck's fascia, allowing a more physiological erection with markedly reduced erosion rates (Gee, 1975). These early prosthetic devices, however, were associated with significant numbers of periprosthetic infections and erosions as a result of poorly tolerated device materials; high infection rates were caused by inadequate antibiotic prophylaxis. The development of silicone-based prosthetic materials in the late 1960s as a result of the space programme furthered the science of human prosthetics and penile prosthetic devices (Habal, 1984). Lash, in 1968, reported 28 patients using a single silicone prosthetic device with good results. Pearman, in 1972, demonstrated the successful use of a single silicone silastic prosthetic rod (Figure 19.1) in 126 patients. These devices were increasingly successful; however, their placement beneath Buck's fascia and stabilization only by the penile suspensory ligament led to significant discomfort, poor physiological penile shape and high extrusion rates.

The era of modern penile prosthetic treatment began with the reports of Small, Carrion and Gordon (1975) and Scott, Bradley and Timm (1973). These early reports defined the two classes of penile prostheses that we continue to implant today. Small, Carrion and Gordon described a pair of silicone implants sized to fill the corpora cavernosa from glans penis to crura. These implants which decreased prosthetic movement and recreated a physiological erection could be sized to the individual patient with two different girths and four different lengths. These implants are sufficient in size and rigidity to simulate normal erection and provide stability adequate for coital activity. Since its introduction, the Small–Carrion penile prosthesis has been the most widely implanted prosthesis ever developed. Initial results from the Small–Carrion penile prosthesis, the archetype of semi-rigid prostheses, varied from 9% to 27% (Small, Carrion and Gordon, 1975; Kramer *et al.*, 1979; Kaufman, Lindner and Raz, 1982; Rossier and Fam, 1984).

The second family of penile prostheses is the inflatable penile prosthesis described by Scott, Bradley and Timm in 1973. Because the inflatable design promised a more physiological erection and natural appearing flaccid state, the Scott inflatable penile prosthesis is widely implanted. The initial

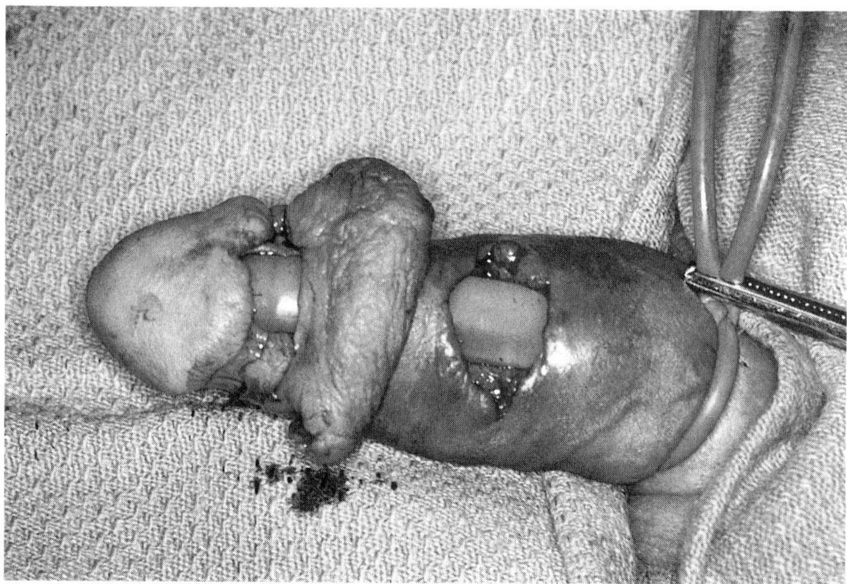

**Figure 19.1** Pearman penile prosthesis implanted beneath Buck's fascia

device and the current inflatable penile prostheses consist of three components. There are paired silastic corporeal cylinders which can be sized to the individual patient, connected to a fluid-filled reservoir placed beneath the anterior abdominal rectus muscle wall. The third component consists of the pump mechanism which was initially two pumps, and subsequently united into a single pump located in the scrotum. Patients can palpate the pump mechanism, inflate the prosthesis, and expect a normal appearing, normal feeling erection. On deflation of the device, a normal flaccid penis will result. The components of the prosthesis are connected by silicone tubes which are tailored and connected by stainless steel suture connectors. Initial results demonstrated excellent erections; however, mechanical malfunction rates were reported in excess of 60% of cases (Scott, Bradley and Timm, 1973; Kessler, 1981; Malloy, Wein and Carpiniello, 1982; Carson, 1983; Joseph, Bruskewitz and Benson, 1984; Dorflinger and Bruskewitz, 1986; Woodworth, Carson and Webster, 1990). Multiple and continued design changes ensued, reducing the malfunction rate continuously.

Current prosthetic devices can be grouped according to the historical background of these devices. Thus, the families of penile prostheses can be separated into those of the inflatable penile prosthesis variety and those of the semi-rigid prosthesis group. Subgroups of each of these families have recently been introduced.

## Semi-rigid penile prostheses

Since Small, Carrion and Gordon described their prosthesis and reported their results in 1975, a variety of semi-rigid prostheses of different designs has been developed and extensively used (Figure 19.2). These prostheses which use the same basic concept to provide erectile function have been modified to address the problems of concealment beneath clothing and the flaccid state.

The first of these modifications was developed by Finney and reported in 1977. His semi-rigid device, subsequently marketed as the Flexi-Rod and the more recent Flexi-Rod II (Figure 19.2c), is composed of silicone with a less rigid 5 cm segment positioned at the penile base to allow the prosthesis to 'hinge' and enhance concealment. In order to decrease operating room inventory, the Flexi-Rod consists of a trimmable proximal end for sizing. This proximal end allows 0.5 cm segments to be trimmed from the device. The distal-most portion of this prosthesis is more cone-shaped and is less blunt-shaped to enhance its fit beneath the glans penis. The Flexi-Rod II is available in diameters of 9, 10.5 and 12 mm with 0.5 cm trimmable lengths at the proximal portion of the device. Because the 'hinge' must be positioned at the base of the penis, an additional measurement between the mid-glans and pubis must be made exactly at the proximal pendulous penis.

In an effort to further improve the concealability

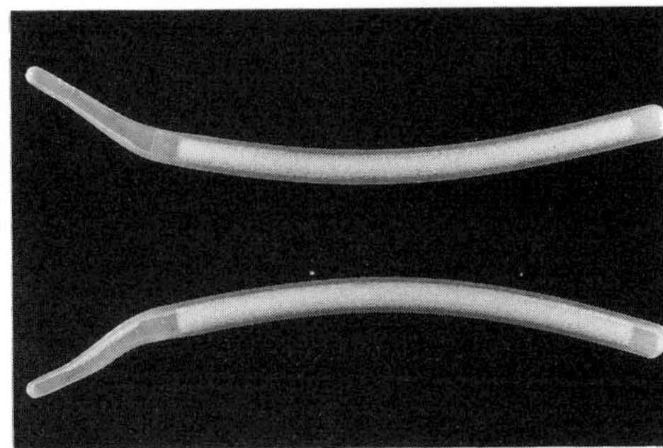
(a)

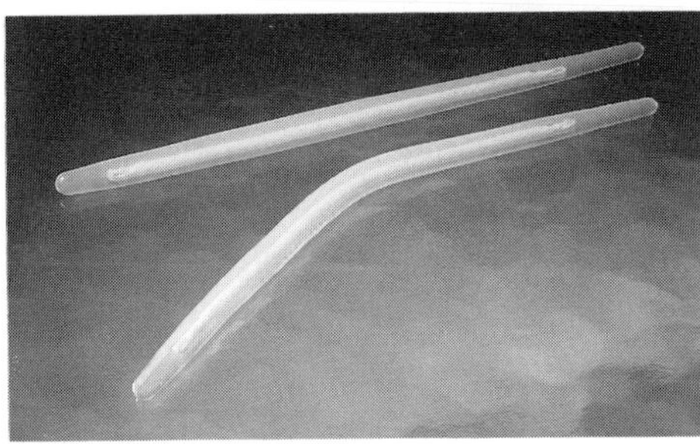
(b)

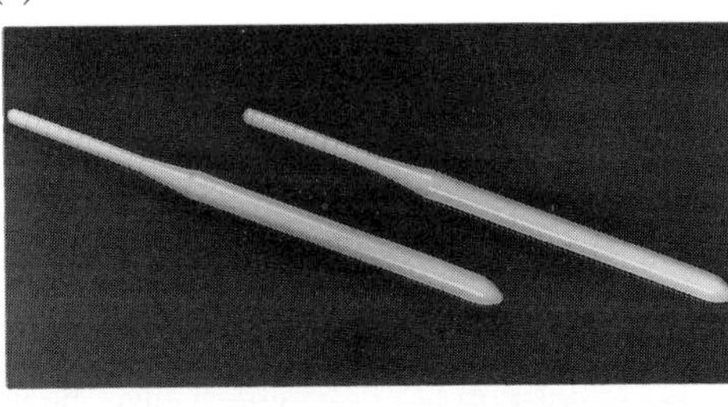
(c)

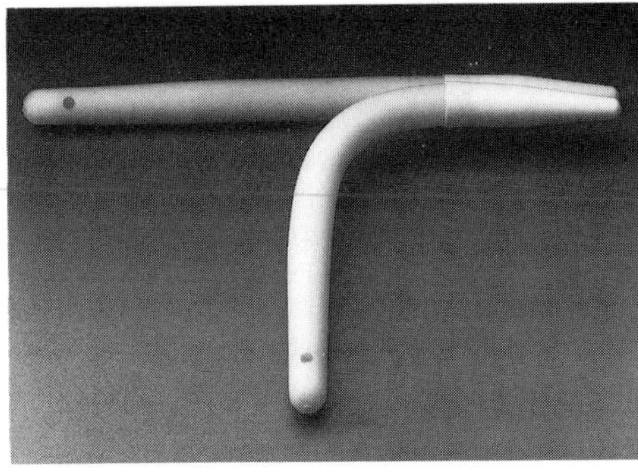
(d)

**Figure 19.2** Semi-rigid rod penile prostheses: (a) Small–Carrion penile prosthesis (Mentor); (b) Jonas penile prosthesis (Bard) (courtesy of C. R. Bard Inc, Covington, GA); (c) Flexi-Rod II penile prosthesis (Surgitek) (courtesy of Surgitek, Racine, Wis); (d) AMS malleable 600 penile prosthesis (American Medical Systems) (courtesy of American Medical Systems, Minnetonka, MN)

of the semi-rigid rod penile prosthesis, Jonas and Jacobi (1980) designed a silicone semi-rigid rod prosthesis containing a braided silver wire embedded within the core of the prosthesis (Figure 19.2b). This braided silver wire was designed to maintain the penis in a dependent position for improved concealment. Subsequently, American Medical Systems introduced a malleable prosthesis called the 'AMS 600' (Figure 19.2d), also designed with a silicone cylinder containing stainless steel wires in a helical configuration wrapped in a synthetic fabric (Moul and McCleod, 1986). The wires are capped at the ends with stainless steel and have an eye for suture passage to allow pull-through insertion. They further improved the design of the malleable-type penile prosthesis by placing a removable external silicone jacket around the prosthesis, allowing a 13 mm diameter with the jacket in place and an 11 mm diameter when the jacket is removed. Lengths of the AMS malleable 600 are adjusted by placing 1, 2 or 3 cm rear tip extenders to adjust the three base lengths of 12, 16 and 20 cm to a range from 12 to 26 cm.

The Mentor Corporation has also designed a malleable prosthesis consisting of silicone rods with an inner double-coiled silver wire wrapped in a teflon sheath. For inventory control, these prostheses are trimmable within 4–5 cm of the distal tip of the rod and are available in 9.5, 11 and 13 mm diameters. The distal portion is trimmed away from the wire and a silicone cap is added to finish the trimmed portion of the prosthesis. If excessive trimming is performed, a longer cap can be placed.

The most recent subgroup of semi-rigid rod penile prostheses are mechanical penile prostheses designed by Dacomed as the 'Omniphase' and 'Duraphase' penile prostheses (Krane, 1986) (Figure 19.3). Each of these prostheses consists of two cylinders each composed of a distal tip, proximal tip and central body portion in 10 and 12 mm diameters. Distal segments are available in 1–7 cm lengths and proximal segments are available in 2–7 cm lengths. The middle or body portion is 13 cm in length. The Omniphase prosthesis body consists of a spring-loaded cable which allows the penis to be rendered flaccid on flexion. The body of this Omniphase penile prosthesis consists of polysulfone cylinders which fit together in a ball and socket fashion articulating to each other. A stainless steel cable runs through these cylinders and is stabilized at one end. The opposite end of the cable is attached to a switch mechanism. The body mechanism is covered by a polytetrafluoroethylene (PTFE) covering with an outer silicone layer. The switch or activator mechanism consists of a spring mechanism which shortens and lengthens the cable. When the penis is pushed to a greater than 90° angle the switch is activated, shortening the cable and providing tension upon the articulated cylinders. With these

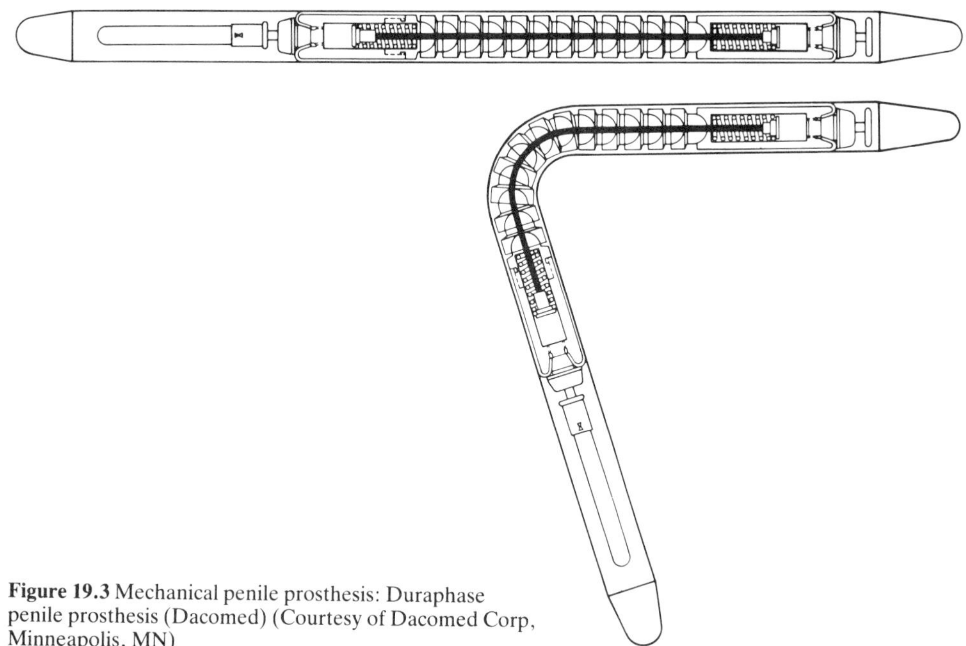

**Figure 19.3** Mechanical penile prosthesis: Duraphase penile prosthesis (Dacomed) (Courtesy of Dacomed Corp, Minneapolis, MN)

cylinders pulled tightly together, the penis becomes rigid. When the switch is again activated, the cable lengthens, allowing the cylinders to become loosely attached and the penis to become flaccid. Because of the risk of cable breakage, the newer Duraphase penile prosthesis was designed in a similar fashion but without the activator mechanism. With the Duraphase, a heavier cable is present and the attached spring allows the prosthesis to be positioned in a dependent fashion for enhanced concealability. When the prosthesis is extended, adequate rigidity and erectile function can be expected. Cable breakage with this design has been minimal and patient acceptance satisfactory.

## Inflatable penile prostheses (Figure 19.4)

The original inflatable penile prosthesis design of Scott has now been extended and modified to include the original three-piece inflatable prosthesis, a two-piece penile prosthesis design, and a single self-contained inflatable penile prosthesis design which can also be termed a hydraulic hinge.

### Three-piece inflatable penile prosthesis

The three-piece inflatable penile prosthesis is currently available from the Mentor Corporation and from American Medical Systems (AMS). These devices are similar in design and function as well as reliability (Carson, 1983; Engel, Smoler and Hackler, 1986; Gerstenberger, Osborn and Furlow, 1986; Merrill, 1986, 1989; Woodworth, Carson and Webster, 1990). Each of these prostheses consists of a fluid-containing reservoir with a 65 ml volume (AMS) or a 40 and 125 ml volume (Mentor). Tubing connects this reservoir to a pump placed in the scrotum for activation and deflation of the device. The Mentor and AMS pumps are similar in function, but different in shape. The pump connects to two inflatable cylinders placed in the corpora cavernosa of the penis. Length modification using 1, 2 and 3 cm rear tip extenders is designed with each company's prosthesis. These rear tip extenders allow direct perpendicular exit of the input tubing from the corporotomy incision. AMS 700 CX cylinders are available in lengths of 12, 15, 18 and 21 cm and Mentor cylinders are available in 1 cm increments from 12 to 28 cm. The major difference between these prosthetic devices is in the material used for the construction of the cylinders themselves. AMS 700 CX cylinders consist of an inner silicone cylinder surrounded by a woven fabric of controlled expansion and finally coated by a second layer of silicone. These controlled expansion cylinders, while providing less expansion than earlier models, are much more reliable, have fewer fluid leaks and virtually no aneurysmal dilatation (Woodworth, Carson and Webster, 1990). The Mentor penile prosthetic cylinder is constructed of Bioflex polyurethane. This material, which is quite

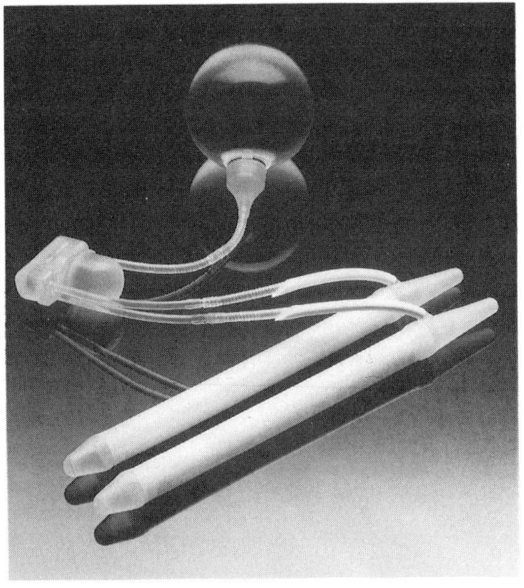
(a)

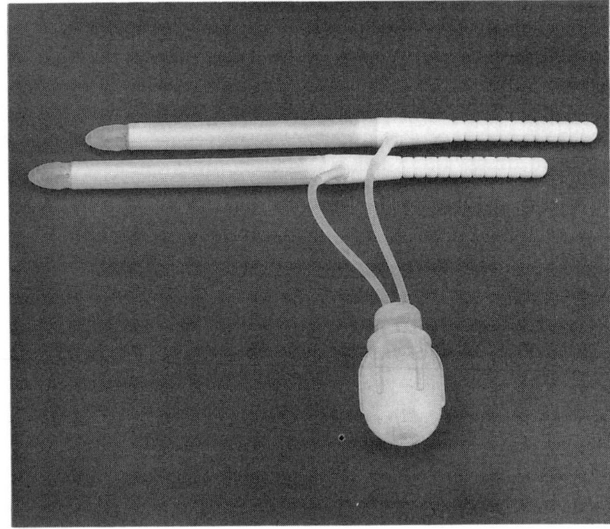
(b)

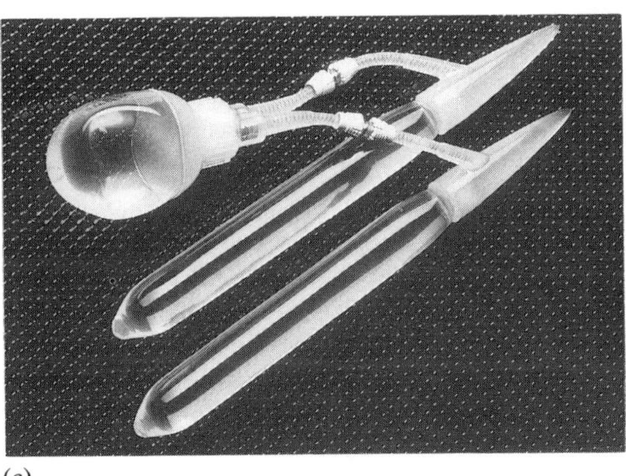
(c)

**Figure 19.4** Inflatable penile prostheses: (a) AMS 700 inflatable penile prosthesis (AMS) (courtesy of American Medical Systems, Minnetonka, MN); (b) Mentor GFX inflatable penile prosthesis (Mentor); (c) Uni-Flate 1000 inflatable penile prosthesis (Surgitek) (courtesy of Surgitek, Racine, Wis)

biocompatible, also has defined expansion diameter and is free from aneurysmal dilatation and demonstrates limited numbers of fluid leaks (Merrill, 1989).

The functional and cosmetic results of these inflatable penile prostheses remain the most desirable of prosthetic devices available. The ease of inflation, completeness of the flaccid condition, and excellent erection attest to the versatility of these devices. Patient and partner satisfaction is generally excellent (Gerstenberger, Osborn and Furlow, 1986; Steege, Stout and Carson, 1986). Patients who have changed prosthetic devices from inflatable to non-inflatable devices have usually been dissatisfied with the results of these non-inflatable prostheses and have frequently requested return to an inflatable device. With design evolution of the Mentor and AMS inflatable penile prostheses, reliability can be expected to be similar to that of a semi-rigid rod penile prosthesis.

## Two-piece inflatable penile prosthesis

More recent modifications of the inflatable penile prosthesis have incorporated the pump and the reservoir into one unit. These two-piece inflatable penile prostheses available from Surgitek (Uni-Flate 1000) or from Mentor (GFS) have simplified the implantation of an inflatable penile prosthesis and decreased the number of parts in an effort to improve reliability without sacrificing the inflatable penile prosthesis results. The elimination of the reservoir component has simplified surgical implantation and eliminated the difficulty of dissection in patients with previous extensive abdominal surgery. The cylinders of the Uni-flate 1000 penile prosthesis are similar in construction to those of the Flexi-Flate and Flexi-Flate II penile prostheses. These cylinders consist of an inner non-expansile cylinder which becomes rigid on fluid filling and an outer expansile cylinder which allows increased expansion and promotes penile rigidity and increased girth. This double cylinder is durable and is associated with few fluid leaks or mechanical complications and an expected excellent rigid and flaccid state. The Uni-Flate 1000 is prefilled and has a needle injection port at the base of the pump reservoir which allows for adjustment of the fluid volume for increased rigidity or flaccidity as needed. If later extensive expansion occurs and additional fluid is necessary for full rigidity, it can be added by injection through the skin and injection port. The single-piece construction without tubing connectors and factory pre-filled prosthesis decreases the possibilities of mechanical malfunction by eliminating tubing connection and facilitates implantation by decreasing pre-insertion prosthesis preparation. The Mentor GFS prosthesis is also a two-piece prosthesis with a pump reservoir capacity of approximately 20–25 ml and cylinders constructed in a fashion similar to those previously described as the Mentor inflatable penile prosthesis. Sizing and rear tip extenders are identical. The major disadvantage of the two-piece inflatable penile prosthesis is its incomplete deflation as a result of limited reservoir capacity. While this generally is a minimal problem, few patients report difficulties from this incomplete deflation. Some patients who have had both the three-piece inflatable and Uni-Flate 1000, however, find the Uni-Flate 1000 to be equal to the three-piece inflatable prosthesis in both inflation and deflation but somewhat superior in the ease of pump design and manipulation.

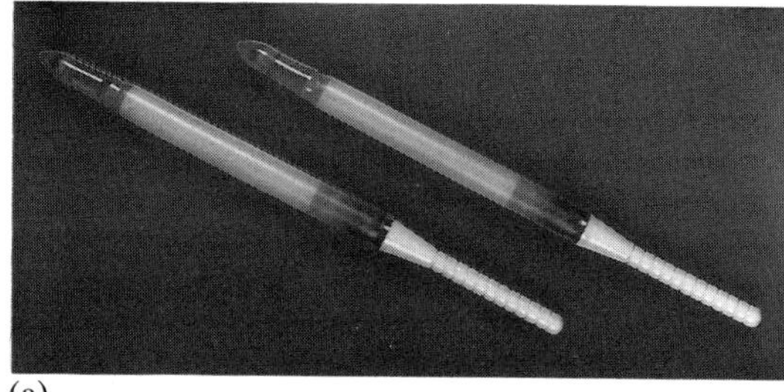

(a)

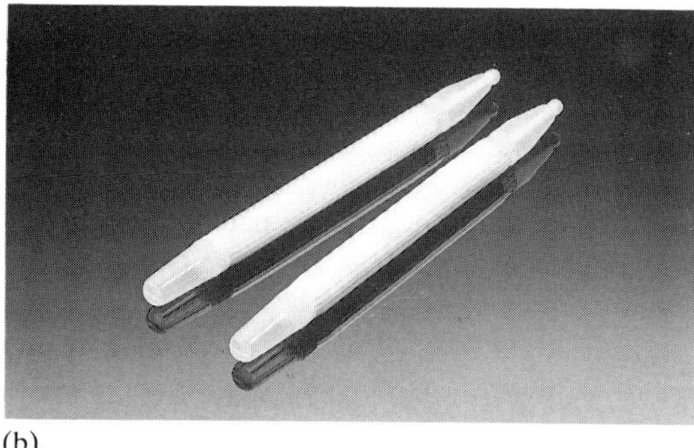

(b)

**Figure 19.5** Hydraulic hinge penile prostheses: (a) Flexi-Flate II penile prosthesis (Surgitek) (courtesy of Surgitek, Racine, Wis); (b) Dynaflex penile prosthesis (American Medical Systems) (courtesy of American Medical Systems, Minnetonka, MN)

## Self-contained inflatable penile prosthesis (Figure 19.5)

An additional modification of inflatable penile prosthesis technology is the development of the self-contained inflatable penile prosthesis by American Medical Systems and Surgitek. The AMS Hydroflex and Dynaflex and Surgitek Flexi-Flate II penile prostheses consist of paired cylinders placed within the corpora in a fashion similar to placement of semi-rigid rod penile prostheses. Each of these cylinders, however, contains a pump, reservoir and inflation chamber to allow inflation and deflation of the device. The pump in each of these devices is located at the distal portion of the cylinder. The Hydroflex and Dynaflex penile prostheses contain a fluid reservoir located in the proximal segment of the cylinder while the Flexi-Flate prosthesis has its reservoir in a distensible external chamber. The pump in these prostheses is palpated just proximal to the glans penis. Pressure on each cylinder inflates the prosthesis. Deflation of the Hydroflex prosthesis is performed by pressure on a release valve just proximal to the pump portion of the prosthesis. Digital compression of this release valve allows return to the flaccid state. The Flexi-Flate and Dynaflex cylinders are deflated by bending the prosthesis in the middle. Increased pressure within the inflation chamber allows spontaneous deflation of the device. The Dynaflex prosthesis has a built-in 10 s delay to avoid deflation during coitus. Because these devices are self-contained, only a small amount of fluid is actually moved between inflation and deflation states. As a result, deflation flaccidity is generally poor in comparison with the two- and three-piece inflatable penile prostheses. Similarly, the erect state does not result in enough girth expansion to produce a result similar to a multi-piece inflatable penile prosthesis and the rigid inflation is similar to that produced by a semi-rigid rod penile prosthesis, thus these may be more accurately termed hydraulic hinged prostheses.

The Flexi-Flate prosthesis, like the Uni-Flate 1000 and Flexi-Rod II has a trimmable proximal portion for sizing and 11 and 13 mm widths. In order to enhance fit from pubis to mid glans, cylinder lengths are available in 10, 12 and 14 cm lengths. The AMS Hydroflex and Dynaflex prostheses are available in 11 mm and 13 mm widths. Lengths consist of 13, 16, 19 and 22 cm with 1 and 2 cm rear tip extenders for increased versatility. These prostheses have had few mechanical failures (Finney, 1986; Fishman, 1986; Kabalin and Kessler, 1989).

## Prosthesis selection

The most appropriate penile prosthesis for an individual patient will vary with the patient's needs, anatomy and impotence aetiology. While the multiple component inflatable penile prostheses are the most physiological, these devices may not be appropriate in patients with limited manual dexterity, severe corpus cavernosum fibrosis, or those patients concerned with mechanical malfunction.

It is most important to discuss the advantages and disadvantages of each prosthesis category with the patient and his partner when possible. We discuss each type of prosthesis with each patient, allowing him to choose the type of prosthesis he prefers with physician counselling and advice. Most patients choose an inflatable variety of penile prosthesis because of a desire for a more naturally appearing flaccid penis and an increase in penile girth during erection. Because the mechanical malfunction rate of inflatable penile prostheses has declined to an acceptable level, patients choosing malleable penile prostheses have declined in the past several years. Any patient discussion, however, should include other possible forms of treatment for erectile dysfunction as well as the complications of penile prosthetic implantation such as infection, mechanical malfunction, extrusion and postoperative pain.

## Surgical implantation

Penile prostheses can be implanted through a variety of surgical approaches. Initially, malleable penile prostheses were implanted through a perineal approach. This approach has been largely abandoned as a result of its complexity and morbidity. Currently, at Duke University Medical Center, semi-rigid rod penile prostheses are implanted through a dorsal sub-coronal approach while inflatable penile prostheses are generally implanted through an infrapubic incision. Semi-rigid rod and self-contained inflatable prostheses can also be implanted through a dorsal penile shaft, ventral penile shaft, penoscrotal, perineal or suprapubic approach. Inflatable penile prostheses can be implanted through a penoscrotal as well as an infrapubic approach. Once the incision has been made, however, the principles of penile prosthesis implantation are similar despite the incision chosen. The infrapubic incision for implantation of inflatable penile prostheses has the advantage of minimal postoperative scarring and excellent cosmetic result. Surgical exposure for both surgeon and assistant is excellent. Furthermore, revision of inflatable penile prostheses with the infrapubic approach is facilitated and electrical prosthesis testing is simpler through this approach. Reservoir placement is under direct vision and careful dissection beneath the rectus sheath in patients with postoperative scarring allows for safe reservoir placement. With the placement of any prosthetic device, gentle surgical technique, careful attention to minimal dissection, and exquisite sterile technique must be maintained to minimize the possibility of postoperative infection. Perioperative infection with prosthetic devices results in disastrous consequences in many cases. As a result, frequent irrigation of the surgical wound with antibiotic solution containing bacitracin and an aminoglycoside antibiotic agent as well as limiting operating room traffic, operating time and postoperative bleeding will decrease perioperative infections. A careful 10 min preoperative scrub using antiseptic solutions is critical. Postoperative wound management and inspection are also keys to limiting perioperative infection.

The infrapubic incision is a horizontal type in slim patients and low midline in more obese patients. Once the skin inicision is carried out, careful dissection is performed to expose the corpora cavernosa bilaterally. The tissue between the corpora cavernosa is preserved to avoid the midline neurovascular bundle and the small sensory nerves which course in this area. Unless significant phimosis or redundant foreskin is present, we avoid circumcision at the time of penile prosthesis implantation to avoid the increase in infection attendant to this combined procedure (Fallon and Ghanem, 1989). Once the corpora cavernosa are identified, Buck's fascia is dissected free and the tunica albuginea exposed and secured with stay sutures. A longitudinal incision is carried out between the stay sutures and the corpora are opened. Scissor dissection is used to initiate the tunnels both proximally and distally within the corpora cavernosa. Dilation is then carried out proximally and distally, carefully maintaining the dilation instruments within the corpus and avoiding crossing into the contralateral corpus cavernosum. Dilation must be performed both proximally and distally to dilate completely to the ischial tuberosities and into the area just below the glans penis distally. Inadequate dilation results in the placement of an excessively short prosthesis cylinder and migration of that prosthesis postoperatively with a resultant inadequate support of the glans penis, allowing the glans to fall ventrally on insertion, making vaginal penetration uncomfortable. Gentle dilation using Hegar dilators or the Dilamazensert must be performed, however, as puncture of the corpus cavernosum proximally or distally may result in prosthesis extrusion postoperatively. Fibrotic corpora can be dilated using an Otis urethrotome for incision, avoiding the Otis away from the inferior quadrant of the corpus cavernosum to preserve the urethra. Large Kelly clamps can also be used to facilitate this dilation. Most corpora cavernosa can, however, be dilated using Hegar dilators.

Following adequate corporeal dilation, careful sizing must be carried out to fit the individual patient appropriately. The Furlow insertion tool is an excellent device for this purpose. Cylinders must be chosen which will lie flat in the corpus cavernosum without kinking, but will fill the dilated corpus cavernosum completely. Once the appropriate cylinder size and rear tip extenders are chosen, the prosthesis is placed using a suture at the distal-most portion of the cylinder and a Keith needle with the Furlow insertion tool or Dilamezensert. The cylinders are then placed in the corpora cavernosa and the corporotomy incisions closed with interrupted sutures placed prior to cylinder placement to limit the possibility of cylinder puncture. Pouches are then created beneath the rectus muscle and within the right scrotum for the reservoir and pump respectively. Once these components are placed, input tubing is tailored, the reservoir filled, and the tubes connected with non-suture connecting devices available from AMS or Mentor. A subdartos scrotal pouch is created for the pumps and the pumps placed in the most dependent portion of the scrotum for best results. While the GFS and Uni-Flate pumps are somewhat larger than the three-piece pumps, little difficulty has been associated with this increase in size in patients with a normal size scrotum. Once tubing connection has been completed, inflation and deflation of the device should be carried out to evaluate penile shape, cylinder position and adequacy of size. Changes in size or position should be carried out if necessary. Thorough antibiotic irrigation of all components of the device is then performed and closure carried out. A suction drain can be placed in those patients with some corporeal bleeding after prosthesis placement. Subcuticular skin closure will facilitate early hospital discharge and decrease postoperative wound infection. A Foley catheter may be placed for 24 h for urine drainage as necessary.

## Perioperative care

Perioperative antibiotic treatment is critical in diminishing the incidence of perioperative infections and prosthetic removal (Carson, 1980). An initial preoperative dosage of an aminoglycoside with a first-generation cephalosporin 1–2 h prior to surgery followed by a 48 h course of aminoglycoside and cephalosporin is preferred. Patients are then discharged for 7 days of first-generation cephalosporin antibiotic. The penile prosthesis remains deflated for 4 weeks while healing occurs. Prior to activation, the patient is advised to retract the pump into his scrotum on a daily basis and tight underwear or athletic supporters are avoided to maintain pump position. A return office visit for activation of the device is carried out. Patients are then advised to inflate and deflate their device on a daily basis for 3 weeks to allow tissue expansion around the prosthesis. Most patients can then begin use of their device immediately.

## Postoperative complications

The most worrisome postoperative complication is postoperative infection. Fortunately, this complication occurs in fewer than 5% of patients (Montague, 1987; Thomalla *et al.*, 1987; Carson, 1989). Perioperative prosthetic infections can, however, occur at any time in the postoperative period and patients with penile or other prosthetic devices continue to be at risk for haematogenously seeded infections from gastrointestinal, dental or urological manipulations as well as remote infectious processes. Patients must be counselled to request antibiotic coverage for these manipulative devices throughout the rest of their lives (Carson and Robertson, 1988). Most periprosthetic infections are caused by Gram-positive organisms such as *Staphylococcus epidermidis* but Gram-negative organisms such as *E. coli* and *Pseudomonas* are also common culprits (Fallon and Ghanem, 1989). Severe gangrenous infections with a combination of a Gram-negative and anaerobic organism have also been identified and frequently result in significant disability and tissue loss (Carson, 1983; McClellan and Masih, 1985). Patients at increased risk for perioperative infections include diabetics, patients undergoing penile straightening procedures or circumcision with prosthetic implantation, patients with urinary tract bacterial colonization, and immunocompromised patients such as post-transplant patients (Walther *et al.*, 1987). While these patients are at increased risk, their risk of infection continues to be less than 10% and is, in most cases, quite acceptable (Carson, 1983; Fallon and Ghanem, 1989). Spinal cord injury patients have been reported to be at especially increased risk with infection rates reported as high as 15% (Fallon and Ghanem, 1989). Because of decreased sensation, an increased risk of extrusion of semi-rigid rod prostheses have been reported in this group of patients.

Appropriate treatment of periprosthetic infection requires early and immediate identification with institution of parenteral antibiotic therapy and early prosthesis removal (Montague, 1987). Conservative treatment would dictate a healing period of 3–6 months followed by repeat prosthesis implantation (Carson, 1983). Excellent results with prosthesis removal, a 5–7 day course of antibiotic irrigation followed by additional replacement can also be attempted (Fishman, Scott and Selim, 1987; Furlow and Goldwasser, 1987). Reports have also appeared proposing antibiotic irrigation and drainage alone in an attempt to salvage part or all of the penile prosthesis. Several thorough reviews of the problem of penile prosthesis infection and its treatment have been published (Carson, 1983; Montague, 1987; Fallon and Ghanem, 1989).

The most common complication of inflatable penile prosthesis is mechanical malfunction. Mechanical malfunction has declined from rates as high as 61% to a level below 5% since the late 1970s (Kesler, 1981; Joseph, Bruskewitz and Benson, 1984; Woodworth, Carson and Webster, 1990). Aneurysmal dilatation of the inflatable cylinders, tubing kinking and reservoir leakage have been eliminated by device modifications.' Fluid leak, However, continues to be a problem in many inflatable penile prostheses. These mechanical malfunctions require replacement of the leaking portion of the inflatable penile prosthesis after intraoperative diagnostic procedures such as electrical testing.

Semi-rigid rod penile prostheses are associated with few mechanical problems and the most common complication associated with these prostheses is cylinder erosion through the skin or urethra (Montague, 1984; Benson, Patterson and Barrett, 1985). Prosthesis fracture and breakage have been occasionally reported (Agastin, Farrer and Raz, 1986; Tawil and Gregory, 1986). This problem is most marked in spinal cord injured patients, especially those requiring urinary management with catheter placement or condom collection.

## Conclusion

The implantation of penile prostheses is a commonly performed and successful procedure in most urological centres. A knowledge of the types of prostheses available, their advantages and disadvantages, and a variety of implantation techniques, is necessary for skilled prosthetic management of erectile impotence. Careful discussion of types of prostheses available and their advantages and disadvantages, providing a choice of devices available, optimizes patient satisfaction. Patients should be allowed to choose a prosthesis from each of the classifications of prostheses currently available. With careful patient selection, prosthesis choice, and with the currently available reliable prosthetic devices, the urologist can expect excellent patient and partner satisfaction with low morbidity.

### References


Agastin, E. H., Farrer, J. H. and Raz, S. (1986) Fracture of semi-rigid penile prosthesis: a rare complication. *Journal of Urology,* **135**, 376

Benson, R. C., Patterson, D. E. and Barrett, D. M. (1985) Long term results with Jonas malleable penile prosthesis. *Journal of Urology,* **134**, 899

Bergman, R. T., Howard, A. H. and Barnes, R. W. (1948) Plastic reconstruction of the penis. *Journal of Urology,* **59**, 1174

Carson, C. C. (1980) Prophylactic antibiotics in urologic surgery. *Urology, Weekly Update,* **2**, 26

Carson, C. C. (1983) Inflatable penile prosthesis: experience with 100 patients. *Southern Medical Journal,* **76**, 1139

Carson, C. C. (1989) Infections in genitourinary prostheses. *Urologic Clinics of North America,* **16**, 139

Carson, C. C. and Robertson, C. N. (1988) Late hematogenous infection of penile prosthesis. *Journal of Urology,* **139**, 112

Dorflinger, T. and Bruskewitz, R. (1986) AMS malleable penile prosthesis. *Urology,* **18**, 480

Engel, R. M. E., Smolev, J. K. and Hackler, R. (1986) Experience with Mentor inflatable penile prosthesis. *Journal of Urology,* **135**, 1181

Fallon, B. and Ghanem, H. (1989) Infected penile prostheses incidence and outcomes. *International Journal of Impotence Research,* **1**, 175

Finney, R. P. (1977) New hinged silicone penile implant. *Journal of Urology,* **118**, 585

Finney, R. P. (1986) Flexi-flate penile prosthesis. *Seminars in Urology,* **4**, 244

Fishman, I. J. (1986) Experience with the Hydroflex penile prosthesis. *Seminars in Urology,* **4**, 239

Fishman, I. J., Scott, F. B. and Selim, A. M. (1987) Rescue procedure: an alternative to complete removal for treatment of infected penile prosthesis. *Journal of Urology,* **137**, 202A

Furlow, W. L. and Goldwasser, B. (1987) Salvage of the eroded inflatable penile prosthesis: a new concept. *Journal of Urology,* **138**, 312

Gee, W. F. (1975) A history of surgical treatment of impotence. *Urology,* **5**, 401

Gerstenberger, D. I., Osborn, E. D. and Furlow, W. L. (1986) Inflatable penile prosthesis: follow-up study of patient–partner satisfaction. *Urology,* **14**, 239

Goodwin, W. E., Scardino, P. L. and Scott, W. W. (1981) Penile prosthesis for impotence: case report. *Journal of Urology,* **126**, 409

Habal, M. B. (1984) The biologic basis for the clinical application of the silicones. *Archives of Surgery,* **119**, 843

Jonas, U. and Jacobi, G. H. (1980) Silicone-silver penile prosthesis: description, operative approach and results. *Journal of Urology,* **123**, 865

Joseph, D. B., Bruskewitz, R. C. and Benson, R. C. (1984) Long term evaluation of inflatable penile prosthesis. *Journal of Urology,* **131**, 670

Kabalin, J. N. and Kessler, R. (1989) Experience with the Hydroflex penile prosthesis. *Journal of Urology,* **141**, 58

Kaufman, J. J., Lindner, A. and Raz, S. (1982) Complications of penile prosthesis surgery for impotence. *Journal of Urology,* **128**, 1191

Kessler, R. (1981) Complications of inflatable penile prostheses. *Urology,* **18**, 470

Kramer, S. A., Anderson, E. E., Bredeal, J. J. *et al.*

(1979) Complications of Small–Carrion penile prosthesis. *Urology,* **13**, 49

Krane, R. J. (1986) Omniphase penile prosthesis. *Seminars in Urology,* **4**, 247

Loeffler, R. A. and Sayegh, E. S. (1960) Perforated acrylic implants in the management of organic impotence. *Journal of Urology,* **84**, 559

Lowsley, O. S. and Bray, J. L. (1936) The surgical relief of impotence. *Journal of the American Medical Association,* **107**, 2029

Macht, D. and Teagarden, E. (1923) Rejuvenation experiments with vas ligation in rats. *Journal of Urology,* **10**, 407

Malloy, T. R., Wein, A. J. and Carpiniello, V.L. (1982) Improved mechanical survival with revised model inflatable penile prosthesis using rear tip extenders. *Journal of Urology,* **128**, 489

McClellan, D. S. and Masih, B. K. (1985) Gangrene of the penis as a complication of penile prosthesis. *Journal of Urology,* **133**, 862

Merrill, D. C. (1986) Clinical experience with Mentor inflatable penile prosthesis in 206 patients. *Urology,* **28**, 185

Merrill, D. C. (1989) Mentor inflatable penile prostheses. *Urologic Clinics of North America,* **16**, 51

Montague, D. K. (1984) Experience with Jonas malleable penile prosthesis. *Urology,* **23**, 83

Montague, D. K. (1987) Periprosthetic infections. *Journal of Urology,* **138**, 68

Moul, J. W. and McCleod, D. G. (1986) Experience with the AMS 600 malleable penile prosthesis. *Journal of Urology,* **135**, 929

Pearman, R. O. (1972) Insertion of a silastic penile prosthesis for the treatment of organic sexual impotence. *Journal of Urology,* **107**, 802

Rossier, A. B. and Fam, B. A. (1984) Indication and results of semi-rigid penile prostheses and spinal cord injury patients: long term follow-up. *Journal of Urology,* **131**, 59

Scott, F. B., Bradley, W. E. and Timm, G. W. (1973) Management of erectile impotence – use of implantable inflatable prosthesis. *Urology,* **2**, 80

Small, M. P., Carrion, H. M. and Gordon, J. A. (1975) Small-Carrion penile prosthesis: a new implant for management of impotence. *Urology,* **5**, 479

Steege, J. F., Stout, A. L. and Carson, C. C. (1986) Patient satisfaction in Scott and Small–Carrion penile implant recipients: a study of 52 patients. *Archives of Sexual Behaviour,* **15**, 393

Tawil, E. A. and Gregory, J. G. (1986) Failure of the Jonas prosthesis. *Journal of Urology,* **135**, 703

Thomalla, J. V., Thompson, S. T., Rowland, L. D. *et al.* (1987) Infectious complications of penile prosthetic implants. *Journal of Urology,* **138**, 65

Walther, P. J., Andriani, R. T., Maggio, M. I. and Carson, C. C. (1987) Fournier's gangrene: a complication of penile prosthetic implantation in a renal transplant patient. *Journal of Urology,* **137**, 299

Woodworth, B. W., Carson, C. C. and Webster, G. D. Long term survival of inflatable penile prostheses. *Urology* (in press)

Wooten, J. S. (1902) Ligation of the dorsal vein of the penis as a cure for atonic impotence. *Texas Medical Journal,* **18**, 325

# 20

# Venous leak and its correction

G. Williams

## Introduction

At the beginning of the century Wooten (1902) and Lydston (1908) demonstrated the importance of venous drainage of the penis during an erection and the benefit of ligation of the deep dorsal vein in the restoration of potency. The first report of a venous contribution to erectile dysfunction was by Lowsley and Bray (1936). However, the importance of venous outflow restriction in the maintenance of an erection was largely ignored until Wagner's observation that an abnormal venous shunting between the glans and corpora cavernosa can be a cause of impotence (Wagner, 1979). This observation was followed by that of Wagner and Uhrenholdt (1980) who demonstrated that there is a decrease in venous return from the penis in human volunteers during visualization of erotic motion pictures. Recent dynamic vascular studies have clearly demonstrated that venous outflow restriction is essential for both initiating and maintaining an erection (Lue *et al.*, 1983, 1984; Juenemann, Lue *et al.*, 1986; Fournier *et al.*, 1987; Aboseif *et al.*, 1989). Failure of the venous system can now be clearly demonstrated with dynamic cavernosography using a saline infusion to induce an erection (Virag, 1982). More recently, pharmacocavernosography and pharmacocavernosometry, using a combination of intracavernosal vasoactive drugs and saline infusion, have been used to identify abnormalities of venous outflow restriction, which may be amenable to surgery (Lue *et al.*, 1986; Dickinson and Pryor, 1989).

Many surgical techniques have been described to deal with these leaking veins from simple ligation of the deep dorsal vein (Wespes and Schulman, 1985), spongiolysis (Gilbert and Stief, 1987) to more radical excision of the deep dorsal veins, circumflex veins and cavernosal veins (Williams *et al.*, 1988). None of these surgical techniques is entirely satisfactory as surgical access to leaking cavernosal veins is difficult and many patients have, in addition, abnormalities of arterial inflow and psychogenic disorders (McLoughlin *et al.*, 1990).

## Role of the venous system in a penile erection

### Venous anatomy

The penis is drained by three systems of veins – the superficial, intermediate and deep – in addition to emissary, circumflex and unnamed communicating vessels (Newman and Northup, 1981; Aboseif *et al.*, 1989).

#### Superficial system

This consists of a network of subcutaneous veins which join to form the superficial dorsal vein at the root of the penis. This vessel is usually single and empties into the left saphenous vein, but may be multiple and can empty into the right saphenous vein, epigastric or femoral veins. The superficial dorsal vein may receive communicating veins from the intermediate system.

#### Intermediate veins

These vessels are deep to Buck's fascia and consist of the deep dorsal vein, which is usually single, but occasionally multiple. It receives numerous vessels from the glans and, in addition, in the distal two-thirds of the penis, 3–10 circumflex veins which arise from the undersurface of the corpora spongiosa and track around the corpora cavernosa to empty into the deep dorsal vein lying in the dorsal groove between the two corpora cavernosa. The deep dorsal vein passes backwards under the pubic arch to drain into the periprostatic plexus. There are, in addition, small venae commitantes running with the dorsal arteries of the penis.

#### Deep veins

The emissary veins are short channels passing through the corpora cavernosa draining directly into the intermediate set of veins. The cavernous veins arise from the dorsomedial aspect of each corpus in the area of the separation of the crus and drain either into the internal pudendal system, but frequently drain into the periprostatic plexus. Small crural veins arise directly from the crura and drain into the internal pudendal veins.

### Venous physiology

The mechanism of erection has been extensively investigated both in animals and human volunteers. In the flaccid state the penile arterioles are constricted and the sinusoids of the corpora contracted. While the sinusoids are contracted, the large intramedullary venules and those lying in the periphery between the sinusoidal wall and the corpora drain freely into the emissary veins. During an erection the sinusoidal smooth muscle relaxes allowing an increase in arterial flow and sinusoidal distension resulting in compression of the venules between the sinusoids and the inelastic tunica albuginea (Lue and Tanagho, 1987).

## Clinical features and classification of venous leak

It has been estimated that up to 30% of men suffering from erectile dysfunction will have venous incompetence either as the sole or contributing cause of their impotence (Virag, 1984).

In younger men with no risk factors such as hypertension, smoking, diabetes or neurological disease who present with primary impotence, there is a high possibility of a significant venous leak being the aetiology of their erectile dysfunction. Most men, however, present with secondary impotence and give a 2–3-year history of progressive difficulty of obtaining an erection with rapid detumescence without ejaculation, or the ability to achieve a partial erection only. Some men complain of a rapid detumescence with change in penile position. A history of diabetes, antihypertensive drug therapy or a neurological disorder does not preclude the diagnosis of a venous leak (Williams *et al.*, 1988).

The diagnosis is made by cavernosography and cavernosometry, but this should only be performed on those patients who have failed to respond with a full erection to at least two separate injections of papaverine 30–60 mg and phentolamine 1 mg. Only patients with severe arterial inflow abnormalities or cavernosal fibrosis will fail to respond to such an injection. The remainder will have a venous leak. Papaverine alone is not as effective as a combination of papaverine and phentolamine in inducing an erection and is not as useful a screening test for a venous leak (Sheikh *et al.*, 1990). It is essential when intracavernosal injections of vasoactive drugs are administered that the patient is supine. Up to 50% of those with a venous leak will develop facial flushing and/or hypotension after an intracavernosal injection of papaverine and phentolamine.

### Classification of venous leaks

There is no ideal classification as the exact aetiology of this condition is unkown. However, from the clinical features the following classification is suggested.

#### Congenital

This usually presents with primary impotence in young men and is frequently due to the presence of a large tortuous vein exiting directly from the corpora cavernosa (Figure 20.1). Shunts between the distal corpora cavernosa and corpora spongiosa may also be congenital in origin.

#### Iatrogenic

Following the creation of a shunt between the glans and corpora cavernosa, or corpora cavernosa and corpora spongiosa, or corpora cavernosa and saphenous vein for the treatment of priapism, the patient will usually remain impotent until such a shunt is taken down.

#### Acquired abnormalities of the tunica albuginea

In Peyronie's disease the tunica albuginea becomes stretched and may result in incompetence of the venous occlusive mechanism.

#### Ischaemia

Prolonged ischaemia results in degeneration and fibrosis of the corporeal smooth muscle leading to an inability of those muscles to relax and occlude the venous sinuses.

#### Lack of neurotransmitters

An almost complete absence of the neurotransmitter vasoactive intestinal polypeptide has been found in the corpora cavernosa of impotent diabetics (Gu *et al.*, 1984) and, since up to one-third of impotent diabetics may have a venous leak, the lack of a neurotransmitter may be part of its aetiology.

## Functional evaluation of the venous system

### Cavernosography and cavernosometry

Virag (1982) was the first to use dynamic cavernosography. Using this technique, saline at 37°C is infused into the corpora cavernosa at increasing flow rates. In a normal male a flow of less than $120\,\mathrm{ml\,min^{-1}}$ will induce an erection and less than $50\,\mathrm{ml\,min^{-1}}$ will be required to maintain the erection. In a patient with a venous leak an erection may not be achieved even with flows up to $300\,\mathrm{ml\,mm^{-1}}$. Using this technique, diluted contrast media can be infused into the corpora and the sites of venous leakage determined radiologically. In a normal male, such an infusion will result in an erection with minimal contrast outlined in the deep dorsal vein and no filling of the pelvic veins (Figure

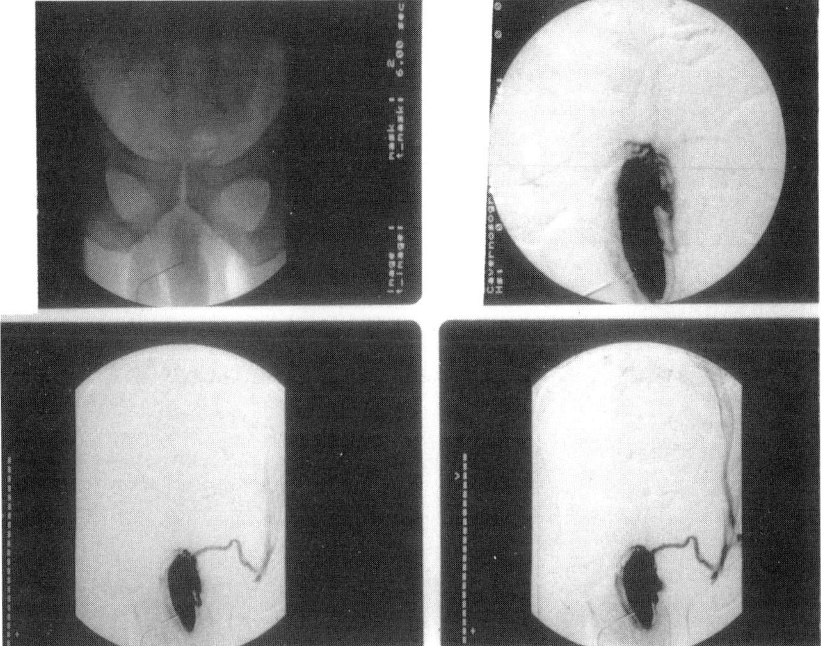

**Figure 20.1** A presumed congenital venous leak with no erection during cavernosography, but with a large single incompetent vein draining into the superficial venous system

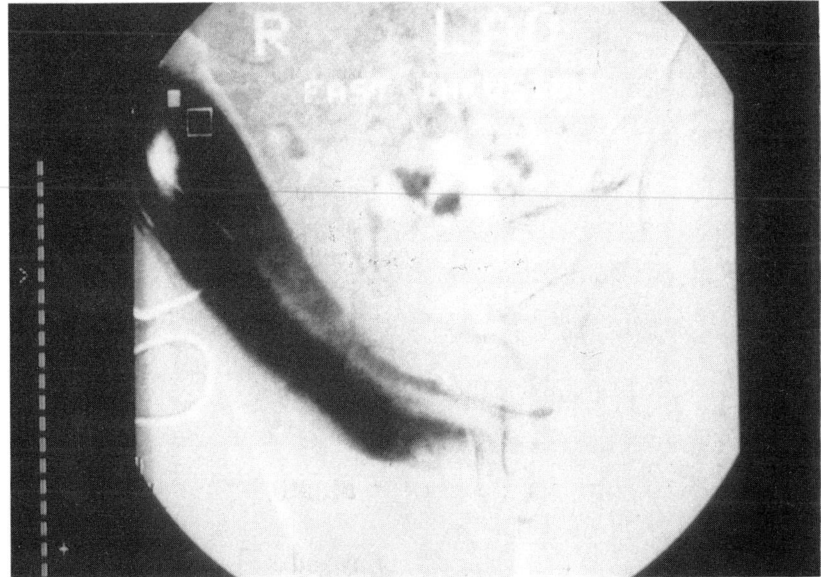

**Figure 20.2** Digital subtraction dynamic cavernosography in a normal volunteer showing a full erection with minimal filling of the deep dorsal vein

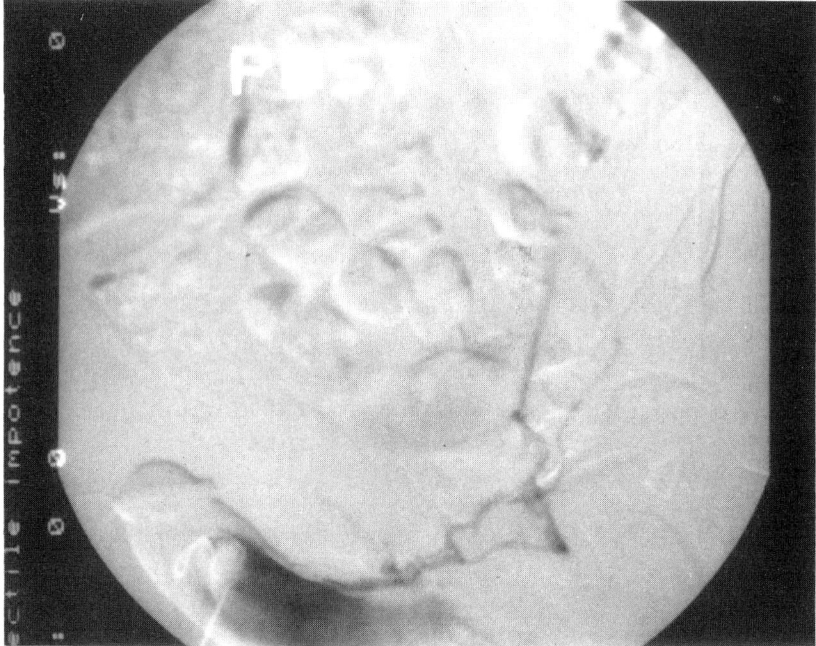

**Figure 20.3** Digital dynamic subtraction cavernosography. Patient required an inflow infusion of 250 ml $min^{-1}$ to produce the erection. A significant leaking vein is identified

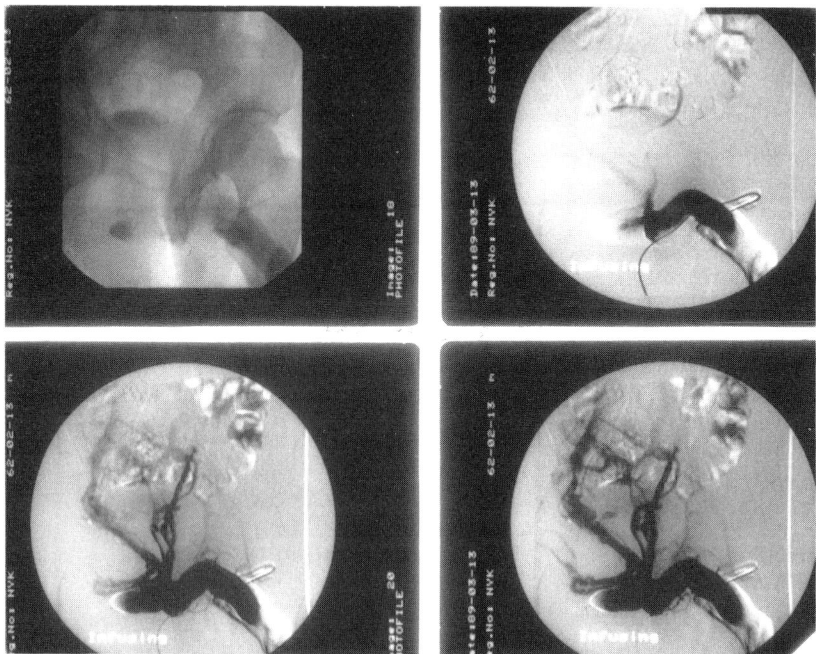

**Figure 20.4** Digital subtraction dynamic cavernosography showing no erection during the infusion phase with significant leaking into the superficial, deep and cavernosal systems

20.2). In a patient with a leak an erection may be achieved, but at much higher flows than in normal men and the site of venous leak can be easily determined (Figure 20.3). In other patients with venous leaks no erection will be achieved and extensive leakage into the deep dorsal, cavernosal and superficial veins will be seen (Figure 20.4)

Such studies have been criticised as being unphysiological in that no smooth muscle relaxation occurs during the test to activate the venous occlusive mechanism, and as a result a venous leak will be over-diagnosed. This is unlikely if such tests are reserved solely for those who fail to respond to an intracavernosal injection of papaverine and phentolamine. However, Desai and Gingell (1988) have reported two patients who were subsequently found to have psychogenic impotence who did not achieve a full erection with a maximal saline infusion. The investigation of choice is now considered to be dynamic pharmacocavernosography and pharmacocavernosometry.

A standardized method of producing maximal smooth muscle relaxation has not yet been determined; for example, should prostaglandin $E_1$, papaverine or papaverine and phentolamine be used and, if so, in what dose? In our own studies we have used a combination of papaverine 30 mg and phentolamine 1 mg and then infused half-strength contrast media taking pictures in the anteroposterior and left and right oblique positions using digital subtraction. In normal males an erection will be induced with a flow of less than 35 ml $min^{-1}$ and a maintenance of less than 5 ml $min^{-1}$ required. The percentage drop in intracavernosal pressure over 5 min after stopping the infusion will be less than 50%. If the patient has a venous leak the induction and maintenance flows will be higher than those in a normal male and will vary according to the degree of leakage. A pressure drop of more than 75% in the 5 min after stopping the infusion can be expected (Aboseif *et al.*, 1989; Dickinson and Pryor, 1989).

## Treatment of venous leakage

From the description of the venous drainage and the extensive venous involvement which may occur in this condition (Figure 20.4), it is clear that no single surgical approach to the penis will be entirely adequate. Most authors have used an infrapubic approach (Wespes and Schulman, 1985; Williams *et al.*, 1988). Lue (1988) has described a peripenile/scrotal approach. Others have used, in addition to these, a perineal approach (Bar-Moshe and Van Dendris, 1987) or a circumferential approach (Gilbert and Stief, 1987). As the failure of the veno-occlusive mechanism appears to be at the level of the corpora cavernosa, operations describing ligation of the internal iliac, internal pudendal and periprostatic plexus will not be described.

### Operative technique

The technique described is that used by the author in a series of 48 patients. All patients received prophylactic antibiotics. The operations have been carried out under general anaesthesia with the patient supine and the table in a head-up tilt position. A 3 inch infrapubic incision is made and all veins in this area carefully dissected back to their origin, ligated with non-absorbable sutures and removed. Buck's fascia is then incised and the deep dorsal vein identified taking care to avoid damage to the dorsal arteries and nerves which lie immediately lateral to it. The deep dorsal vein is exposed distally using fine dissection and all branches identified, ligated and removed. Those arising directly from the corpora cavernosa are oversewn. The deep dorsal vein is transected at the level of the glans penis. Proximally, further exposure of the deep dorsal vein is carried out by division of the suspensory ligament and dissection of the crura from the inferior pubic rami. The deep dorsal vein is ligated as far proximally as possible and removed. The dissection then continues lateral to the dorsal artery and nerves around the corpora cavernosa on both sides, removing all emissary and circumflex veins and those communicating veins passing laterally into the superficial systems. The corpora are then reopposed to the pubic rami, the suspensory ligament repaired and the wound closed in layers with suction drainage. An occlusion dressing is placed around the penis. The patient is usually discharged from hospital 48–72 h later.

### Results of surgery

A summary of the short-term results for venous leakage are presented in Table 20.1. In the author's series of 48 patients the mean follow-up was 28 months with a range of 6–43 months. The mean age of the patients operated on was 58 years and the mean duration of erectile dysfunction 4.5 years. Six patients had had lifetime erectile dysfunction. Fourteen of the 48 patients were diabetic. At 3 months following surgery, 24 patients had erections satisfactory for intercourse and ten were able to achieve erections using intracavernosal injections of either papaverine or papaverine and phentolamine. A further ten had some improvement in their erections with intracavernosal pharmacotherapy but these were insufficient for intercourse, and four had no benefit at all from the operation. Of the 24 patients with full erections, the mean follow-up was 23 months. Six of these patients were diabetic and five of these six have subsequently failed to achieve spontaneous erections at a mean period of 10

**Table 20.1 Short-term results of surgery for venous leakage**

| | *No.* | *Excellent* | *Improved* | *Failed* | *Follow-up* (months) |
|---|---|---|---|---|---|
| Wagenknecht (1985) | 22 | 16 | – | 6 | 4–20 |
| Buvat (1985) | 18 | 5 | – | 13 | – |
| De Sy *et al*. (1985) | 10 | 5 | – | 5 | 26 |
| Wespes *et al*. (1986) | 67 | 31 | 16 | 20 | 26 |
| Anstoni *et al*. (1987) | 234 | – | 150 | – | 3 |
| Steif (1987) | 40 | 15 | 20 | 3 | – |
| Society for Study of Impotence (1987) | 108 | 44 | 20 | 42 | – |
| Williams *et al*. (1988) | 13 | 9 | 1 | 3 | – |
| Lewis (1987) | 50 | 12 | 12 | 17 | 15 |
| Treiber and Gilbert (1989) | 115 | 28 | 39 | 58 | 13 |

Modified from Lewis (1988), *Urological Clinics of North America*, **15**, 119

months following the operation with a range of 6–17 months. However, all five still respond satisfactorily to intracavernosal injections. It is of significance that eight of these 24 patients, despite being able to achieve a full erection, have not had sexual intercourse. Of the ten patients who were able to achieve a full erection following surgery with the addition of pharmacotherapy, two no longer respond adequately to injections; both are diabetic. Of these ten patients two have not had intercourse. Repeat cavernosography has been carried out in 11 of the 14 failures. All have been shown to have persistent leakage from posteriorly placed cavernosal veins or into the most proximal part of the deep dorsal vein (Figure 20.5). In contrast, in 11 of 58 failures in the series reported by Treiber and Gilbert (1989) venous shunts between the corpora cavernosa and corpus spongiosum were identified. Nine of these 11 who underwent spongiolysis and glans lysis reported excellent rigidity; however, five were only able to achieve such rigidity with the use of intracavernosal pharmacotherapy.

Surgery for the treatment of venous leakage is not without complications. The majority of patients will develop penile oedema, which usually resolves over a 3 month period. A significant proportion will develop altered sensation of the penis. Some report a decreased penile length. Others develop penile nodularity secondary to venous thrombosis, and others complain of tethering of the infrapubic scar.

Venous leakage as a significant cause of erectile dysfunction should be suspected in all men who fail to respond to intracavernosal injections of papaverine and phentolamine. The diagnosis can be confirmed using pharmacocavernosography, but such diagnostic methods do not adequately identify those who have in addition abnormalities of arterial inflow, nor significant psychogenic or marital and social disorders. Venous leaks occur in a significant proportion of diabetics. With the current surgical techniques available, approximately 50% of men should have an excellent response following venous ligation and excision. Despite this excellent response and the ability to have intercourse, only 17 of the 27 (64%) who where fully potent at 2 years did so.

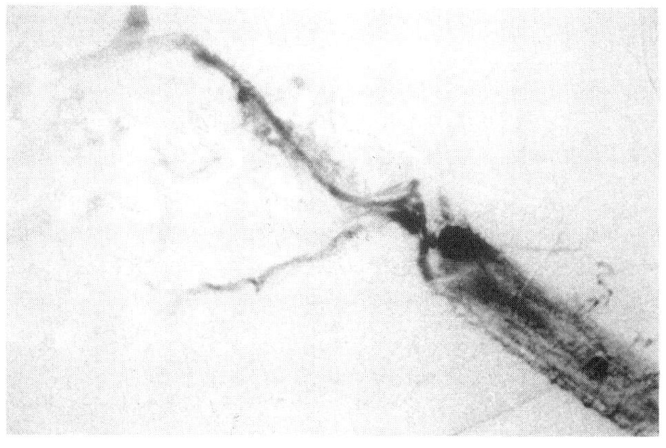

**Figure 20.5** Digital subtraction dynamic cavernosography in a patient who failed surgery for venous leak showing persistent leakage into the crural and most proximal deep dorsal vein

## References


Aboseif, S. R., Breza, J., Lue, T. F. and Tanagho, E. A. (1989) Penile venous drainage in erectile dysfunction. Anatomical, radiological and functional considerations. *British Journal of Urology,* **64**, 183–189

Austoni, E., Bellorofonte, C. and Mantovani, F. (1987) Improved results with intracavernous vasoactive drug infusion following new surgical techniques for vasculogenic impotence. *World Journal of Urology,* **5**, 182–189

Bar-Moshe, O. and Van Dendris, N. (1987) Ligation of crura penis for impotence due to perineal venous leakage. *Journal of Urology,* **137**, Part 2, 185a, Abstract No. 325

Desai, K. M. and Gingell, J. C. (1988) Saline-induced artificial erection without papaverine. A potential source of error in diagnosing cavernosal venous leakage. *British Journal of Urology,* **62**, 176–178

Dickinson, I. K. and Pryor, J. P. (1989) Pharmacocavernometry: a modified papaverine test. *British Journal of Urology,* **63**, 539–545

Fournier, G. R. Jr., Juenemann, K-P., Lue, T. F. and Tanagho, E. A. (1987) Mechanisms of venous occlusion during canine penile erection: an anatomic demonstration. *Journal of Urology,* **137**, 163–167

Gilbert, P. and Stief, C. (1987) Spongiolysis: a new surgical treatment of impotence caused by distal venous leakage. *Journal of Urology,* **138**, 784–786

Gu, J., Lazarides, M., Pryor, J. P. *et al.* (1984) Decrease of vasoactive intestinal polypeptide (VIP) in the penises from impotent men. *Lancet,* **ii**, 315–317

Juenemann, K.-P., Luo, J. A., Lue, T. F. and Tanagho, E. A. (1986) Further evidence of venous outflow restriction during erection. *British Journal of Urology,* **58**, 320–324

Lewis, R. W. (1988) Venous surgery for impotence. *Urologic Clinics of North America,* **15**, 115–121

Lowsley, O. S. and Bray, J. L. (1936) The surgical relief of impotence; further experiences with a new operative procedure. *Journal of the American Medical Association,* **107**, 2029–2035

Lue, T. F. (1988) Treatment of venogenic impotence. In *Contemporary Management of Impotence and Infertility* (eds E. A. Tanagho, T. F. Lue and R. D. McClure), Williams and Wilkins, Baltimore, pp. 175–177

Lue, T. F., Hricak, H., Schmidt, R. A. and Tanagho, E. A. (1986) Functional evaluation of penile veins by cavernosography in papaverine-induced erection. *Journal of Urology,* **135**, 479–482

Lue, T. F., Takamura, T., Schmidt, R. A. *et al.* (1983) Haemodynamics of erection in the monkey. *Journal of Urology,* **130**, 1237–1241

Lue, T. F., Takamura, T., Umraiya, M. *et al.* (1984) Haemodynamics of canine corpora cavernosa during erection. *Urology,* **24**, 347–352

Lue, T. F. and Tanagho, E. A. (1987) Physiology of erection and pharmacological management of impotence. *Journal of Urology,* **137**, 829–836

Lydston, G. F. (1908) The surgical treatment of impotency. *American Journal of Clinical Medicine,* **15**, 1571–1573

McLoughlin, J., Asopa, R. and Williams, G. (1990) Surgical treatment of venous leakage: medium term follow-up. *European Journal of Urology,* (In press)

Newman, H. F. and Northup, J. D. (1981) Mechanism of human penile erection: an overview. *Urology,* **17**, 399–408

Sheikh, N., Downey, G. and Williams, G. (1990) Diabetic impotence and its treatment. *British Journal of Urology,* (In preparation)

Treiber, U. and Gilbert, P. (1989) Venous surgery in erectile dysfunction. A critical report on 116 patients. *Urology,* **34**, 22–27

Virag, R. (1982) Arterial and venous haemodynamics in male impotence. In *Management of Male Impotence* (ed. A. H. Bennett), Williams and Wilkins, Baltimore, pp. 108–176

Virag, R. (1984) Impotence: a new field in angiography. *International Angiology,* **3**, 217–219

Wagner, G. (1979), A. L'impuissance par anomalie veineuse des corps caverneux. *Contracep-Fertil-Sexual,* **8**, 593–596

Wagner, G. and Uhrenholdt, A. (1980) Blood flow measurement by clearance methods in the human corpus cavernosum in the flaccid and erect states. In *Vasculogenic Impotence* (Proceedings of the First International Conference on Corpus Cavernosum Revascularization) (eds. A. Zorgniotti and G. Rossi), Charles C. Thomas, Springfield, pp. 42–48

Wespes, E. and Schulman, C. C. (1985) Venous leakage: surgical treatment of a curable cause of impotence. *Journal of Urology,* **133**, 796–798

Williams, G., Mulcahy, M. J., Hartnell, G. and Kiely, E. (1988) The diagnosis and treatment of venous leakage, a curable cause of impotence. *British Journal of Urology,* **61**, 151–155

Wooten, J. S. (1902) Ligation of the dorsal vein of the penis as a cure for atonic impotence. *Texas Medical Journal,* **18**, 325–326

# 21

# Arterial revascularization

J. S. P. Lumley

Less than 5% of patients presenting in an impotence clinic have focal arterial disease. However, it is important to identify those that do, since their problems may be amenable to effective therapy. These measures can avoid the inconveniences of intracavernous self-injection or the potential complications of prosthetic devices. The outcome depends on patient selection, the choice of bypass procedure and the skill with which the treatment is undertaken.

## Aetiology

Erection is dependent on an adequate pressure within the corpora cavernosa and this is, to a large extent, related to the integrity of a normal arterial supply as considered elsewhere in this volume (Chapter 2). The arterial input may be compromised by disease at any site from the aorta to the peripheral penile vessels. In 1923 Leriche first described impotence in patients with occlusive disease of the lower aorta and iliac arteries. The syndrome also included buttock pain and lower limb claudication.

The angle of erection declines with age as noted in the Kinsey (1948) report. However, no equivalent population survey has been undertaken to determine whether these changes are likely to be due to peripheral arterial disease or other defects in the erectile mechanism. Specific questionnaires in a peripheral vascular clinic have yielded an incidence of between 21% and 73%. This wide range may be related to the depth of questioning or the definition of impotence, both by the questioner and the patient. Older patients vary considerably with respect to their expectation of potency.

The vast majority of large vessel diseases causing impotence are atheromatous in origin. Common and internal iliac artery disease has to be severe and bilateral to produce impotence. In the presence of widespread aortoiliac stenotic disease, flow in the pudendal arteries can be reduced on exercise, be this lower limb or specifically of the gluteal muscles, the so-called pelvic steal syndrome (Michal, Pospichal and Blazkova, 1978).

Arterial surgery of large vessel disease can improve impotence but it can also precipitate this symptom by a number of mechanisms. Dissection of iliac vessels involving the presacral region can damage the pelvic parasympathetic plexuses controlling erection. Bilateral lumbar sympathectomy produces retrograde ejaculation and these factors must be taken into account in large vessel surgery. In this group of patients, embolism of debris into the pudendal vessels may also produce impotence, the so-called 'trash pelvis'. Such debris can accumulate in the arterial lumen during endarterectomy and other forms of reconstructive surgery and then be flushed into the pelvic arterial tree on reperfusion.

Arterial bypass from the aorta to the external iliac or femoral vessels can exclude the internal iliac arteries. End-to-side anastomosis of the graft onto the aorta or distal vessels may mean that the internal iliac arteries are still perfused antegradely or retrogradely, provided the internal iliac and its peripheral branches are not totally occluded. Much of the evidence in relation to impotence with large vessel surgery is anecdotal, but Queral *et al.* (1979) studied the haemodynamics of pelvic flow after 38 aortoiliac reconstructions. The high (71%) preoperative impotence level emphasized the magnitude of the problem which is uncovered by detailed history taking in this group of patients. The varied response to surgery was also documented by these workers, in that the penile arterial pressures were increased in 37% of patients and reduced in 21% after surgery.

The dramatic reduction in surgery for aortoiliac occlusive disease, due to the widespread use of percutaneous transluminal angioplasty, makes it more difficult to currently assess the relative value of different surgical approaches; these factors are considered again later in the chapter.

Bilateral internal iliac artery disconnection, such as in bilateral renal transplantation, may give rise to impotence. However, this is unpredictable since brachiopenile arterial pressure indices were not reduced in 55% of patients in this group. Disease of the pudendal and penile arteries is not routinely looked for in the assessment of lower limb peripheral vascular disease and the incidence of coexistent proximal and distal disease is poorly documented.

Bilateral focal pudendal and penile vascular disease is not infrequently encountered in an impotence clinic. The aetiology of these lesions is usually assumed to be atheromatous in nature, although patients are often in the third and fourth decade and may have no marked associated proximal disease. The lesions are usually bilateral and symmetrical and particularly involve the distal pudendal arteries. These vessels and other collateral pelvic arteries may be damaged in severe pelvic fractures, impotence becoming apparent as a late sequel of these events. Impotence has also been reported in cyclists, the saddle presumably pressing on the internal pudendal arteries in the pudendal canals.

## Assessment

Assessment of patients with arterial impotence, as with all forms of impotence, commences with a detailed history and examination. It is important to establish whether a patient has ever had normal erectile function as this is closely linked with the patient's expectations from any therapeutic measures. Arterial impotence is suggested by the slow onset of tumescence and failure to reach rigidity. Progression of the arterial disease is accompanied by decreasing potency until erection disappears completely. This contrasts with venous impotence in which erections usually develop promptly but do not reach full rigidity or rapidly disappear. However, both of these problems may coexist and there may be superadded neuropathic disease, such as in the diabetic patient.

The preservation of normal early morning erections suggests that there is no significant vascular disease. Similarly, intermittent problems are unlikely to be vascular-mediated. The history should include a full vascular survey, this encompassing lower limb symptoms of intermittent claudication or rest pain, angina or myocardial infarction, and cerebrovascular symptoms such as transient ischaemic attacks and strokes. All risk factors, such as hypertension, smoking and diabetes, should be noted. Examination includes a thorough assessment of the genitalia and lumbosacral nervous system. Cardiovascular examination pays particular attention to lower limb pulses and the nutrition of the feet. Bruits are sought over the carotid and subclavian vessels in the neck, the abdominal aorta and iliac vessels in the abdomen and the femoral arteries along the length of each thigh. It is sometimes difficult to feel a penile pulse in a normal individual and the presence or absence of this sign is not a good diagnostic indicator.

It is our practice to undertake an endocrine screen on patients with impotence although it rarely identifies unsuspected abnormalities. Of prime importance is to check for glycosuria and a raised blood sugar. The screen includes testosterone, prolactin, FSH and LH. Our next screening test is an intracorporeal injection of 30–60 mg papaverine, the dosage depending on the degree of impotence reported. A normal response is interpreted as indicating competent arterial and venous systems and no further vascular investigations are undertaken.

If the response to papaverine is reduced or short-lived, further studies are undertaken. Our initial research programme included sleep laboratory testing and visual erotic stimulation. While these were valuable in establishing the baselines against which to assess other investigations, they were not of sufficient discriminatory value to include as routine studies. Similarly isotope penile blood flow techniques were initially developed and found of value in diagnosing large vessel abnormalities but were less discriminatory for small vessel disease. The technique used in these investigations was deconvolution analysis of penile artery isotope transit times.

Ultrasound has revolutionized the non-invasive assessment of peripheral vascular disease, including its use in vasculogenic impotence. Abelson (1975) was one of the first to measure penile blood pressure in impotent patients. A more valuable measure is the penile/brachial pressure index, since this takes the systemic pressure into the equation (Kempczinski, 1979). Indices below 0.6 are a useful indicator of severe arterial disease. However, values between 0.6 and 0.9 are less sensitive or specific in the diagnosis of arterial impotence (Metz and Bengtsson, 1981).

The superficial dorsal arteries of the penis can be assessed easily with a hand-held Doppler probe but flow in the deeper arteries is difficult to identify with this instrument. In recent years, attention has been directed at duplex scanning of penile arteries (Lue *et al.*, 1985). The duplex instrument provides a means of assessing the deep arteries as well as the dorsal and is currently the only reliable non-invasive measure for assessing flows in these vessels (Robinson, Woodcock and Stephenson, 1989). The duplex instrument also enables waveform analysis of all penile vessels (Shabsigh and Fishman, 1988), providing information on arterial flow.

The combination of an intracorporeal injection of papaverine and ultrasonic assessment provides an indication of the presence of arterial disease and enables the decision to be made as to the necessity of progressing to angiography. The latter not only provides supportive evidence of arterial disease, but also identifies the site of any lesions and enables the planning of a treatment regime. If there is suggestion of a venous component to a patient's impotence, preliminary venous studies are advisable. This usually takes the form of cavernosometry and cavernosography; these techniques are considered elsewhere.

## Angiography

Arteriography is undertaken in patients in whom arterial disease has been identified by non-invasive studies and who would consider undergoing reconstructive arterial surgery. It should not be carried out without valid reason, since it can produce focal vascular and systemic complications. If the history and clinical findings are suggestive of major aortoiliac disease, the study is primarily to visualize these large vessels. The usual procedure is a retrograde femoral aortogram or, in severe occlusive disease, an intravenous digital subtraction arteriogram. The latter is preferred to translumbar or transbrachial catheterization.

In most impotent patients being considered for reconstructive surgery, the lesions are more distally sited and selective demonstration of the internal iliac tree is required. Even in these patients a preliminary flush aortogram is advised to identify coexistent large vessel disease.

The penile arteries are not visualized on routine aortography and cannulation of the internal pudendal arteries can be technically difficult and is prone to artefact. Initial studies (Michal, Pospichal and Blazkova, 1978; Struyven *et al.*, 1979) were undertaken under general anaesthesia to overcome some of the problems of spasm. However, improvements and modifications have made it possible to undertake the procedure under local anaesthetic (Delcour *et al.*, 1989). Bilateral disease is present in these patients and views are required of both internal pudendal arteries. Conversely, if the first side examined shows a completely normal study, there is little to be gained from proceeding to investigation of the second side. Cannulation is usually via the femoral artery in the groin and it may be possible to cannulate both internal iliac and internal pudendal arteries through a single access site. As with pharmacocavernosography, improved results are obtained by preliminary intracorporeal injection of 40 mg papaverine (Bookstein *et al.*, 1987). The procedure has been further facilitated by improvements in catheter and guidewire design, primarily due to developments in the coronary artery field. The amount of contrast medium can be reduced using digital subtraction techniques: low osmolality contrast agents further reduce pain and associated spasm.

Positioning of the patient is important. The penis is placed horizontally across the contralateral thigh, views are taken anteroposteriorly after tilting the pelvis to 45 degrees. In the latter view, the internal pudendal artery crosses the head of the femur but its branches are not overlain by bony structures and abnormalities are more clearly demonstrated. A volume of 20–30 ml of contrast is required to demonstrate the iliac and 10 ml the internal pudendal arteries. Typical injection rates are 3 ml $s^{-1}$, the timing and number of films depending on blood flow rate and available apparatus. Decisions on surgical management can only be made after the bilateral anatomy and any abnormalities of the pudendal arteries have been demonstrated.

Absence of a dorsal or deep artery on one side does not in itself constitute the cause of arterial impotence, since congenital anomalies are common. However, bilateral focal occlusive or stenotic lesions in the internal pudendal artery, or the deep or dorsal arteries, and the presence of collateral vessels are suggestive of arteriogenic causes of impotence.

## Surgical procedures

Although the relation of arterial disease to impotence has been recognized since Leriche's original report, the surgical management of these lesions was slow to follow. The problems and unpredictability of aortoiliac reconstruction has already been referred to and, when appropriate, percutaneous transluminal angioplasty presents a much more satisfactory alternative for large vessel occlusive disease. Common, external and internal iliac stenoses can be effectively catheterized and dilated with minimal morbidity and without the risk of pelvic denervation.

The incidence of distal embolization after angioplasty is surprisingly low, in view of the unstable surfaces observed at operation. In our experience it has also been possible to negotiate and successfully dilate over half the occluded common iliac arteries currently encountered in peripheral lower limb disease. Selective cannulation and dilatation of the distal internal iliac arteries is more difficult, and occlusive lesions in the pudendal artery and its penile branches do not currently lend themselves to this technique. In view of this, some form of bypass has to be considered.

One of the first reported operative procedures was direct surgery to the pudendal artery, using a vein bypass from the femoral artery (Michal, Kramer and Bartak, 1974). Subsequent reports for most of the next decade were towards revascularization of the corpora cavernosa. Michal's group was again actively involved in these procedures. Vein grafting from a femoral artery to a window in the tunica albuginea was an early procedure of choice. The main complication of this approach was a high incidence of priapism. A smaller bypass vessel was therefore considered necessary: the inferior epigastric became the donor vessel of choice.

Michal *et al.* (1977) reported initial success with the latter procedure; however, long-term follow-up bypass procedures to the corpora cavernosa were unsatisfactory. Hawatmeh *et al.* (1982) demonstrated a high incidence of fibrous thickening of the septum and, to a lesser extent, the cavernous tissue following long saphenous vein, femoral to cavernous bypass. They considered these effects were due to the high pressure within the intracavernous tissue. Metz and Frimodt-Moller (1983) assessed the long-term results in nine patients in whom they had undertaken epigastric to cavernous anastomoses. Only two of the anastomoses were patent, these being at 12 and 24 months following surgery. This team considered the operation to be an unsatisfactory procedure in the management of arterial impotence.

A novel alternative approach was introduced by Virag *et al.* (1981) who reported improvement of erectile function after arterializing the deep dorsal vein. Furlow (1979) modified the approach by proximal ligation of the arterialized segment, together with ligation of the cirucumflex veins, but leaving the perforator veins intact. Virag later extended the latter modification by arterializing the corpora cavernosa from the arterialized segment of vein, by a side-to-side anastomosis to a window in the tunica albuginea. This Virag V procedure was accompanied by less priapism than a femorocavernous vein bypass.

Current trends have returned to Michal's original principle of revascularizing the arteries normally supplying penile blood flow, i.e. the internal pudendal and the deep and dorsal penile arteries. On physiological grounds the deep artery is the most appropriate vessel to revascularize, since it feeds directly into the cavernous vascular plexuses, and is most likely to re-establish normal erection. The deep artery, however, is relatively inaccessible. The terminal portion of the internal pudendal artery is deeply placed in the perineum and there is no convenient adjacent artery for bypass. A vein bypass is therefore required and the denervated free graft has less satisfactory characteristics in terms of size and physiological control compared with a natural artery.

The deep artery of the penis can be exposed in the corpora cavernosa at the base of the penis (Figure 21.1). The tunica albuginea is incised and a blunt nerve hook is swept transversely from lateral to medial, gently lifting out the deep artery. The artery is medially placed within the corpora cavernosa and can be stretched to the dorsal surface for end-to-side anastomosis with a donor vessel. The procedure has a number of disadvantages. The tunica is opened and has to be left unsutured, at least in part, to allow passage of the donor vessel; locating the deep artery can be difficult as it is variable in size and may be congenitally absent, resulting in technical problems; re-establishment of normal flow may be unsuccessful. Dissection invariably involves local destruction of cavernous tissue and the tumescence mechanisms at this site.

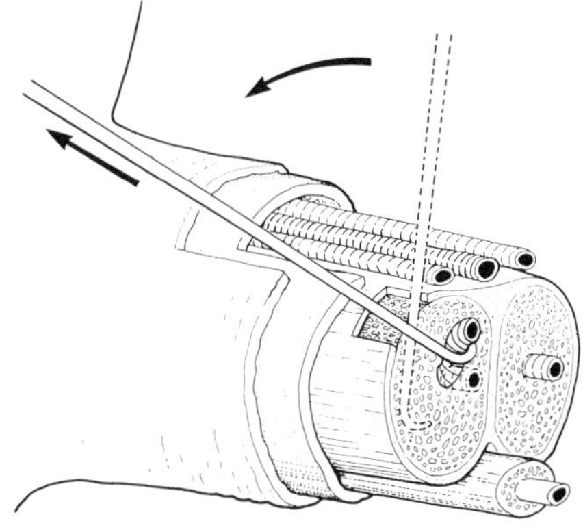

**Figure 21.1** Dissection of the deep (cavernosal) artery of the penis. The tunica albuginea is divided longitudinally, on one side of the midline, at the base of the penis. A blunt hook is inserted into the lateral aspect of the corpus cavernosum. The hook is then gently swept medially to engage the deep artery, which is lifted to the surface for anastomosis

These comments are based on the disappointing personal experiences of the author, since the technical details and results of this procedure are poorly documented in the literature. Generally they have been incorporated in an overview of the surgical practice of individual surgeons and specific technical details and results are not available.

The dorsal penile arteries are more readily accessible for surgical bypass than the deep. However, they carry physiological disadvantages as their terminal supply is predominantly to the glans penis. They do have branches to the corpora cavernosa but these are ill-defined and inconsistent, and are probably of little importance in normal erection. The justification for their use in revascularization is therefore based on retrograde flow to the origin of the vessels and thence to the deep penile artery. This in turn is dependent on normal vessels back to and including the bifurcation of the internal pudendal artery, and the presence of a normal deep penile artery on the side of anastomosis. These features may have been demonstrated radiologically, filling through collaterals beyond proximal disease; however, occasionally this information is not available until peroperative and postoperative assessment.

Goldstein (1986) advocated end-to-end anastomosis of the inferior epigastric to the proximal cut end of one or both dorsal penile arteries (Figure 21.2). This serves to ensure maximum retrograde

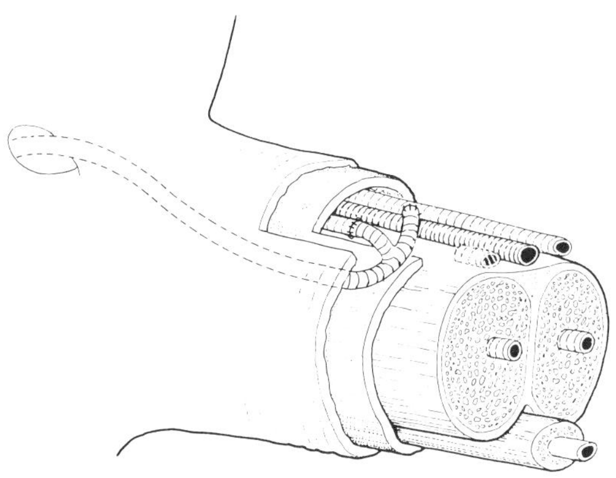

**Figure 21.2** Inferior epigastric to bilateral dorsal artery anastomoses. The cut end of the inferior epigastric artery has been anastomosed end-to-side onto the left dorsal artery of the penis. A large muscular branch of the donor artery has been anastomosed end-to-end onto the proximal right dorsal artery of the penis, because of distal occlusion of the latter vessel

flow in the dorsal arteries and from thence to the deep penile arteries.

The flow in a vessel is dependent on the pressure gradient across a vascular bed. Microanastomoses are therefore more likely to remain patent if the donor artery, providing blood at systemic pressure, is anastomosed to a vessel with a low peripheral resistance. This is demonstrated by the remarkably consistent high patency rates in transcranial revascularization, when these procedures have been undertaken in patients with a low cerebral blood flow. Resistance in the cavernous plexus falls during the initial phase of erection but is high during full tumescence and may also be relatively high in the resting phase. The concept of shunt vessels as proposed by Wagner *et al.* (1982) does provide a physiological means of lowering peripheral resistance although the mechanism remains uncertain. To overcome potential peripheral resistance problems, a useful addition to the dorsal artery revascularization procedure is a concomitant arteriovenous fistula as proposed by Hauri (1985).

## Technical considerations

The author favours revascularization through an inferior epigastric to dorsal penile artery anastomosis. This is usually an end-to-side anastomosis onto the penile vessel with an additional side-to-side anastomosis to the second dorsal artery, if two satisfactory vessels are located. A concomitant arteriovenous fistula is fashioned to the deep dorsal vein of the penis.

### Inferior epigastric artery as a donor vessel

The inferior epigastric artery has to be mobilized from the deep inguinal ring to the level of the umbilicus to provide an adequate length for bypass. At the latter site the major component of the artery enters the deep surface of the rectus abdominus muscle; its continuation for anastomosis to the superior epigastric artery is less suitable for anastomosis.

The vessel is exposed by a longitudinal lower abdominal incision, onto and then through the rectus sheath. A paramedian incision allows exposure of the inferior epigastric artery, but the rectus muscle requires a good deal of lateral retraction and the proximal dissection of the vessel has to pass deep to the muscle and then beyond its lateral edge. A lateral pararectal incision is therefore more convenient. The rectus sheath is incised near the lateral border of the rectus muscle and the muscle retracted medially (Figure 21.3). The lower thoracic nerves

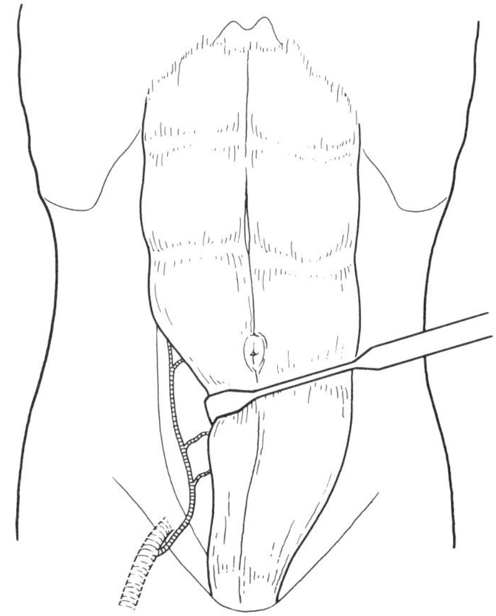

**Figure 21.3** Exposure of the inferior epigastric artery. The skin, superficial abdominal fascial layers and the anterior rectus sheath have been divided along the lateral border of the right rectus muscle. After distal division of the artery, the cut end is passed anterior to the conjoint tendon and through the superficial inguinal ring to the root of the penis

supplying the rectus abdominis muscle are often ill-defined, but when identified must be carefully preserved. The inferior epigastric artery is mobilized together with its venae commitantes. Separating the artery from these one or two veins is difficult and carries the potential of arterial damage; it is unnecessary. Small branches can be coagulated with a bipolar instrument away from the main vessel. Two or three larger branches passing to the deep surface of the rectus abdominis muscle are best ligated with a 6/0 tie. The large branch entering the muscle at the level of the umbilicus is identified, but only ligated and divided with the main vessel when it is needed for bypass.

The proximal end of the inferior epigastric artery dissection passes to within a centimetre of the deep ring, beneath the conjoined tendon. No attempt is made to define its origin, since this is usually surrounded by fatty tissue and the vessel can be easily damaged at this site. While the penile dissection is being undertaken the inferior epigastric artery is left in continuity. The vessel is kept moist and a few drops of papaverine or an alpha-blocking agent may be placed on it to relieve any spasm. When ready for anastomosis the distal vessel is transected at approximately the level of the umbilicus preserving the last perforating rectus muscle branch as this may be larger than the main trunk, or two ends may be needed for revascularization.

The route to the dorsum of the penis is through the superficial inguinal ring. Gentle blunt dissection is used to fashion a pathway from the abdominal wound through to the incision over the base of the penis, in a deep subcutaneous plane. In closing the abdominal incision, care must be taken not to damage the pedicle when suturing the lower extremity of the divided anterior rectus sheath. Usually bleeding is minimal at the time of closure and in this case it is unnecessary to drain the wound.

## Exposure of dorsal penile vessels

The incision at the base of the penis is approximately 2.5 cm long and may be transverse or longitudinal. Even if the skin incision is transverse, the fascial incision and vessel dissection is longitudinal. Approximately 1 cm of at least one dorsal artery is required for satisfactory anastomosis and a similar length of deep dorsal vein when a fistula is being fashioned. The incision is deepened onto these vessels by a mixture of blunt and sharp dissection, particular attention being paid to preservation of neuronal and vascular structures. Magnification must be used during this procedure but ×2–4 surgical loupes are usually sufficient at this stage. A surprising number of fascial layers are encountered in the search for suitable vessels, but careful gentle dissection starting from the midline and working first to the side of the abdominal incision and then to the contralateral side is usually rewarded by the definition of a satisfactory length of dorsal penile artery on at least one side.

Normal dorsal penile arteries are to be expected in patients following pelvic trauma or bilateral renal transplant. However, occasionally in the elderly patient an occluded atheromatous dorsal vessel is present on one side and stenosed artery on the other. Following these vessels proximally may allow the definition of a more normal segment which, on transection, produces a weak forward flow. End-to-end anastomosis is the procedure of choice in this situation, preferably using both dorsal arteries, possibly using the last rectus branch of the inferior epigastric artery to provide two end-to-end anastomoses.

When at least one normal dorsal penile artery is present, the author's preference is to undertake a single end-to-side anastomosis. With such a normal vessel it is also possible to incorporate the arterio-venous fistula within the single anastomosis (Figure 21.4). The dorsal artery and vein are mobilized and brought alongside each other and subsequent manoeuvres carried out under a dissecting microscope. At this stage the adequacy of the tunnel for the donor artery is checked and the inferior epigastric is drawn into the penile wound. A microvascular clip is applied to the divided artery and bleeding veins bipolar coagulated or ligated. Care is taken to secure the distal cut ends, since a considerable haematoma can ensue if these ligatures come off.

Micro-Mayfield clips are applied proximally and distally to the adjacent dorsal penile artery and vein. Adventitial strands and residual adherent tissues must be teased out and divided from the segments to ensure they are not pulled into the anastomosis during suture. Equal ellipses of adjacent walls are removed with curved micro-scissors, firmly picking up the centre of each ellipse with a forceps. The length of anastomosis is approximately 2 mm. Pulling up on a forceps allows the length of the incision to be carefully judged. Care must be taken not to remove more than a quarter of the circumference of either vessel since this will leave inadequate vessel wall for suture without a stenosis. Incisions can be made with a diamond knife or other microblades; however, the anastomosis is facilitated by removal of the ellipse.

The posterior adjacent walls of the incised artery and vein are sutured first. A continuous 10/0 monofilament nylon suture can be used, but long loops cannot be visualised under the microscope and can catch adjacent tissues. This will exert excessive traction on the anastomosis or break the suture. An interrupted anastomotic technique is therefore usually undertaken. The first stitch is placed in the middle of the back wall, the knot being tied on the outside of the lumen. Subsequent stitches are placed on either side of the first until the two corner sutures are in place.

The divided end of the inferior epigastric artery is now brought alongside the anastomosis. It is usually 1 mm in diameter and therefore will need to be divided slightly obliquely to match the length of the

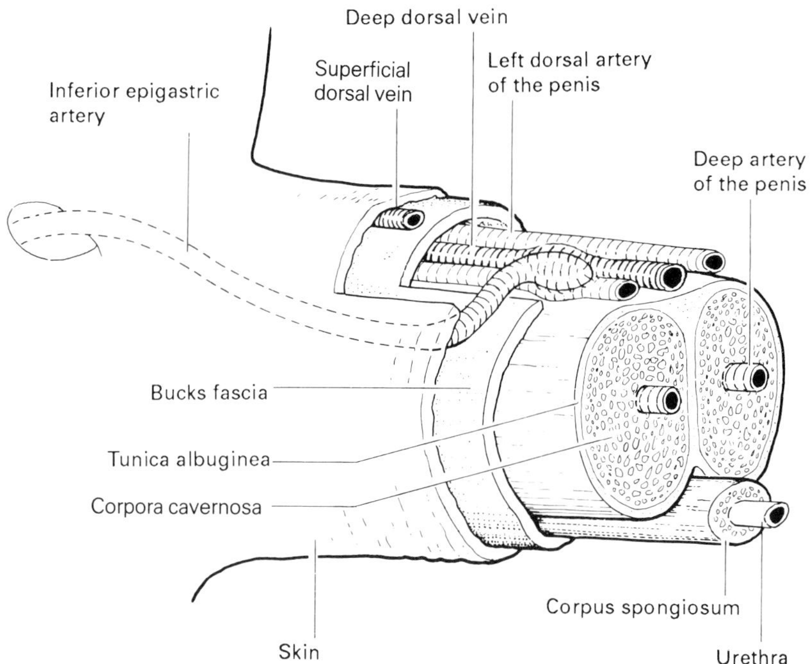


**Figure 21.4** The Hauri operation. The inferior epigastric artery is anastomosed over the site of a dorsal artery to deep dorsal vein arteriovenous fistula

anastomosis. Excessive adventitia must be removed to expose at least 1 mm of clearly dissected normal vessel end. The anastomosis is completed between the donor vessel and the dorsal penile vein on one side, and the dorsal penile artery on the other, using interrupted sutures. On completion of the anastomosis the micro-clips are first removed from the deep dorsal vein, blood being allowed to flow across the anastomosis to check for obvious leaks. If these are absent or once they have been sutured, the clips are removed from the dorsal artery, haemostasis rechecked, and a swab placed over the anastomosis while the clamp is removed from the donor artery. The swab is left in place for 2–3 min. The clamp may require replacement to deal with a spurting leak but stitch holes should be gently covered until haemostasis is obtained.

Following this procedure there should be no stenoses and flow should be demonstrable in all limbs of the anastomosis. This may be tested by gently occluding each limb with a forceps and milking out the blood from the adjacent segment with a second forceps: on release of the first forceps the milked segment should fill across the anastomosis. If this is not so, gentle manipulation of the vessels and removal of all adventitial strands is necessary.

At all times the dissection must be kept moist with heparinized saline. Systemic heparinization is not required in these micro-anastomoses but debris must be washed away from the lumen before completion, using a stream of heparinized saline from a syringe and needle. The operator must be confident that the anastomosis and the fistula are patent before wound closure. If back bleeding was present from the dorsal penile artery and pulsatile forward flow from the inferior epigastric artery prior to anastomosis, primary patency should be obtainable. Occlusion of the deep dorsal vein on the proximal side of the anastomosis may be seen to improve pulsation in the dorsal artery and it may be appropriate to ligate one limb of the fistula. If there is any doubt about patency, however, it is wise to omit this manoeuvre.

In the absence of a suitable dorsal penile artery a Virag V procedure is recommended. In this a 2.5 cm length of deep dorsal vein is mobilized and an adjacent length of tunica aluginea over the dorsal aspect of one corpora cavernosa is freed of adherent tissue. The incision in the tunica is approximately 12 mm long, removing a 1.5 mm strip of the wall with a pointed scalpel or micro-knife. The segment of vein is occluded proximally and distally with micro-clips, and an ellipse of venous wall of equivalent length and adjacent to the tunica defect is removed with curved micro-scissors. A fine probe is passed distally along the vein to destroy the two or three valve cusps along the length of the penis, but preserving the valve adjacent to the glans penis. A venocavernous anastomosis is undertaken using 10/0 monofilament suture. A cutting needle is appropriate to suture the thick tunica wall. The inferior epigastric artery is anastomosed end-to-side onto the vein, proximal to the first anastomosis. The proximal limb of the venous fistula can be ligated at a later stage once flow and an erectile pattern have been established.

Operative complications from these various procedures are minimal. The patient can leave hospital after 2–3 days and stitches can be removed after 8–9 days. Sexual activity is encouraged but intercourse should be delayed for 5–6 weeks.

## Outcome

The results of these various procedures have been variously reported. The disappointing outcome of the vein bypasses and direct anastomses to the corpora cavernosa have already been referred to. Other figures are complex, including many procedures and ill-defined lengths of follow-up. Important factors such as aetiology and age are often difficult to analyse. In our own series, procedures were initially undertaken on severe arteriopaths and results were disappointing. However, this may also have been linked to development of the techniques and choice of operative procedure. In our first reported 12 patients followed up over a period of 4 years, only six showed prolonged improvement. The four most recent cases using the Hauri fistula technique, however, have all shown marked improvement of erectile status and anastomotic patency has been retained by the addition of the arteriovenous fistula.

Goldstein (1986) reported the results of 130 procedures followed from 6 months to 5 years with a return of coitus rate of 54%. Classification into atherosclerotic, idiopathic and traumatic vasculogenic groups obtained return of coitus rates respectively in 24%, 40% and 81% of patients. One may still question whether an overall 50% success for a revascularization procedure is an acceptable figure. However, penile prostheses are not an acceptable alternative for all patients and the long-term complication rate remains a problem. Of prime importance, therefore, is patient selection. Traumatic, and to a lesser extent congenital, anomalies of the internal pudendal artery are of prime importance since, in these patients, return of erectile function can be expected.

The reliability of the techniques is partly dependent on experience and the expertise of the clinical team managing the assessment. It is also essential to have the full understanding of the patient with regard to possible failure and realistic expectation of outcome. Retention of the natural mechanism of erection is a desirable aim, particularly as it does not damage the normal sensation of erection. Revascularization does not prevent subsequent implant insertion, whereas this is not true for the reverse situation. Further research should be directed towards the understanding of the natural physiological mechanism involved in the erectile response, selection of patients for operative procedures, methods of bringing a physiologically controlled alternative blood supply to the penis and the factors influencing the long-term patency of revascularization procedures.

### References


Abelson, D. (1975) Diagnostic value of the penile pulse and blood pressure: a Doppler study of impotence in diabetes. *Journal of Urology,* **113**, 636–639

Bookstein, J. J., Valji, K., Parsons, L. and Kessler, W. (1987) Pharmacoarteriography in the evaluation of impotence. *Journal of Urology,* **133**, 39–41

Delcour, C., Katoto, R. M., Richoz, B. *et al.* (1989) Penile arteriogrpahy: technical improvements. *International Journal of Impotence Research,* **1**, 43–47

Furlow, W. L. (1979) Therapy of impotence. *Clinical Neuro-Urology* (ed. R. J. S. Krane), Little Brown, Boston pp. 213–218

Goldstein, I. (1986) Arterial revascularization procedures. *Seminars in Urology,* **4**, 252–258

Hauri, D. (1985) Anastomose des arterielle epigastrica inferiore mit der arterielle dorsalis penis und zusatzlieben AV-Shunt zur V dorsalis penis produnda. *Proceedings of the Leiden Urological Foundation Symposium on Controversy in Diagnosis and Treatment of Erectile Impotence,* p. 12

Hawatmeh, J. S., Houttuin, E., Gregory, J. G. *et al.* (1982) The diagnosis and management of vasculogenic impotence. *Journal of Urology,* **127**, 910–914

Kempczinski, R. F. (1979) Role of the vascular diagnostic laboratory in the evaluation of male impotence. *American Journal of Surgery,* **138**, 278

Kinsey, A. C., Pomeroy, W. and Martin, C. (1948) Age and sexual outlet. In: *Sexual Behaviour in the Human Male* (eds A. C. Kinsey, W. B. Pomeroy, C. E. Martin), W. B. Saunders, Philadelphia, pp. 297–325

Leriche, R. (1923) Des obliterations arterielles hautes comme cause d'une insuffisance circulatoire des membres inferieurs. *Bull. Soc. Chirurgie,* **49**, 1404

Lue, T. F., Hricak, H., Marich, K. W. and Tanagho, E. A. (1985) Vasculogenic impotence evaluated by high-resolution ultrasonography and pulsed Doppler spectrum analysis. *Radiology,* **155**, 777–781

Metz, P. and Bengtsson, J. (1981) Penile blood pressure. *Scandinavian Journal of Urology and Nephrology,* **15**, 161–164

Metz, P. and Frimodt-Moller, C. (1983) Epigastrico-cavernous anastomosis in the treatment of arteriogenic impotence. *Scandinavian Journal of Urology and Nephrology,* **17**, 271–275

Michal, V., Kramer, R., Pospichal, J. and Hejhal, L. (1977) Arterial epigastrico–cavernous anastomosis for the treatment of sexual impotence. *World Journal of Surgery,* **1**, 515–520

Michal, V., Kramer, R. and Bartak, V. (1974) Femoro-pudendal bypass in the treatment of sexual impotence. *Journal of Cardiovascular Surgery,* **15**, 356

Michal, V., Pospichal, J. and Blazkova, J. (1978) Phalloarteriogrpahy in the diagnosis of erectile impotence. *World Journal of Surgery,* **2**, 239–247

Queral, L. A., Whitehouse, W. M., Flinn, W. R. *et al.* (1979) Pelvic haemodynamics after aortoiliac reconstruction. *Surgery,* **86**, 799–809

Robinson, L. Q., Woodcock, J. P. and Stephenson, T. P. (1989) Duplex scanning in suspected vasculogenic impotence: a worthwhile exercise? *British Journal of Urology,* **63**, 432–436

Shabsigh, R. and Fishman, I. J. (1988) Evaluation of erectile impotence. *Urology,* **32**, 83–90

Struyven, J., Gregoir, W., Giannakopoulos, X. and Wauters, E. (1979) Selective pudendal arteriography. *European Urology,* **5**, 233–242

Virag, R., Zwang, G., Dermange, H. and Legman, M. (1981) Vasculogenic impotence: a review of 92 cases with 54 surgical operations. *Journal of Vascular Surgery,* **15**, 9–17

Wagner, G., Willis, E. A., Bro-Pasmussen, F. and Nielsen, M. H. (1982) New theory on the mechanism of erection involving hitherto undescribed vessels. *Lancet,* **i**, 416–418

# Section Four

# Specific problems in erectile dysfunction

# 22

# Surgically induced erectile dysfunction and its prevention

R. S. Kirby

Erectile impotence is a common disorder and, when naturally induced by ageing, is often borne with fortitude by the sufferer. By contrast, when the condition occurs as a result of surgery the patient is often less sanguine, especially if he has not been fully informed of the possible consequences preoperatively. The exact incidence of surgically-induced erectile impotence is unknown. However, it has been estimated that about 14% of men who have organic impotence suffer this condition as a direct result of nerve and/or blood vessel injury during surgery or radiotherapy.

## Pathogenesis

Normal erectile and ejaculatory function depends on the functional integrity of the central nervous system and its peripheral connections. The sympathetic outflow from the T10–L1 spinal segments, the parasympathetic outflow from S2–S4 segments, and the somatic afferent and efferent fibres running in the pudendal nerves may all be injured during pelvic or retroperitoneal surgery. Recently, careful documentation of the exact anatomical course of the nerves supplying the corpora cavernosa (Walsh and Donker, 1982) has thrown new light on the nature of these injuries, and the methods of their prevention.

The hypogastric nerves run caudally anterior to the aorta and cross the iliac vessels (Figure 22.1) to merge with the parasympathetic plexus in the pelvis anterolateral to the rectum (Figure 22.2). Injury to these sympathetic fibres may occur during aortic surgery and, more importantly because of the age group concerned, during retroperitoneal lymph node dissection for non-seminomatous testicular malignancies.

The pelvic ganglia lying lateral to the rectum are important relay stations for the innervation of both the bladder and corpora cavernosa. In addition there is evidence from studies in cats that they may be involved in the interaction of the sympathetic and parasympathetic innervation of the bladder and genitalia (De Groat *et al.*, 1979). Injury to these structures may occur during abdominoperineal resection of the rectum or low anterior resection of rectal tumours as well as during pan-proctocolectomy. The pelvic plexus provides visceral branches that innervate the seminal vesicles, prostate, rectum, membranous urethra and corpora cavernosa. In addition, branches that contain somatic motor axons probably travel through the pelvic plexus to supply the levator ani, coccygeus and the striated urethral musculature. The nerves innervating the prostate travel outside the capsule of the prostate and Denonvillier's fascia until they perforate the capsule and enter the prostate. The branches to the membranous urethra and corpora cavernosa ('nerves of Walsh') also travel outside and behind the prostate capsule in the lateral pelvic fascia. Near the apex of the prostate these nerves come to lie a little further anteriorly on the lateral surface of the membranous urethra in the 3 o'clock and 9 o'clock positions respectively; here they are particularly vulnerable during radical prostatectomy, cystoprostatectomy and transpubic urethroplasty (Lepor *et al.*, 1985). After piercing the urogenital diaphragm they pass behind the dorsal penile artery and dorsal penile nerve on each side to enter the corpora on their medial aspect (Lue *et al.*, 1984).

Potency also critically depends on an intact arterial blood supply. Equally vulnerable to injury during pelvic surgery are the arterial vessels supplying the corpora. Both internal iliac arteries are deliberately ligated by some surgeons during cystectomy – a manoeuvre very likely to induce vasculogenic impotence. The terminal branches of the internal iliac arteries pass posterolateral to the prostate in close association with the nerves described above forming the 'neurovascular bundles'. In addition, the veins draining the corpora may be affected by radical prostatic surgery for cancer, since the dorsal vein complex is always ligated and divided in the retropubic space. Other surgical causes of erectile impotence include bilateral orchidectomy undertaken to reduce androgen stimulation of prostate cancer. Psychological causes of post-operative loss of potency must also be taken into account as surgery, especially when undertaken in the later decades of life, constitutes a significant 'life event' to which other phenomena such as age-related impotence may incorrectly be attributed.

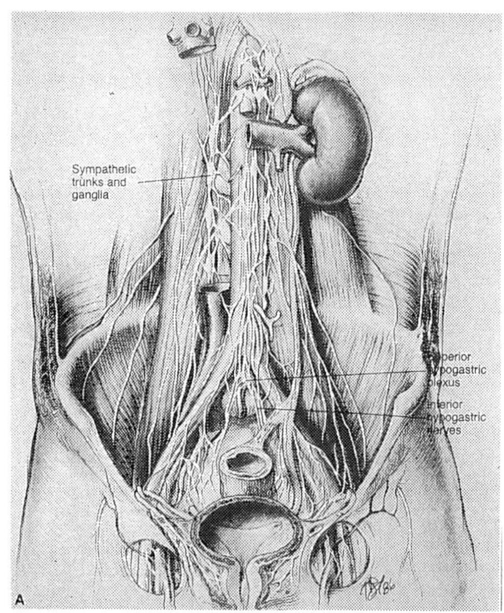


**Figure 22.1** The sympathetic pathways to the pelvis. From Skinner and Lieskovsky (1988) with permission of the publishers

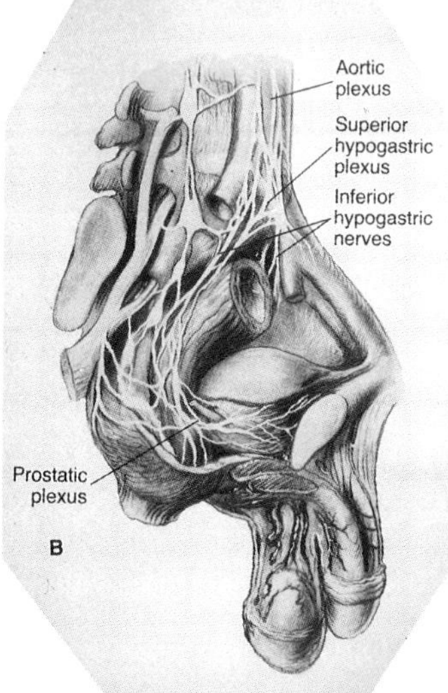


**Figure 22.2** The sympathetic and parasympathetic pathways merge in the pelvis. From Skinner and Lieskovsky (1988) with permission of the publishers

## Individual operations which may result in impotence

### Abdominoperineal resection of the rectum

Abdominoperineal resection, pan-proctocolectomy and low anterior resection of the rectum, especially the former, are all operations which may result in injury to the pelvic plexus. This may be either a slowly resolving neuropraxis or a more permanent neurotmesis. Postoperatively erectile impotence is often accompanied by prolonged bladder dysfunction, including difficulty with voiding and occasionally stress incontinence. Urodynamic studies reveal a reduction of bladder compliance and detrusor areflexia. Neurophysiological investigations confirm the presence of abnormal motor units (Kirby *et al.*, 1986) and either prolongation or absence of the sacral reflex latency (bulbocavernosus reflex analogue).

Avoidance of these complications of rectal surgery depends on the careful preservation of the pelvic plexus lateral to the rectum. However this, of course, has to be balanced against the need for adequate local cancer clearance (impotence and bladder dysfunction are more common after resection of more locally extensive lesions) and the patient should be counselled to this effect before surgery.

If urinary retention does develop following extirpative rectal surgery, caution should be exercised before proceeding to transurethral surgery. If the cause is a neural injury rather than the usually assumed bladder obstruction due to benign prostatic hyperplasia, then there may also be a partial denervation of the external (distal) urinary sphincter. Resection of the bladder neck and prostate will destroy the proximal continence mechanisms and leave the patient dependent on a distal sphincter which may not be totally competent. Urinary incontinence may therefore be the result. An alternative to transurethral prostatectomy, at least in the immediate postoperative period, is intermittent self-catheterization or suprapubic catheterization, in combination with judicious doses of an α-adrenoceptor blocker such as prazosin, which will reversibly reduce bladder neck and prostatic tone and can be stopped when full recovery occurs or if incontinence supervenes.

### Radical prostatectomy

Radical excision of the prostate, either by the perineal or retropubic route, has historically been associated with an incidence of postoperative erectile impotence that approached 100%; in addition, a proportion of patients suffer urinary incontinence after this form of surgery. The observations of Walsh and Donker (1982), however, have led to the development of a modified retropubic procedure in which the neurovascular bundles are carefully preserved (Walsh, Lepor and Eggleton, 1983).

For fuller details of this technique the reader is referred to the beautifully illustrated publications of Walsh (1986, 1987), but the essentials of the procedure will be briefly reiterated here. The patient is positioned supine on the operating table in slight Trendelenburg tilt and a urethral catheter inserted. A midline lower abdominal incision is made and the retropubic space explored. The peritoneum is maintained intact and both vasa are divided just beyond their entry to the abdomen, through the internal ring. This manoeuvre allows medial retraction of the bladder and facilitates the dissection of the internal iliac lymph nodes on each side which are sent for frozen section. This also allows exposure and temporary occlusion of the internal iliac arteries (Figure 22.3). Attention is then paid to the apex of the prostate beneath the pubis. Incisions are made bilaterally into the endopelvic fascia to allow the apex of lateral prostate to be palpated and the puboprostatic ligaments are then divided. The key to the operation is the securing of the dorsal vein complex, which is a much bulkier structure than usually imagined. The avascular shelf between it and the urethra can clearly be palpated, with the aid of an 18 Fr urethral catheter, and a right-angled or curved Satinsky clamp passed behind the structure to allow the complex to be ligated with a strong silk or Dexon suture (Figure 22.4). The complex is then divided with a long-handled scalpel; additional sutures may be necessary if this ligature slips. The urethra itself can then be encircled with a right-angled clamp and a silicone tube passed posteriorly to provide gentle traction. Because of the extreme proximity of the neurovascular bundles at the apex of the prostate, great care must be taken at this point to avoid injury to the tissues lateral to the urethra, either by dissection or diathermy. The urethra is then divided at the apex of the prostate and the urethral catheter clamped and divided; this manoeuvre permits the use of the catheter as a retractor for the prostate. The rectourethralis muscle is then divided and the lateral fascia is dissected away stepwise from the posterolateral prostate bilaterally. This releases the neurovascular bundles laterally and maintains their integrity (Figure 22.5). Towards the base of the prostate the seminal vesicles with their overlying fascia are by now easily identified.

Attention is then turned to the prostato-vesical junction and an incision is made into the bladder. Once the ureteric orifices have been visualized and catheterized to protect them from inadvertent injury, the incision is carried round to the junction of the trigone and prostate. Deepening the incision at this point exposes the seminal vesicles and the ampullary portions of the vasa from their cranial

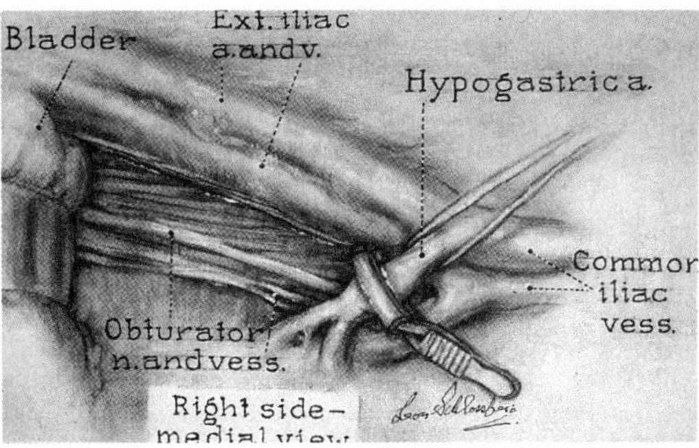


**Figure 22.3** The internal iliac arteries are temporarily occluded with a bulldog clamp. From Walsh (1986) with permission of the publishers

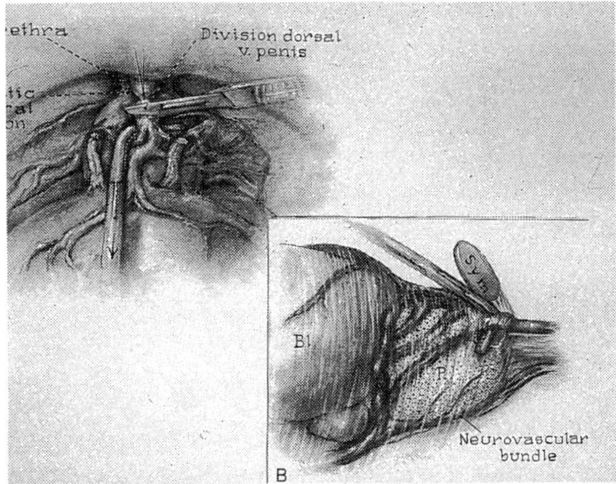


**Figure 22.4** The dorsal vein complex is secured. From Walsh (1986) with permission of the publishers

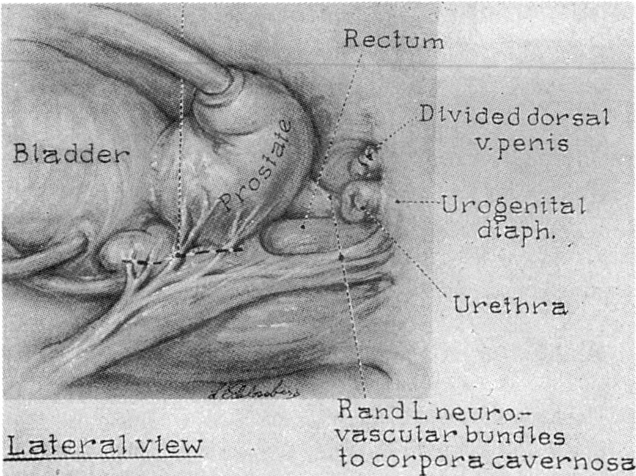


**Figure 22.5** The prostate is reflected cranially and the lateral pedicles divided close to the capsule. From Walsh (1986) with permission of the publishers

aspect. These may then be secured and the vasa and vessels supplying the seminal vesicles divided to permit removal of the specimen, which includes the entire prostate and seminal vesicles. At this point the corporeal vessels which provide macroscopic markers for the microscopic autonomic nerves can usually be visualized running in the posterolateral extensions of the wound, lying on the surface of the rectum. The bladder neck is then reconstructed in a tennis racket fashion and tightened to a diameter whereby it will accept the terminal phalanx of the fifth digit. In order to ensure circumferential mucosa to mucosa apposition at the urethrovesical anastomosis, the mucosa of the bladder neck is everted using fine Dexon sutures. An anastomosis is then created without tension between the bladder and urethra over an 18 Fr silicone urethral catheter using four fine absorbable sutures in the 1, 5, 7 and 11 o'clock positions (Figure 22.6).

Postoperatively the catheter is left in for 3 weeks although the patient need not stay in hospital this long. On its removal some degree of stress incontinence is usual. This rapidly settles, however, although minor stress leakage may persist. Potency also takes time to return, but Walsh and Mostwyn (1984) have reported that nearly 80% of patients undergoing radical prostatectomy by his nerve-sparing technique eventually have return of erections of sufficient rigidity to accomplish intercourse. Age does not seem to be a significant factor in this, but the pathological stage of the resected prostatic tissue has been shown to influence the chances of eventual restoration of potency. This reflects the fact that, in more advanced but still localized lesions, the neurovascular bundle often has to be sacrificed to achieve adequate cancer clearance. Walsh, Epstein and Lowe (1987) have reported that potency may be preserved in some individuals even after one neurovascular bundle has been deliberately excised, but in our experience this is not always the case.

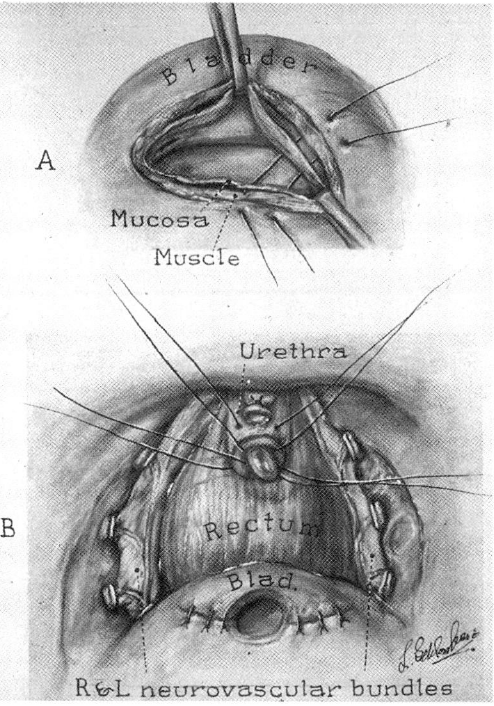


**Figure 22.6** The bladder neck is reconstructed and an anastomosis created between the bladder and urethra. From Walsh (1986) with permission of the publishers

## Radical cystoprostatectomy

As mentioned above, the original descriptions of radical cystoprostatectomy advocated ligation in continuity of both internal iliac arteries to reduce bleeding during the pelvic dissection. Although this manoeuvre does not always result in erectile impotence (potency has been preserved in some individuals in whom the internal iliac arteries have been deliberately ligated bilaterally to prevent excessive bleeding after retropubic prostatectomy), it will certainly reduce arterial inflow to the corpora. In addition, the neurovascular bundles lying lateral to the prostate and membranous urethra are almost always sacrificed during the ligation of the lateral pedicles as performed in the traditional operation. As in radical prostatectomy, the observations of Walsh and Donker (1982) have allowed modifications of the operative technique which permit preservation of the neurovascular bundles (Schlegel and Walsh, 1987). The internal iliac nodes are dissected as in the operation for radical prostatectomy and any nodes in the obturator fossa excised. The superior vesical and obliterated umbilical arteries are then clearly seen branching anteriorly from the internal iliac artery and are ligated and divided. Next the plane between the bladder and the rectum is developed by incising the peritoneum in the rectovesical pouch. Gentle (and it *must* be gentle because it is possible at this stage to tear the rectum) blunt dissection is used to separate the rectum from the bladder down to the level of Denonvillier's fascia. During this dissection some vessels inferior to the superior vesical artery are ligated and divided, but the lateral dissection is not carried down as far as the inferior vesical vessels for fear of injuring the cavernosal nerves.

At this point, with a view to maintaining the integrity of the neurovascular bundles, one of two methods is employed: either the urethra is divided and the prostate removed retrogradely as described above for radical prostatectomy (Walsh, 1986), or the procedure continues from above in the following manner. Once Denonvillier's fascia and the tips of the seminal vesicles have been identified, attention is paid to the inferior vesical pedicle. As shown in Figure 22.2, the cavernous nerves travel to the posterolateral surface of the prostate posterior to the seminal vesicles. Therefore if these structures are used as landmarks and the posterior prostatic pedicles ligated stepwise on their lateral aspects, the neurovascular bundles should be preserved. The only drawback of this method is that, on occasion, during the dissection beside the seminal vesicles, Santorini's plexus may be entered at which point considerable venous bleeding is encountered. If this occurs the remedy is to gain control of the dorsal venous complex in the manner described above. Once the dorsal vein has been secured the urethra is isolated and a ligature passed posteriorly to prevent spillage of urine after the urethra has been divided. The urethra is then transected and the clamped end of the catheter used to provide traction on the prostate and bladder. The rectourethralis muscle is divided in the midline and gentle blunt dissection used to separate the prostate from the rectum. The prostate may then be retracted gently superiorly and to one side and a right-angled clamp passed between the prostatic capsule and the transparent lateral pelvic fascia on the contralateral side. This manoeuvre helps to identify the site of division of the fascia anterior to the neurovascular bundle. The residual branches of the bundle are secured and divided, freeing the prostate from all attachments. By now the neurovascular bundle is visible along the anterolateral surface of the rectum to its point of exit from the pelvis at the urogenital diaphragm. Schlegel and Walsh (1987) have reported potency rates of 83% using this technique when performing cystoprostatectomy alone. In those undergoing cystoprostatectomy and simultaneous urethrectomy, however, the potency rate was only 40%.

Recently the Johns Hopkins group has reported a modification of urethrectomy which may allow preservation of corporeal innervation (Brendler, Schlegel and Walsh, 1990). This technique depends on keeping the dissection of the membranous urethra as close as possible to the midline and minimizing the use of diathermy to avoid damage to the neurovascular bundles. By these means potency may even be maintained in patients undergoing cystoprostatectomy and urethrectomy for extensive transitional cell disease. The critical question of course, which only time and careful comparative evaluation will settle, is whether these nerve-sparing modifications in fact compromise the efficiency of the procedures in terms of complete cancer excision. Even if the local recurrence rate does eventually prove slightly higher with these operations, many patients may opt for preservation of sexual function which is so important for the individual's overall wellbeing and self-esteem.

## Transpubic urethroplasty

Pelvic fractures in the male are not uncommonly associated with partial or complete disruption of the urethra at the prostatomembranous junction. This is, of course, precisely the location in which the cavernous nerves are in closest apposition to the urethra and it is therefore not surprising that the majority of patients suffer some degree of erectile dysfunction after this injury which, in a proportion of cases, may be permanent.

Unfortunately the procedures designed to restore continuity between the prostatic urethra and bulbar urethra (transpubic or perineal prostatobulbar urethroplasty) may often compound the neurovascular injury to the corpora. Thus, while freeing the patient of his suprapubic catheter they may make the erectile dysfunction, which may initially be only partial, in effect worse. There is no certain way of avoiding this complication but the principles of Walsh employed in cystoprostatectomy may be applied at the time of perineal or abdominoperineal urethroplasty and thus damage to the cavernous nerves and vessels minimized.

When a patient presents with a fractured pelvis and an associated injury to the membranous urethra, a decision has to be made as to whether to undertake primary or delayed repair. Although primary repair has been advocated by some, there are a number of reasons why delayed repair (usually at 3–6 months after the initial injury) is to be preferred. Firstly, patients with pelvic fractures and urethral disruption have commonly suffered other associated injuries such as major abdominal, chest or head and neck trauma. To subject such an individual to prolonged anaesthesia and complex reconstructive surgery risks compounding the original injury by inducing complications such as shock lung syndrome and renal failure. Secondly, the restoration of urethral continuity in the acute situation is usually undertaken in surgically suboptimal circumstances which compromises the quality of the prostato-urethral anastomosis and risks development of a post-repair membranous urethral stricture, which may necessitate further surgery later. Finally, the incidence of erectile impotence is probably greater after primary rather than delayed repair. The explanation for the last point lies in the improved anatomical definition which is available after a delay of 3–6 months, during which time the pelvic fracture haematoma has time to largely reabsorb. At the time of delayed repair the urethra is explored either through synchronous retropubic and perineal incisions or simply a perineal approach. The perineal dissection and mobilization of the bulbar urethra does not risk injury to the cavernous nerves, but the creation of the tunnel between the crura of the corpora and up to the apex of the prostate may further damage the site of entry of

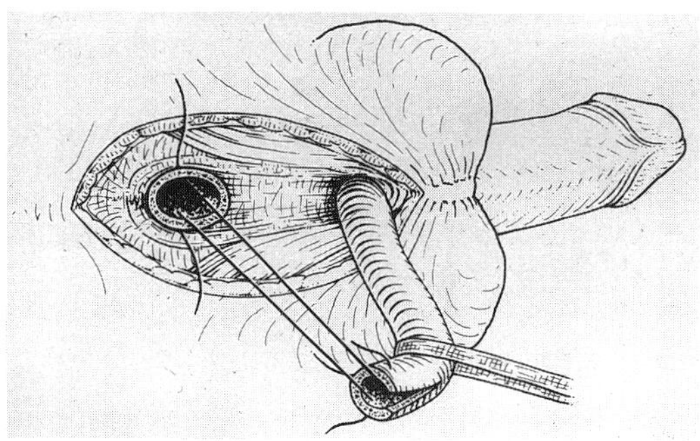

**Figure 22.7** A bulboprostatic anastomosis is created to resolve a stricture of the membranous urethra after a pelvic fracture

neurovascular bundles to the corporeal bodies at the level of the pelvic floor. There is no certain way to avoid this, but the dissection should be kept near to the midline and the tissues gently displaced laterally before the bulbar urethra is brought up to create the spatulated bulbo-prostatic anastomosis (Figure 22.7). The bulbar urethral arteries should be controlled with Ligaclips or ties rather than diathermied to avoid injury to the internal pudendal arteries from which the bulbar urethral arteries arise and which provide the arterial supply to the corpora cavernosa. An omental wrap as advocated by Turner-Warwick gives added security to the anastomosis and reduces the incidence of anastomotic leaks and fistula formation but obviously requires abdominal exploration.

Impotence after pelvic fractures with urethral disruption often does not respond to papaverine pharmacotherapy, which suggests that the dominant cause of the problem is vascular insufficiency although there is usually associated neural injury. In these patients colour Doppler evaluation and arteriography is indicated since a localized block of the pudendal artery may be amenable to revascularization and these are among the group of patients who do best after vascular reconstruction.

## Surgery for benign enlargement of the prostate

That some degree of sexual dysfunction may follow either open or transurethral surgery for benign prostatic hyperplasia (BPH) is not disputed, but the frequency and nature of these disorders remain controversial. When one considers that nearly 380 000 transurethral prostatectomies (TURPs) were performed in the USA in 1988 it is surprising that we have so little accurate data on this subject. Those studies that are available are listed in Table 22.1; unfortunately many of them do not clearly differentiate between ejaculatory dysfunction – which might be expected to be almost universal after prostatectomy – and erectile dysfunction, which should be rare. Moreover, many of the reports are based on patient questionnaires without corroboration from the partner or spouse. Those few investigators who have used objective criteria to assess erectile potency before and after surgery have seldom demonstrated any very definite differences.

### Ejaculatory disturbances after prostatectomy

The neurophysiological basis of ejaculation has been described in Chapter 3. This reflex, which is mediated by the sympathetic nervous system, involves rhythmic contractions of the vasa, seminal vesicles and prostate. The bladder neck closes tightly to direct semen antegradely down the urethra past the relaxed distal sphincter. The pulsatile nature of ejaculation is mainly provided by reflex contractions of the bulbocavernosus and bulbospongiosus muscles. After most forms of prostatectomy the bladder neck is rendered incompetent and this provides the mechanism for retrograde ejaculation which usually follows. Rather surprisingly not all patients undergoing TURP actually suffer retrograde ejaculation – the proportion doing so is nearer to 60% in most studies; however, the explanation for this is unclear. Certainly when a patient who initially has post-TURP retrograde ejaculation subsequently begins to ejaculate antegradely again, this often indicates either recurrent prostatic outflow obstruction or a bladder neck stricture. A much smaller proportion of patients complain of painful ejaculation after prostatectomy. There have been no scientific studies to elucidate the cause of this but the presumption must be that prostatectomy may result in stenosis of the prostatic and ejaculatory ducts.

### Erectile dysfunction after prostatectomy

The exact incidence of erectile problems after prostatectomy is still uncertain, and there is no consensus in the literature on this subject (see Table 22.1). The neurovascular bundles could conceivably be compromised by spread of diathermy current or extravasation of irrigant, especially at the apex of the prostate during TURP.

Padma-Nathan and Krane (1990) have reported veno-occlusive insufficiency in their cases who suffered erectile dysfunction after TURP, but the mechanism by which this could be incurred is obscure. Significantly, Zohan *et al.* (1976) have demonstrated that the incidence of sexual dysfunction after prostatic surgery may be reduced by the simple expedient of preoperative sexual counselling. Time should be taken to clearly explain the implications of the operation in terms of ejaculation and the patient should be reassured that an effect on libido, sensation of orgasm or erectile ability is unusual.

**Table 22.1 Incidence of impotence after prostatectomy**

| *Study* | *Type of operation* | *Postoperative impotence (%)* |
|---|---|---|
| Hargreave and Stephenson (1977) | TURP | 5 |
| | Retropubic | 0 |
| Hauri (1982) | TURP | 8 |
| | Open | 20 |
| Finkle and Moyers (1966) | TURP | 5 |
| | Suprapubic | 14 |
| Moller-Nielsen *et al.* (1985) | TURP | 31 |
| So *et al.* (1982) | TURP | 0 |
| Zohar *et al.* (1976) | TURP with explanation | 0 |
| | TURP without explanation | 63 |

TURP, transurethral prostatectomy

## Retroperitoneal lymph node dissection

Erectile impotence is uncommon after either thoracoabdominal or transabdominal lymph node dissection for non-seminomatous testicular cancer; however, loss of ejaculation is not infrequent. In a disease which affects young men with cure rates currently well in excess of 90%, ejaculatory disturbances and infertility are obviously a major consideration (Donahue and Rowland, 1981).

A number of reports (Lange, Narayan and Fraley, 1984; Richie and Garrick, 1985) have suggested ejaculatory function may be retained by modified procedures in which the lumbar sympathetic chains are preserved. The margins of dissection, however, vary somewhat between reports. Lange, Narayan and Fraley (1984) recommended preservation of lumbar sympathetic chains bilaterally, carefully dissecting the tissue overlying them. The dissection extended to the lateral aspect of the contralateral great vessel above the inferior mesenteric artery but remained ipsilateral below it, carefully avoiding the tissue between the iliac arteries. They reported that 51% of their patients with early stage disease experienced spontaneous recovery of ejaculation. Fossa *et al.* (1984) suggested avoiding the suprahilar regions and limiting the dissection to the mid-aorta for both right and left-sided tumours. In a series of 36 patients she reported preservation of ejaculation in 78%; however, it seems likely that a proportion of potentially positive nodes remain *in situ* with this procedure. Pizzacaro *et al.* (1985) performed a similar dissection with preservation of recovery of ejaculation in 87% of patients. Here again the dissection did not include the inter-aortocaval area. However, this limited dissection appears to result in a slightly higher relapse rate than in those series using more extended lymph node dissections. A recent report from Donahue and associates (1990), however, provided evidence for a relapse rate with a nerve-sparing technique comparable with more extensive procedures.

It is still not entirely clear which nerves must be preserved to maintain ejaculatory function. Unilateral lumbar sympathectomy seldom disturbs ejaculation and even bilateral sympathectomy from T12 and L3 leaves half the patients able to ejaculate. However, resection of the hypogastric plexus in the presacral area between the iliac arteries – the final common pathway for sympathetic innervation – invariably results in dry ejaculation. A recent anatomical study has delineated the exact location of the lumbar first to fourth sympathetic ganglia and demonstrated how they may be preserved surgically (Colleselli *et al.*, 1990).

The place of retroperitoneal lymph node dissection for residual disease after adequate chemotherapy for non-seminomatous testicular malignancy is not contested but its role in early disease is still controversial. Peckham *et al.* (1982) have championed the alternative course of close surveillance with CT scans and tumour marker levels every 3 months after orchidectomy, and this is the most commonly employed management in the UK. Donahue *et al.* (1988), however, have stressed the not infrequent occurrence of patients presenting with advanced disease who have defaulted from surveillance – a position it is not always possible to salvage even with the state of the art of chemotherapy and surgery. In the USA retroperitoneal lymph node dissection is still a commonly performed procedure carried out through either a transabdominal (Donahue, 1977) or a throaco-abdominal approach (Scardino, 1982), either of which will provide satisfactory access to the retroperitoneum.

## Conclusions

This chapter has reviewed the ways in which modifications of surgical technique may preserve sexual function. A careful explanation of any surgical procedure and its likely sequelae is always important, but nowhere more so than in the realms of sexual dysfunction. Without careful counselling patients may often wrongly assume that an operation has rendered them impotent or infertile, when in fact normal function is likely to return. The critical question is often whether nerve-sparing modifications of radical surgery in fact compromise effective cancer clearance, and in most cases this issue is still to be resolved. Probably at this juncture the best course is to explain to the patient that possibilities of preservation of sexual function now exist – many younger patients will opt for this and accept that the chances of local recurrence may be marginally increased.

### References


Brendler, G. B., Schlegel, P. N. and Walsh, P. C. (1990) Urethrectomy with preservation of potency. *Journal of Urology,* **144**, 270–273

Colleselli, K., Poisel, S., Schachtner, W. and Bartsch, G. (1990) Nerve-preserving bilateral retroperitoneal lymphadenectomy: anatomical study and operative approach. *Journal of Urology,* **144**, 293–298

De Groat, W. C., Booth, A. M., Krier, J. (1979) Interaction between sacral parasympathetic and lumbar sympathetic inputs to pelvic ganglia. In: *Intergrative functions of the autonomic nervous system.* (eds Brooks, C. M., Koizani, K., and Sato, A.) University of Tokyo Press, 234–247

Donahue, J. P., Foster, R. S., Rowland, R. G. *et al.* (1990) Nerve sparing retroperitoneal lymphadenectomy with preservation of ejaculation. *Journal of Urology,* **144**, 287–292

Donahue, J. P. and Rowland, R. G. (1981) Complications of retroperitoneal lymph node dissection. *Journal of Urology,* **125**, 338–340

Donahue, J. P., Rowland, R. G. and Bihrle, R. (1988) Transabdominal retroperitoneal lymph node dissection. In: *Genitourinary cancer.* (eds Skinner, D. G. and Leiskovsky, G.) Saunders, Philadelphia, pp. 802–816

Finkle, A. L. and Moyers, T. G. (1966) Sexual potency in ageing males: status of private patients before and after prostatectomy. *Journal of Urology,* **84**, 1952

Fossa, S. D., Klepp, O., Ous, S. *et al.* (1984) Unilateral retroperitoneal lymph node dissection in patients with non-seminomatous testicular malignancy in clinical stage 1. *European Urology,* **10**, 17–23

Hargreave, T. B. and Stephenson, T. P. (1977) Potency and prostatectomy. *British Journal of Urology,* **49**, 683

Hauri, D. (1982) Life after prostatectomy. *Urologia Internationalis,* **37**, 271

Kirby, R. S., Fowler, C. J., Gosling, J. A. *et al.* (1986) Bladder muscle biopsy and urethral sphincter EMG in patients with peripheral nerve injury to the bladder. *Journal of the Royal Society of Medicine,* **79**, 270–273

Lange, P. H., Narayan, P. and Fraley, E. E. (1984) Fertility issues following therapy for testicular cancer. *Seminars in Urology,* **2**, 264–274

Lepor, H., Gregerman, M., Crosby, R. *et al.* (1985) Precise localization of the autonomic nerves from the pelvic plexus to the corpora cavernosa: a detailed study of the adult male pelvis. *Journal of Urology,* **133**, 207

Lue, T. F., Zeineh, S. J., Schmidt, R. A. and Tanagho, E. M. (1984) Neuroanatomy of penile erection: its relevance to iatrogenic impotence. *Journal of Urology,* **131**, 273

Moller-Neilsen, C., Landhus, E. and Moller-Madsen, B. (1985) Sexual life following minimal and 'total' transurethral prostatic resection. *Urologia Internationalis,* **40**, 3

Padma-Nathan, H. and Krane, R. J. (1990) Impotence and prostate surgery. In *The Prostate* (eds J. M. Fitzpatrick and R. J. Krane), Churchill Livingstone, Edinburgh, p. 197

Peckham, M. J., Barrett, A., Husband, J. E. and Hendry, W. F. (1982) Orchidectomy alone in testicular stage 1 non-seminomatous germ cell tumours of the testis. *Lancet*, 678–686

Pizzocaro, B., Zanori, F., Salvioni, R. *et al.* (1985) Surveillance or lymph node dissection in clinical stage 1 non-seminomatous germinal testis cancer. *British Journal of Urology,* **57**, 759–762

Richie, J. P. and Garrick, M. (1985) Modified lymph node dissection in clincial stage 1 disease. *Société Internationale d'Urologie,* Abstract 79

Scardino, P. T. (1982) Thoracoabdominal retroperitoneal lymphadenectomy for testicular cancer. In *Genitourinary Cancer Surgery* (eds E. D. Crawford and T. A. Border), Lea and Febiger, Philadelphia, pp. 271–289

Schlegel, P. N. and Walsh, P. C. (1987) Neuroanatomical approach to radical cystoprostatectomy with preservation of sexual function. *Journal of Urology,* **138**, 1402

Skinner, D. G. and Lieskovsky, G. (eds) (1988) *Diagnosis and Therapy of Genitourinary Tumours,* W. B. Saunders, Philadelphia, pp. 782–783

So, E. B., Ho, P. C., Bodenstab, W. and Parson, C. L. (1982) Erectile impotence associated with transurethral prostatectomy. *Urology,* **19**, 259

Walsh, P. C. (1986) Radical retropubic prostatectomy. In *Campbell's Urology,* Vol. 3, 5th edn (eds P. C. Walsh, R. F. Gitters, A. D. Permutter and T. A. Stamey), W. B. Saunders, Philadelphia, p. 2769

Walsh, P. C. (1987) Radical prostatectomy, preservation of sexual function, cancer control. *Urologic Clinics of*

*North America,* **14**, 663

Walsh, P. C. and Donker, P. J. (1982) Impotence following radical prostatectomy: insight to aetiology and prevention. *Journal of Urology,* **128**, 492

Walsh, P. C., Epstein, J. I. and Lowe, F. C. (1987) Potency following radical prostatectomy with wide unilateral excision of the neurovascular bundle. *Journal of Urology,* **138**, 823

Walsh, P. C., Lepor, H. and Eggleton, J. C. (1983) Radical prostatectomy with preservation of sexual function: anatomical and pathological considerations. *Prostate,* **4**, 473

Walsh, P. C. and Mostwyn, J. L. (1984) Radical prostatectomy and cystoprostatectomy with preservation of sexual potency. Results using a new nerve-sparing technique. *British Journal of Urology,* **56**, 694

Zohar, J., Meiroz, D., Maoz, B. and Durst, N. (1976) Factors influencing sexual activity after prostatectomy: a prospective study. *Journal of Urology,* **116**, 332

# 23

# Priapism and post-priapism potency problems

C. C. Carson

Priapism is defined as persistent painful erection involving only the corpora cavernosa, not necessarily accompanied by sexual stimulation or desire. Voiding difficulty caused by priaprism may be encountered, but is not generally the rule. Priapism has been recorded in all age groups, with many different aetiologies (Table 23.1). Appropriate management of priapism continues to be controversial and has changed significantly with further clarification of the physiological mechanisms of erection and pharmacological treatment of erectile dysfunction. Despite these advances, however, varied regimens for management have been proposed and erectile impotence is a frequent sequel. As a result of erectile dysfunction caused by priapism, the condition carries significant medicolegal importance.

The aetiologies of priapism can be divided into patients with primary or idiopathic causes and patients with priapism secondary to other conditions or disease processes (Table 23.1). Prior to the use of pharmacological agents for the production of erections, idiopathic priapism was the most common aetiology (Bertram, Webster and Carson, 1985). The most common aetiologies for secondary priapism include: sickle cell anaemia, anticoagulant therapy, haematological malignancies such as leukaemia, perineal and pelvic trauma, penile infiltration by solid tumours such as prostatic carcinoma or penile carcinoma, alcoholism, psychotropic medications such as trazodone, antihypertensive medications, especially those with central or peripheral vasodilatation effects, other thromboembolic diseases such as atrial fibrillation or fat emboli, and neurogenic causes such as autonomic neuropathy and other lesions of the spinal cord (Nelson and Winter, 1977; Wasmer *et al.*, 1981; Bertram, Webster and Carson, 1985; Lue *et al.*, 1986). Keyes, in 1903, stated that ‘prolonged mental exertion, over-anxiety, and other conditions capable of reducing the tone of the nervous system are attended by priapism’. Hinman in 1914 collected the first large series of patients with priapism, describing 170 cases of priapism, the majority of which were caused by ‘systemic disease’. Young, in 1926, ascribed the aetiology of priapism to systemic disease, ‘local irritation of the lower genital tract, or neurologic lesions’.

**Table 23.1 Causes of priapism**

| |
|---|
| Medications: |
| Vasoactive agents (α-adrenergic blockers) |
| Anticoagulants |
| Psychotropic agents |
| Anticonvulsants |
| Total parenteral nutrition |
| Androgen replacement |
| Haematological conditions: |
| Sickle cell disease |
| Leukaemia |
| Multiple myeloma |
| Other haematological disorders |
| Neurological conditions and trauma |
| Genitourinary inflammation and infection |
| Pelvic and perineal trauma |
| Haemodialysis |
| Neoplasms |
| Idiopathic |

## Aetiology

Since the introduction of pharmacological agents to induce erections by Virag in 1984 and Brindley in 1983, the use of medications by injection to induce erections has become a widespread practice. With this widespread use of pharmacological erection agents, the incidence of complications such as prolonged erections and priapism has markedly increased. In the past 5 years at the Duke University Medical Center, only eight patients with priapism caused by idiopathic or secondary priapism other

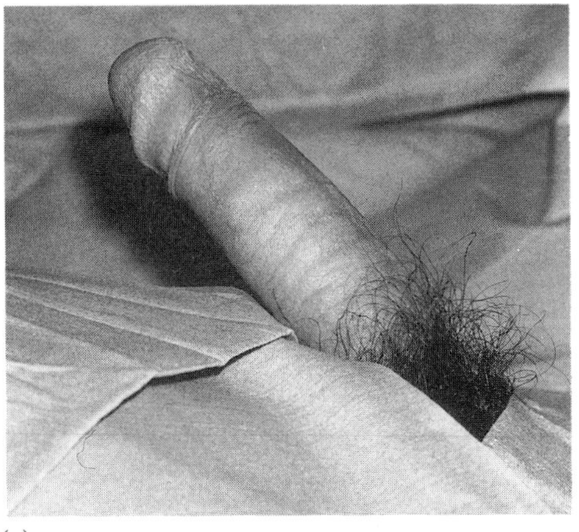

(a)

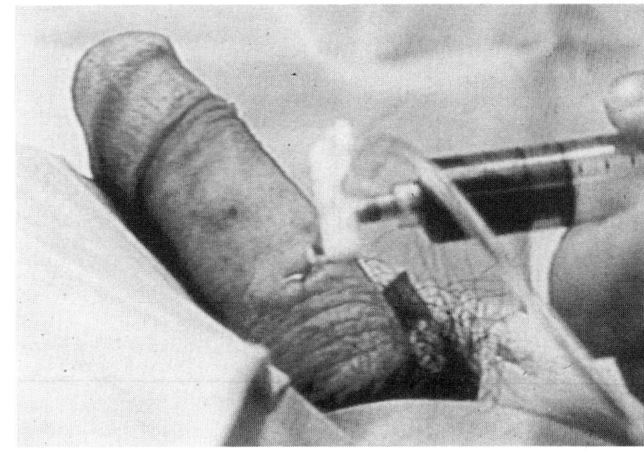

(b)

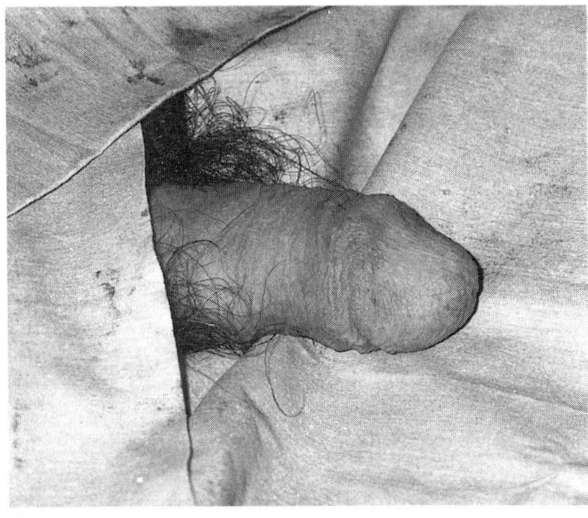

(c)

**Figure 23.1** (a) Post-papaverine/phentolamine injection priapism of 6 h duration; (b) corpus cavernosum aspiration using a 19 gauge needle, syringe and three-way stopcock connected to irrigation solution of 10 mg phenylephrine in 500 ml normal saline; (c) flaccid penis after lavage and aspiration

than that associated with injection therapy have been treated. On the other hand, 28 episodes of priapism associated with injection therapy have been treated. While many of these latter patients had prolonged erections of less than 8 h duration, they were treated as cases of priapism (Figure 23.1a and b).

Pohl, Pott and Kleinhaus (1986), in their series from the UK, identified 21% of patients with priapism from alcohol abuse or drug therapy, 12% from perineal trauma, and 11% with sickle cell anaemia. One-third of Pohl's group were idiopathic. Since the aetiology of priapism is distinctly dependent upon the population surveyed, US series with larger numbers of black patients usually have more patients with sickle cell disease. In our series from Duke University Medical Center, 31% of patients had associated sickle cell anaemia and 46% of patients were identified as idiopathic (Bertram, Webster and Carson, 1985). Nelson and Winter (1977) similarly reported 46% of patients with idiopathic priapism and 23% of adult cases associated with sickle cell disease. In their series, a majority of patients demonstrated multiple episodes of priapism prior to presentation. Because sickle cell disease affects almost 10% of black Americans, sickle cell anaemia is the most common cause of priapism in the paediatric age group, accounting for 6.4% incidence in the series reported by Tarry, Duckett and Snyder (1987).

## Pathophysiology

Recently, differentiation between two aetiologies of priapism has been identified (Witt *et al.*, 1990). The two types of priapism which can be identified are veno-occlusive or low-flow priapism, and high-flow or arterial priapism. The classic and most common form of priapism is caused by abnormalities in the veno-occlusive mechanism of the penis and a low or decreased venous outflow. This decreased venous outflow may be produced at the penile sinusoidal level with 'sludging of blood' in conditions such as sickle cell disease or hypercoagulable haematological states or as a result of penile embolism. This veno-occlusive priapism may also occur from external compression caused by such conditions as large solid tumours, hematoma or oedema secondary to pelvic trauma, or other forms of corpus cavernosum compression. Similarly, neurogenic causes of abnormal corpus cavernosum smooth muscle relaxation may result in stasis within the corpora cavernosa and subsequent low-flow priapism.

Experimental evidence of the physiological and haemodynamic function of the cavernosal bodies lends some theoretical basis to the cause of priapism. It has been well established by Lue, Goldstein and others that erectile function begins with relaxation of the smooth arteriolar muscles within the corpus cavernosum. Subsequent relaxation of the sinusoidal spaces with increased sinusoidal compliance results in a decrease in inflow resistance raising the flow of blood through the internal pudendal artery into the corpora cavernosa. This increase in flow results in distension of the sinusoidal spaces and thus the corpora cavernosa with secondary compression of emissary veins beneath the tunica albuginea. This compression results in decreased but not absent venous outflow. As intracorporeal pressure increases and perineal musculature contracts, intracorporeal pressure rises and venous outflow further diminishes. The decrease in venous outflow during the erect state and diminished flow within the sinusoidal spaces during erection account for the observation that priapism frequently develops following normal erection. In the normal penis, resolution of erection begins with an increase in inflow resistance from contraction of the cavernous and arteriolar smooth muscles. This contraction results in decreased pudendal artery blood flow, decreased sinusoidal compliance, and thus decreased intracavernosal pressure. As the cavernosal pressure diminishes, emissary veins are decompressed and venous flow returns to the detumescent state. If smooth muscle relaxation is accentuated pharmacologically as with papaverine or prostaglandin $E_1$ or if venous outflow resistance is artificially maintained, prolonged erection or priapism will ensue.

High-flow priapism is a less common cause of priapism usually associated with penile or pelvic trauma. High-flow priapism was described by Hauri *et al.* (1983) and Witt *et al.* (1990). Their decription of traumatically induced high-flow priapism is similar to that identified in the post-surgical setting from penile revascularization procedures as detailed by Michal *et al.* (1977). In these procedures, the inferior epigastric artery is anastomosed directly to a window in the tunica albuginea. As a result of high flow from these surgical procedures, priapism was identified in many cases with treatment directed at ligation of the previously placed inferior epigastric artery. Thus, arterial inflow without regulation from smooth muscle cavernosal vessels, if allowed to remain unchecked, produces pressures high enough within the corpora cavernosa to result in prolonged erection. In this form of priapism, arterial abnormalities allow uncontrolled arterial inflow, bypassing the helicine arteries and their smooth muscle control mechanisms with entry of arterial flow directly into the sinusoidal spaces. These spaces then distend under direct pressure and are unable to initiate detumescence by smooth muscle contraction. Thus, continued high inflow results in prolonged high venous outflow and subsequent pooling of blood within the corpora cavernosa. While this form of priapism is uncommon, it is important diagnostically to differentiate high-flow and low-flow priapism for appropriate therapeutic planning.

The histological consequences of prolonged erections or priapism may define the causes of abnormal erectile function which are frequent sequelae of priapism. Hinman (1960) noted the presence of dark, unclotted blood within the corpora cavernosa after priapism. Light microscopy demonstrated that the septa of the corpora cavernosa were thickened and oedematous following prolonged erection. Subsequent studies using electron microscopy have demostrated significant interstitial oedema of these trabecula after 12 h of low-flow priapism. Within 24 h the endothelium of the sinusoids is profoundly altered with thrombocyte adherence to the basement membranes. Within 48 h, necrosis of smooth muscle cells and fibroblastic proliferation within the sinusoids are identified (Spycher and Hauri, 1986). Subsequent fibrosis and even calcification have been identified clinically (Vapnek and Lue, 1989). These rapid histological changes, as a result of prolonged erection, stress the concept that priapism is a urological emergency. While idiopathic priapism is the most common cause of this abnormality, its diagnosis suggests that current diagnostic methods have yet to identify a precise aetiology. In patients with idiopathic priapism, a careful history and physical examination must be undertaken in an attempt to uncover an otherwise unsuspected cause. Careful diagnostic evaluation of these patients must be performed to plan a therapeutic approach.

The most common cause of priapism with newer approaches to the treatment of impotence is the use of intracavernous injections of pharmacological agents. Prolonged erections or priapism are well recognized complications and sequelae of excessive dosage of these medications. This complication occurs in 8–10% of patients treated with papaverine, papaverine/phentolamine combination, or prostaglandin $E_1$ (Lue *et al.*, 1986; Shantha, Finnerty and Rodriguez, 1989). Patients with normal vascular supply to the penis are at highest risk for these prolonged erections. Such patients with neurogenic or psychogenic impotence are most sensitive to injection medication. In our series of more than 350 patients, the incidence of prolonged erections in neurogenic or psychogenic patients is approximately 18% compared with an 8% incidence overall. The majority of these prolonged erections occur with the first injection, requiring the treating physician to carefully observe patients before discharging them after intial intercavernous injection. treatment of these patients without sequelae is easily carried out with corporeal aspiration and injection or lavage with dilute vasoconstrictors. Similarly, in patients undergoing dynamic infusion cavernosography and cavernosometry, many patients will have prolonged erections which must be treated with aspiration and vasoconstrictor infusion. Since this is a common sequel of cavernosal studies, one must be prepared to treat prolonged erections prior to discharging patients.

Trauma to the perineum, penis or groin may be associated with both high and low-flow priapism. While this cause of priapism is infrequent, it has been reported in almost every series of priapism patients. Persky and Kursh (1977) reported seven such patients, all of whom were successfully treated with conservative management. Pohl, Pott and Kleinhaus (1986) identified 12% of patients with trauma as an aetiology for priapism while trauma was associated with 7% of patients in 105 patients reviewed by Winter and McDowell (1988). The probable pathophysiology of traumatic priapism was defined by Witt *et al.* (1990) as previously described, but venous compression by a pelvic haematoma or oedema may also produce low-flow priapism after pelvic or perineal trauma. Trauma caused by intracavernous injection therapy must also be listed with those patients. A similar aetiology can be suspected with surgically-induced priapism as in those patients reported by Michal *et al.* (1977), after arterial revascularization (Bennett, 1988).

Neurological causes for priapism have long been described. Keyes, in 1903, described neurological injuries and stated that 'death by hanging is often accompanied by partial erection'. Other neurological conditions such as lumbar disc disease, seizure disorders, cerebrovascular disease and other diseases of the nervous system have been associated with priapism. These conditions, which are probably produced by continuous abnormal stimulation of the central nervous system, frequently require surgical treatment.

Haematological conditions which produce priapism occur frequently. The most frequent causes are the sickle cell haemoglobinopathies (Kinney *et al.*, 1975). Priapism has been reported in 2.5–5% of male patients with sickle cell disease (Tarry, Duckett and Snyder, 1987). Conversely, Hasen and Raines (1962) found that 80% of the black males hospitalized with priapism had sickle cell disease. Many of these patients were in the pediatric age group. Nelson and Winter (1977) support these data, noting that 50% of black males with priapism had sickle cell disease, of which more than 60% were children. The majority of patients with sickle cell priapism will report multiple episodes of prolonged erections throughout their childhood, frequently beginning with the onset of puberty. Many patients report frequent prolonged erections following nocturnal erections. In some cases the result of these repeated episodes of priapism is a markedly enlarged penis with fibrotic corpora, presenting with complete impotence in late adolescence or early adulthood. Because of the low-flow characteristics of the corpora cavernosa during erection, sickle cell disease is especially prone to sludging of blood within the penis during erection, producing priapism and subsequent progressive corporeal fibrosis. Exchange transfusions and intensive hydration have been helpful in treating these patients when rapid, spontaneous resolution has not occurred (Seeler, 1973). Sickle cell trait and other sickle associated haemoglobinopathies may also produce priapism in some patients. In addition to sickle cell disease, primary thrombocytopenia, haemoglobin C disease and thalassaemia have been associated with sporadic reports of priapism (Leifer and Leifer, 1979; Walker *et al.*, 1984).

Haematological malignancies such as leukaemia and multiple myeloma can present with priapism (Jaffe and Kim, 1969; Vadakan and Ortega, 1972; Schreibman, Gee and Grabstald, 1974; Altebarmakin *et al.*, 1980). Most often granulocytic leukaemia is associated with priapism and probably results from malignant leukaemic cells infiltrating the corpora cavernosa in a method similar to their infiltration into other organ systems (Schreibman, Gee and Grabstald, 1974). Treatment of leukaemia-associated priapism is directed at the primary disease using systemic chemotherapy and local radiation therapy to the penis although shunt procedures have been successful in some patients (Altebarmakin *et al.*, 1980). Similarly, multiple myeloma may be associated with priapism as reported by Rosenbaum, Thompson and Glassberg (1978). Detumescence can be expected with plasmapheresis and hydration.

Solid tumours have also been associated with malignant priapism. The most often associated tumours are those of the genitourinary system, primarily prostate, bladder, kidney and testis (Krco, Jacobs and Lawson, 1984; Witters, Cornelissen and Vereeckern, 1985). Treatment of this malignant priapism using radiation therapy or systemic chemotherapy may be effective. This most painful form of priapism will frequently be refractory to conservative methods for management.

Infections and 'inflammation' of the genitourinary system have also been associated with priapism since early descriptions by Keyes and others. Since effective antibiotic treatment of genitourinary infections has become commonplace, recent series have demonstrated few patients with causes related to inflammatory diseases of the prostate or genitalia. In our series, no patients demonstrated genitourinary tract infections as a possible aetiology for priapism (Bertram, Webster and Carson, 1985). Amyloidosis has been associated with occasional priapism (Lapan *et al.*, 1980).

Perhaps the most important causes for priapism include drugs and medications. Many prescription medications as well as illegal drugs and chemical substances may be associated with prolonged erections or priapism. While discontinuation of drugs or medications may eliminate future episodes of priapism, the immediate cause of the episode of priapism must be treated in addition to discontinuation of the offending medication.

Anticoagulants including intravenous heparin and oral anticoagulant treatment have been associated with priapism. In most reported cases, priapism occurred following discontinuation of the anticoagulant medication, suggesting a possible rebound hypercoaguability or hyperviscosity associated with the withdrawal of treatment with these medications. Similarly, patients on haemodialysis may suffer priapism as a result of hypercoaguability and rebound from heparin treatment (Port *et al.*, 1974; Singhal, Lynn and Scharschmidt, 1986). Priapism has also been identified in patients undergoing total parenteral nutrition associated with intravenous fat emulsion infusion: five such patients have been reported (Ekstrom and Olsson, 1987). Possible causes include hyperviscosity and a decrease in blood coagulability, perhaps associated with fat embolism. Treatment of these patients should be by surgical aspiration. Prevention of this form of priapism is effective by use of fat emulsion formulae containing a less than 10% solution (Kline, Montague and Steiger, 1985).

Psychotropic medications are very commonly associated with prolonged erections. The most commonly reported are the phenothiazines and trazodone (Dormen and Schmidt, 1976; Abber *et al.*, 1987; Carson and Mino, 1988). Other medications commonly associated with priapism include antihypertensive medications such as prazosin, guanethidine, and hydralazine and testosterone replacement therapy (Zelissen and Stricker, 1988). The most likely cause for this side effect of these medications is the α-adrenergic antagonist properties common to all of these medications. This may also suggest the cause for priapism identified in some patients taking yohimbine. Thus, treatment using α-adrenergic agonists may be the most appropriate method for treatment in these individuals (Carson and Mino, 1988).

## Diagnosis of priapism

Prior to the initiation of therapy for priapism, adequate evaluation to identify the cause and type of priapism is essential to appropriate management. The medical history is of great importance in differentiating high and low-flow priapism. Patients should be questioned with regard to medication and drug use, haematological history, previous surgery, trauma and recent sexual activity. Evaluation should then continue with Doppler ultrasound examination of the penis. Cavernosal arterial blood flow can be identified and quantitated using Doppler ultrasound and is best evaluated using colour Doppler. The presence of arterial pulsations by Doppler is consistent with, but not diagnostic of, high-flow priapism. The presence of arterial pulsations does, however, suggest the stage to which priapism has progressed. If the Doppler blood flow study fails to reveal normal arterial blood flow through the cavernous arteries, the possibility of severe cavernosal ischaemia is suggested. In these patients the prognosis for recovery of adequate sexual function is poor. Following Doppler evaluation, corporeal aspiration should be carried out with determination of intracavernosal blood gas values. The aspiration of dark appearing blood which is markedly hypoxic, acidotic and hypercapnic is diagnostic of veno-occlusive priapism. In high-flow priapism, blood gas determinations will demonstrate normal oxygen and carbon dioxide levels consistent with arterial blood.

In some cases of partial, episodic priapism, additional studies may help to clarify the differential diagnosis. Computed tomographic scanning and ultrasonography may be helpful in these cases. Partial priapism may occur as a result of trazodone medication, trauma or idiopathic aetiologies. Patients with perineal pain and possible priapism may be differentiated by the use of a computed tomographic scan (Burkhalter and Morano, 1985; Carson and Mino, 1988).

If aspirated blood pH is less than 7.25, $p\text{O}_2$ less than 30 mmHg and $p\text{CO}_2$ is above 60 mmHg, ischaemic priapism is highly probable (Gibel, Reiley and Borden, 1985).

Patients who have significant arterial pulsation by Doppler ultrasound and blood gas determinations consistent with arterial blood should undergo irrigation with α-adrenoceptor substances in an effort to further differentiate high- and low-flow priapism. If rapid retumescence occurs after irrigation, or if there is a significant history of penile or pelvic trauma, selective internal pudendal arteriography should be performed to eliminate the possiblity of high-flow priapism. An abnormal selective pudendal arteriogram consistent with high-flow priapism is best treated by selective arterial embolization (Puppo *et al.*, 1985; Pohl, Pott and Kleinhaus, 1986).

## Management of priapism

While the diagnosis of priapism has been refined and improved in recent years, the management of priapism has markedly changed since the days when Hugh Hampton Young suggested incision of a corpus cavernosum as the only treatment for priapism. Since priapism is frequently associated with significant superficial penile oedema and deep pelvic, perineal and penile pain, treatment of pain and anxiety should be undertaken initially and the patient treated for his priapism as a urological emergency in an effort to rapidly restore arterial inflow and venous outflow by decreasing intracavernosal pressure (Figure 23.2). Conservative initial therapy with narcotic analgesics should be carried out immediately, followed by evaluation of a complete blood count, sickle cell preparation, chest X-ray, urine analysis, coagulation profile and serum electrolytes. In addition, a thorough physical examination including an examination of the prostate, perineum and genitalia should be carried out. In the past, conservative management has consisted of hot or cold water enemas, prostatic massage, spinal anaesthesia, penile compression or milking and the liberal administration of oestrogen medications. These methods of 'conservative treatment' are unproven and represent a loss of valuable time with a delay in appropriate management. The success of these treatments is probably a result of spontaneous resolution of priapism rather than direct effect of these manipulations.

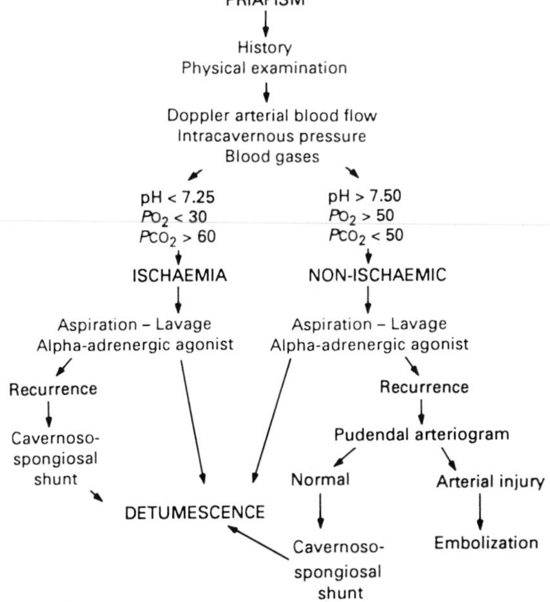


**Figure 23.2** Algorithm for diagnosis and treatment of priapism. Modified from Lue *et al.* (1986)

**Table 23.2 Alpha-adrenergic agonists for priapism therapy**

| *Agent* | *Dosage* |
|---|---|
| Phenylephrine | 0.5–1 mg injection<br>10 mg/500 ml normal saline lavage |
| Adrenaline | 0.05–0.1 mg injection |
| Noradrenaline | 10–50 g injection |
| Ephedrine | 50–100 mg injection |
| Metaraminol | 1 mg/4 ml normal saline injection |

Initial treatment, therefore, should be aimed at decreasing intracavernosal pressure through corpus cavernosum aspiration and pharmacological lavage (Table 23.2). Intracavernosal pressure can be monitored through a 23 gauge scalp vein needle connected to an arterial monitor placed in one corpus cavernosum. Intracavernosal pressures above 50 mmHg suggest the probability of progressive ischaemia (Lue *et al.*, 1986). Using general or local anaesthesia, a 19 gauge scalp vein needle is placed into one corpus cavernosum, aspirating a sample of blood for blood gas determination. Further aspiration is carried out followed by aspiration and irrigation of the corpus cavernosum using normal saline and dilute solutions of noradrenaline, terbutaline, adrenaline, metaraminol, phenylephrine and other similar α-adrenergic agents. Lavage should be continued until detumescence has been established. Blood pressure, pulse and electrocardiogram should be monitored during this lavage in patients with established priapism. Complications with these small doses of α-adrenergic agents are unusual but those patients with previous history of cardiac disease must be carefully monitored during any α-adrenergic medication administration. Beneficial effects of intracavernosal injection of streptokinase in refractory priapism has been reported as an adjunct to aspiration and saline lavage (Gibel, Reiley and Borden, 1985).

Following detumescence with aspiration and irrigation, a firm dressing should be applied, incorporating a 2 cm pediatric blood pressure cuff for compression and decompression on a regular basis (Bertram, Webster and Carson, 1985). This blood pressure cuff can be connected to an anaesthesia blood pressure monitoring unit and set at a level between systolic and diastolic blood pressures to detumesce the penis without occluding arterial inflow. Careful monitoring of the tumescence of the penis must be carried out during the follow-up phase.

Priapism of more than 24–36 h duration, or that priapism refractory to α-agonists, must be considered for surgical intervention. The goal of surgical intervention is to shunt venous blood from the corpus cavernosum to the corpus spongiosum. Shunting procedures can be performed through a Winter's shunt using a Tru-Cut biopsy needle or a scalpel as described by Ebbehoj (1975) and Winter (1978). Using thse techniques, a biopsy needle or scalpel is passed through the glans penis creating a shunt between the glans penis and the corpus cavernosum. This shunt or fistula depends on removing a section of tunica albuginea allowing venous drainage. After a penile block has been established using local anaesthesia, an 18 gauge needle is passed through the glans penis into a corpus cavernosum aspirating as much blood as possible, and irrigating with normal saline. When blood return has changed to a lighter colour, the 18 gauge needle is replaced by a Tru-Cut biopsy needle pushing the biopsy needle to the junction between the corpus cavernosum and corpus spongiosum. Removing cores of tissue at this location opens a fistula between the corpus cavernosum and corpus spongiosum through the fibrous septum between the glans penis and corpus cavernosum. Winter (1978) suggests at least four similar cores to provide adequate shunting. The puncture holes in the glans skin are then closed with single absorbable sutures. He reported four of five patients successfully treated using this technique. Our own results with the Winter technique have been mixed, with successful results in three of five patients so treated (Bertram, Webster and Carson, 1985).

The Al Ghorab procedure described by Ercole (1987) uses a principle similar to that described by Winter. A small incision is created on the dorsal aspect of the glans penis approximately 1 cm from the corona penis. Dissecting beneath the glans penis, the corpora cavernosa are easily identified and a small segment of tunica albuginea is removed from each corpus cavernosum using sharp dissection. Tissue of the underside of the glans penis is likewise opened and the corpora cavernosa are drained into the corpus spongiosum through these incisions. Following detumescence, the glans penis is returned to its normal position and the shunt maintained in an open position using sutures of 4/0 polyglycolic acid. Ercole, Pontes and Pierce (1981) have described four of five patients adequately treated with this technique with preservation of potency postoperatively.

Other options for shunting include proximal corporospongiosum shunts as described by Quakles (1964). These procedures demonstrate a greater potential for postoperative erectile dysfunction. In our experience, corporospongiosum shunting is associated with retained potency in only 24% of patients (Bertram, Webster and Carson, 1985). This shunting procedure is performed by the creation of an anastomosis between the corpora cavernosa and the corpora spongiosum along the penile shaft. The safest area for performing this procedure is in the perineal region where the spongiosum is thickest to avoid inadvertent urethral damage. A longitudinal incision in the tunica albuginea of the corpus cavernosum is approximated to a similar incision in the corpus spongiosum creating a fistula. These fistulae are maintained patent by opposing the walls of the corpora with continuous sutures of 5/0 polyglycolic acid.

Grayhack *et al.* (1964) have described a method for shunting the corpus cavernosum with the saphenous vein. In 50 patients who underwent this procedure reported by Cosgrove and Larocque (1974), 62% remained potent when unilateral shunts were performed. This shunting procedure is more difficult surgically than the previously described ones, but appears to be effective in creating detumescence.

Recently, repeated partial priapism has been reported. In this condition, usually caused by trauma, sickle cell disease or psychotropic agents, priapism may occur as often as daily. Oral treatment with $\alpha$ stimulators such as ephedrine (Ornade) or phenyl propanolamine, and self-injection with dilute phenylephrine may be helpful in maintaining detumescence and avoiding severe priapism.

## Complications

Priapism and its subsequent surgical treatment most commonly results in erectile dysfunction. Surgical shunting procedures have been associated with penile gangrene as well as other tissue necrosis (Fortuno and Carriollo, 1972; Cosgrove and Larocque, 1974; Weiss and Ferguson, 1974). The risk of postoperative infection must be anticipated and adequate perioperative antibiotics administered. Urethral damage and fistulae have also been reported (Robbins, Crawford and Lackner, 1984).

Treatment of high-flow priapism is best performed with pudendal artery selective angiography and embolization as described by Witt *et al.* (1990) and Puppo *et al.* (1984). This treatment will eliminate arteriovenous fistulization and, in the cases reported, be likely to preserve erectile function.

Patients with prolonged or repetitive episodes of priapism are likely to suffer erectile dysfunction after resolution of their condition (Figure 23.3). Impotence occurred in 15 of 28 patients with prolonged priapism in our series. Hinman (1960) stated that 'treatment is generally not effective, impotency is the usual result'. Impotence in other studies is based upon duration of priapism, aetiology of priapism, and method of treatment. In most series, postoperative potency varies from 54% to 57%. Traumatic priapism appears to have the best prognosis whereas patients in the older group with

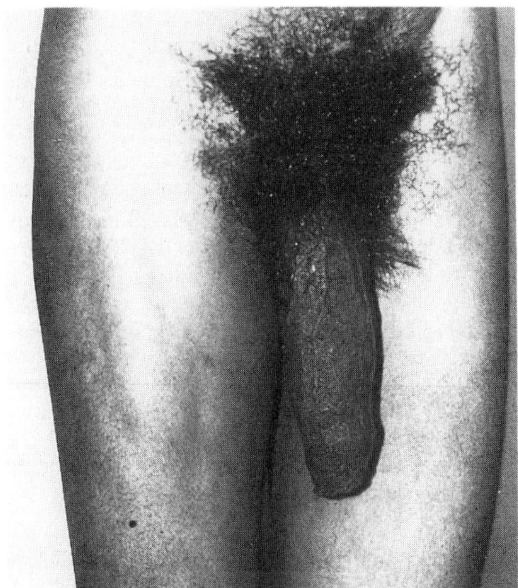

**Figure 23.3** Penile enlargement in a 24-year-old black patient impotent after multiple episodes of priapism caused by sickle cell disease

priapism secondary to antihypertensive therapy and those patients with repeated episodes of priapism from sickle cell anaemia have a poor prognosis for future potency.

Post-priapism treatment using implantation of a penile prosthesis has been described. Since priapism, especially if repeated, results in severe corporeal fibrosis, prosthesis implantation may be somewhat difficult. Placement of a penile prosthesis with this severe corporeal fibrosis may be surgically difficult and require initial sharp channelling into the corpora cavernosa with active dilation using Hegar dilators, and in some cases, corpora cavernosa incision using an Otis urethrotome. Occasionally, inflatable prostheses cannot overcome the rigidity of the severe fibrosis and a semi-rigid rod prosthesis may be necessary. In most cases, however, if adequate corporeal dilation can be undertaken, placement of an inflatable penile prosthesis can be successfully performed. Priapism, either prolonged or repeated, should not be considered a contraindication to implantation of a penile prosthesis.

## Conclusion

The aetiology, diagnosis and treatment options for the management of patients with prolonged erections and priapism have evolved greatly in the past several years. Causes of priapism from newer psychotropic medications to intracavernosal injection therapy have increased the numbers of patients with priapism presenting to the urologist. A more thorough knowledge of the pathophysiology of priapism and the differentiation of high and low-flow states have significantly changed the diagnostic protocol for these individuals. Doppler evaluation and blood gas determinations must be carried out in all patients who present with priapism. Early intervention with corpus cavernosum aspiration and pharmacological manipulation must not be delayed by older 'conservative measures'. Priapism must be considered a urological emergency.

## References


Abber, J. C., Lue, T. F., Luo, J. A. *et al.* (1987) Priapism induced by chlorpromazine and trazodone: mechanism of action. *Journal of Urology,* **137**, 1039

Altebarmakin, V. K., Rabinowitz, R., Rana, S. R. *et al.*, (1980) Transglandular cavernosum-spongiosum shunt for leukemic priapism in childhood. *Journal of Urology,* **123**, 287

Bennett, A. H. (1988) Venous arterialization for erectile impotence. *Urologic Clinics of North America,* **15**, 111

Bertram, R. A., Webster, G. D. and Carson, C. C. (1985) Priapism: etiology, treatment and results in a series of 35 presentations. *Urology,* **26**, 229

Bertram, R. A., Carson, C. C. and Webster, G. D. (1985) Implantation of penile prosthesis in patients impotent after priapism. *Urology,* **26**, 325

Brindley, G. S. (1983) Cavernosal alpha blockade: a new technique for investigating and treating erectile impotence. *British Journal of Psychiatry,* **143**, 332

Burkhalter, J. L. and Morano, J. U. (1985) Partial priapism: the role of CT in its diagnosis. *Radiology,* **156**, 159

Carson, C. C. and Mino, R. D. (1988) Priapism associated with trazodone therapy. *Journal of Urology,* **139**, 369

Cosgrove, M. D. and Larocque, M. A. (1974) Shunt surgery for priapism: review of results. *Urology,* **4**, 1

Dormen, B. W. and Schmidt, J. D. (1976) Association of priapism in phenothiazine therapy. *Journal of Urology,* **116**, 51

Ebbehoj, J. A new operation for priapism. *Scandinavian Journal of Plastic and Reconstructive Surgery,* **8**, 241

Ekstrom, B. and Olsson, A. M. (1987) Priapism in patients treated with total parenteral nutrition. *British Journal of Urology,* **59**, 170

Ercole, C. J. J., Pontes, J. E. and Pierce, J. M. (1981) Changing surgical concepts in the treatment of priapism. *Journal of Urology,* **125**, 210

Fortuno, R. F. and Carrillo, R. (1972) Gangrene of the penis following cavernospongiosum shunt in a case of priapism. *Journal of Urology,* **108**, 752

Gibel, L. J., Reiley, E. and Borden, T. A. (1985) Intracorporal cavernosa streptokinase as adjuvant therapy in the delayed treatment of idiopathic priapism. *Journal of Urology,* **133**, 1040

Grayhack, J. T., McCullough, W., O'Conor, V. J. *et al.* (1964) Venous bypass to control priapism. *Investigative Urology,* **1**, 509

Hasen, H. B. and Raines, S. (1962) Priapism associated

with sickle cell disease. *Journal of Urology,* **88**, 71

Hauri, D., Spycher, M. and Bruhlmann, W. (1983) Erection and priapism: a new physiopathological concept. *Urologia Internationalis*, **38**, 138

Hinman, F. (1914) Priapism, review of 170 cases. *Annals of Surgery,* **4**, 689

Hinman, F. Jr. (1960) Priapism: reasons for failure of therapy. *Journal of Urology,* **83**, 420

Jaffe, N. and Kim, B. S. (1969) Priapism in acute granulocytic leukemia. *American Journal of Diseases of Children,* **118**, 619

Keyes, E. L. and Keyes, E. L. Jr. (1903) Priapism. In *Surgical Diseases of the Genitourinary Organs* (ed. E. L. Keyes), D. Appleton and Company, New York, p. 807

Kinney, T. R., Harris, M. B., Russell, M. O. *et al.* (1975) Priapism in association with sickle hemoglobinopathies in children. *Journal of Pediatrics,* **86**, 241

Kline, E. A., Montague, D. K. and Steiger, E. (1985) Priapism associated with the use of intravenous fat emulsion: case reports and postulated pathogenesis. *Journal of Urology,* **133**, 587

Krco, J. J., Jacobs, S. C. and Lawson, R. K. (1984) Priapism due to solid malignancy. *Urology,* **23**, 264

Lapan, D. I., Graham, A. R., Bangert, J. L. *et al.* (1980) Amyloidosis presenting as priapism. *Urology,* **15**, 167

Leifer, W. and Leifer, G. (1979) Priapism caused by primary thrombocytohemia. *Journal of Urology,* **121**, 254

Lue, T. F., Helstrom, W. J. G., McAninch, J. W. *et al.* (1986) Priapism: a refined approach to diagnosis and treatment. *Journal of Urology,* **136**, 104

Michal, V., Kramar, R., Pospichal, J. and Hejhal, L. (1977) Arterial epigastricocavernous anastomosis for the treatment of sexual impotence. *World Journal of Surgery,* **1**, 515

Nelson, J. H. and Winter, C. C. (1977) Priapism: evolution of management in 48 patients in a 22 year series. *Journal of Urology,* **117**, 455

Persky, L. and Kursh, E. (1977) Post-traumatic priapism. *Journal of Urology,* **118**, 397

Pohl, J., Pott, B. and Kleinhaus, G. (1986) Priapism: a three phase concept of management according to aetiology and prognosis. *British Journal of Urology,* **58**, 113

Port, F. K., Hecking, E., Fiegel, P. *et al.* (1974) Priapism during regular hemodialysis. *Lancet,* **ii**, 1287

Puppo, P., Belgrano, E., Germanile, F. *et al.* (1985) Angiographic treatment of high flow priapism. *European Urology,* **11**, 397

Puppo, E. B., Quattrin, I. S., Trombetta, C. *et al.* (1984) Percutaneous temporary embolization of the internal pudendal arteries and idiopathic priapism: two additional cases. *Journal of Urology,* **131**, 756

Quackles, R. (1964) Cure of a patient suffering from priapism by cavernosospongiosal anastomosis. *Acta Urologica Belgica,* **32**, 5

Robbins, E. M., Crawford, E. D. and Lackner, H. L. (1984) Late development of urethrocavernous fistula after cavernosospongiosum shunt for priapism. *Journal of Urology,* **132**, 126

Rosenbaum, E. H., Thompson, H. E. and Glassberg, A. B. (1978) Priapism in multiple myeloma, successful treatment with plasmapheresis. *Urology,* **12**, 201

Schreibman, S. M., Gee, T. S. and Grabstald, H. (1974) Management of priapism in patients with chronic granulocytic leukemia. *Journal of Urology,* **111**, 786

Seeler, R. A. (1973) Intensive transfusion therapy in boys with sickle cell anemia. *Journal of Urology,* **110**, 360

Shantha, T. R., Finnerty, D. P. and Rodriguez, A. P. (1989) Treatment of persistent penile erection and priapism using terbutaline. *Journal of Urology,* **141**, 1427

Singhal, P. C., Lynn, R. I. and Scharschmidt, L. A. (1986) Priapism and dialysis. *American Journal of Nephrology,* **6**, 358

Spycher, M. A. and Hauri, D. (1986) The ultrastructure of erectile tissue in priapism. *Journal of Urology,* **135**, 142

Tarry, W. F., Duckett, J. W. and Snyder, H. (1987) Urological complications of sickle cell disease in the pediatric population. *Journal of Urology,* **138**, 592

Vadakan, V. V. and Ortega, J. (1972) Priapism in acute lymphoblastic leukemia. *Cancer,* **30**, 373

Vapnek, J. and Lue, T. F. (1989) Heterotopic bone formation in the corpus cavernosum: a complication of papaverine-induced priapism. *Journal of Urology,* **142**, 1323

Virag, R., Frydman, D., Legman, M. *et al.* (1984) Intracavernous injection of papaverine as a diagnostic and therapeutic method in erectile failure. *Angiology,* **35**, 79

Walker, E. M., Mitchum, E. N., Rous, S. N. *et al.* (1984) Automated erythrocytopheresis for relief of priapism in sickle cell hemoglobinopathies. *Journal of Urology,* **126**, 912

Wasmer, J. M., Carrion, H. M. Mekras, G. *et al.* (1981) Evaluation of treatment and priapism. *Journal of Urology,* **125**, 204

Weiss, J. N. and Ferguson, D. (1974) Priapism: the danger of treatment with compression. *Journal of Urology,* **112**, 616

Winter, C. C. (1978) Priapism cured by creation of fistulas between glans penis and corpora cavernosa. *Journal of Urology,* **119**, 227

Winter, C. C. and McDowell, G. (1988) Experience with 105 patients with priapism: update review of all aspects. *Journal of Urology,* **140**, 980

Witt, M. A., Goldstein, I., Saenz de Tajeda, I. *et al.* (1990) Traumatic laceration of intracavernosal arteries: the pathophysiology of non-ischemic, high flow arterial priapism. *Journal of Urology,* **143**, 129

Witters, S., Cornelissen, M. and Vereeckern, I. L. (1985) Malignant priapism. *European Urology,* **11**, 431

Young, H. H. (1926) Priapism. In *Young's Practice of Urology* (ed. H. H. Young), W. B. Saunders, Philadelphia, p. 714a

Zelissen, P. M. J. and Stricker, B. H. (1988) Severe priapism as a complication of testosterone substitution therapy. *American Journal of Medicine,* **85**, 273

# 24

# Sexual function in congenital anomalies

C. R. J. Woodhouse

## Introduction

In the major congenital anomalies of the genitourinary system, sexual function may be compromised for six possible reasons:

1. The penis may be grossly malformed (e.g. exstrophy and micropenis).
2. The penis may be a little deformed but the patient's perception may so exaggerate the deformity that sexual function is impaired (e.g. hypospadias).
3. Obstructive lesions of the bladder outlet may cause back pressure on the prostate leading to ejaculatory failure and seminal abnormalities (e.g. posterior urethral valves).
4. Developmental failure may impair hormonal or ejaculatory function (e.g. prune belly syndrome).
5. Penile innervation may be incomplete (e.g. spina bifida) or destroyed by pelvic surgery.
6. Embarrassment about some aspect of the general abnormalities may prevent the formation of a partnership in which intercourse can take place (e.g. an external urinary diversion).

The general trend in all these groups of patients is a far more active sex life than would be imagined. It should always be assumed that erectile function and intercourse are desired and possible until proved otherwise. It is astonishing how severe handicaps can be overcome and how little a penis is necessary for apparently satisfactory intercourse.

## Exstrophy and epispadias

### Penile anatomy

The typical exstrophy penis is short and broad. When seen in the flaccid state it certainly does not 'dangle'. Its shortness is emphasized by the normal size of the scrotum and the recession of the lower abdominal wall.

The orientation of the inferior pubic rami and the attachments of the deep parts of the corpora are unlike those of normal males. The findings by cavernosogram, by computerized tomography and at surgery are consistent (Woodhouse and Kellett, 1984). The symphysis is not only open but the pelvis is rotated caudally so that the inferior pubic ramus is parallel to the floor when the patient is standing.

The penis, although attached to the inferior pubic rami in the usual way, is not short because of the divarication of the pelvic bones, but because the corpora are deficient in length.

### Erectile deformities

All exstrophy males complain of dorsal chordee on erection (Figure 24.1). The degree of chordee is variable. In some the angle is such that sexual intercourse is possible either in the conventional position or in one that brings the female introitus in more direct apposition to the penis, such as with the female sitting astride the supine male. Cavernosogram in these cases shows that the site of the maximum curvature is at the point where the corpora emerge from the perineum.

A more complex deformity occurs when one or both of the corpora are abnormal. If one corpus fails to fill on erection it acts as a 'bow-string' on the other and causes lateral deviation in addition to the dorsal chordee (Figure 24.2).

If both corpora are rudimentary, the visible or exophytic part of the penis is normal except that it is a little higher than usual on the abdomen. On cavernosography the corpora appear to have no attachment to the pubic rami. Erection is very limited and the penis unstable.

The author believes that these rudimentary corpora were normal (for exstrophy) at birth and were damaged at the reconstructive surgery (Woodhouse and Kellett 1984; Brzezinski *et al.*, 1986). The three main types of erectile deformity identified by the author are shown in Table 24.1.

If a young man with exstrophy has a short penis that is otherwise normal and has no chordee, there is nothing that can be done. A review from the Mayo Clinic suggests that modern techniques of reconstruction do lead to just this situation: a short but

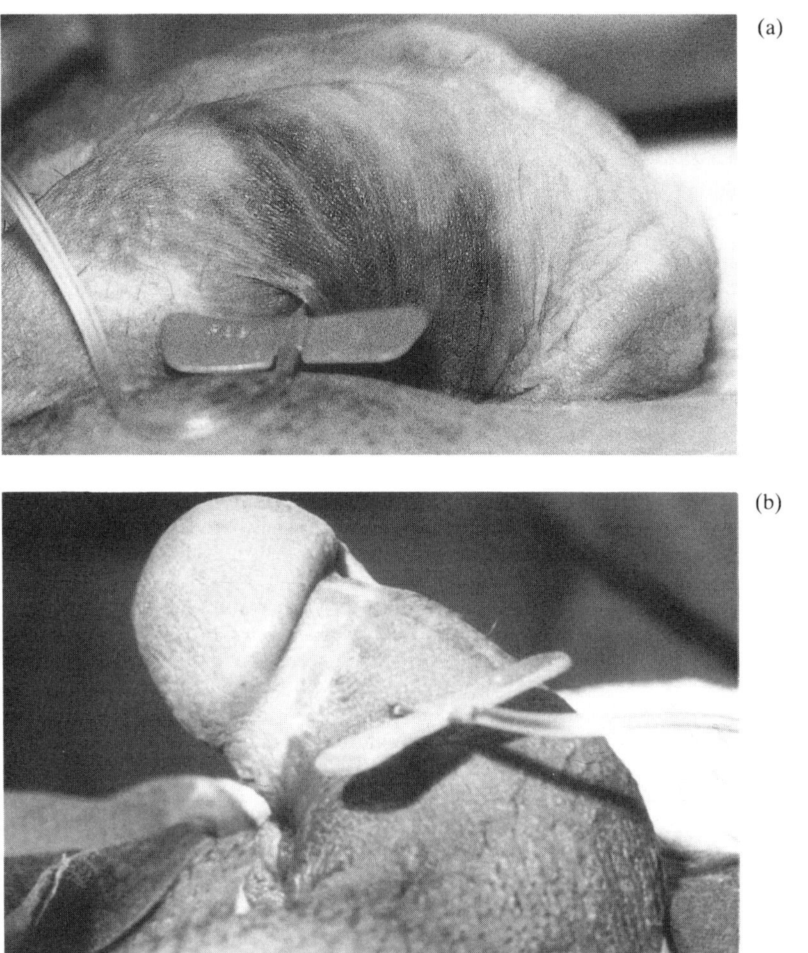

(a)

(b)

**Figure 24.1** Artificial erection showing the tight dorsal chordee that is the commonest erectile deformity in exstrophy; (b) artificial erection after surgical correction

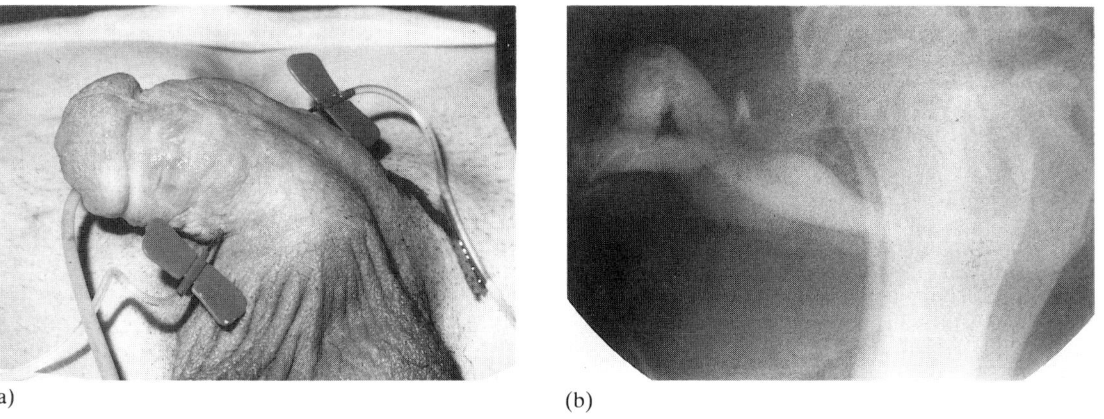

(a) (b)

**Figure 24.2** (a) Clinical photograph of an exstrophy penis showing deviation to the right on artificial erection; (b) cavernosogram of the same patient showing a rudimentary right corpus that fails to fill and acts as a 'bow-string' on the left corpus

**Table 24.1 Distribution of types of erectile deformity in exstrophy and epispadias (Woodhouse and Kellet, 1984)**

| *Deformity* | *Number* |
|---|---|
| Dorsal chordee | 27 |
| Unilateral rudimentary corpus | 3 |
| Bilateral rudimentary corpora | 5 |

normal penis (Mesrobian, Kelalis and Kramer, 1986). Thus the management in adolescence in the future may only be concerned with helping the boys to adjust to their abnormality. However, the author's experience with patients who are now young adults is that nearly all have an erectile deformity.

## Lengthening procedures

The anatomical evidence outlined above shows that the corpora are deficient in length. Increase in the length of the visible penis can only be achieved by making the best use of the corpora distal to their attachment to the inferior pubic rami. Additional length is not achieved by osteotomy to close the pubic symphysis (Johnston, 1974). However, it has been pointed out that the penis is longer if the divarication of the pubic bones is 3 cm or less and it is shorter if the divarication is 4 cm or more (Schillinger and Wiley, 1984). Whatever the situation in infants, pelvic osteotomy does not seem to be a very attractive option for adults.

In some patients the corpora may have been 'concertina-ed' by contraction and scarring of the urethral plate and pericorporeal tissue. Considerable lengthening can be achieved in children by clearing it all away and cleaning the corpora (Hendren, 1979). This dissection is the first step in chordee correction but in the author's experience in adults it has not allowed any penile lengthening; it may be that by this stage in life secondary and irreversible changes have occurred in the corpora.

The horizontal plane in which the inferior pubic rami lie prevents the lengthening of the penis by partial detachment of the corpora. Some length is gained by dissection from the body of the pubis but it is useless to continue it posterior to the junction with the inferior ramus. Complete detachment of the corpora from the inferior pubic rami is said to have given good lengthening in nine of 11 children (Kelley and Eraklis, 1971; King, 1984) but there has been no follow-up.

Thus it seems that in adolescents and adults there is no worthwhile procedure to lengthen the penis.

## Correction of erectile deformities

The techniques of chordee correction are described in detail elsewhere (Woodhouse, 1986, 1988).

The base of the penis and the junction of the corpora with the pubis are exposed. The urethra in these older patients still lies on the dorsum; it is mobilized, divided as far distally as possible and retracted cranially. All the scar tissue is then cleared from the dorsum of the corpora. The superficial neurovascular bundles which are not in the usual position must be identified and protected (Hurwitz, Woodhouse and Ransley, 1986).

In only one case has this dissection been found to be sufficient to eliminate the chordee, though others have found that the chordee is relieved at this stage (Spehr and Melchior, 1985).

Until recently the author has lengthened the concavity on the dorsum of the penis by inserting a gusset of lyophilized human dura. Unfortunately it has now been discovered that viruses can be transmitted by dura (*JAMA* Editorial, 1987) and so rectus sheath is now used. Each corpus is incised transversely, the penis straightened and the implant sutured into the resulting elliptical defect.

An alternative to insertion of any material is a caverno-cavernostomy which might be considered a variation of the Koff procedure (Koff and Eakins, 1984; P.G. Ransley, personal communication, 1987). After the corpora have been incised they are rotated towards each other and the cavernotomies sutured to each other face to face. The curvatures of each corpus will then cancel out. In effect each corpus is incised transversely and sutured longitudinally. The urethra is brought through to the ventrum of the penis. If there is sufficient good skin a urethroplasty is done straight away but usually is left to a second stage.

### Results

The author's series consists of 30 phalloplasties of which 20 are assessable with a 1–5 year follow-up. Thirteen had an excellent result on the first occasion and three only after a revision (Figure 24.1b). Three were improved and two were unchanged.

Caverno-cavernostomy has been done on five adolescents or children over 10 by Woodhouse and Ransley. It has proved technically satisfactory and chordee has been corrected in all cases in the immediate postoperative period. There is no long-term follow-up and no conclusions can be drawn.

## Complex erectile deformities

When the penis is deviated to one side, the fault lies in a rudimentary corpus which does not fill and acts as a 'bow-string' on the normal side. If possible the rudimentary corpus should be reconstructed with an implant as described above. It should not be divided as the resulting erection is straight but unstable: a proper erection requires the two corpora to support each other like the gables of a house.

When both corpora are rudimentary they have no attachment to the pubic rami. The venous drainage is into the superficial veins and not into the pudendal vein through Alcock's canal; the arterial supply presumably follows the same route. Penile surgery is likely to damage that little blood supply which remains and thus abolish any erection. Complete reconstruction, as is done for female to male gender reassignment, would be a possibility but has not been attempted on any of the author's patients.

### Sexual function

With or without surgical correction, the men appear to have a normal libido. They have fewer casual sexual partners than would be expected. They appear to form very stable partnerships with normal women and have normal family life. Of 43 in the author's series for whom full information is available, 33 have been married or lived with a partner. The remaining patients of all ages do not admit to any sexual contact and for many of them the combination of abnormal genitalia and an external urinary diversion seems to be too overwhelming. They have normal erections and orgasms. Internal continent diversions may help such patients. For the next generation a working bladder and counselling of children and parents may further improve sexual function.

### Ejaculation and paternity

Ejaculation has been assessed continuously during follow-up. In the first review of adult patients all but two of 31 patients ejaculated (Hanna and Williams, 1972). Absence of ejaculation is still rare in spite of the more extensive reconstructions that are done, but the emission that does occur is slow and may continue over several hours after orgasm. Some patients describe a more or less continuous urethral discharge of semen-like fluid. In another series 16 of 25 patients had ejaculation but its quality was not recorded (Mesrobian, Kelalis and Kramer, 1986). Although the genital tract up to the veru montanum is normal, there is a high incidence of poor or absent sperm. It is not known whether this is due to obstruction or repeated infection.

Seven patients in the author's series have initiated one or two pregnancies from which there have been five children. A further 13 are known to be infertile. These figures are broadly in line with those reported elsewhere. The main cause of infertility appears to be repeated prostatic and bladder infections. Thus, ironically, the boys who underwent early urinary diversion have the best record for fertility (Lattimer, MacFarlane and Puchor, 1979; Mesrobian, Kelalis and Kramer, 1986).

## The small penis

It is generally agreed that a small penis must have normal anatomy but be more than 2 or 2.5 standard deviations below the normal stretched length. Thus it ranges from 1.75 cm to 2.7 cm at birth (Feldman and Smith, 1975; Flatau *et al.*, 1975). Growth curves have been constructed from which the normal penile lengths can be derived at any age (Schonfeld, 1943).

The andrologist may be asked to see a neonate or adult with a small penis for whom endocrine treatment is impossible or has failed. The questions that then arise are what use will the present organ be, can it be made any bigger and, in an extreme case, should a gender resassignment be made?

### Sexual function with a small penis

Reilly has investigated the male role in 20 patients who had a small penis from a variety of causes (eight pre-pubertal and 12 post-pubertal). Patients were included only if their penis, at the time of review, conformed to the standard definition of 'micropenis' even though some had previously had hypospadias. In spite of the very short length of penile shaft, sexual function was satisfactory (Figure 24.3).

It is interesting to compare the pre-pubertal and post-pubertal groups of micropenis patients as they were the offspring of different generations of parents. Half of the older group remembered unhappy experiences of teasing by their peers because of their small penis. In the younger group all eight were able to change and shower without comment from their peers. This difference was atributed to better counselling of parents.

The most surprising feature of these patients was the firmness with which they were established in the male role and the success that they had in sexual relationships. In the adult group all had heterosexual interests, erections and orgasms; 11 of 12 had ejaculates. Three-quarters had had sexual intercourse. The mean age of sexual debut was 16.4 years (range 13.5–20 years) while the normal is 16.2. All claimed to find intercourse enjoyable though their partners' views were unknown. One patient had a wife and a mistress. The partnerships were stable and long-lasting, a situation that some patients attributed to the extra attention that had to be paid to intercourse because of the short penis. Although vaginal penetration was usual, there was an experimental attitude to positions and methods. One patient was the father of a child (Reilly and Woodhouse, 1989).

There is little supportive evidence for these data from other units. However, the data are sufficiently consistent that it seems safe to conclude that even the possession of the very small penis illustrated in Figure 24.3 is compatible with a normal male role, especially with proper parental support.

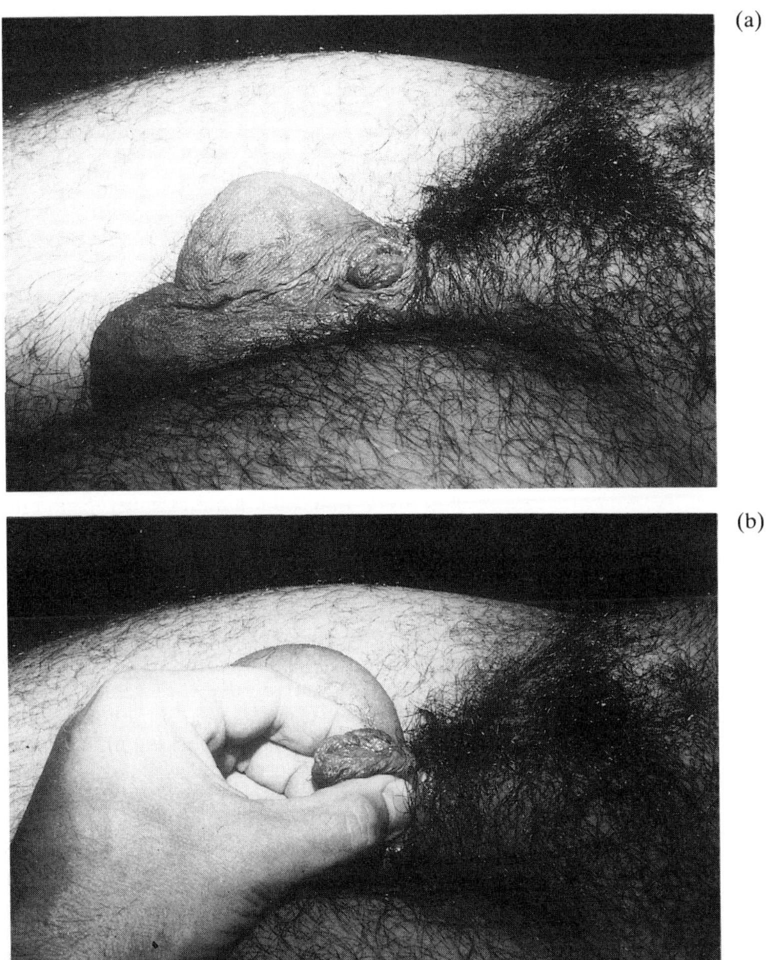


**Figure 24.3** (a) and (b) Clinical photographs of micropenis in an adult

## Medical treatment of the small penis

It cannot be emphasized too strongly that a small penis may be the only presenting sign of a specific endocrine anomaly (Salisbury *et al.*, 1984). Correct treatment may restore the child and his penis to normality.

There remains a group of boys with a small penis who are either of undefined diagnosis or who lack definitive treatment. The role of hormone treatment is uncertain. If there is good volume of erectile tissue and no androgen insensitivity, the penis will grow with testosterone or human chorionic gonadotrophin (HCG) treatment. There is no doubt that early treatment has a role in defining responsiveness of the genitalia to testosterone. The resulting growth encourages the parents to persevere with upbringing in the male gender. From the young boy's point of view, the improved growth usually brings the penis into the normal range of size.

The late results of this treatment are much less clear. The follow-up in most series is short. It would seem from the author's patients that the position on the penile growth curve is not maintained. Treatment probably only achieves that which puberty would achieve anyway and the adult ends up with a small penis. Late treatment of a 12-year-old and a 17-year-old boy have been reported but the responses were poor (Klugo and Cerny,1978).

## Surgical treatment of the small penis

Small penis is not a condition that lends itself to surgical correction. No operation has yet been devised to make the corpora of the truly small penis longer. Theoretically the techniques used for female to male gender re-assignment could be used. They would certainly not appeal for the infant as the phallus created would not grow. They seem to be also of limited appeal for the adult who will have his small but sexually sensitive penis replaced by a large but insensitive and inert object.

The male with a small penis can have satisfactory sexual function and surgery should be avoided. Patients may need help to come to terms with the abnormality if they have been badly counselled in childhood.

## Hypospadias

The repairs done from 1950 to about 1970 had satisfactory results for chordee correction but often left an external urinary meatus that was not terminal and a less than perfect penile appearance. Although these patients have normal erectile mechanisms, some have been left with erectile dysfunction either through residual chordee or for psychiatric reasons.

### Surgical results

Taken at their best, the results of the Denis Browne repair, the most popular operation of the 1950s, are very good. Johanson has reviewed his own cases at a mean age of 18.4 years and at a mean of 7.1 years from the last operation. All of 220 cases had a straight erection, a formed stream with normal flow rate and a urethra that had grown appropriately with the rest of the penis; 142 patients had reached 'fertile age' and apparently had a normal ejaculate; seven had a hypoplastic penis but four of them had other causes of developmental failure (Johanson and Avellan, 1980).

Looking at later operations, Summerlad attempted to trace 113 patients operated on in one unit who would have been aged 17 years or more. Sixty were actually found and seen: 30 had had a Denis Browne repair and 24 an Ombredanne for a distal meatus; six had had a meatotomy alone. Thirteen penises were not straight in the flaccid position, but only 10 patients complained of chordee on erection, two of whom had a straight penis when examined flaccid.

Sexual intercourse was difficult because of pain in four patients and because of hypoplasia of the penis in two (one of whom also had chordee). Twenty patients had weak or incomplete ejaculation (Summerlad, 1975).

### Psychological results

Several authors have suggested that there might be psychological consequences from hypospadias or from its treatment. There have been few formal studies of adults.

Summerlad found that, of 60 patients, 21 avoided changing in public and 31 admitted to anxieties during adolescence, mainly about sexual function and fertility; 43 thought that their penis was abnormal. Two patients who could not be interviewed (and were not part of the series) were in prison, both for sexual offences (Summerlad, 1975).

The difficulty of following up these patients is illustrated by the series from Great Ormond Street where many of the cases had been personally operated on by Denis Browne. Of 351 patients only 82 could be contacted as adults. The main object of this review was to assess the patients' sexual function. Unlike the Berg and Berg survey (see below), sexual function was largely normal and in particular the age of sexual debut was normal (41% by the age of 18 years). Four of five patients who had sexual difficulties had residual chordee as the cause and only one had psychological problems (Kenawi, 1976).

A very extensive psychoanalysis has been made of 33 men who were operated on for hypospadias as children. Thirty-six men who had had an appendicectomy were investigated as controls. The patients who had hypospadias fared badly. They had lower ego strength and poor utilization of mental resources. They had reduced capacity for social and emotional relationships. Their levels of hostility, general anxiety and castration anxiety were higher and they had lower self-esteem. The severity of these abnormalities was not related to the original severity of the hypospadias. In childhood the patients had been shy, timid, isolated and mobbed. As adults they were prone to neurotic (but not psychotic) disturbances and abnormal social relationships. They were less secure in their gender identity, had delayed sexual debut and a smaller number of sexual partners. Eventually they settled down in secure and lasting sexual partnerships. In the long run, they had less rewarding and less demanding jobs. The modern jargon for such men might be 'under-achievers' (Berg, Berg and Svensson, 1982; Berg *et al.*, 1983a, b; Berg and Berg, 1983a, b).

These studies are open to several criticisms, both of method and case selection. The control subjects did not have remotely similar problems to the index patients. The patients clearly did not have a good result from their surgery: 13 had a spraying stream, five had poor flow and five had residual chordee, one of whom could not have intercourse as a result (Svensson and Berg, 1983).

Nonetheless, these are very detailed and important studies and their results cannot be dismissed without proper thought. If patients treated for hypospadias have psychological problems we should seek the reasons and try to correct them.

The suggestion of Berg and Berg is that the abnormalities are the consequence of the malformed penis. If we accept that the appendicectomy control group did not have comparable surgery, it is possible that the series of operations suffered by the hypospadiacs is the cause. Berg and Berg stress the fact that hypospadias surgery was started at 3–4 years of age when the ego is particularly vulnerable. If either of these explanations is correct, single-stage surgery in infancy (assuming the surgical results are excellent) should solve the psychological problems. Likewise better counselling of the parents would improve their attitudes and so produce better orientated patients.

It is also possible, as Berg and Berg considered, that the psychological disturbances are a part of a syndrome which includes hypospadias. An endocrine failure might cause both. In searching for such a cause, Berg and colleagues found low serum 5α-reductase levels in hypospadiacs (Berg *et al.*, 1983b). Poor sperm quality has also been reported in 50% of a series of adult hypospadiacs (Zubowska *et al.*, 1979). If hypospadias is more than just an example of target organ failure and is a part of a more complex syndrome, the psychological abnormalities will continue to be seen.

### Late surgical problems

Even when a patient has not had a perfect result from hypospadias repair, he may not have sufficient symptoms to want further surgery. In some cases he may develop symptoms many years after a successful repair: up to 50 years has been reported (Flynn, Johnston and Blandy, 1980).

Symptoms are usually of stricture or fistula but some patients may have disabling chordee. Although the problems may, at first sight, appear simple, it should be assumed that all have a total inadequacy of the repair until proved otherwise. Many may be described as 'hypospadiac cripples' with a neo-urethra that is too short, too narrow and of poor material. No specific type of primary repair is particularly associated with this disastrous complication (Stecker *et al.*, 1981).

Chordee may occur with a urethra of normal calibre. Correction of the deformity by excision of the ventral chordee tissue will result in a urethra that is too short and further urethroplasty will be needed. If the penis is of adequate length, the patient may be content with a dorsal Nesbitt's procedure rather than risk yet more reconstruction.

The site of chordee may be easy to identify, being opposite the neo-urethra. Occasionally, the deformity has been found to be more proximal (Figure 24.4; Svensson and Berg, 1983). In difficult cases an artificial erection will clarify the problem. This should be achieved either by intracorporeal injection of papaverine or by the infusion technique. If a tourniquet is put around the penis at scrotal level and saline injected into the corpora, the chordee may be missed.

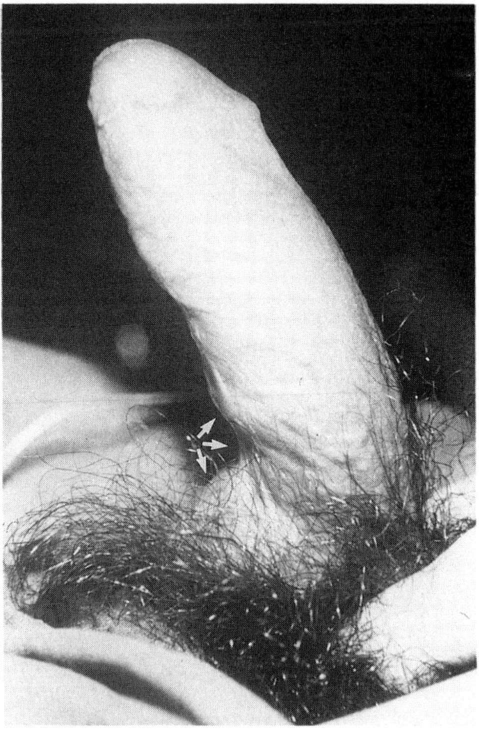

**Figure 24.4** Chordee in a erect penis operated on for hypospadias in childhood. Although the original hypospadias was distal, the chordee is now proximal (arrowed)

## Myelomeningocoele

Even the most crippled spina bifida patient has sexual desires. Normal sexual intercourse, pregnancy and delivery are quite possible even when life is spent largely in a wheel chair. It is very disappointing to find that, in spite of the openness of the 'swinging sixties', 23% of adolescents in one series did not know how babies were concieved and many more had no knowledge of contraception (Dorner, 1977).

In a series of 52 post-pubertal males 70% claimed to have erections, in most cases supported by parental observation. Erections occurred in all patients with a positive anocutaneous reflex and in 64% of those with a negative reflex and a sensory level at or below the sympathetic outflow (D10–L2). Only 14% of males with higher lesions and absent reflex had erections (Diamond, Rickwood and Thomas, 1986). It is not known whether these erections were in response to appropriate sexual stimuli; in the most severely affected patients it seems more likely that they were reflex. Likewise, it is not known how many were able to ejaculate or to have intercourse. It is reasonable to think that the 20% of myelomeningocoele patients who have normal bladder funtion will also have normal sexual function (Diamond, Rickwood and Thomas, 1986).

In a smaller series of men, ejaculation and orgasm were recorded in two of three with lesions at L2 and above, three of five with intermediate lesions and all of four with lesions at S1 or below. Six were having intercourse, one of whom was a father of three normal children (Cass, Bloom and Luxenberg, 1986).

Translating theory into practice is altogether more difficult. In Dorner's series 80% of adolescents expressed interest in the opposite sex but only 28% had dated. In the males only those with minimal handicaps had dated, none had established a steady relationship and none had had intercourse (Dorner, 1977).

The situation improves as the patients get older. In a review of 49 adults it was found that nine had steady partners and 22 were married. Of the others, ten were under 20 years of age, two were mentally handicapped and two had over-protective parents. It could, therefore, be said that 88% of those with realistic prospects were married or had a steady partner. Many of the patients were severely handicapped and incontinent which seemed no bar to their achievements (Laurence and Beresford, 1975).

Patients who are impotent or do not ejaculate should be investigated along conventional lines. Although there have been no studies specifically on these patients, it is known that patients with spinal cord defects can be managed with intracorporeal injections of papaverine and other agents with appropriate dose reductions (Lue and Tanagho, 1987). Electro-ejaculation may have a role in a few patients (Brindley, 1981).

Combined series of spina bifida offspring have shown an increased risk of neural tube defects as high as 4%. The risk is the same whether the affected parent is male or female, but daughters have a one in 13 incidence while the risk for sons is only one in 50 (Laurence and Beresford, 1975). Diagnosis *in utero* by ultrasound and α-fetoprotein estimation is now routine.

## References


Berg, G. and Berg, R. (1983a) Castration complex, evidence from men operated for hypospadias. *Acta Psychiatrica Scandinavica*, **68**, 143–153

Berg, R. and Berg, G. (1983b) Penile malformation, gender identity and sexual orientation. *Acta Psychiatrica Scandinavica*, **68**, 154–166

Berg, R., Berg, G., Edman, G. *et al.* (1983a) Androgens and personality in normal men and men operated for hypospadias in childhood. *Acta Psychiatrica Scandinavica*, **68**, 167–177

Berg, R., Berg, G. and Svensson, J. (1982) Penile malformation and mental health. *Acta Psychiatrica Scandinavica*, **66**, 398–416

Berg, R., Svensson, J., Astrom, G. *et al.* (1983b) Social and sexual adjustment of men operated for hypospadias during childhood: a controlled study. *Journal of Urology*, **125**, 313–317

Brindley, G. S. (1981) Electro-ejaculation: its technique, neurological implications and uses. *Journal of Neurological and Neurosurgical Psychiatry*, **44**, 9–18

Brzezinski, A. E., Homsy, Y. L. and Laberge, I. (1986) Orthoplasty in epispadias. *Journal of Urology*, **136**, 259–261

Burstein, S., Grumbach, M. M. and Kaplan, S. L. (1979) Early determination of androgen responsiveness is important in the management of microphallus. *Lancet*, **ii**, 983–986

Cass, A. S., Bloom, B. A. and Luxenberg, M. (1986) Sexual function in adults with myelomeningocoele. *Journal of Urology*, **136**, 425–426

Diamond, D. A., Rickwood, A. M. K. and Thomas, D. G. (1986) Penile erections in myelomeningocoele patients. *British Journal of Urology*, **58**, 434–435

Dorner, S. (1977) Sexual interest and activity in adolescents with spina bifida. *Journal of Childhood Psychology and Psychiatry*, **18**, 229–237

Editorial (1987) Update: Creutzfeld-Jacob disease in a patient receiving a cadaveric dura mater graft. *Journal of the American Medical Association*, **258**, 309–310

Feldman, K. W. and Smith, D. W. (1975) Fetal phallic growth and penile standards for newborn male infants. *Journal of Pediatrics*, **86**, 395–398

Flatau, E., Josefsberg, Z., Reisner, S. H. *et al.* (1975) Penile size in the newborn infant. *Journal of Pediatrics*, **87**, 663–664

Flynn, J. T., Johnston, S. R. and Blandy, J. P. (1980) The late sequelae of hypospadias repair. *British Journal of Urology*, **52**, 555–559

Hanna, M. K. and Williams, D. I. (1972) Genital function in males with vesical exstrophy and epispadias. *British Journal of Urology*, **44**, 169–174

Hendren, W. H. (1979) Penile lengthening after previous repair of epispadias. *Journal of Urology*, **121**, 527–534

Hurwitz, R. S., Woodhouse, C. R. J. and Ransley, P. G. (1986) The anatomical course of the neurovascular bundles in epispadias. *Journal of Urology*, **136**, 68–70

Johanson, B. and Avellan, L. (1980) Hypospadias: a review of 299 cases operated 1957–1969. *Scandanavian Journal of Plastic and Reconstructive Surgery*, **14**, 259–267

Johnston, J. H. (1974) Lengthening of the congenital or acquired short penis. *British Journal of Urology*, **46**, 685–687

Kelley, J. H. and Eraklis, A. J. (1971) A procedure for lengthening the phallus in boys with exstrophy of the bladder. *Journal of Pediatric Surgery*, **6**, 645–649

Kenawi, M. M. (1976) Sexual function hypospadiacs. *British Journal of Urology*, **47**, 883–890

King, L. R. (1984) Editorial – exstrophy and epispadias.

*Journal of Urology*, **132**, 1159–1160

Klugo, R. C. and Cerny, J. C. (1978) Response of the micropenis to topical testosterone and gonadotrophin. *Journal of Urology*, **119**, 667–668

Koff, S. A. and Eakins, M. (1984) The treatment of penile chordee using corporeal rotation. *Journal of Urology*, **131**, 931–932

Lattimer, J. K., Macfarlane, M. T. and Puchor, P. J. (1979) Male exstrophy patients: a preliminary report on the reproductive capability. *Transactions of the American Association of Genito-Urinary Surgeons*, **70**, 42–46

Laurence, K. M. and Beresford, A. (1975) Continence, friends, marriage and children in 51 adults with spina bifida. *Developmental Medicine and Childhood Neurology*, **17**, (Suppl. 35), 123–128

Lue, T. F. and Tanagho, E. A. (1987) Physiology of erection and pharmacological management of impotence. *Journal of Urology*, **137**, 829–836

Mesrobian, H-G. J., Kelalis, P. P. and Kramer, S. A. (1986) Long-term follow-up of cosmetic appearance and genital function in boys with exstrophy: review of 53 patients. *Journal of Urology*, **136**, 256–258

Reilly, J. M. and Woodhouse, C. R. J. (1989) Small penis and male sexual role. *Journal of Urology*, **142**, 569–571

Salisbury, D. M., Leonard, J. V., Dezateux, C. A. and Savage, M. O. (1984) Micropenis: an important early sign of congenital hypopipuitarism. *British Medical Journal*, **288**, 621–622

Schillinger, J. F. and Wiley, M. J. (1984) Bladder exstrophy penile lengthening procedure. *Urology*, **24**, 434–437

Schonfeld, W. A. (1943) Primary and secondary sexual characteristics. *American Journal of Diseases of Childhood*, **65**, 535–549

Spehr, Ch. and Melchior, C. (1985) Operative correction of the penis deformity in bladder exstrophy. In *XXth Congress of the International Society of Urology*, (Vienna), Abstract 1008, pp. 320

Stecker, J. F., Horton, C. E., Devine, C. J. and McCraw, J. B. (1981) Hypospadias cripples. *Urologic Clinics of North America*, **8**, 539–544

Summerlad, B. C. (1975) A long-term follow-up of hypospadias patients. *British Journal of Plastic Surgery*, **28**, 324–330

Svensson, J. and Berg, R. (1983) Micturition studies and sexual function in operated hypospadiacs. *British Journal of Urology*, **55**, 422–426

Woodhouse, C. R. J. (1986) The management of erectile deformity in adults with exstrophy and epispadias. *Journal of Urology*, **135**, 932–935

Woodhouse, C. R. J. (1988) Dural phalloplasty in exstrophy and epispadias. In *Current Operative Surgery – Urology*, (ed. A. R. Mundy), Bailliere Tindall, London, pp. 106–118

Woodhouse, C. R. J. and Kellett, M. J. (1984) Anatomy of the penis and its deformities in exstrophy and epispadias. *Journal of Urology*, **132**, 1122–1124

Zubowska, J., Jankowska, J., Kula, K. *et al.* (1979) Clinical, hormonal and semiological data in adult men operated in childhood for hypospadias. *Endokrynologia Polska*, **30**, 565–573

# 25

# Diabetic impotence

**I. Eardley, E. Gale and R. S. Kirby**

## Introduction

In 1798, Rollo first noticed the association between diabetes mellitus and erectile impotence and, in 1906, Naunyn observed that impotence was one of the commonest clinical features of diabetic men. Diabetes mellitus is certainly the commonest single cause of impotence seen in clinical practice, and may account for up to 28% of men who present to an impotence clinic (Maatman, Montague and Martin, 1987). In recent years interest has centred upon the pathogenesis of erectile dysfunction in these patients, and psychological, endocrine, neurological and vascular causes have all been suggested. Although this question has not yet been finally answered, a variety of epidemiological, clinical, biochemical, neurophysiological and pathological studies have increased our understanding of the means by which erectile dysfunction arises, and have suggested ways in which it may be prevented and treated.

## Epidemiology

The prevalence of erectile impotence in men with diabetes has been reported to be between 23% and 59% (Rubin and Babbott, 1958; Schoffling *et al.*, 1963; Ellenberg, 1971; Kolodny *et al.*, 1974; McCulloch *et al.*, 1980), which is significantly greater than the prevalence in the general population (Frank, Anderson and Rubinstein, 1978; Newman and Marcus, 1985). Although erectile dysfunction usually develops later in the course of the disease, it may sometimes be the presenting symptom (Deutsch and Sherman, 1980) and in one study, when patients attending an impotence clinic were screened for glucose intolerance, 11.1% were found to have previously unrecognized diabetes (Maatman, Montague and Martin, 1987).

It has been suggested that the likelihood of developing impotence is related to the duration of the diabetes (Schoffling *et al.*, 1963; McCulloch *et al.*, 1980; Newman and Marcus, 1985) although other studies have not confirmed this (Rubin and Babbott, 1958; Kolodny *et al.*, 1974). Similarly, while some have shown that the development of erectile dysfunction is related to the quality of diabetic control (McCulloch *et al.*, 1984), other groups disagree (Rubin and Babbott, 1963; Ellenberg, 1971).

Most studies do show, however, that the type of diabetes and the mode of treatment do not influence the likelihood of developing impotence (Schoffling *et al.*, 1963; Kolodny *et al.*, 1974), although in one small study Lehman and Jacobs (1983) found an increased incidence of erectile dysfunction in men with insulin-dependent diabetes.

## Aetiology

It was originally supposed that many diabetic men were impotent for psychological reasons, but by the 1960s interest had centred upon the role of testosterone in the pathogenesis of diabetic impotence. Only in recent years has the importance of diabetic neuropathy and arteriopathy been recognized and, although it is now accepted that these are the most important factors, it is still not clear how they interact with each other to produce erectile dysfunction.

### Endocrine factors

Schoffling and his colleagues (1963) undertook an extensive endocrinological study of impotent diabetics and found both a decrease in the amount of urinary gonadotrophin and a reduction in the urinary levels of the metabolites of testosterone when compared with controls. They concluded that many impotent diabetics had a degree of hypogonadotrophic hypogonadism as the underlying cause of the impotence. On this basis, they treated a group of young impotent diabetics with chorionic gonadotrophin and testosterone, reporting improvement or total cure of the impotence in all but one case. In older diabetics they treated the impotence with testosterone alone, and reported improvement of erectile function in 76% of their patients.

These findings have not been substantiated in subsequent studies. While Maatman, Montague and Martin (1987) reported a low serum testosterone in 11.8% of their patients, in another large study Ellenberg (1971) found that serum testosterone levels were normal. In addition he found that treatment with testosterone had no therapeutic benefit. Similarly Kaiser and Korenman (1988) found that low serum testosterone levels were no more frequent than in control subjects and it thus seems that endocrine factors only play a marginal role in the pathogenesis of diabetic impotence.

## Neurogenic factors

Several lines of evidence have suggested that diabetic neuropathy is related to the development of erectile impotence. This neuropathy primarily affects small myelinated and unmyelinated fibres (Said, Slama and Selva, 1983) and affects the longest fibres first, to produce the typical glove and stocking peripheral sensory loss. It is, however, small myelinated and unmyelinated fibres which mediate penile erection in man (see Chapter 3), and it has been suggested that damage to these nerve fibres may be the underlying cause of impotence in diabetes.

Several studies have demonstrated a correlation between erectile impotence and clinical signs of neuropathy. For instance, Ellenberg (1971) reported that 82% of impotent men had evidence of neuropathy compared with only 12% of potent diabetics. Kolodny and his colleagues (1974) also demonstrated an increased incidence of neuropathy in impotent diabetics.

Studies of bladder function in diabetics have also revealed a correlation between urodynamic evidence of autonomic dysfunction and the presence of erectile dysfunction. Ellenberg and Weber (1967) studied a group of diabetics with clinical neuropathy but with no urinary symptoms and found a high incidence of urodynamic abnormalities which in turn were commonly associated with impotence. Similarly, Faerman *et al.* (1971) also found a high incidence of impotence in a group of young men with urodynamic evidence of bladder neuropathy. However, Buvat *et al.* (1985) found that cystometrography did not discriminate between impotent and potent diabetics.

Neurophysiological studies have confirmed that a large proportion of impotent diabetics have evidence of neuropathy (Ertekin and Reel, 1976; Desai *et al.*, 1988). However, these groups tested only the sacral reflex arc, which is mediated by large diameter myelinated fibres, and which accordingly is affected relatively late in the disease. Both Robinson, Woodcock and Stephenson (1987) and Fowler and her colleagues (1988) attempted to rectify this by studying the thermal thresholds of a group of impotent diabetics. Temperature sensation is carried by small myelinated and unmyelinated fibres, and thus should be a more sensitive indicator of diabetic neuropathy. Indeed, both groups found a high incidence of neuropathy in diabetics with impotence which on clinical grounds was thought to be of neurogenic origin.

Some pathological studies have demonstrated neuropathy in patients with erectile impotence secondary to diabetes. Both Faerman *et al.* (1974) using light microscopy, and de Tejada and Goldstein (1988) with electron microscopy, found evidence of neuropathy in this group. Interestingly the former group only found evidence of microangiopathy in one patient although, as shall be seen later, Jevtich, Kass and Khawand (1985) found a rather higher incidence in a group of patients undergoing insertion of penile prostheses.

Finally, several groups have investigated the levels of neurotransmitters within the penis. Melman and Henry (1979) found a reduction in the levels of noradrenaline in insulin-dependent diabetics, although the level in patients whose diabetes was controlled by diet or oral agents was normal. They concluded that this reflected a sympathetic neuropathy. Lincoln *et al.* (1987) confirmed this finding and also found a reduction in the amount of VIP-like reactivity and the amount of acetylcholinesterase staining in nerves associated with corporeal smooth muscle. Since these neurotransmitters are associated with parasympathetic nerves, it seems likely that the neuropathy of diabetes affects both sections of the autonomic nervous system.

In conclusion, there is evidence from clinical, urodynamic, neurophysiological, pathological and biochemical studies that neuropathy does play a significant role in the development of impotence in diabetic men.

## Arteriogenic factors

Diabetes mellitus causes both large and small vessel disease. In large arteries, atherosclerosis appears more frequently and at an earlier age than in non-diabetics, and in smaller vessels there is a characteristic angiopathy characterized by thickening of the basement membrane. It has been suggested that both these phenomena may be causally related to the development of impotence in diabetes mellitus.

One of the easiest ways of diagnosing small vessel disease in diabetics is by examination of the retina, and several groups have found an association between diabetic retinopathy and erectile impotence. Schoffling *et al.* (1963) found an increased incidence of angiopathy in impotent diabetics compared with potent controls, while McCulloch *et al.* (1980) found that erectile impotence was significantly associated with the presence of retinopathy. A later study (McCulloch *et al.*, 1984) showed that retinopathy was a predictive factor for the subsequent development of erectile dysfunction in potent diabetics, as was peripheral vascular disease as characterized by intermittent claudication. Arteriography has also supported an association between large vessel disease in diabetics and impotence, since Herman, Adar and Rubinstein (1978) found an increased incidence of internal pudendal artery stenosis in impotent diabetics compared with their potent counterparts.

With the advent of techniques to assess penile blood flow non-invasively (Abelson, 1975; Jevtich, 1980; Lue *et al.*, 1985; Desai *et al.*, 1987), several groups have used Doppler studies to assess impotent diabetics. Using Doppler to record penile blood pressure, Abelson (1975) found that abnormal pressures were more common in diabetics, while Jevtich *et al.* (1982), using penile Doppler with waveform analysis, found that over 90% of their patients had obstructive penile vascular changes. Lehman and Jacobs (1983) also concluded that vascular changes were important following their studies of the penobrachial index in diabetics, and these findings were confirmed by Maatman, Montague and Martin (1987) who found that 37% of their patients had a penobrachial index below 0.7.

In recent years it has become clear that investigations using papaverine are more accurate in diagnosing arteriogenic impotence, and several groups have applied these principles to the investigation of the impotent diabetic. Robinson, Woodcock and Stephenson (1987), using duplex scanning with papaverine, found that peak flow in the penile arteries was impaired in most of their patients, while Desai *et al.* (1988), using Doppler waveform analysis, found that 49% of their patients had abnormal penile haemodynamics.

Finally, Jevtich, Kass and Khawand (1985) have shown in histological studies that vascular changes may underlie the erectile impotence of diabetics. They assessed corporeal tissue from ten diabetics undergoing penile prosthesis insertion and found almost universal evidence of endothelial proliferation, intimal fibrosis and perivascular fibrosis with endarteritis obliterans. In contrast they found little or no evidence of damage to the nerve fibres of the corpora.

### Psychological factors

While most groups have emphasized organic factors leading to impotence in diabetic men, others have suggested that psychogenic factors may contribute to the development of erectile dysfunction in some. Karacan *et al.* (1977) found that in a minority of impotent diabetics there were normal nocturnal erections, while both Renshaw (1978) and El-Bayoumi, El-Sherbani and Mostafa (1984) found significant subgroups of patients who responded, at least partially to psychological or sexual therapy.

As with other organic forms of impotence, secondary psychogenic factors may contribute to the erectile dysfunction of diabetes. However the proportion of diabetics who have primary psychogenic impotence is probably small, and it seems likely that most have organic problems.

### Conclusion

In conclusion, there is evidence that both vascular and neurological factors play a role in the development of diabetic impotence. Both vascular and neurological impairment is present in many patients (Robinson, Woodcock and Stephenson, 1987) and while in some vascular disease may be more important, in others neurological factors seem to predominate. The early suggestion that endocrine factors are important has largely been disproved, but secondary psychological factors may be involved in some patients.

## Clinical features

Diabetic impotence may present in two ways. Firstly, there may be a transient period of erectile dysfunction, usually at the onset of the disease. This is probably related to systemic malaise due to untreated diabetes and is comparable with the impotence often seen with other debilitating illnesses. With control of the diabetes it usually resolves (Rubin and Babbott, 1958; Fairburn *et al.*, 1982).

However, the majority of patients develop irreversible erectile dysfunction later in the course of the disease with a gradual onset over a period of 6–12 months (Ellenberg, 1971; Kolodny *et al.*, 1974). There is initially a reduction in the strength and duration of the erections (Karacan *et al.*, 1977), leading to complete impotence with a secondary loss of libido (Fairburn *et al.*, 1982).

## Management

### Evaluation

The evaluation of the impotent diabetic is similar to the evaluation of any other patient with erectile dysfunction. A thorough history and examination is mandatory. Some 30–50% of middle-aged diabetics are taking antihypertensive medication and this may, in some instances, contribute to the erectile dysfunction. Advice to restrict alcohol intake is sometimes also needed. The examination should take account of evidence of peripheral neuropathy in the form of absent ankle jerks and sensory neuropathy. Retinopathy and proteinuria due to diabetic nephropathy will suggest widespread microangiopathy, whereas evidence of peripheral vascular disease will indicate the likelihood of arterial disease.

In our clinic a hormonal screen is undertaken to exclude any other associated endocrine abnormalities. The next step is to test the response to intracorporeal papaverine, and a dose of 20–40 mg is typically used which may be increased to 80 mg in patients with a poor response at the lower dosage.

Non-responders then undergo pharmacocavernometry (Eardley *et al.*, 1990) to identify venous leakage. In those patients who require a low infusion rate to initiate and maintain an erection, isotope phallography (Blacklay, 1986) and selective pudendal arteriography are performed to identify those suitable for reconstructive arterial surgery.

### Treatment

Occasionally, diabetic patients have impotence due to endocrine abnormalities or venous leakage, but in the majority neuropathy or arterial disease are responsible. Treatment is thus similar to the treatment of other patients with neurogenic or arteriogenic impotence.

Many diabetic patients have a good response to intracorporeal pharmacotherapy either with papaverine alone, or in combination with phentolamine (Zorgniotti and Lefleur, 1985; Sidi *et al.*, 1986; Williams, Mulcahy and Kiely, 1987). Accordingly, many are suitable for self-injection therapy, and those who are already injecting themselves with insulin easily learn the technique of intracavernous self-injection. Quite large doses of papaverine (with or without phentolamine) are required in some patients who presumably have a degree of vascular insufficiency. A few patients are not able to cope with self-injection therapy, and some may benefit from the use of suction devices.

Many patients do not respond at all to intracorporeal pharmacotherapy and these are often found to have vascular insufficiency. This may be amenable to reconstructive microvascular surgery, or alternatively to the insertion of penile prostheses. Although the results of prosthetic surgery are generally good, diabetics have been shown in several series to be at particular risk of infection (Kaufman, Lindner and Raz, 1982; Wilson, Wahman and Lange. 1988; Fallon and Ghanem, 1989). This may be minimized by good perioperative diabetic control, careful surgical technique and prophylactic antibiotics.

In a small proportion of patients there may be evidence of large vessel atherosclerosis which may be associated with intermittent claudication, and here reconstructive aortoiliac surgery may be appropriate.

Finally, as was suggested above, psychological problems are not uncommon in diabetic patients and it is the responsibility of the physician to be alert to this, so that appropriate emotional and psychological support can be provided in conjunction with treatment for organic problems.

### Prevention

There has been some controversy about whether good diabetic control can prevent the onset of diabetic impotence, but probably the largest study by McCulloch *et al.* (1984) demonstrated that poor glycaemic control was correlated with the subsequent development of impotence in diabetics. Interestingly they also showed that alcohol intake correlated well with the development of impotence, and they concluded that moderation of alcohol consumption and better glycaemic control might diminish the prevalence of impotence in diabetic men.

## Conclusion

Impotence is a common complication of diabetes mellitus and is probably due to either vascular insufficiency or peripheral neuropathy, or both. Management is aimed at identifying those patients who respond to intracorporeal pharmacotherapy and, in the rest (who usually have severe arterial disease), the erectile dysfunction may be managed by penile revascularization or penile prosthesis insertion.

### References


Abelson, D. (1975) Diagnostic value of the penile pulse and blood pressure: a Doppler study of diabetic impotence. *Journal of Urology*, **113**, 636–639

Blacklay, P. J. (1986) *MS Thesis*, London University

Buvat, J., Lemaire, A., Buvat-Herbaut, M. *et al.* (1985) Comparative investigations in 26 impotent and 26 non-impotent diabetic patients. *Journal of Urology*, **133**, 34–38

Desai, K. M., Dembny, K., Morgan, H. *et al.* (1988). Neurophysiological investigation of diabetic impotence. Are sacral reflex studies of value? *British Journal of Urology*, **61**, 68–73

Desai, K. M., Gingell, J. C., Skidmore, R. and Follett, D. H. (1987) Application of computerised penile waveform analysis in the diagnosis of arteriogenic impotence. An initial study in potent and impotent men. *British Journal of Urology*, **60**, 450–456

de Tejada, I. S. and Goldstein, I. (1988) Diabetic penile neuropathy. *Urologic Clinics of North America*, **15**, 17–22

Deutsch, S. and Sherman, L. (1980) Previously unrecognised diabetes mellitus in sexually impotent men. *Journal of the American Medical Association*, **244**,

2430–2432

Eardley, I., Vale, J., Holmes, S. *et al.* (1990) Pharmacocavernometry in the assessment of erectile impotence. *Journal of the Royal Society of Medicine*, **83**, 22–24

El-Bayoumi, M., El-Sherbani, O. and Mostafa, M. (1984) Impotence in diabetics: organic versus psychogenic factors. *Urology*, **24**, 459–463

Ellenberg, M. (1971) Impotence in diabetes: the neurologic factor. *Annals of Internal Medicine*, **75**, 213–219

Ellenberg, M. and Weber, H. (1967) The incipient assymptomatic diabetic bladder. *Diabetes*, **16**, 331–335

Ertekin, C. and Reel, F. (1976) Bulbocavernosus reflex in normal men and patients with neurogenic bladder and/or impotence. *Journal of Neurological Science*, **28**, 1–15

Faerman, I., Glocer, L., Fox, D. *et al.* (1974) Impotence and diabetes. Histological studies of the autonomic nervous fibres of the corpora cavernosa inpotent diabetic males. *Diabetes*, **23**, 971–975

Faerman, I., Maler, M., Jadzinsky, M. *et al.* (1971) Asymptomatic neurogenic bladder in juvenile diabetics. *Diabetologia*, **7**, 168–172

Fairburn, C. G., Wu, F. C. W., McCulloch, D. K. *et al.* (1982) The clinical features of diabetic impotence: a preliminary study. *British Journal of Psychiatry*, **140**, 447–452

Fallon, B. and Ghanem, H. (1989) Infected penile prostheses: incidence and outcomes. *International Journal of Impotence Research*, **1**, 175–181

Fowler, C. J., Ali, Z., Kirby, R. S. and Pryor, J. P. (1988) The value of testing for unmyelinated fibre, sensory neuropathy in diabetic impotence. *British Journal of Urology*, **61**, 63–67

Frank, E., Anderson, C. and Rubinstein, D. (1987) Frequency of sexual dysfunction in 'normal' couples *New England Journal of Medicine*, **299**, 111–115

Herman, A., Adar, R. and Rubinstein, Z. (1978) Vascular lesions associated with impotence in diabetic and non-diabetic arterial occlusive disease. *Diabetes*, **27**, 975–981

Jevtich, M.J. (1980) Importance of penile arterial pulse sound examination in impotence. *Journal of Urology*, **124**, 820–824

Jevtich, M. J., Edson, M., Jarman, W. D. and Herrera, H. H. (1982) Vascular factors in erectile failure among diabetics. *Urology*, **19**, 163–168

Jevtich, M. J., Kass, M. and Khawand, N. (1985) Changes in the corpora cavernosa of impotent diabetics: comparing histological with clinical findings. *Journal d'Urologie*, **91**, 281–285

Kaiser, F. E. and Korenman, S. G. (1988) Impotence in diabetic men. *American Journal of Medicine*, **85**, (Suppl. 5A), 147–151

Karacan, I., Brantley Scott, F., Salis, P. J. *et al.* (1977) Nocturnal erections, differential diagnosis of impotence and diabetes. *Biological Psychiatry*, **12**, 373–380

Kaufman, J. J., Lindner, A. and Raz, S. (1982) Penile prosthesis surgery for impotence. *Journal of Urology*, **128**, 1192–1194

Kolodny, R. C., Kahn, C. B., Goldstein, H. and Barnett, D. M. (1974) Sexual dysfunction in diabetic men. *Diabetes*, **23**, 306–309

Lehman, T. P. and Jacobs, J. A. (1983) Etiology of diabetic impotence. *Journal of Urology*, **129**, 291–294

Lincoln, J., Crowe, R., Blacklay, P. F. *et al.* (1987) Changes in the VIPergic, cholinergic and adrenergic innervation of human penile tissue in diabetic and non-diabetic impotent males. *Journal of Urology*, **137**, 1053–1059

Lue, T. F., Hricack, H., Marich, K. W. and Tanagho, E. A. (1985) Vasculogenic impotence evaluated by high resolution ultrasonography and pulsed Doppler spectrum analysis. *Radiology*, **155**, 777–781

Maatman, T. J., Montague, D. K. and Martin, L. M. (1987) Erectile dysfunction in men with diabetes mellitus. *Urology*, **29**, 589–592

McCulloch, D. K., Campbell, I. W., Wu, F. C. *et al.* (1980) The prevalence of diabetic impotence. *Diabetologia*, **18**, 279–283

McCulloch, D. K., Young, R. J., Prescott, R. J. *et al.* (1984) The natural history of impotence in diabetic men. *Diabetologia*, **26**, 437–440

Melman, A. and Henry, D. (1979) The possible role of catecholamines of the corpora in penile erection. *Journal of Urology*, **121**, 419–421

Naunyn, B. (1906) *Der diabetes mellitus*, 2nd edn, Alfred Holder, Vienna

Newman, H. F. and Marcus, H. (1985) Erectile dysfunction in diabetes and hypertension. *Urology*, **26**, 135–137

Renshaw, D. C. (1978) Impotence in diabetes. In *Handbook of Sex Therapy* (eds J. Lopiccolo and L. Lopiccolo), Plenum Press, New York

Robinson, L. Q., Woodcock, J. P. and Stephenson, T. P. (1987) Results of investigation of impotence in patients with overt or probable neuropathy. *British Journal of Urology*, **60**, 583–587

Rubin, A. and Babbott, D. (1958). Impotence and diabetes mellitus. *Journal of the American Medical Association*, **168**, 498–500

Said, G., Slama, G. and Selva, J. (1983) Progressive centripetal degeneration of axons in small fibre diabetic neuropathy. *Brain*, **106**, 791–807

Schoffling, K., Federlin, K., Ditschuneit, H. and Pfeiffer, E. F. (1963) Disorders of sexual function in male diabetics. *Diabetes*, **12**, 519–527

Sidi, A. A., Cameron, J. S., Duffy, L. M., and Lange, P. H. (1986) Intracavernous drug-induced erections in the management of male erectile dysfunction: experience with 100 patients. *Journal of Urology*, **135**, 704–706

Williams, G., Mulcahy, M. J. and Kiely, E. A. (1987) Impotence: treatment by autoinjection of vasoactive drugs. *British Medical Journal*, **295**, 595–596

Wilson, S. K., Wahman, G. E. and Lange, J. L. (1988) Eleven years experience with the inflatable penile prosthesis. *Journal of Urology*, **139** 951–952

Zorgniotti, A. W. and Lefleur, R. S. (1985) Auto-injection of the corpus cavernosum with a vasoactive drug combination for vasculogenic impotence. *Journal of Urology*, **133**, 39–41

# 26

# Neurogenic impotence

I. Eardley and R. S. Kirby

## Introduction

Intact neural pathways are essential for normal penile erection to occur, and damage to a wide range of different loci within the central and peripheral nervous system may result in erectile impotence. Given the relatively young age of many of the men who are afflicted by neurological disease, there is often a considerable demand for treatment of related potency difficulties. However, the advances in diagnosis and treatment which have been made over recent years, especially in the field of pharmaco-erection, mean that many of them can now avoid the necessity for prosthetic implants.

However, neural damage to the pathways concerned with erectile function is not the only way in which neurological disease can result in impotence. Particularly in patients with central nervous system disorders, disorders of mobility may restrict the patient's ability to have successful sexual relations. Similarly, patients with indwelling catheters which are being used to treat coexistent voiding disorders are unable to participate in normal sexual intercourse. Finally, the psychological effect of having a progressive neurological disease which is often incurable may result in psychogenic impotence. Accordingly, in treating the patient with neurogenic impotence, the clinician must address these other problems in addition to providing a penile erection.

In this chapter we will describe some of the more common neurological causes of impotence and then discuss the management of patients with neurogenic impotence. A more complete list of those disorders which can cause impotence is outlined in Table 26.1.

**Table 26.1 Neurological causes of impotence**

Peripheral nervous system:
- Pelvic nerve injury, e.g. pelvic surgery, pelvic fracture
- Peripheral small fibre neuropathies, e.g. diabetes mellitus, alcoholic neuropathy, Fabry's disease, hereditary amyloidosis
- Cauda equina lesions

Central nervous system:
- Spina bifida
- Spinal cord injury
- Cord compression, e.g. secondary to tumours of the spinal cord
- Transverse myelitis
- Subacute combined degeneration of the cord
- Tabes dorsalis
- Multiple sclerosis
- Idiopathic Parkinson's disease
- Multiple system atrophy
- Temporal lobe epilepsy

## Disorders of the peripheral nervous system

### Pelvic nerve injury

The most common cause of pelvic nerve injury which can result in impotence is radical pelvic surgery, and this subject is dealt with more fully in Chapter 22. The nerves most at risk are the cavernous nerves which pass from the sacral segments, around the rectum, and then pass lateral to the prostate before curving anteriorly to pierce the pelvic diaphragm. The cavernous nerves are most commonly damaged during radical excision of the rectum, bladder and prostate, unless specific measures are taken to avoid them. For instance, the anatomical studies of Walsh and Donker (1982) demonstrated that the cavernous nerves pass posterolaterally to the capsule of the prostate before swinging anteriorly to reach the urethra. Accordingly, the technique of nerve-sparing radical prostatectomy was devised which does not compromise surgical resection margins but which does preserve potency (Walsh, Lepor and Egglestone, 1983).

Pelvic fractures are also known to result in impotence in a proportion of cases (King, 1975) although the exact pathogenesis is often not clear. Trafford (1955) proposed that the impotence had a neurogenic aetiology, suggesting that the cavernous nerves were either damaged at the time of injury or secondary to a subsequent thrombosis. However, there are reports of successful treatment of impotence in cases of pelvic fracture by reconstructive microvascular surgery (Goldstein, 1988), and most studies have concluded that the impotence that follows pelvic fracture has a multifactorial aetiology (Gibson, 1970; Ellison, Timberlake and Kerstein, 1988).

### Peripheral neuropathy

The peripheral neuropathies which most comonly result in impotence are the small fibre neuropathies which affect the small myelinated and unmyelinated nerves which mediate erection in man. By far the commonest of these is the autonomic neuropathy which accompanies diabetes mellitus, and diabetic impotence is dealt with more fully in Chapter 25. However, there are several other causes of small fibre neuropathy, all of which may cause impotence. Some of these are listed in Table 26.1.

Assessment and diagnosis of small fibre neuropathy has recently been much improved by the development of techniques to measure cutaneous warming and cooling (Fowler *et al.*, 1988), and this is dealt with more fully in Chapter 12.

### Cauda equina lesions

Lesions of the cauda equina, such as prolapsed intervertebral discs or tumours of the cauda equina, can result in impotence (Fairburn and Stewart, 1955; Shafer and Rosenblum, 1969). Velcek (1989) reported a series of 20 patients with lumbar disc prolapse associated with impotence, finding that preoperative nocturnal penile tumescence studies were normal in many patients. He proposed that these erections were of psychogenic origin and that they were mediated via sympathetic pathways. Furthermore, he found that surgical treatment of the disc prolapse resulted in restoration of potency in those patients with normal vasculature.

Accordingly, the diagnosis of lumbar disc prolapse must always be considered in patients presenting with impotence and low back pain, particularly if there are also urinary or bowel symptoms, since if a diagnosis can be made, then surgical treatment does seem to offer the possibility of a cure.

## Disorders of the central nervous system

### Spinal cord injury

Following spinal cord injury, so-called 'psychogenic' erections may still occur, provided that the lesion is below T9 (Bors and Comarr, 1960) and these are thought to be mediated via sympathetic pathways. Similarly, reflex erections will also occur provided that the sacral nerve roots are intact (Comarr, 1970) although these erections are seldom adequate for normal intercourse (Bors and Comarr, 1960). The afferent limb of this reflex is probably carried via the pudendal nerve with the efferent limb within the nervi erigentes.

### Multiple sclerosis

Although erectile dysfunction is rarely the presenting complaint in patients with multiple sclerosis, surveys have shown that up to 60% of men with multiple sclerosis are impotent (Ivers and Goldstein, 1963; Miller, Simpson and Yeates, 1965; Vas, 1969). There are probably many sites within the central nervous system which can result in erectile impotence, but in most cases the lesions lie within the spinal cord, of which cervical demyelination is the most common (Oppenheimer, 1978). Indeed sacral demyelination is relatively rare (Philp, Read and Higson, 1980), and certainly it is our experience that erectile impotence is never seen unless there are abnormal clinical signs within the legs.

However, multiple sclerosis may also cause impotence by demyelination within the higher centres of the brain which are involved in penile erection, and it has also been suggested that the general psychological effects of having a severe progressive neurological disease such as multiple sclerosis may account for the impotence of some patients (Miller, Simpson and Yeates, 1965).

Kirkeby *et al.*, (1988) found that a large proportion of patients with impotence related to multiple sclerosis had nocturnal erections. This may well be another manifestation of the psychogenic erections found in spinal cord injured patients with injuries below T9 (see above). Interestingly, they also found that the degree of disability produced by the multiple sclerosis was not related to either the presence of nocturnal erections or the results of neurophysiological testing.

### Parkinsonism and multiple system atrophy

In 1960, Shy and Drager reported the first cases of a syndrome including postural hypotension, urinary incontinence and impotence. Since then it has become clear that the Shy–Drager syndrome is but one manifestation of a more widespread disease of the nervous system known as multiple system atrophy (MSA). This disease may present in a variety of ways including parkinsonism, cerebellar ataxia and autonomic failure, but it is our experience that erectile impotence often precedes the development of other symptoms by several years. This is probably due to a progressive cell loss in the intermediolateral column of the spinal cord (Oppenheimer, 1980) from which most of the parasympathetic outflow arises.

Another prominent pathological feature of the disease is a progressive cell loss in the motor nucleus of the striated urethral and anal sphincters (Sung, Mastri and Segal, 1979). This observation is reflected in the highly abnormal electromyographic activity recorded from the urethral sphincter (Kirby *et al.*, 1986) and has been used as a diagnostic test to differentiate those patients with MSA from those who have idiopathic Parkinson's disease (Eardley *et al.*, 1989). Certainly this diagnosis should be considered in any patient with erectile impotence associated with voiding difficulties, postural hypotension or parkinsonism.

### Temporal lobe epilepsy

There is a well recognized relationship between erectile impotence and temporal lobe epilepsy (TLE) (Johnson, 1965; Hierons and Saunders, 1966). This is probably related to the role of the temporal lobe in modulating sexual and reproductive function, which has been demonstrated in animals (Spark, Wills and Royal, 1984). The temporal lobe is also involved in the control of hypothalamic neuroendocrine function, and Spark and his colleagues (1984) found that in a group of patients with impotence and TLE (which was confirmed by EEG), associated neuroendocrine abnormalities such as hypogonadotrophic hypogonadism and hyperprolactinaemia were common. Treatment with anticonvulsants followed by the appropriate endocrine therapy resulted in a restoration of potency.

## Management

### Clinical assessment

Clinical assessment in the patient with neurogenic impotence has two roles. Firstly it is important to make a firm neurological diagnosis. If the patient has previously seen a neurologist a diagnosis may have already been reached, but in some cases the impotence is the presenting symptom and it is important for the clinician to bear in mind the possibility of neurological disease. Secondly the cause of the erectile dysfunction must also be elucidated. This may simply be due to neural damage to the pathways which control erectile function, but it may also be due to problems of mobility or micturition, as was discussed above.

Accordingly a careful history and examination is essential, and if a neurological diagnosis is suspected then further investigation will be necessary.

### Treatment

#### Treatment of the disease

In a few cases of neurogenic impotence, treatment of the underlying condition may lead to restoration of normal potency. As was described above, a proportion of patients with lumbar disc disease will respond to surgical treatment (Velcek, 1989) and it may be that, in a few other cases where the clinical picture is secondary to a surgically remediable cause, potency may be restored. Similarly medical treatment with anticonvulsants in patients with temporal lobe epilepsy will also restore potency in many cases (Spark, Wills and Royal, 1984). However, in the majority of patients with neurological disease the impotence is irreversible, and other means of treatment must be used.

#### Pharmacotherapy

The finding that intracorporeal injection of a variety of substances could produce an erection in impotent men (Virag, 1982; Brindley, 1983) was of great importance to the treatment of neurogenic impotence since it soon became clear that patients with neurogenic impotence were amongst the most sensitive to intracorporeal pharmacotherapy (Sidi *et al.*, 1986). Indeed, the dose required to produce an erection is somewhat less than in cases of impotence of different aetiologies, while the risk of prolonged erections is somewhat higher. Because of this, Sidi and his colleagues (1987) advised that a small dose of papaverine (e.g. 7.5 mg) is the most suitable initial dose for patients with neurological disease. The dose may then be increased if necessary, and in a few cases it may be necessary to add phentolamine to the mixture. In those patients who fail to respond to even this combination, it is likely that there is another coexistent vascular cause for the impotence.

In addition to the short-term risk of prolonged erections, in a small proportion of patients there are long-term side effects of repeated papaverine injection including corporeal fibrosis (Juenemann and Alken, 1989). In recent years prostaglandin $E_1$ ($PGE_1$), which is both more efficacious and also has a lower incidence of prolonged erections, has gained increasing popularity (Ishii, Watanabe and Irisawa, 1989; Lee, Stevenson and Szasz, 1989). Since many patients with neurogenic impotence are relatively young, they can expect to self-inject for many years, and such considerations are of importance. However, there is as yet no long-term follow-up of the side effects of intracorporeal $PGE_1$ and it is still our policy to use papaverine alone in most patients with neurogenic impotence.

#### Other forms of treatment

Because of the efficacy of intracorporeal pharmacotherapy in the treatment of neurogenic impotence, it has become the mainstay of treatment. However, in a few cases the patient may be unwilling or unable to self-inject and other forms of treatment may be necessary, such as vacuum devices

(Nadig, Lindner and Blumoff, 1986) or penile prostheses (Montague, 1989).

One interesting approach for patients with a spinal cord injury is the use of an anterior root nerve stimulator. These stimulators were originally designed to improve micturition and achieve continence in patients with disorders of the central nervous system (Brindley, Polkey and Rushton, 1982). However, in 38 men with spinal cord injuries who received one of these devices, 26 were able to produce implant-driven erections via stimulation of the S2 or S3 nerve root (Brindley *et al.*, 1986). They were able to achieve successful coitus, and although there was a gradual deterioration of the erections in a few patients, others maintained good erections for a considerable period of time.

## Conclusion

In patients with generalized neurological disease or with disease confined to the sacral segments, erectile impotence is relatively common. Moreover, in a few patients it may even be the presenting feature of the disease. It behoves the clinician to whom such a patient presents to be aware of the possibility of a neurological disorder. Correct diagnosis is the first stage of management, and then appropriate treatment of the erectile dysfunction is required. Currently, the mainstay of treatment in these patients is intracorporeal pharmacotherapy, although such treatment is not suitable for all. In addition, it is important to recognize the effects of neurological disease upon the patient as a whole, and in some patients it may be necessary to liaise with other specialists such as neurologists, physiotherapists and sex therapists, in order to adequately treat the patient.

### References

Bors, E. and Comarr, A. E. (1960) Neurological disturbances of sexual function with special reference to 529 patients with spinal cord injuries. *Urological Survey*, **10**, 191–222

Brindley, G. S. (1983) Cavernosal alpha-blockade: a new technique for investigating and treating erectile impotence. *British Journal of Psychiatry*, **143**, 332–337

Brindley, G. S., Polkey, C. E. and Rushton, D. N. (1982) Sacral anterior nerve root stimulators for bladder control in paraplegia. *Paraplegia*, **20**, 365–381

Brindley, G. S., Polkey, C. E., Rushton, D. N. and Cardozo, L. (1986) Sacral anterior root stimulators for bladder control in paraplegia: the first 50 cases. *Journal of Neurology, Neurosurgery and Psychiatry*, **49**, 1104–1114

Comarr, A. E. (1970) Sexual function among patients with spinal cord injury. *Urology International*, **25**, 134

Eardley, I., Quinn, N. P., Fowler, C. J. *et al.* (1989) The role of urethral sphincter EMG in the differential diagnosis of parkinsonism. *British Journal of Urology*, **64**, 360–362

Ellison, M., Timberlake, G. A. and Kerstein, M. D. (1988) Impotence following pelvic fracture. *Journal of Trauma*, **28**, 695–696

Fairburn, B. and Stewart, J. M. (1955) Lumbar disc protrusion as a surgical emergency. *Lancet*, **ii**, 319–321

Fowler, C. J., Ali, Z., Kirby, R. S. and Pryor, J. P. (1988) The value of testing for unmyelinated fibre, sensory neuropathy in diabetic impotence. *British Journal of Urology*, **61**, 63–67

Gibson, G. R. (1970) Impotence following fractured pelvis and urethral rupture. *British Journal of Urology*, **42**, 86–88

Goldstein, I. (1988) Penile revascularisation. In *Current Operative Surgery. Urology*, (ed. A. R. Mundy), Baillière Tindall, London, 97–105

Hierons, R. and Saunders, M. (1966) Impotence in patients with temporal lobe lesions. *Lancet*, **ii**, 761–764

Ishii, N., Watanabe, H. and Irisawa, C. (1989) Intracavernous injection of prostaglandin $E_1$ for the treatment of erectile impotence. *Journal of Urology*, **141**, 323–325

Ivers, R. R. and Goldstein, N. P. (1963) Multiple sclerosis: a current appraisal of symptoms and signs. *Proceedings of the Mayo Clinic*, **38**, 457–466

Johnson, J. (1965) Sexual impotence and the limbic system. *British Journal of Psychiatry*, **111**, 300–303

Juenemann, K. P., and Alken, P. (1989) Pharmacotherapy of erectile dysfunction. *International Journal of Impotence Research*, **1**, 71–93

King, J. (1975) Impotence after fractures of the pelvis. *Journal of Bone and Joint Surgery*, **57-A**, 1107–1109

Kirby, R. S., Fowler, C. J., Gosling, J. D. and Bannister, R. (1986) Urethrovesical dysfunction in progressive autonomic failure with multiple system atrophy. *Journal of Neurology, Neurosurgery and Psychiatry*, **49**, 554–562

Kirkeby, H. J., Poulson, E. U., Petersen, T. and Dorup, J. (1988) Erectile dysfunction in multiple sclerosis. *Neurology*, **38**, 1366–1370

Lee, L. M., Stevenson, R. W. and Szasz, G. (1989) Prostaglandin $E_1$ versus phentolamine/papaverine for the treatment of erectile impotence: a double blind comparison. *Journal of Urology*, **141**, 549–550

Miller, H., Simpson, C. A. and Yeates, W. F. (1965) Bladder dysfunction in multiple sclerosis. *British Medical Journal*, **i**, 1265–1269

Montague, D. K. (1989) Penile prostheses. An overview. *Urologic Clinics of North America*, **16**, 7–12

Nadig, P. W., Lindner, A. and Blumoff, R. (1986) Non-invasive device to produce and maintain an erection like state. *Urology*, **27**, 126–131

Oppenheimer, D. R. (1978) The cervical cord in multiple sclerosis. *Neuropathology and Applied Neurobiology*, **4**, 151–162

Oppenheimer, D. R. (1980) Lateral horn cells in progressive autonomic failure. *Journal of the Neurological Sciences*, **46**, 393–404

Philp, T., Read, D. J. and Higson, R. H. (1980) The urodynamic characteristics of multiple sclerosis. *British Journal of Urology*, **53**, 672–675

Shafer, N. and Rosenblum, J. (1969) Occult lumbar disc causing impotency. *New York State Journal of Medicine*, **69**, 2465–2470

Shy, G. M. and Drager, G. A. (1960) A neurological syndrome associated with orthostatic hypotension. *Archives of Neurology (Chicago)*, **3**, 511–527

Sidi, A. A., Cameron, J. S., Duffy, L. M. and Lange, P. H. (1986) Intracavernous drug-induced erections in the management of male erectile dysfunction: experience with 100 patients. *Journal of Urology*, **135**, 704–706

Sidi, A. A., Cameron, J. S., Dysktra, D. D. *et al.* (1987) Vasoactive intracavernous pharmacotherapy for the treatment of erectile impotence in men with spinal cord injury. *Journal of Urology*, **138**, 539–542

Spark, R. F., Wills, C. A. and Royal, H. (1984) Hypogonadism, hyperprolactinaemia and temporal lobe epilepsy in hyposexual men. *Lancet*, **i**, 413–417

Sung, J. H., Mastri, A. R. and Segal, E. (1979) Pathology of the Shy–Drager syndrome. *Journal of Neuropathology and Experimental Neurology*, **38**, 353–368

Trafford, H. S. (1955) Traumatic rupture of the posterior urethra with a review of thirty-two civilian cases. *British Journal of Urology*, **27**, 163–171

Vas, C. J. (1969) Sexual impotence and some autonomic disturbances in men with multiple sclerosis. *Acta Neurologica Scandinavica*, **45**, 166–182

Velcek, D. (1989) Discogenic impotence. *International Journal of Impotence Research*, **1**, 95–113

Virag, R. (1982) Intracavernous injection of papaverine for erectile failure. *Lancet*, **ii**, 938

Walsh, P. C. and Donker, P. J. (1982) Impotence following radical prostatectomy. Insight into etiology and prevention. *Journal of Urology*, **128**, 492–497

Walsh, P. C., Lepor, H. and Egglestone, J. C. (1983) Radical prostatectomy with preservation of sexual function: anatomical and pathological considerations. *Prostate*, **4**, 473–485

# 27

# Potency problems in cardiac patients and arteriopaths

A. W. Zorgniotti

## Arterial disease as a cause for impotence

In the mid 1970s Jean-François Ginestie (1976), a French radiologist, and Vaclav Michal (1976), a Czechoslovak vascular surgeon, independently performed selective pudendal arteriography demonstrating obstructive arterial disease in impotent patients. A further step was taken when Michal, Kramar and Bartak, (1974) reported the first inferior epigastric artery to corpus cavernosum microsurgical bypass, reversing impotence. A shift in thinking toward vascular disease as the primary cause of impotence had begun in earnest.

A relationship between impotence and vascular disease is corroborated by an increase in impotence with ageing (Kinsey, Pomeroy and Martin, 1948). Arteriosclerosis is generally accepted as also increasing with age, although proof of such a correlation has been elusive. Ruzbarsky and Michal (1977) and Cohen *et al.* (1980) have demonstrated age-related sclerotic changes on biopsies of the corpus cavernosum. More recently, a study of selective pudendal arteriograms in impotent males (ages ranging from 26 to 73 years) showed that 89% of the cavernosal arteries, which provide blood to the erectile body, showed radiographic evidence of arterial disease (Washecka, and Zorgniotti, 1988).

## Similarities between the cavernosal and coronary arteries

The cavernous arteries resemble the coronary arteries mainly in that they are 'end' arteries without collateral circulation. The resemblance may end when we consider how function is altered by arterial narrowing and loss of elasticity. With initiation of erection, the cavernous bodies need very high arterial flow. Observations by Dorr and Brody (1967) on stimulation of the nervi erigentes in dogs and penile artery diameter with blood velocity studies after intracavernous papaverine in humans (Lue *et al.*, 1985) have provided objective data for this increase. Flow through a tubular structure is subject to Poiseuille's law, i.e. a two-fold increase in vessel diameter results in a sixteen-fold increase in flow. Although matters are not so simple, there being other factors which affect blood flow, Poiseuille's law may offer an explanation why relatively minor narrowing or loss of compliance in penile arteries can radically impair flow. Poiseuille's law also operates when diameter decreases by the same order of magnitude, hence flow may fall below the critical level required to initiate erection.

## Shared risk factors for impotence and ischaemic heart disease (IHD)

Epidemiological studies have identified the same principal risk factors for impotence and IHD, namely ageing, hypertension, diabetes, smoking and hyperlipidaemia (Virag, Bouilly and Frydman, 1985). Public health programmes aimed at preventing IHD could produce a parallel decrease in impotence although this does not appear to be part of any study protocols.

### Smoking

Stopping smoking is necessary in patients who are to undergo penile bypass revascularization or start pharmacological erection. If a man is unable to stop smoking, a penile implant may be the preferred course. It is not uncommon for a patient to discount smoking as the cause for his impotence on the ground that he has stopped. Another question also arises: will stopping restore function? Although my observation has been that no patient has a return of potency after stopping, we can look at IHD epidemiological studies for some idea of when benefit might be achieved. Excess risk of IHD death persists for years after stopping cigarette smoking and it may be as much as 15 years before this excess risk begins to approach that of non-smokers (Doll and Peto, 1976).

### Hypogonadism

The effect of androgens to influence the growth and development of the male repoductive system and secondary sexual characteristics has long been known. The effect of testosterone on erection is not as clearly defined and therein lies a common misconception with regard to the treatment of impotence.

Hypogonadism in the ageing adult is common to both sexes although more obvious in the female. In a detailed review (Swartz, 1988), attention was focused on hypogonadism as an important but little understood factor in ischaemic heart disease in men and women. Among the observations in men was the fact that administration of testosterone has been shown to relieve angina. Another was a relationship between low morning testosterone levels and a history of myocardial infarction. Also, high levels of serum testosterone may protect against myocardial infarction. But is hypogonadism a major factor in impotence?

Many older men have serum testosterone levels at or below the laboratory limits of normal (Vermeulen, Rubens and Verdonck, 1972). In clinical practice, taking blood samples at any time other than around 8.00 a.m. will result in false low values. 'Low testosterone' has become a *faute de mieux* diagnosis and the patient is administered an androgen which, more often than not, has no effect on erectile function but does improve the sense of well-being and increases libido. 'Low testosterone' can become fixed in the patient's mind and may result in his taking testosterone for several years, a treatment which carries other risks. The relationship between hypogonadism and impotence remains unresolved although there is one report of an increase in nocturnal erectile activity with such replacement therapy (Kwan *et al.*, 1983).

### Sleep disorders

Obstructive sleep apnoea is invariably accompanied by heavy snoring and is characterized by arterial hypoxia, hypercapnia and ultimately pulmonary hypertension and systemic hypertension (Guilleminault, Cummisky and Motta, 1976). Impotence is a frequent complaint in men with obstructive sleep apnoea, and needs to be identified by the clinician. Heavy snoring, extreme daytime fatigue (hypersomnolence) and obesity are important clues for this entity. A simple way to identify this is to recruit the patient's partner to stay awake and observe him during sleep. If suspected, sleep studies are in order and very effective corrective measures are available which include positive pressure breathing and pharyngeal surgery. The urologist who treats impotence has a duty to identify this disorder.

## Problems specific to cardiac failure and arteriopathy

These fall into three overlapping categories:

1. Problems intrinsic to cardiovascular disease and its treatment.
2. Problems related to diagnosis of impotence.
3. Problems encountered in the pharmacological treatment of impotence.

### Problems intrinsic to cardiovascular disease and its treatment

Impotence is as much a medical problem as it is a quality of life issue and it is in the presence of diseases of varying life-threatening severity that this calls for judicious thought. There is always the risk of worsening a precarious clinical state owing to the physical effort involved; some patients are simply too sick to think about sex. In this regard, patients who have had myocardial infarction are concerned about sudden death during coitus. This is a very rare occurrence; in a Japanese study of 5559 sudden deaths, only six were associated with the stress of intercourse (Ueno, 1963). This viewpoint may be furthered by the clinician's attitude toward the ominous connotations of heart disease. Patients still may be able to enjoy spontaneous or pharmacologically assisted intercourse depending upon the degree of disability present. It is common to see vigorous men who have recovered from myocardial infarction and heart bypass surgery who have returned to productive work and physical activities in an impotence practice. Cooperation between cardiologist and urologist can result in successful outcome for patients who would otherwise be sexual 'invalids' by selecting those patients with minimum risk and advising them to be prudent about coitus when fatigued or after a heavy meal or heavy drinking

#### Implantation risks

Most surgical penile prosthesis implanations can be performed in under 90 min by an experienced operator. These surgeries require massive intravenous antibiotics. There is, in spite of this, risk of infection of the prosthesis. In general implantation should be avoided in all men who are at risk for infection of heart valves and arterial prostheses. Risk of infection with pharmacological erection is very slight, so that when these occur they are reported in the literature.

## Drug-related impotence

### *Antihypertensives*

The *Medical Letter* (Anonymous, 1980) gave a long list of drugs implicated in impotence and the anonymous author concluded that all antihypertensive drugs can have an adverse effect on sexual function when administered. Some antihypertensive drugs cause dysfunction in a high percentage of users such as clonidine (24%) (Onesti, 1971) and methyldopa (53%) (Alexander and Evans, 1975). It is not uncommon to encounter men who give a history of loss of erection after commencing antihypertensive drug therapy and the public is well aware of this. Curiously, very few report that potency returned with discontinuation or a switch to another agent(s). Examination of these men will usually uncover a vascular explanation for the impotence. Before undertaking a prolonged evaluation a trial without the agent is worthwhile if blood pressures remain at safe levels. Many treating physicians prefer that this not be done as a result of the risks of increased blood pressure without medication, in which case it is better to allow the patient to continue the antihypertensive drug and to treat the impotence.

Oral antihypertensive drugs can be classified by their primary site or mechanism of action as follows (modified from Goodman and Gilman, 1985):

1. Diuretics:
   (a) Thiazides and related agents (hydrochlorothiazide, chlorthalidone, etc.).
   (b) Loop diuretics (furosemide, bumetanide, ethacrynic acid).
   (c) Potassium-sparing diuretics (triamterene, spironolactone, amiloride).
   (d) Carbonic anhydrase inhibitors (acetazolamide).
2. Sympatholytic drugs
   (a) Centrally acting agents (methyldopa, clonidine, guanabenz, guanfacine).
   (b) Beta-adrenergic antagonists (propranolol, metaprolol, etc.).
   (c) Alpha-adrenergic antagonists (prazosin, phenoxybenzamine).
   (d) Mixed antagonists (labetalol).
   (e) Adrenergic neurone blocking agents (guanethidine, guanadrel, reserpine).
   (f) Ganglionic blocking agents (mecamylamine).
4. Vasodilators
   (a) Arterial (hydralazine, minoxidil, calcium channel blockers)
5. Angiotensin-converting enzyme inhibitors (captopril, enalapril).
6. 5-Hydroxytryptamine antagonist (ketanserin).
7. Monoamine oxidase inhibitor (pargyline).

The antihypertensive agents least likely to be associated with impotence include the calcium channel blocking agents, vasodilators such as minoxidil, and angiotensin-converting enzyme inhibitors such as captopril and enalapril.

### *Cardiac drugs*

Digitalis (digoxin) administration which is known to produce gynaecomastia can have an effect on sexual function. The chemical structure of digitalis closely resembles that of the sex hormones and digitalis can exert oestrogenic activity (Hoffman and Bigger, 1985). It is unlikely that this drug can be discontinued for the purpose of restoring sexual function in most instances.

Two frequently prescribed anti-arrhythmic agents have been reported as causing impotence, namely dysopyramide (McHaffie, Guz and Johnston, 1977) and verapamil (King *et al.*, 1983).

## Problems related to the diagnosis of impotence

There are two important risks to cardiac patients in the diagnosis of impotence: those resulting from cavernosometry and those resulting from intracorporeal injections.

### Cavernosometry

With the rapid increase of interest in veno-occlusive dysfunction, older men are being studied for this entity. This applies to those who, after a period of successful pharmacological injection, no longer obtain sufficient erection for penetration. In the author's practice, such patients are being investigated and operated for veno-occlusive dysfunction with recovery of erection. The diagnosis requires cavernosometry and cavernosography following intracorporeal injection of papaverine hydrochloride. Cavernosometry calls for rapid infusion of heparinized saline into the corpus cavernosum in order to produce erection and to measure intracavernous pressures. In the presence of a veno-occlusive disorder, the fluid passes directly into the circulation and the volume injected can reach 700–1000 ml over a few minutes. This sudden hypervolaemia can have disastrous consequences so that this step should not be performed. The investigator would be better advised to proceed directly to cavernosography which requires an infusion of 100 ml of low osmolar contrast and carries a lesser risk.

### Intracorporeal injection of pharmacological agents

These are discussed below.

## Problems encountered in the pharmacological treatment of impotence

A major advance in the treatment of impotence occurred when Virag (1982) reported on the effect of intracavernosal papaverine hydrochloride in producing erection. The concept of self-injection was furthered when Brindley (1983) demonstrated erections using intracavernosal injection of phenoxybenzamine. Soon after, Zorgniotti and Lefleur (1985) proposed the use of a mixture of papaverine hydrochloride and phentolamine mesylate which produced improved erectile rigidity. Worldwide, this combination is the most commonly used agent, although recently prostaglandin $E_1$ has been introduced (Ishii *et al.*, 1986). It is becoming apparent that combinations of all three agents produce even better results where the indivual components have failed to produce an erection. Patients with severe arterial disease or veno-occlusive disorder do not respond well to pharmacological erection.

The pharmacological agents used both in diagnosis and treatment have the potential of producing systemic side effects. The appearance of side effects is not necessarily indicative of the presence of veno-occlusive dysfunction when injected into the corpus cavernosum. These can be: vasovagal episode, syncope, hypotension and non-specific transitory ECG changes (the latter in a patient who may have had an idiosyncrasy to papaverine). It is obvious that unstable cardiacs, or those who might be at risk from ischaemia produced by hypotension, will require detailed evaluation beforehand. For reasons that are not clear, side effects usually occur with the first injection and are much less likely to occur with subsequent administration making it possible to offer self-injection, provided the practitioner consults with the patient's cardiologist and is organized to treat an emergency should it occur. In high-risk patients, prostaglandin $E_1$ may be safer than papaverine and phentolamine and it would be best to start with a small amount (5.0 μg), being sure to occlude the base of the penis with a rubber band for 2–3 min to allow the agent to become fixed in the corporeal tissues.

The treatment of the complication of prolonged penile erection which can occur with the initial injection also poses a special risk to cardiac patients. This risk consists of intracavernous injection of a vasoconstrictor and aspiration of the corpora. The agent of choice for all patients is phenylephrine (0.1 mg $ml^{-1}$ of saline) which produces the least cardiogenic effect while giving adequate vasoconstriction, although it can produce bradycardia which can be reversed with atropine. Dopamine hydrochloride, properly diluted, is the second agent of choice as it has a short half-life in plasma and has also proved effective in de-erecting when phenylephrine has failed. Adrenaline is much less suitable and, along with metaraminol which also has a strong cardiogenic effect, should be avoided. The practitioner has to be thoroughly familiar with the management of these agents and have emergency supplies at hand

In cardiac patients these agents should only be administered with careful monitoring of blood pressure and pulse and electrocardiogram.

## Conclusions

Cardiac disease is not necessarily a contraindication to the treatment of associated sexual dysfunction. Diagnosis and treatment require extra care in order to avoid a potentially disastrous outcome. It is important that the urologist and cardiologist cooperate not only to achieve success but to share the onus of refusing treatment when this appears necessary. Informed consent plays an important role in the diagnosis and treatment of impotence and should be insisted upon. In this regard, the rules have changed and all informed consents must now include information on Benefits, Risks and Alternative Treatment (BRAT).

### Addendum

It has come to the attention of the author that revascularization had been performed earlier than 1974. In 1970, Gruber anastomosed the inferior epigastric artery to the tunica albuginea in a procedure which was intended to prevent impotence in a patient who was operated upon for priapism. Other than this one instance, there is no doubt that Michal pursued revascularization on a large number of impotent patients (Gruber, (1972).

### References

Alexander, W. D. and Evans, J. I. (1975) Side effects of methyldopa. *British Medical Journal*, **ii**, 501

Anonymous (1980) Drugs that cause sexual dysfunction. *Medical Letter*, **22**, 25–26

Brindley, G. (1983) Cavernosal alpha-blockade: a new technique for investigating and treating erectile impotence. *British Journal of Psychiatry*, **143**, 332–337

Cohen, M. S., Sharpe, W., Warner, R. *et al.* (1980) Morphology of the corpus cavernosum arterial bed in impotence. In *Vasculogenic Impotence*, (eds A.W.Zorgniotti and G. Rossi), Charles C. Thomas, Springfield, Illinois, pp. 103–111

Doll, R. and Peto, R. (1976) Mortality in relation to smoking: 20 years observation on male British doctors. *British Medical Journal*, **ii**, 1525–1536

Dorr, L. D. and Brody, M. J. (1967) Hemodynamic mechanism of erection in the canine penis. *American Journal of Physiology*, **213**, 1526–1531

Ginestie, J.-F. and Romieu, A. (1976) *L'Exploration Radiologique de l'Impuissance*, Maloine, Paris

Goodman and Gilman (eds) (1985) *The Pharmacologic Basis of Therapeutics*, 7th edn, Macmillan, New York, p. 785

Gruber, H. (1972) The treatment of priapism: use of the inferior epigastric artery. A case report. *Journal of*

*Urology,* **108**, 882–886

Guilleminault, C., Cummiskey, J. and Motta, J. (1976) Chronic obstructive airflow disease and sleep studies. *American Review of Respiratory Diseases*, **122**, 397–406

Hoffman, B. F. and Bigger, T. J. Jr. (1985) Digitalis and allied cardiac glycosides. In Goodman and Gilman's *The Pharmacologic Basis of Therapeutics*, 7th edn, Macmillan, New York, p. 741

Ishii, N., Watanabe, H., Irisawa, C. *et al.* (1986) Studies on male sexual impotence. Report 18. Therapeutic trial with prostaglandin $E_1$ for organic impotence. *Japanese Journal of Urology*, **77**, 954–959

King, B. D., Pitchon, R. and Stein, E. H. (1983) Impotence during therapy with verapamil. *Archives of Internal Medicine,* **145**, 1248–1249

Kinsey, A., Pomeroy, W. and Martin, C. (1948) *Sexual Behaviour in the Human Male*, W.B. Saunders, Philadelphia, pp. 235–238

Kwan, M., Greenleaf, W., Mann, I. *et al.* (1983) The nature of androgen action on male sexuality: a combined laboratory-self report study in hypogonadal men. *Journal of Clinical Endocrinology and Metabolism*, **57**, 557–562

Lue, T. F., Hricak, H., Marich, K. W. and Tanagho, E. A. (1985) Vasculogenic impotence evaluated by high resolution ultrasonography and pulsed Doppler spectrum analysis. *Radiology*, **155**, 777–781

McHaffie, D. J., Guz, A. and Johnston, A. (1977) Impotence in patients on disopyramide. *Lancet*, **i**, 859

Michal, V., Pospichal, J. and Lachman, M. (1976) Penile arteries occlusions in erectile impotence. A new type of angiography – phalloarteriography. *Casopis Lekaru Ceskych*, **115**, 1245–1247

Michal, V., Kramar, R. and Bartak, V. (1974) Femoropudendal bypass in the treatment of sexual impotence. *Journal of Cardiovascular Surgery*, **15**, 356–359

Onesti, G. (1971) Clonidine: new antihypertensive agent. *American Journal of Cardiology*, **28**, 74–81

Ruzbarsky, V. and Michal, V. (1977) Morphologic changes in the arterial bed of the penis with aging: relationship to the pathogenesis of impotence. *Investigative Urology*, **15**, 149–199

Swartz, C. M. (1988) Low serum testosterone: a cardiovascular risk in elderly men. *Geriatric Medicine Today*, **7**, 39–49

Ueno, M. (1963) The so-called coital death. *Japanese Journal of Legal Medicine*, **17**, 330–334

Vermeulen, A., Rubens, R. and Verdonck, L. (1972) Testosterone secretion and metabolism in male senescence. *Journal of Clinical Endocrinology and Metabolism*, **34**, 730–735

Virag, R. (1982) Intracavernous injection of papaverine for erectile failure. *Lancet*, **ii**, 938

Virag, R., Bouilly, P. and Frydman, D. (1985) Is impotence an arterial disorder? A study of arterial risk factors in 440 impotent men. *Lancet*, **i**, 181–184

Washecka, R. and Zorgniotti, A. W. (1988) Non-correlation of penile brachial index to angiograms. *Proceedings of the 6th Biennial International Symposium for Corpus Cavernosum Revascularization and Third Biennial World Meeting of Impotence*, Boston University School of Medicine, p. 31

Zorgniotti, A. W. and Lefleur, R. (1985) Auto-injection of the corpus cavernosum with a vasoactive drug combination for vasculogenic impotence. *Journal of Urology*, **133**, 39–41

# 28

# Penile reconstruction for trauma, intersex and gender reassignment

W. J. Barwick

## Introduction

As the preceding chapters have demonstrated, penile erectile function is a complex blend of emotional, hormonal and neurovascular factors. All of these mechanisms may operate perfectly, yet the individual must still have an organ upon which they can act. The penis may be absent for several reasons including congenital absence, trauma, neoplasia, iatrogenic injuries, and in transsexuals.

Congenital absence of the penis in a genetic male is extremely rare. Although many would argue that agenesis of the phallus should more properly be treated by orchiectomy and rearing as a female, Gillies and Harrison (1948) reported on two individuals with congenital absence of the penis who had been reared as males. He reconstructed the penis using a multi-stage operation that will be discussed subsequently.

Trauma to the external genitalia can occur as a result of industrial accidents, gunshot or stab wounds, self-inflicted injury, or other iatrogenic trauma. High-speed rotational machinery catches the clothing of the individual, quickly tearing it loose along with the external genitalia. Many times skin alone is avulsed from the penis and scrotum, but occasionally the entire genitalia are avulsed. The penis may also be injured on purpose, either as a result of domestic violence or self-mutilation.

Infection can occasionally result in penile loss. Fournier's gangrene is a synergistic infection usually related to the genitourinary tract that may cause loss of all or part of the penis and scrotum. The exact aetiology of Fournier's gangrene remains obscure (Bejanga, 1979).

Carcinoma of the penis occurs in approximately 0.3% of reported cancers in the United States (Boxer, 1975). The treatment usually involves penectomy, many times with associated radiation therapy or regional lymph node dissection. These are usually poor candidates for reconstruction, due either to ongoing disease or poor general health.

Gender reassignment surgery is being done more frequently now. It is recognized that male-to-female transsexual operations are technically easier and the results better than female-to-male. However, the techniques described in this chapter have been used with some success in creating male genitalia in transsexuals. These patients are usually more interested in the ability to have intercourse than the ability to urinate while standing, so reconstruction of the urethra is usually not done.

## History

Unlikely many reconstructive procedures, total phalloplasty is a product of the 20th century. Rogers (1973) states that Ambrose Pare created an external conduit to allow males with missing penises to void while standing. Further attempts to reconstruct the penis awaited the development of the tubed pedicle flap by Filatov and Gillies just after World War I.

Borgoras (1936) first used a tubed pedicle flap for reconstruction of the penis. Modifications of this technique included the use of an autogenous cartilage graft for stiffness (Frumkin, 1944) and formation of a neourethra by using a tubed split thickness skin graft within the tubed flap (McIndoe, 1948). Maltz (1946) described the use of a small tubed pedicle flap for neourethra inside a larger tubed pedicle flap for the body of the penis. This technique was later modified by Gillies and Harrison (1948) and became the standard multi-stage procedure. Failures were common in these early reconstructions due to stricture, fistula formation or hair within the urethra.

A similar technique of creating a 'tube within a tube' was devised by Goodwin and Scott (1952). In their procedure, both the inner tube (with the cutaneous side inward) and the outer tube (with the cutaneous side outward) were created from scrotal tissue. A modification of this technique that gave more stiffness utilized an upper medial thigh flap to cover and eventually surround the neourethra, created from the scrotum (Kaplan and Wesser, 1971). This was the first reconstructive procedure to give some sensation to the neophallus, since the terminal branch of the ilioinguinal nerve supplies this area.

The advent of microsurgery has brought a new dimension to penile reconstructive surgery. In many cases, a penis can now be constructed in one stage with urethral continuity, a baculum and the potential for sensation. This compares well with, for example, the case described by Orticochea (1972) which had a fine end result, but took five stages and some 2 years to complete.

In the half century since Borgoras performed the first penile reconstruction, there have been many techniques of phalloplasty published. This attests to the inability of any single procedure to consistently achieve the desired result.

## Objectives in penile reconstruction

The goals in reconstruction of the penis are quite simple. The reconstructed organ should look like a penis, feel like a penis and function like a penis. Unfortunately the achievement of these goals is time-consuming and frequently falls far short of the desired result. It is obviously vital to discuss thoroughly with the patient which goals are more important as well as the likelihood of achieving these goals.

That the neophallus should be aesthetically acceptable to the patient is obvious, although no reconstructed penis will ever withstand close inspection. A useful goal, however, as Dubin, Sato and Laub (1979) have stated, is a penis that will appear normal to a casual observer from a distance, for example a man standing at the next urinal in a public restroom.

The reconstructed penis should also feel like a penis – that is, to the patient himself. Most of the multi-staged reconstructions provide a penile shaft that is totally devoid of sensation, except in the unusual case where some penile tissue remains and can be incorporated into the reconstructed penis. This is a distinct advantage of the more recent one-stage reconstructions using free tissue transfers that have the potential for sensation.

The reconstructed penis should also function as a penis. In general the function of the penis is two-fold. It provides a conduit for urine so that a man may urinate in a standing position. It also functions as an erectile organ for penetration during sexual intercourse. The ideal result obviously should have enough stiffness for penetration and also a skin-lined tube for urination. The achievement of both of these goals is difficult. In procedures that are done primarily for the restoration of urination, fistulae are a frequent complication. Thus, where the primary goal is sexual penetration, as in gender reassignment surgery, no attempt is made to create a neourethra (Boxer and Miller, 1976; Puckett and Montie, 1978; Dubin, Sato and Laub, 1979).

One of the chief limiting factors in phallic reconstruction is that the erectile tissue of the penis is unique – there is no substitute which can be borrowed from anywhere else in the body. A flaccid skin tube, which may look like a penis but which has neither erectile nor urinary function, is a useless appendage that would have been better left unreconstructed.

The following sections will describe some of the techniques that are useful in reconstructing the penis. Multi-stage procedures that have stood the test of time will be included as will newer, one- or two-stage procedures that show promise. No attempt has been made to include all the reported techniques. However, the ones presented here should be within the capabilities of most urologists and plastic surgeons.

## Multi-stage procedures

### Gillies procedure

The Gillies operation (Gillies and Harrison, 1948) is a variation of the procedure first devised by Maltz (1946) that makes use of two tubed abdominal flaps. One flap is tubed so that the skin side is to the inside and the other is tubed so that the skin side is to the outside. The inside tubed flap resides on the inside of the outside tubed flap and this creates a 'tube within a tube' that functions as the urethra and shaft of the penis, respectively. It is a multi-stage procedure and a brief description will be given of each stage.

#### Stage 1

The first stage creates the skin flaps that become the two abdominal tubes. Three parallel incisions are made in an oblique direction on the lower lateral abdominal wall. The most lateral incision measures approximately 9–10 cm in length. The two medial incisions both measure approximately 14 cm in length. The distance between the lateral two incisions is 2.5 cm and between the medial two incisions is approximately 6 cm (Figure 28.1a).

The lateral two incisions are made first. The intervening strip of skin is formed into a tube with the cutaneous side inward and the tube open at both ends. This creates a raw surface area which is then covered by a bipedicle flap that is created by incising the remaining medial incision, elevating the intervening abdominal skin and advancing it laterally to cover the neourethra. The medial defect is

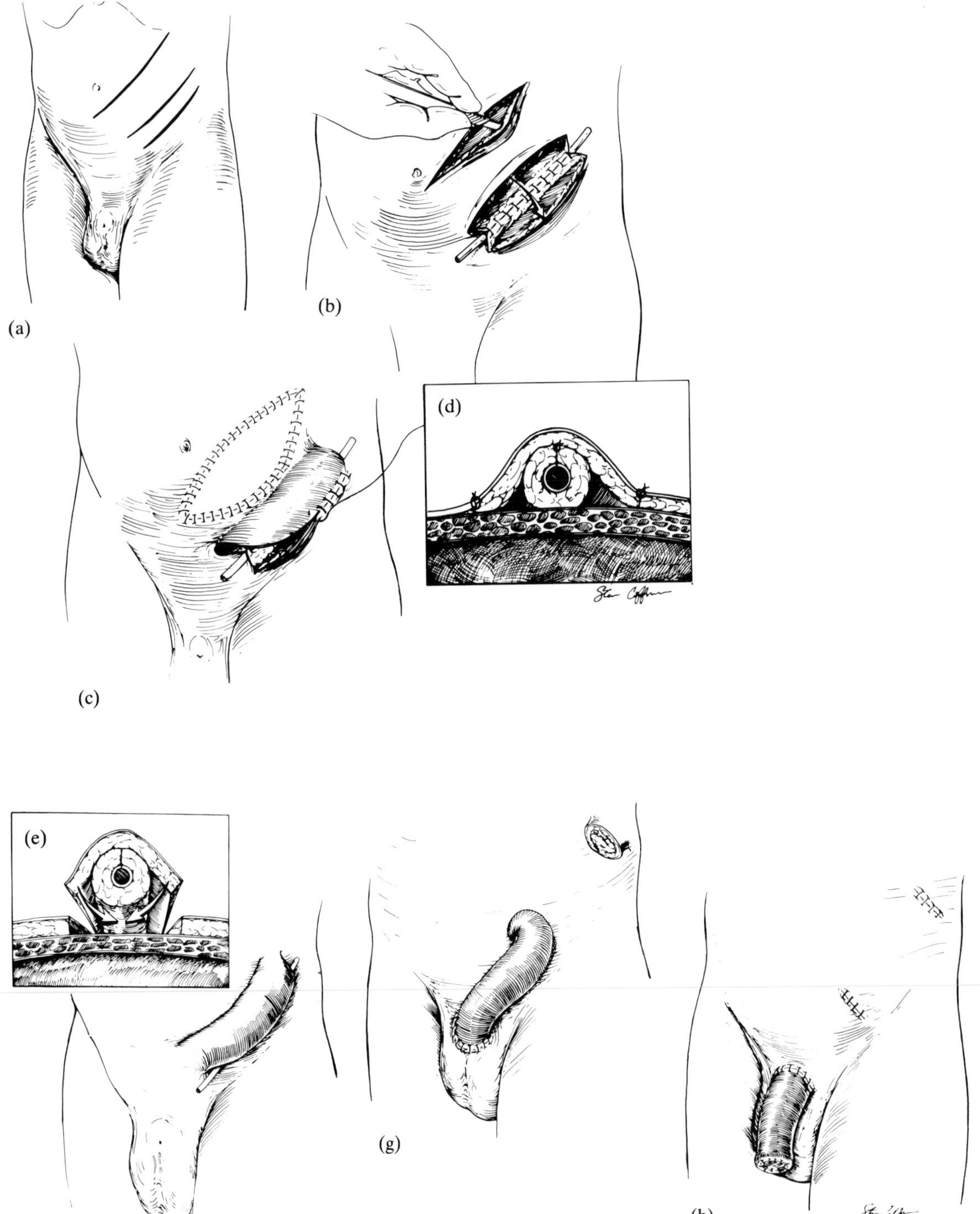


**Figure 28.1** The multi-stage Gillies procedure: (a)–(d) stage 1; (e) and (f) stage 2 – the inner tube and outer tube are now created; (g) stage 3 – division of the superior end of the flap with implantation into the perineal area; (h) fourth stage division of the lower end of the tube and completion of the neophallus

covered with a split thickness skin graft. This is allowed to heal for 4 weeks before proceeding to the second stage.

### Stage 2

The medial bipedicle flap is again elevated and this time is fashioned into a tube surrounding the lateral tube. The attachment of the bipedicle flap over the inverted lateral tube is not disturbed. After forming the large tube the reconstruction now consists of a double tube with the inside tube with its cutaneous side inward and the outside tube with its cutaneous side outward. If necessary, the defect has an additional skin graft placed on it (Figure 28.1b). It is important to allow the tubed reconstruction to heal for at least 6–8 weeks before the next stage.

### Stage 3

During this stage the flap is transferred to the groin area. The easiest way to do this is to divide the superior portion of the tube, flip that end down, and attach that to the stump of the penis. The internal tube is anastomosed to the remnant of the urethra using everting stitches. The remainder of the external tube is then sutured around the corpora cavernosa if any portion of this structure remains. If this is a female-to-male transsexual, the penile location is determined and the superior end of the tube is attached into this area. If a baculum was inserted in the second stage, this is anchored either on the pubis or in the remnants of the corpora cavernosa. This is allowed to heal for at least 2–3 months in its new position.

### Stage 4

The time between the third and fourth stages is generally the longest time, because once the remaining abdominal attachment of the tube is divided, the entire blood supply to the reconstructed penis will be coming through vascular connections that have developed from the insertion of the superior end of the tube into the pubic area or penile remnant.

A useful procedure at this stage is to place a constricting band around the abdominal end of the tube and leave this is place for 30–60 min three times a day. This will help train the blood supply to develop from the perineal end. Another technique is to use a monitor such as the laser Doppler or the transcutaneous $pO_2$ monitor. While constricting the abdominal end of the flap, readings can be obtained with laser Doppler or transcutaneous $pO_2$ that will let the reconstructive surgeon know whether adequate blood flow is coming through the newly attached end. When these studies show that adequate blood supply is present, the abdominal end may be divided. The neophallus now hangs in its new position (Figure 28.1d). The divided end is shaped into a glans.

Before allowing urination it is advisable to look at the urethrocutaneous anastomosis with a cystoscope. Assuming normal healing, the urinary diversion may be removed and the patient may begin to urinate through the neophallus. If there is any question, urinary diversion should be maintained for an additional 2–3 weeks.

In the original Gillies operation, the urethral tube was medial to the penile shaft tube. However, placing this tube in the lateral position is better because the lateral skin is more likely to he hairless. Another variation uses a piece of autogenous rib cartilage as a baculum. Others have advised against inserting the cartilage at this stage (Noe, Birdsell and Laub, 1974; Boxer and Miller, 1976).

The Gillies procedures is a time-honoured procedure. However, there are drawbacks. If hair is present on the abdominal wall this may result in infection or stone formation in the urethra. Strictures and fistulae are also common. If no baculum has been used the neophallus will eventually become flaccid as the scar tissue softens. If cartilage is used for a baculum, the penis stays in the erect position all the time.

## Goodwin–Scott procedure

This procedure (Goodwin and Scott, 1952) makes use of scrotal tissues to form both the urethra and penile shaft. It is a two-stage procedure and has the advantage of simplicity and the use of readily available local tissue.

### Stage 1

The neourethra is constructed of midline scrotal skin by making a tennis racket-shaped incision around the penile stump. This is usually done over a catheter that passes through the urethral stump into the bladder. The tube is closed with the cutaneous side inward and the remaining scrotal skin is then advanced to cover the raw surface thus created (Figure 28.2a). At least 2 months, and preferably 3 months, should elapse before the second stage.

### Stage 2

In the second stage the new urethra is separated from the scrotum and surrounded by scrotal skin flaps to construct the body of the penis (Figure 28.2b). Two incisions are outlined, each approximately 2.5 cm lateral to the previously closed scrotal skin and joined inferiorly. By these two incisions, scrotal skin flaps are elevated that are based proximally and medially. As the urethra is separated from the scrotum, these flaps then drape around and join each other on the new ventral surface of the neophallus. These incisions are made in a zigzag fashion (Figure 28.2b) so the closure on the ventral surface of the new penis will not have a straight line that might result in contracture.

One limitation of the Goodwin–Scott procedure is that it produces a structure which has very little diameter or bulk. Moreover, even if a strip of skin can be found in the midline of the scrotum that does not contain hair, most certainly the body of the new penis will be covered with hair. It will also continue to resemble scrotal skin. It is extremely difficult for any kind of a baculum to be inserted in this type of reconstructed penis. This procedure, however, has the advantage of the elimination of a urethrocutaneous anastomosis and the advantage of using tissues that are usually readily available locally.

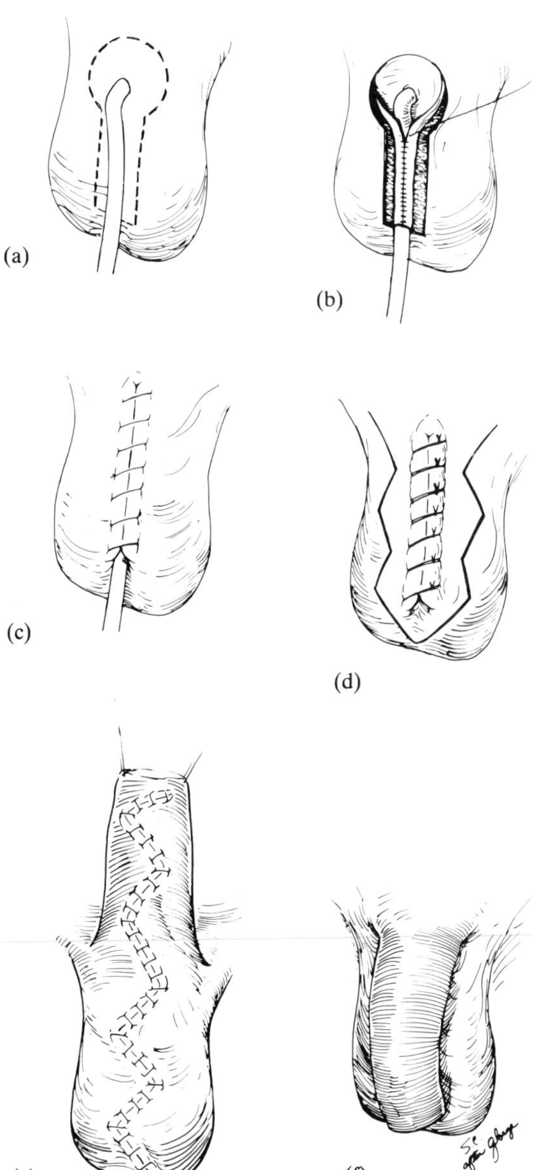


**Figure 28.2** Goodwin–Scott procedure: (a)–(c) stage 1 – the neourethra is created and the scrotal tissue reapproximated over this; (d)–(f) separation of the neourethra and construction of scrotal skin flaps to surround this creating the neophallus

An improvement on the Goodwin–Scott procedure is the Kaplan–Wesser procedure (1971) in which a skin flap from the superomedial thigh is used to cover a neourethra that is constructed in the same fashion as in the Goodwin–Scott procedure. The flap from the superomedial thigh is based on direct cutaneous arteries from the femoral artery. In most cases this is the deep external pudendal artery. Thus, the flap can be elevated as an arterialized flap having greater length than width. In the first stage of the Kaplan–Wesser procedure, the thigh flap is elevated and transposed to cover the neourethra. Several weeks later the flap with the neourethra inside it is elevated again and the flap tubed. This creates a bulkier penis than in the Goodwin–Scott procedure, and it has the additional advantage of sensation as long as the terminal branches of the ilioinguinal nerve are left intact. The ilioinguinal nerve accompanies the spermatic cord and sends terminal branches into this area of the superomedial thigh. One problem with this procedure, however, is that the neophallus is covered with hair which may be fairly dense in some individuals.

## One-stage procedures

One of the main drawbacks of the traditional multi-stage procedures was the length of time necessary to complete the reconstruction. Most cases take many months to complete. The trend in recent years has been toward one-stage reconstruction of the penis. In particular, the use of musculocutaneous flaps and free flap transfers have greatly facilitated the ability of reconstructive surgeons to create a penis that is sensate, functional and aesthetically pleasing. Several promising procedures will be described in the following sections.

### Reconstruction of the penis and urethra using a single cutaneous flap

Chang and Hwang (1984) reported on seven patients in whom the radial forearm flap was used as a one-stage reconstruction of both penis and urethra. The forearm flap is supplied by septocutaneous perforators from the radial artery as it passes through the forearm. In the distal portion of the forearm where the radial artery is close to the skin, there are numerous small branches that pass from the radial artery to the skin. If these are preserved, the entire forearm skin can be raised as a flap based on the radial artery which can extend as a pedicle all the way to the division of the brachial artery. The venous drainage of the flap is the venae commitantes of the radial artery or the superficial venous system of the forearm. The radial nerve accompanies the radial artery and should not be sacrificed due to its important sensory distribution in the hand. However, the lateral antebrachial cutaneous nerve supplies this area and can be included in the flap as a sensory nerve. The flap is drawn as shown in Figure 28.3a and is located over the radial surface of the distal forearm. It measures 12 cm in length and 14 or 15 cm in width. On the hairless side of the flap a strip of skin 3 cm in width and running the entire length of the flap is outlined. This will become the neourethra. On the opposite side of the flap a strip of skin 10 cm wide will become the body of the penis. Between these two cutaneous areas, a 1 cm strip is de-epithelialized to allow closure of the large flap around the small neourethra flap. Koshima, Tai and Yamasaki (1986) have recommended adding another small area of de-epithelialized skin on the other side of the neourethra to facilitate closure without fistula.

It is possible to include a portion of radius as a vascularized baculum. If this is done, the minute arterial branches from the radial artery into the radius must be carefully preserved. The periosteum should not be elevated from the radius. The portion of radius that is to be used as the baculum can be removed using sharp osteotomes or a vibrating saw.

After the flap is elevated, the parts that will be buried are de-epithelialized (Figure 28.3a). Now there are two cutaneous paddles separated by a de-epithelialized segment. The narrow skin paddle is tubed over a Foley catheter with the cutaneous side inward (Figure 28.3b). Next, the entire neourethral segment is surrounded by the remaining skin paddle. It is sutured back to itself over the de-epithelialized segment (Figure 28.3c).

This entire unit is then transferred to the perineal area where the artery and vein are anastomosed to a suitable recipient vessel. This may be either the femoral artery and vein, or the deep inferior epigastric artery and vein. With this flap there is generally enough pedicle length to hook into either one of these sets of vessels. If the flap is to be innervated, which is desirable, the recipient nerve is located. In traumatic penile loss, the stump of the dorsal nerve of the penis may be used. In a female-to-male transsexual, the internal pudendal nerve is used.

The neourethra is joined to the remnant of the penile urethra. This portion of the procedure is quite important. The stitches must evert the edges of the anastomosis. Horizontal mattress sutures are useful in this manoeuvre.

In the published reports of this technique, complications have been frequent. Gilbert *et al.* (1987) reported urethrocutaneous fistulae in both patients in whom they tried this technique. Matti, Matthews and Davies (1988) felt their results were disappointing. They used the radial forearm flap in five cases of female-to-male transsexuals. Three of the patients had complete failure due to vascular thrombosis and the remaining two developed a urethrocutaneous fistula. The Chinese experience is better, however. Chang and Hwang (1984) only had one fistula in their seven cases. Kao *et al.* (1984) reported three cases with no complications. The superior results in the Chinese and Japanese cases may reflect the fact that the forearm skin contains less hair than Western forearms.

To overcome the problem of hairiness of the radial forearm, different areas of the body have been used with the same technique for penile reconstruction. A forearm flap based on the ulnar artery (Glasson, Lovie and Duncan, 1986) has been used for phalloplasty, the advantage being that the ulnar skin of the forearm contained less hair than the radial side.

The lateral arm flap is a septocutaneous flap that is based on the posterior radial recurrent artery, which is the terminal branch of the deep brachial artery. This flap is located in the lateral upper arm with its longitudinal axis directly over the lateral intermuscular septum. Upton *et al.* (1987) reported the use of this flap for penile reconstruction. Sensation was provided by the lateral brachial cutaneous nerve which is a branch of the radial nerve. The problem of hairy skin may be obviated in other ways. Shenaq and Dinh (1989) used a tissue expander in the lateral arm area to increase the amount of hairless skin available. This increases the length of time necessary for reconstruction and requires two or more stages.

## One-stage reconstruction using musculocutaneous flaps and free flap in combination

A musculocutaneous flap is a composite flap of muscle and skin in which the skin gets its blood supply through perforators passing from the muscle into the skin. If the muscle has a single or dominant vascular pedicle, the musculocutaneous flap may be used either as an island pedicle flap or as a free flap. A technique which has produced good results involves the use of an island rectus abdominis musculocutaneous flap for the neourethra combined with a free vascularized innervated cutaneous flap for penile skin coverage.

Gilbert *et al.* (1987) presented two patients in a series of 12 phallic reconstructions in which the rectus abdominis musculocutaneous flap was used for neourethra and external coverage by a free

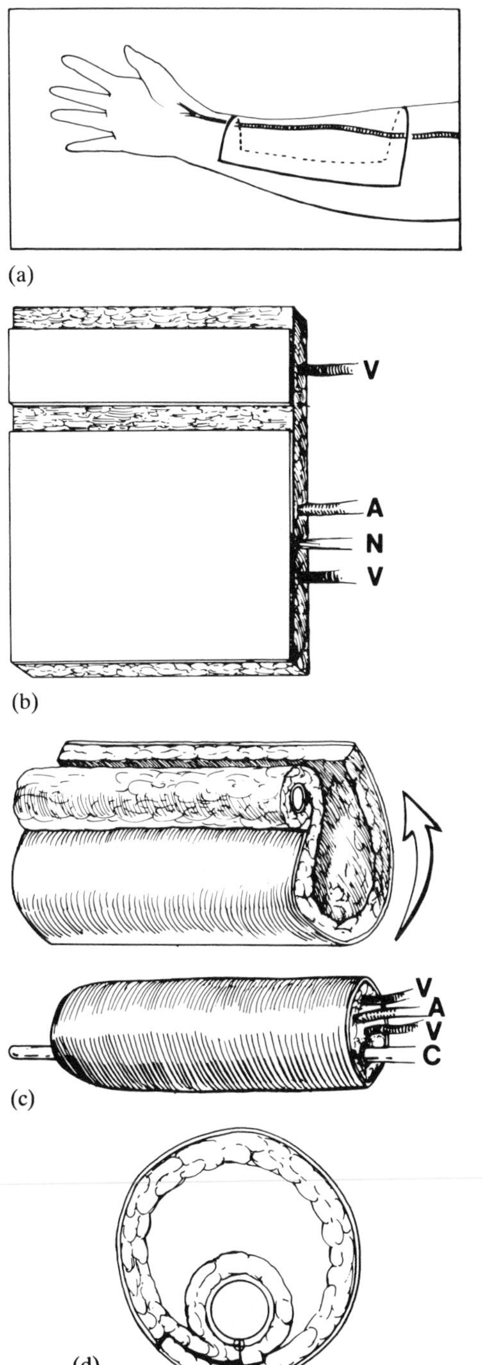


**Figure 28.3** One-stage reconstruction using the radial forearm flap: (a) location of the flap on the radial side of the forearm; (b) construction of the flap showing the areas of de-epithelialization; (c) the small strip of skin is tubed inward and the large strip of skin is tubed outward to surround this; (d) and (e) the neophallus is created with a catheter (C) running through the inner tube

innervated cutaneous flap. They reported no incidence of permanent fistula formation. The technique is illustrated in Figure 28.4. The cutaneous paddle is outlined over the rectus abdominis muscle. This cutaneous paddle is tubed on itself to form a skin-lined tube. It is then carried along with the rectus abdominis muscle, which is based on the deep inferior epigastric artery, into the perineum where this skin-lined tube is joined to the remnant of the penile urethra. The rectus abdominis muscle is tubed around the neourethra. A free dorsalis pedis flap is harvested. This flap is based on the anterior tibial artery and vein with sensation provided by the superficial peroneal nerve. This flap is then draped around the rectus muscle and the anterior tibial artery and vein are joined to the contralateral deep inferior epigastric artery and vein. The superficial peroneal nerve is joined to the internal pudendal nerve. This procedure has much to recommend it. A vascularized skin tube is used for the neourethra, and this is separated from the external skin covering by a vascularized muscle. Even though the muscle will eventually atrophy resulting in some loss of bulk of the neophallus, a penile prothesis can be inserted at a later date. Obviously a quantity of hairless skin must be available in the midline of the abdomen. The choice of dorsalis pedis flap for external covering provides a flap that is thin and supple with an excellent nerve supply in the superficial peroneal. Unfortunately, there are occasional problems with donor site morbidity with the dorsalis pedis flap. Other potential donor sites for use in this technique include the radial forearm flap or the lateral arm flap, which have been discussed previously.

The vascularized groin flap has also been used as a free flap in penis reconstruction. Puckett, Reinisch and Montie (1982) reported on the use of a free groin flap in three transsexuals. Urethra reconstruction was not done and there was one failure. In these patients an inflatable prosthesis was inserted at a later date. The iliac crest can be included with the lateral portion of the groin flap (Sun and Huang, 1985). This produces a neophallus that is permanently rigid.

In spite of the continued difficulties and frequency of complications, the trend continues to be toward the use of free vascularized, innervated tissue transfers in penile reconstruction. Regardless of whether a urethroplasty is done, or a baculum inserted, the improved blood supply to the neophallus using these techniques should make them preferable to the older multi-stage techniques in which the reconstructed penis has a random blood supply.

A functioning urethra without fistula or stricture formation remains an elusive goal. A technique that appears promising and may be combined with many other techniques is the use of a long bladder flap for urethral reconstruction. Edgerton *et al.* (1984)

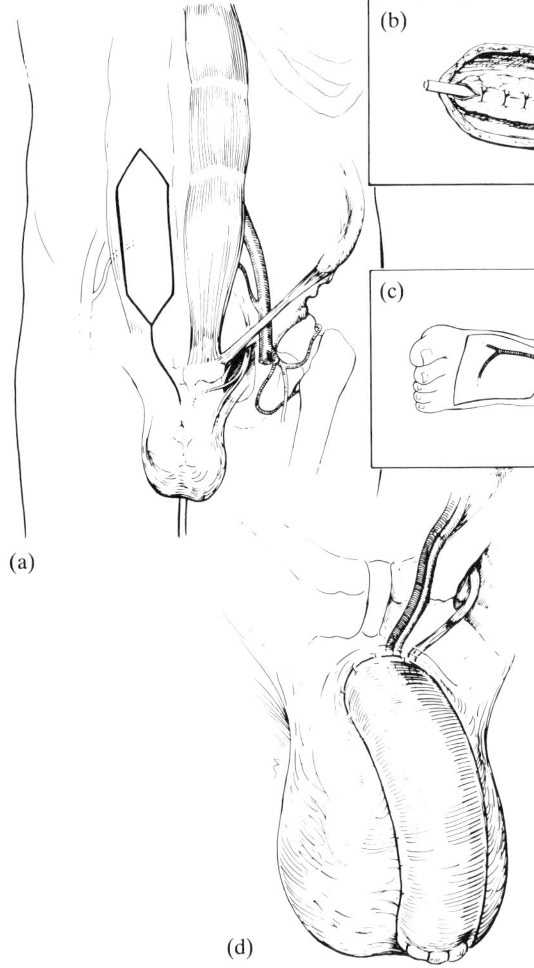


**Figure 28.4** One-stage reconstruction using pedicled rectus abdominis musculocutaneous flap for inner tube (a) and (b) with a free innervated dorsalis pedis flap for the outer tube (c) and (d)

described this technique in which a 4 × 28 cm strip of bladder is obtained with its base anteriorly. The strip is tubed and passed through the neophallus. The advantages of this technique are that it provides a well-vascularized flap of tissue lined with transitional epithelium which eliminates the need for a circular anastomosis within the penile urethra.

## Conclusions

Penile reconstruction is a challenging and difficult job. The limitations of the techniques currently available must be accepted by both the patient and the surgeon at the outset. Although techniques are available which provide both orthostatic micturition and sexual penetration, the surgeon and patient frequently need to decide which of these is more important and concentrate on that at the expense of the other.

## References

Bejanga, B. I. (1979) Fournier's gangrene. *British Journal of Urology*, **51**, 312–316

Borgoras, N. (1936) Über die volle Plastische Wieden herstellung eines zum Koitess Fahigen Penis (Peniplastica totalis). *Zentralblatt Chirurgie*, **63**, 1271

Boxer, R. J. (1975) Reconstruction of the male genitalia. *Surgery, Gynecology and Obstetrics*, **141**, 939–944

Boxer, R. J. and Miller, T. A. (1976) Penile reconstruction in the irradiated patient. *Urology*, **7**, 403–408

Chang, T. S. and Hwang, W. Y. (1984) Forearm flap in one-stage reconstruction of the penis. *Plastic and Reconstructive Surgery*, **74**, 251–258

Dubin, B. J., Sato, R. M. and Laub, D. R. (1979) Results of phalloplasty. *Plastic and Reconstructive Surgery*, **64**, 163–170

Edgerton, M. T., Gillenwater, J. Y., Kenney, J. G. and Horowitz, J. (1984) The bladder flap for urethral reconstruction in total phalloplasty. *Plastic and Reconstructive Surgery*, **74**, 259–266

Frumkin, A. P. (1944) Reconstruction of the male genitalia. *American Review of Soviet Medicine*, **2**, 14

Gilbert, D. A., Horton, C. E., Terzis, J. K. *et al.* (1987) New concepts in phallic reconstruction. *Annals of Plastic Surgery*, **18**, 128–136

Gillies, H. D. and Harrison, R. J. (1948) Congenital absence of the penis. *British Journal of Plastic Surgery*, **1**, 8–20

Glasson, D. W., Lovie, M. J. and Duncan, G. M. (1986) The ulnar forearm free flap in penile reconstruction. *Australian and New Zealand Journal of Surgery*, **56**, 477–479

Goodwin, W. E. and Scott, W. W. (1952) Phalloplasty. *Journal of Urology*, **68**, 903

Kao, X. S., Kao, J. H., Ho, C. L. *et al.* (1984) One stage reconstruction of the penis with free skin flap: report of three cases. *Journal of Reconstructive Microsurgery*, **1**, 149–153

Kaplan, I. and Wesser, D. A. (1971) A rapid method for reconstructing a functional sensitive penis. *British Journal of Plastic Surgery*, **24**, 342

Koshima, I., Tai, T. and Yamasaki, M. (1986) One stage reconstruction of the penis using an innervated radial forearm osteocutaneous flap. *Journal of Reconstructive Microsurgery*, **3**, 19–24

Maltz, (1946) *Evolution of Plastic Surgery*, Frobin Press New York, p. 278

Matti, B. A., Matthews, R. N. and Davies, D. M. (1988) Phalloplasty using the free radial forearm flap. *British Journal of Plastic Surgery*, **41**, 160–164

McIndoe, A. (1948) Deformities of the male urethra. *British Journal of Plastic Surgery*. **1**, 34

Noe, J. M., Birdsell, D. and Laub, D. R. (1974) The surgical construction of male genitalia for the female-to-male transsexual. *Plastic and Reconstructive Surgery*, **53**, 511–516

Orticochea, M. (1972) A new method of total reconstruction of the penis. *British Journal of Plastic Surgery*, **25**, 347–366

Puckett, C. L. and Montie, J. E. (1978) Construction of male genitalia in the transsexual using a tubed groin flap for the penis and a hydraulic inflation device. *Plastic and Reconstructive Surgery*, **61**, 523–530

Puckett, O. L., Reinisch, J. F. and Montie, J. E. (1982) Free flap phalloplasty. *Journal of Urology*, **128**, 294–297

Rogers, B. O. (1973) History of external genital surgery. In *Plastic and Reconstructive Surgery of the Genital Area*, (ed. C. E. Horton), Little, Brown and Company, Boston, pp. 3–47

Shenaq, S. M. and Dinh, T. A. (1989) Total penile and urethral reconstruction with an expanded sensate lateral arm flap: case report. *Journal of Reconstructive Microsurgery*, **5**, 245–248

Sun, G. and Huang, J. (1985) One stage reconstruction of the penis with composite iliac crest and lateral groin skin flap. *Annals of Plastic Surgery*, **6**, 519–528

Upton, J., Mutimer, K. L., Loughlin, K. and Ritchie, J. (1987) Penile reconstruction using the lateral arm flap. *Journal of the Royal College of Surgeons of Edinburgh*, **32**, 97–100

# 29

# Prospects for the development of cavernous tissue biopsy in the assessment of vascular impotence

Eric Wespes

Erectile impotence may be due to psychological problems, neurogenic dysfunction, hormonal alterations or compromised penile blood flow. With a better understanding of the erectile mechanism and with the development of new investigative techniques, recognition of the origin of the impotence has dramatically improved in recent years, indicating that the majority of these patients are impotent due to vascular abnormalities (Lue and Tanagho, 1987).

Intracavernous papaverine injection is a simple and reliable test to evaluate vasculogenic impotence. A positive test confirms good arterial inflow and venous return, but cannot distinguish neurogenic from psychogenic impotence (Virag *et al.*, 1984). Nocturnal penile plethysmography may therefore help distinguish between these diagnoses.

Doppler examination of the penile arteries during the papaverine test studies the arterial inflow better (Virag *et al.*, 1984). Pudendal arteriography should only be done if a surgical procedure is to be performed (Lue *et al.*, 1985). Pharmacocavernometry–cavernography allows determination of the flows necessary to provoke and maintain erection (Wespes *et al.*, 1986). These are the main criteria for evaluation of venous return.

However, a test to assess the intracavernous components is still lacking. The intracavernous structures consist of bundles of smooth muscles, elastic fibres, collagen and loose alveolar tissue with numerous arterioles and nerves. They represent the key to the problem, and demonstration of their alterations could eventually spare patients from reconstructive surgical treatment.

Recently, the Biopty gun, with its spring trigger mechanism, has increased the ability to obtain consistently good cores of tissue relatively painlessly. The use of this method for biopsies of penile erectile tissues is described below.

The biopsy is performed by first infiltrating about 1 ml lignocaine into the skin of the penis in the balanopreputial groove on the dorsolateral side.

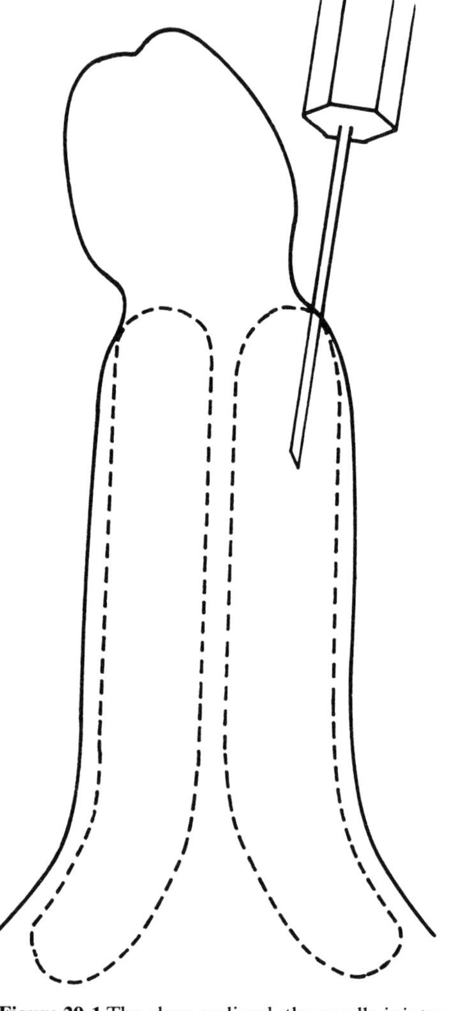

**Figure 29.1** The glans reclined, the needle is introduced through the balanopreputial groove and the tunica albuginea in the penis and the system is fired

After a 2–3 mm skin incision has been made, the biopsy needle is introduced longitudinally through the tunica albuginea into the corpus cavernosum. With one hand, the penis is kept stretched and, with the other hand, the needle is fired from an anterior to a posterior trajectory (Figure 29.1).

More than one pass of the needle can be made to obtain adequate tissue. Needle biopsies have been compared with surgical biopsies taken during penile implants. Cavernous penile arterial Doppler analysis was performed before and after biopsies done with the Biopty gun method.

In all cases, adequate tissue was obtained for histological analysis and the biopsy tissues were similar to those obtained during surgery. Corpus cavernosum tissue was easily identified, with the intracavernous smooth muscle fibres, arteries, nerves and collagen.

None of the patients experienced pain at biopsy or required any postoperative analgesia. No haematoma or significant bleeding was observed. No lesions were observed with the Doppler analysis on the cavernous arteries.

Use of the Biopty gun to perform penile biopsy under local anaesthesia appears to be a simple and reliable method to obtain sufficient tissue for histological analysis. The site of the needle puncture is very important, to avoid secondary subcutaneous haematoma of the penis. The balanopreputial groove is the preferred site, because the glans mucosa of the penile skin, if the patient is circumcized, adheres closely here to the tunica albuginea. The development of haematoma under the skin is therefore impossible. The small hole in the tunica albuginea at this point does not have to be sutured. The needle inserted longitudinally does not damage the intracavernous artery, as demonstrated by Doppler analysis performed before and after puncture, or the urethra. The use of the Biopty system is painless; it is cost-effective and can be done in the surgery under local anaesthesia. The procedure usually lasts less than 10 min. No complication from such a procedure was observed, but it could include bleeding, infection or failure to obtain adequate tissue. Using this ambulatory method or surgical procedures for obtaining cavernous biopsies, an objective decrease of the intracavernous smooth muscle fibres was observed in impotent patients (Wespes *et al.*, in press).

The Biopty gun biopsy also seems to be representative of the entire structures of the penis (Wespes *et al.*, 1991). In cadavers, comparing the percentage of smooth muscle fibres analysed by computer between the small Biopty gun biopsies and larger surgical biopsies taken in different sites of the penis, no significant difference was observed. The value of this new method in the assessment of impotent patients and a definition of the histological criteria in the light of electron microscopic studies is still to be determined; however, the technique holds promise as a method of selecting patients for penile reconstructive vascular surgery.

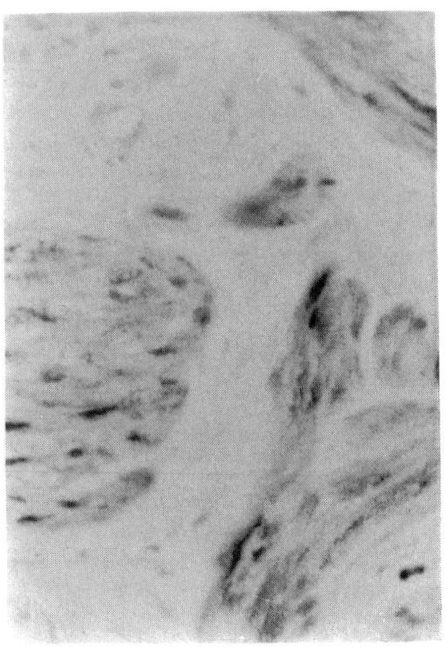

**Figure 29.2** Biopsy of the cavernous body; immunohistochemical staining with desmine–antidesmine. Only smooth muscle cells are stained (black). (×400)

## References


Lue, T. F., Tanagho, E. A. (1987) Physiology of erection and pharmacological management of impotence. *Journal of Urology*, **137**, 829

Lue, T. F., Hricak, H., Marich, K. W., Tanagho, E. A. (1985) Evaluation of arteriogenic impotence with intracorporeal injection of papaverine and the duplex ultrasound scanner. *Seminars in Urology*, **3**, 43

Virag, R., Frydman, D., Legman, M., Virag, H. (1984) Intracavernous injection of papaverine as a diagnostic and therapeutic method in erectile failure. *Angiology*, **35**, 79

Wespes, E., Delcour, C., Struyven, J., Schulman, C. C. (1986) Pharmacocavernometry–cavernography in impotence. *British Journal of Urology*, **58**, 429–433

Wespes, E., Goes, P. M., Schiffmann, S., Depierreux, M., Vanderhaeghen, J. J., Schulman, C. C. (1991) Computerized analysis of smooth muscle fibers in potent and impotent patients. *Journal of Urology*, in press

Wespes, E., Schiffmann, S., Vanderhaeghen, J. J., Schulman, C. C. (1991) Importance of penile biopsy in the assessment of impotent patients. *Journal of Urology*, **145**, 231A73

# 30

# Peyronie's disease

Culley C. Carson

Peyronie's disease is an idiopathic sexually disabling condition of the penis, caused by a fibrotic scar of the tunica albuginea surrounding the corpora cavernosa, which results in a deformity of the penis on erection (Figure 30.1). Although this deformity of the penis was described as early as 1561 by Fallopius, it was the description and publication of this condition in 1743, by Peyronie, which gave us the eponym.[6] Peyronie, who has been called the 'Father of French surgery', helped establish the Royal Academy of Surgery, in Paris, in 1731. In an effort to legitimize the Royal Academy of Surgery, *Archives of Surgery* were begun in an attempt to review common surgical problems and organize surgical techniques for various diseases. In the first volume of these archives in 1743, Peyronie described fibrous cavernositis in a paper entitled. 'Some obstacles preventing the normal ejaculation of semen'.[39] His described treatment for this disease included successful resolution in several patients who took the waters of Bareges. Since that description, many medical, surgical, and other treatment modalities have been suggested to resolve the fibrotic plaque of Peyronie's disease.

Smith, in 1966, hypothesized that the plaque of Peyronie's disease begins as an inflammatory reaction characterized histologically by lymphocytic and plasmacytic infiltration of the perivascular spaces within the areolar tissue of the tunica albuginea.[45] His histologic examination demonstrated that the mature, scarred portion of the Peyronie's plaque is frequently rich in hyaluronic acid. This initial inflammatory process is followed by progressive formation of fibrous tissue associated with a perivascular fibrous collar and production of abnormal elastic fibres. The inelastic scarring shortens one side of the corpus cavernosum, producing curvature toward the area of plaque owing to loss of ipsilateral corpus cavernosum

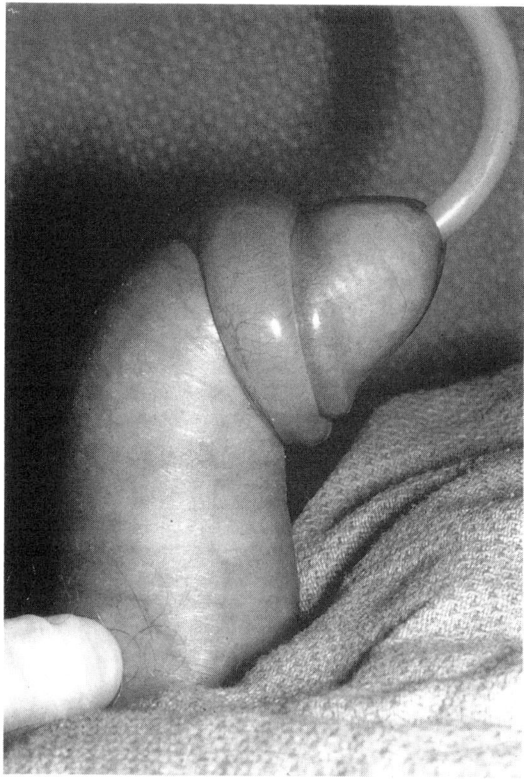

**Figure 30.1** Typical dorsal curvature of Peyronie's disease with an artificial erection

elasticity. As a result of this pathophysiology, medical therapy early in the treatment of Peyronie's disease is focused towards the inflammatory reaction. Later treatment must, however, be concerned with mature fibrosis or calcification.

## Aetiology

The initial inflammatory process associated with subsequent development of fibrosis and Peyronie's plaques may result from a variety of aetiologic processes. The initial inflammation begins in an area between the tunica albuginea and the erectile tissue of the corpora cavernosa. This then becomes generalized, involving the corpora tissue itself as well as the entire thickness of the tunica albuginea, and may include Buck's fascia and structures between Buck's fascia and the tunica albuginea, including the dorsal neurovascular bundle of the penis, the intercorporal septum, or the corpora spongiosa surrounding the urethra. This inflammation may resolve, resulting in complete resolution of the process, or may progress to fibrosis and finally dystrophic calcification within the tunica (Figure 30.2).[20,49] Other similar fibrotic conditions may occur elsewhere in the body. As many as 10% of patients with Peyronie's disease also have Dupuytren's contracture and 3% of males with Dupuytren's contracture also have the plaques of Peyronie's disease. Furthermore, as many as 15% of patients with Peyronie's disease have some evidence of excessive scarring or keloid formation elsewhere in the body. There is also an association with scleroderma.[23] Thus, excessive fibrosis during the healing process may be a congenital or familial trait, and may be associated with the formation of Peyronie's disease in suitable circumstances. Historically, venereal disease and sexual excess have been implicated in Peyronie's disease, although more recent reports have failed to support these factors.[4] Arteriosclerosis, trauma, diabetes mellitus and phlebitis have been mentioned as inciting factors, yet none of these associations have been proven.[7,9,18,33] Various medications have been implicated in Peyronie's disease, including barbiturites and beta-blocking agents such as propranolol and metoprolol.[30,37,53] In 1949, Scardino and Scott noted that vitamin E deficiency interfered with the normal repair of connective tissue, leaving scar tissue in a state of contraction.[43] Although this theory remains unproven, it serves as the basis for the use of vitamin E therapy in patients with Peyronie's disease. Bivens and associates reported that 2 of 6 patients with carcinoid syndrome had Peyronie's disease, and proposed that increased levels of serotonin could be a contributory factor in the fibrosis encountered in the retroperitoneum, endocardium and penises of these patients.[5]

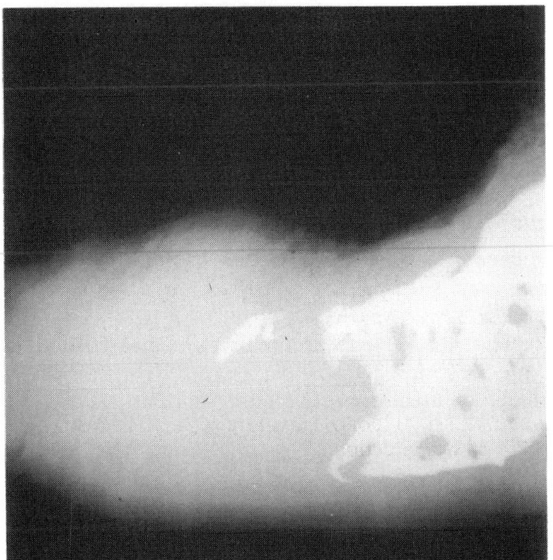

**Figure 30.2** Dystrophic calcification after longstanding Peyronie's disease with impotence

Van de Berg and associates have suggested that Peyronie's disease is an autoimmune response to vascular trauma.[49] Their theory is supported, using scanning and transmission electron microscopy, by the demonstration that the calcification originated from vascular lumina by osteoblastic cells which aligned the calcified plaque (present in 30% of Peyronie's plaques). A familial tendency toward Peyronie's disease was suggested by Willscher and associates, who identified a relationship between Peyronie's disease and the histocompatibility antigens of the B-7 cross-reacting group, and suggested that Peyronie's disease may represent a pathological response to an unidentified infective agent similar to the B-7 antigen.[51] Nyberg and associates studied three families with an inherited form of Peyronie's disease transmitted as an autosomal dominant trait and associated with Dupytren's contracture.[36] These individuals all exhibited HLA-B27 cross-reacting antigens. The occurrence of Dupytren's contracture in 7 of their 9 patients (78%) is in contrast to the 10% normal association in reported sporadic cases and suggests that both conditions are pleiotropic effects of the same gene. These data, however, have been disputed by Leffell and associates, who studied 28 patients with Peyronie's disease and demonstrated no association with any HLA antigen.[28]

One plausible explanation for the initiation of an abnormal fibrotic reaction is associated minimal trauma. Traumatic sexual intercourse, especially with a partially erect penis, in a susceptible individual may result in injury to the penile support structure or corpus cavernosum with subsequent inflammation and fibrosis. Devine has suggested a scenario which could account for the development of Peyronie's disease as a result of trauma.[12] He theorizes that bending the partially rigid penis may generate enough torque on the fibres of the septum or tunica albuginea to 'delaminate' the tunica in the area of stress. Subsequent microvascular injury produces small amounts of haemorrhage within the tunica albuginea, resulting in inflammation and the initiation of the healing process. If an individual has a tendency towards abnormal healing, the blood clot deposition and trapping of fibrin within the tissue space may produce increased scarring as a result of trapped fibrin which is not adequately cleared, producing normal remodelling.[46] This retained fibrin between the layers of the tunica albuginea produces fibroblast activation, proliferation and increased leukocyte deposition. Because the original stimulus and fibrin deposition cannot be cleared adequately, subsequent repeat trauma may be more likely to occur.[47] This concept is supported by ultrastructural work by Dini *et al.*, who have shown that there is intracytoplasmic fibril formation caused by excessive collagen synthesis by fibroblasts.[14] Because younger men have more tissue elasticity, firmer erections, and probably fewer traumatic events, Peyronie's disease is less frequent. In the middle-aged man with less tissue elasticity, heightened fibrin deposition and less firm erections, associated with probably less lubricated partners, there is a heightened tendency toward tissue injury.[32] The association of Peyronie's disease and hypertensive individuals adds further evidence to this theory. Many patients with hypertension have progressive vascular disease, producing less penile rigidity. Devine and associates feel strongly that a diminution in the elasticity of the tunical tissue as patients age produces the major risk factor in the pathogenesis of Peyronie's disease. Another more recent causative factor may be self-injection of pharmacoactive agents for erections.[11] These patients may have scarring from injection trauma which may progress to intracavernosal calcification.

## Patient presentation

Patients with Peyronie's disease can present with a variety of symptoms and signs. The condition usually occurs in patients in the 5th and 6th decades, with a mean age of 53 years.[4,10] Since most patients with Peyronie's disease demonstrate slow progression, the disease symptomatology may evolve during its course, ultimately resolving. Initial symptoms include penile shaft pain at the area of future curvature. This pain may not be present in all patients, but usually resolves as fibrosis progresses and curvature begins, and requires only symptomatic treatment. Pain and discomfort usually resolve within 3–4 months of symptom onset. Palpable plaque formation and penile curvature usually progress simultaneously, most often reaching a maximum within 6 months of onset. While some patients demonstrate initial curvature which appears rapidly and is stable from the outset, most patients note a change in the direction and degree of curvature as the disease progresses. The majority of patients retain the ability to obtain and maintain erections, but may have difficulty with vaginal penetration and sexual activity, as a result of curvature and pain on intromission, and may have coital difficulties as a result of partner dyspareunia. Inadequate erections may occur in as many as 20% of patients with symptomatic Peyronie's disease.[40] In many of these patients, distal penile flaccidity may preclude vaginal penetration. These patients with penile shaft flaccidity distal to the area of curvature and penile plaque formation must be identified prior to suggesting specific surgical treatment. An additional group of patients have been shown to suffer erectile dysfunction as a result of an associated venous leak phenomenon. The increased incidence of venous leak in patients with Peyronie's disease has been recently documented, and its presence must be eliminated prior to selecting definitive surgical intervention.[21]

## Patient management

Initial evaluation and screening should be confined to a history and physical examination. Patients who have minimal curvature and continue to have normal sexual function do not require surgical intervention. Definitive management of Peyronie's disease has eluded urologists since bathing in the Barege spa was recommended by Peyronie in 1743.[39] Many patients will respond to reassurance, and the natural evolution of the disease will result in either resolution of the curvature or diminution sufficient for the maintenance of sexual function. Medical therapy with such agents as corticosteroids, vitamin E and potassium para-aminobenzoate have also been suggested as medical treatment. Most importantly, however, expectant, non-invasive treatment is best maintained for 12 months to allow the progress of the disease to stabilize.[4,10,12,21] At this point, appropriate surgical intervention, if necessary, can be planned if there has been little improvement in the plaque and resultant curvature. Over this period, the curvature and plaque will stabilize and the resultant deformity and sexual disability will be evident. The mere presence of a penile deformity does not, in itself, necessitate correction. In addition, patients with curvature must express a desire to continue sexual activity, since this is obviously the goal of corrective surgery.

Initial treatment with vitamin E, 400 IU daily, may have some effect on symptomatic improvement. One may also add potassium para-aminobenzoate, 4 gm 3–4 times daily, with some expected improvement.[25,54] If patients have continued pain and erectile dysfunction on the basis of that significant discomfort, radiation therapy can reasonably be expected to relieve the symptoms of erectile pain.[7,18] Orthovoltage radiation therapy in doses between 600 and 1600 rads administered in a 10–90-day have been demonstrated to be effective in relieving penile shaft discomfort in 78.5% of patients treated.[7] In this same group of patients, penile plaque was improved in only 13.3% and curvature in only 6.3% of patients treated and followed up for an average of 2 years. Thus, radiation therapy should be restricted to only those patients with severe pain and penile discomfort. While results have been mixed, some advocate ultrasonic treatment for the Peyronie's plaque.[26,34]

Direct injections of medication and enzymes have been tried with mixed success. Injections of corticosteroids and other substances tend to affect only the small portion of plaque injected.[34,52] Trials with clostridial collagenase injection, while showing some promise, have had mixed results.[21,22,24] Reversal of fibrosis with these methods has failed to improve penile curvature or decrease plaque in the series reported. Injection treatment with prostaglandin E for plaque-associated pain, has also been unsuccessful.[48]

## Surgical management

Once Peyronie's disease has stabilized with continued erectile dsyfunction, surgical treatment can be considered. In evaluating patients for possible surgical intervention, it is necessary to identify the abnormality to be treated such that the surgical procedure can be tailored to the individual dysfunction. Initial surgical planning requires identification of the area of curvature. Patients are asked to provide polaroid photographs of their flaccid and erect penis to identify the extent, direction and character of erectile distortion. Pharmacologic injection or suction devices can also be used to create an erection to examine penile curvature. Physical examination with palpation of the stretched penis and its plaque are also helpful in surgical planning. Plane radiographs can identify plaque calcification, and ultrasound images can not only demonstrate calcification but also the depth and extent of the plaque, allowing appropriate planning for plaque excision and grafting (Figure 30.3).[1]

Initial evaluation using nocturnal penile tumescence monitoring studies can be helpful in documenting distal penile flaccidity in patients with severe Peyronie's disease with or without curvature (Figure 30.4). In a patient with complete distal penile flaccidity, implantation of a prosthesis with or without penile straightening should be considered. In patients with moderate erectile dysfunction, dynamic infusion cavernosometry and cavernosography with duplex ultrasound evaluation and pharmacological testing, can help to identify those patients who will respond best to conservative surgical approaches and document Peyronie's associated veno-occlusive disorders (Figure 30.5).[19] The injection of pharmacologically active agents such as papaverine–phentolamine or prostaglandin $E_1$ will produce erectile function and allow direct examination of the erect penis and its associated deformity. Duplex ultrasound following this pharmacoactive injection will allow specific identification of a vascular abnormality. Arterial inflow can be documented before and after administration, and if arterial inflow is adequate, pulsewave analysis will be normal. If adequate erectile function is not observed, veno-occlusive incompetence can be suspected. Cavernosometry can be performed to document the presence of a venous leak. The addition of cavernosography can not only further document the location of a venous leak, but can also identify the filling defect within the corpus cavernosum which corresponds to the Peyronie's plaque.

Initially, 30 mg of papaverine with 1 mg of phentolamine mesylate or 30 μg of prostaglandin $E_1$ are injected into one corpus cavernosum of the penis. Colour Doppler examination is carried out before, and 15 minutes after, injection. At approximately 20 minutes after injection, intracavernosal pressure is measured. If this remains below mean arterial pressure or approximately 90 mmHg, erection can be considered inadequate. At this stage, normal saline is infused with a roller pump to an intracavernosal pressure in excess of 125 mmHg. If arterial flow has been identified as normal and intracavernosal pressure is maintained as previously described, the vascular function of the penis can be assumed to be normal. If the pressure decays and erection is lost rapidly despite saline infusion, veno-occlusive incompetence can be suspected. At this stage, iodinated contrast medium is infused

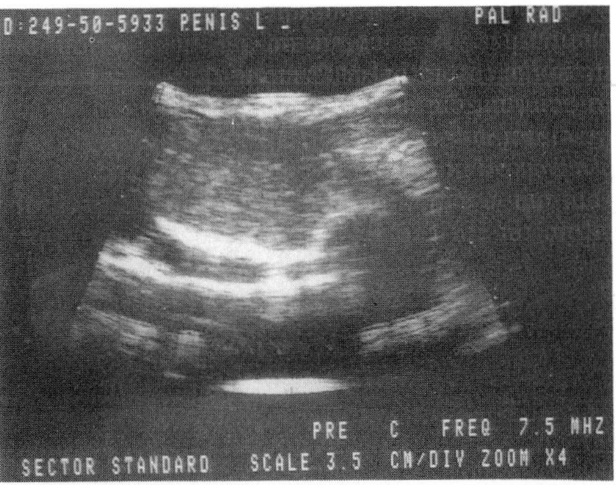


**Figure 30.3** Ultrasound of corpora cavernosa ventrally demonstrating dorsal plaque

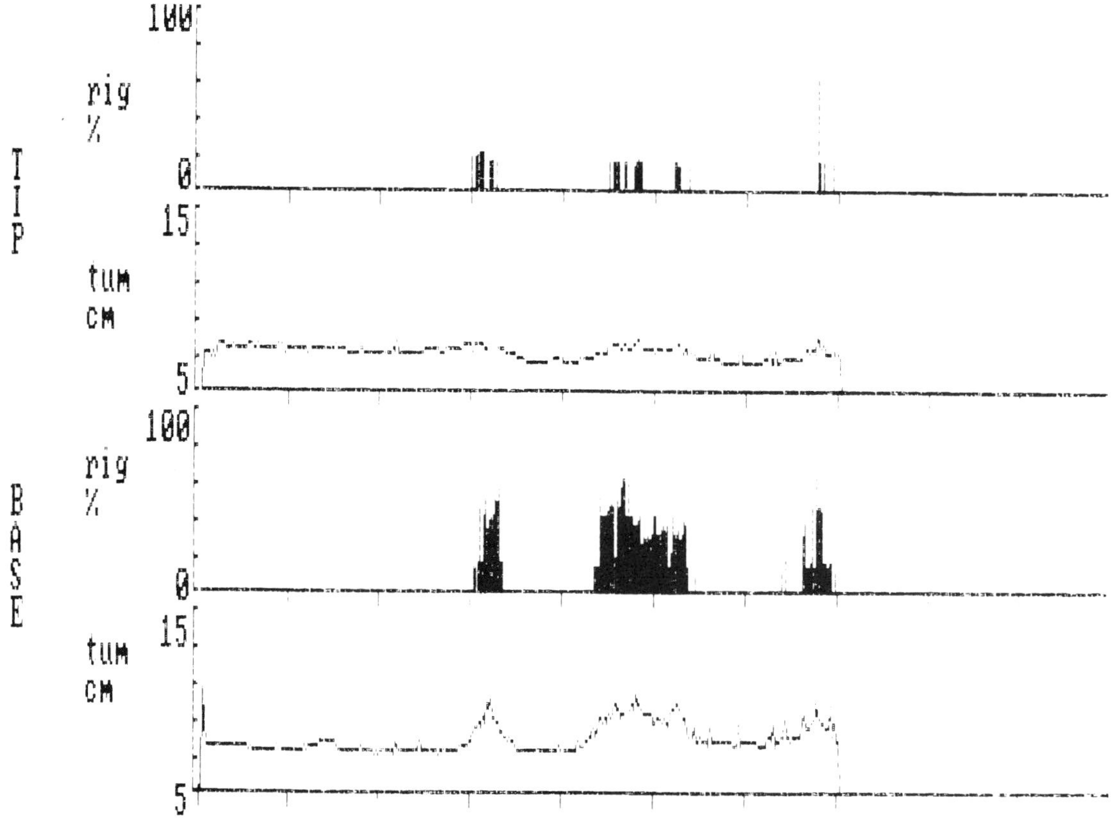

**Figure 30.4** Nocturnal penile tumescence monitoring (Rigiscan) of a patient with Peyronie's disease and penile flaccidity distal to the plaque and curvature

through the roller pump, for fluoroscopic examination. These fluoroscopic images will document the extent and location of venous leak. If leakage is documented as entering the corpus spongiosum or glans penis, venous ligation surgery will be ineffective and patients are best treated with prosthesis implantation, with or without penile curvature correction. If leakage is documented to occur through the deep dorsal vein of the penis and its emissary veins, venous ligation can be carried out simultaneously with plaque excision and grafting, or Nesbitt's procedure.

## Surgical procedures

### Nesbitt's procedure

The Nesbitt procedure is the most conservative method for surgical management and is used in those patients with normal erectile function as documented by nocturnal penile tumescence monitoring studies and cavernosometry.[10] Its use must be

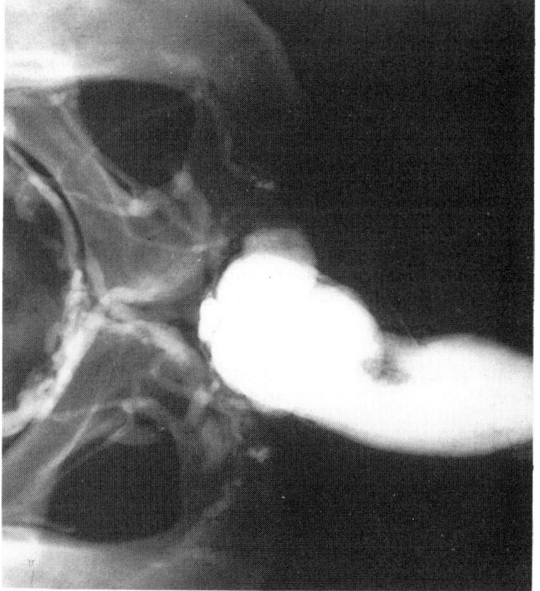

**Figure 30.5** Cavernosogram demonstrates a left cavernosal filling defect from a Peyronie's plaque and associated venous leak

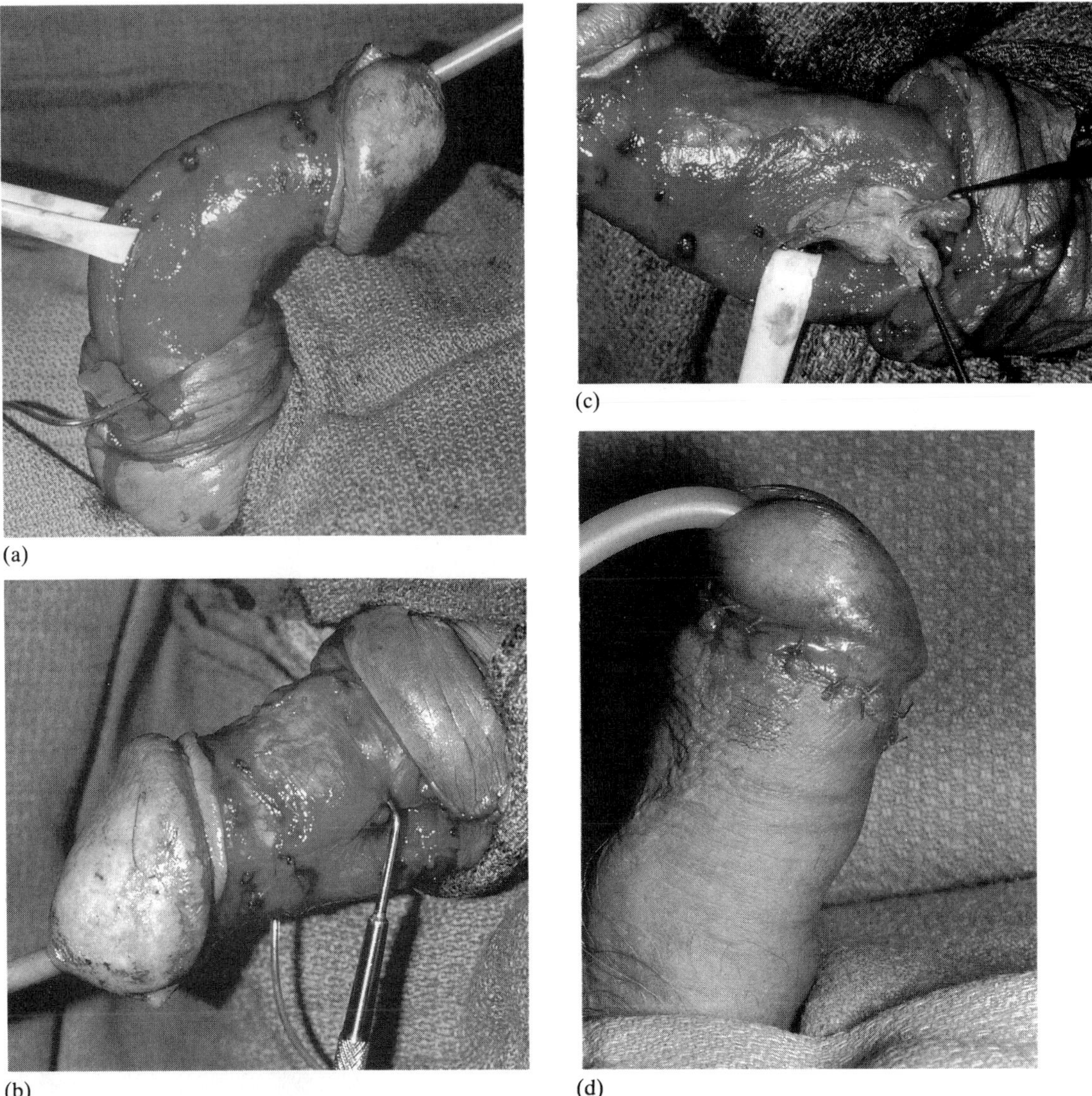

**Figure 30.6** Nesbitt procedure: a) penile skin is retracted. Artificial erection documents dorsal curvature; b) an ellipse of tunica albuginea is removed opposite the maximum curvature; c) corpora cavernosa are closed with a running suture of 4/0 polypropylene suture. Suture line is at nerve hook; d) artificial erection after skin closure

confined to those patients with moderate penile curvature and minimal penile shortening.[35]

An artificial erection is induced once a tourniquet is placed at the base of the penis (Figure 30.6a). Fifty ml of injectable normal saline are inserted into one corpus cavernosum using a 21 gauge scalp vein needle. This artificial erection allows palpation of the Peyronie's plaque and demonstration of the point of maximum curvature, which is then marked using a surgical marking pen. A circumcoronal incision is made and the penile shaft is exposed by retracting the penile skin using sharp and blunt dissection in a sleeving manner. If a very proximal Peyronie's plaque is to be treated, it may be necessary to use a more proximal approach, with a dorsal or ventral midline incision, to allow degloving of the penis. In this situation, artificial erection with a penile tourniquet is difficult. Pressure on the perineum by the surgical assistant may allow for artificial erection in these very proximal penile curvatures. Once the penis has been degloved, it may be necessary to mobilize either the urethra or the dorsal neurovascular bundle to correct a midline deviation. For significant curvature, it is best to excise an ellipse of tunica albuginea at an area opposite the point of greatest curvature (Figure 30.6b). The amount of ellipse to exercise can be decided by approximating Allis clamps proximally and distally to the area to be excised. Once the ellipse has been removed, the defect is closed using a continuous suture of 4/0 polypropylene, or polydiaxanone (PDS) suture can be used (Figure 30.6c). Chromic catgut is not appropriate for this procedure as it may weaken before complete healing can occur. Surgical knots are inverted to preclude postoperative palpation of suture material. Additional artificial erections are then carried out to ensure adequate correction of the deformity. A second ellipse may be necessary for complete correction. In patients with only minimal-to-moderate curvature, the ellipse of tunica albuginea may be eliminated and only surgical plication at various levels may be adequate. Once the surgeon is satisfied that a straight erection has been obtained, the circumcoronal incision is closed in the standard fashion (Figure 30.6d). If a sizable ellipse has been removed, a small suction drain may be left beneath the flap of penile skin to eliminate fluid collection. Usually 24 hours of suction drainage is adequate for healing. A light pressure dressing is applied and a Foley catheter is left in place if the patient had preoperative voiding difficulty. All patients are treated with perioperative broad-spectrum antibiotics.

If venous excision and ligation are to be performed simultaneously with the Nesbitt or the plaque excision procedures, incision should be carried out superior or lateral to the base of the penis such that the dorsal surface of the corporal bodies can be easily exposed. Ligation and excision are carried out as previously described.[12,42]

## Plaque excision and grafting

Initial artificial erection again identifies the area of maximum curvature and Peyronie's plaque. For pendulous penis excisions, a circumcoronal incision is most commonly used. For a more proximal plaque, a dorsal or ventral penile incision may be more useful. For dorsal plaque excision, dissection is begun beneath Buck's fascia lateral to the dorsal neurovascular bundle on each side. Sharp and blunt dissection are carried out, freeing the dorsal neurovascular bundle with its surrounding tissue to preserve these dorsal structures (Figure 30.7a). For ventral plaque excision, the corpus spongiosum and urethra are dissected free from the tunica albuginea. A Foley catheter is placed to facilitate this dissection. The dorsal neurovascular bundle or corpus spongiosum are then mobilized thoroughly approximately 1–2 cm on each side of the plaque to be incised. The tunica albuginea is then exposed. Sharp dissection is frequently necessary as a result of the scarring and inflammation associated with the Peyronie's plaque, which can significantly involve the dorsal neurovascular bundle. The dorsal neurovascular bundle is then isolated with vessel loops and retracted away from the area with the plaque. Maintaining the penile tourniquet during resection of the plaque allows for more accurate dissection. Stay sutures are placed at the most proximal and distal margins of the plaque, as well as at its lateral extent. Full-thickness incision just lateral to the plaque is then carried out in its entirety (Figure 30.7b). The edge of the most distal portion of the plaque is grasped and the plaque is dissected free, carefully preserving the deep erectile tissues. Once the plaque has been excised and removed, four quadrant relaxing incisions are made at the extremities of the excision. These allow for longitudinal extension of the penis and relaxation of any additional curvature. Incision of the plaque must be carried to the level of the intracorporeal septum in order to relax curvature and completely excise the plaque (Figure 30.7c). At this stage, graft material is chosen to fit the defect outline. Artificial materials such as Dacron or Gore-tex can be easily used because of their ready availability and ease of handling.[3,29,31,38,41,44,50] Some authors believe that natural tissues such as tunica albuginea, dermis or dura mater provide a more elastic and normal patch material.[13,16,27] Graft size is defined with the penis on stretch such that the graft is somewhat larger than the size of the flaccid defect. The graft once tailored, is placed and sutured to the tunica albuginea using running 4/0 polypropylene or polydiaxanone (PDS) sutures (Figure 30.7d). Following graft placement, an initial artificial erection is performed to ensure straightening of the penis and a watertight closure. Small leaks are oversewn using figure-of-eight sutures. Closure of the skin is carried out, after satisfactory haemostasis has been achieved, with interrupted sutures of 4/0 chromic catgut. A small plastic surgery drain is placed in the area of graft and a simple minimal compression dressing is applied. A Foley catheter is left in place for 24 hours. The dressing and drain remain in place for approximately 5 days.

Results of the plaque excision and grafting procedure popularized by Horton and Devine have been variable.[31,38,50] Several investigators have reported poor results in subsequent erectile function. In a review by Wild and associates of 52 patients treated with the dermal graft technique, 70% noticed subjective improvement.[50] Surgical failure appeared to correlate with plaque size and previous treatment. Results were worst in patients with large plaques and in those who had received previous radiation therapy or plaque injection

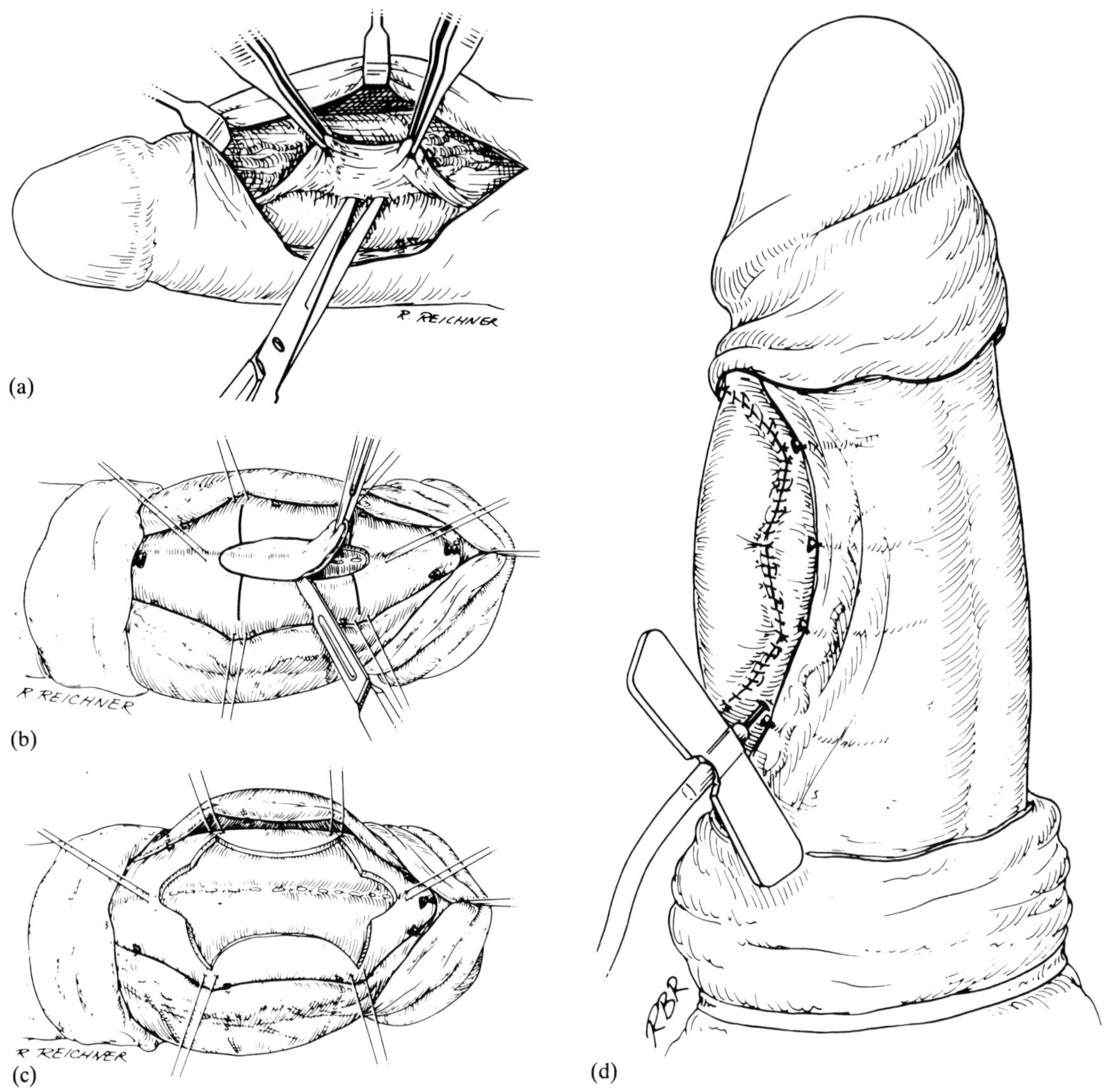


**Figure 30.7** Plaque excision and grafting: a) the dorsal neurovascular bundles are dissected free and retracted from the plaque; b) the plaque is sharply excised, including all septal elements; c) lateral relaxing incisions are performed for expansion; d) graft material is tailored and sutured to the tunica albuginea using 4/0 PDS suture. An artificial erection is repeated to ensure a straight result

treatment with steroids. Unfortunately these patients frequently constitute a significant number of men who eventually require surgical correction for Peyronie's disease.

## Penile prosthesis inplantation in Peyronie's disease

While in many patients simple implantation of a prosthesis will adequately correct the penile curvature and deformity as a result of dilation and cylinder placement, the remaining angulation may require additional surgical modification for adequate results. Prosthesis implantation should be considered in all patients with inadequate erectile function as a result of Peyronie's disease.[8,15,17]

Penile prostheses are implanted as previously described. If significant curvature continues, a modified Nesbitt procedure, glanuloplasty or formal plaque incision with or without grafting can be considered. For curvature at the base of the penis and proximal penile shaft, the previous penoscrotal or infrapubic incision may be extended or retracted

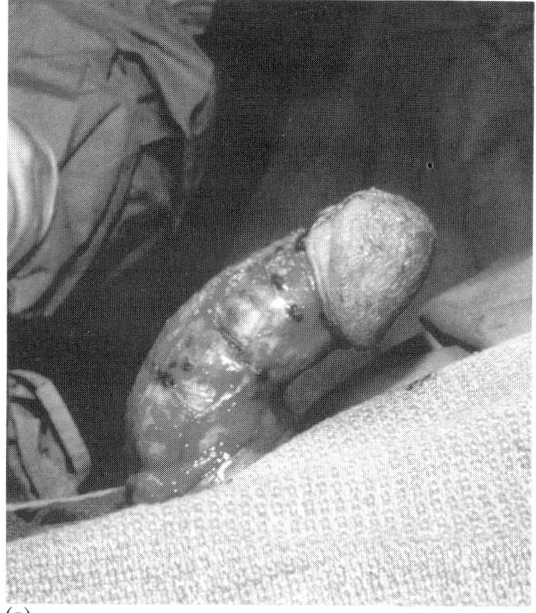
(a)

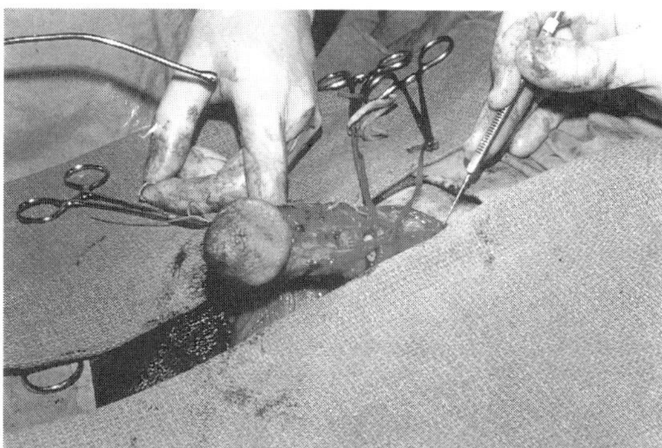
(b)

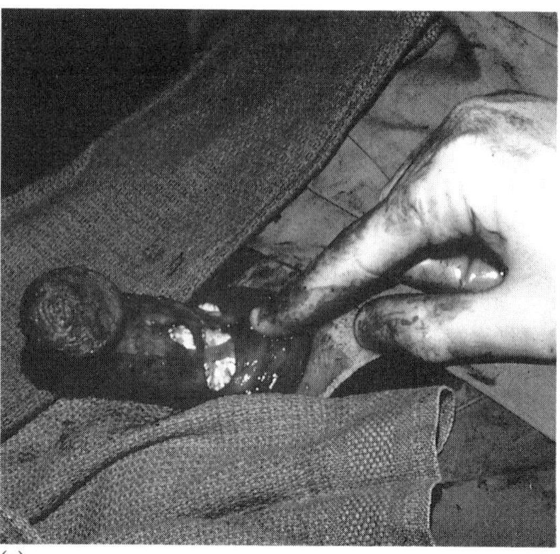
(c)

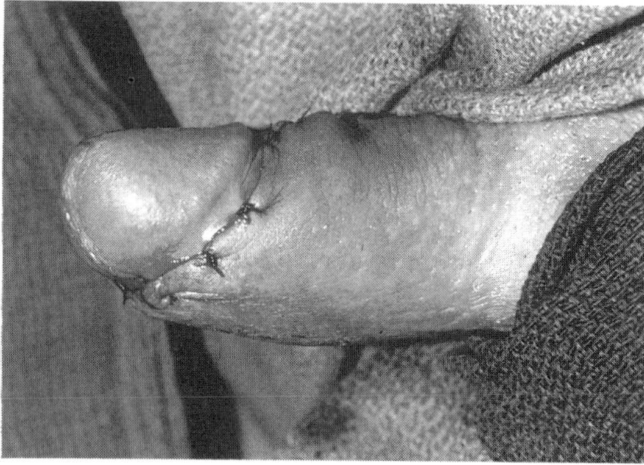
(d)

**Figure 30.8** Penile prothesis implantation with penile straightening: a) penile curvature on maximal prosthesis inflation. Penile skin has been retracted; b) after plaque incision with penile straightening, the prosthesis cylinders are exposed. Note the dorsal neurovascular bundle is protected and retracted; c) Gore-tex is used to patch graft the defect in the tunica albuginea. 4/0 polypropylene or Gore-tex suture is used to fix the graft; d) after closure of the penile skin, the straightening is documented by prosthesis inflation

to expose the area of maximum curvature and Peyronie's plaque. With curvature isolated to the pendulous portion of the penis, the most common presentation, a secondary circumcoronal incision may be necessary to expose the area of maximum curvature for treatment (Figure 30.8a). Dorsal curvature requires dissection of the dorsal neurovascular bundle as previously described. Ventral curvature similarly may require mobilization of the corpus spongiosum and urethra away from the area of maximum curvature. Once penile prostheses are implanted, incision in the area of maximum curvature must be carried out with electrocautery. This is an excellent method for incision of a Peyronie's plaque and will not damage the cylinders of the penile prosthesis during dissection. Once the area of maximum curvature is exposed, an inflatable penile prosthesis is inflated to its maximum rigidity. The dorsal neurovascular bundle or ventral spongiosum are retracted away from the area of curvature using vessel loops. Electrocautery is then used to incise the area of maximum curvature until a complete straightening occurs (Figure 30.8b). This usually requires incision to and through the intracavernosal septum, as the majority of curvature is frequently present at this level. Once complete incision has been carried out, the penis will straighten spontaneously, indicating adequate treatment. Once straightening has been performed, grafting of the remaining defect must be considered. As a result of modifications in the currently available inflatable prostheses, with controlled distension cylinders and bioflex cylinders, aneurysmal distention of the prosthesis cylinders through the defect incised has been eliminated. As a result, grafting is only performed if the defect produced by incision is large enough to be cosmetically objectionable. Fishman suggests that defects of greater than 50% of the corporal circumference should be grafted.[7] The author prefers to graft all those defects which are readily palpable through the replaced skin.[8] Autogenous or synthetic grafts may be used as previously described in the plaque excision and grafting technique. The author prefers vascular Gore-tex for this procedure (Figure 30.8c). The graft is again measured with the penis on greatest stretch, and is tailored approximately 25% larger than the size of the defect to allow for graft contraction and penile extension. The graft is tailored to the size and shape of the defect, and secured in place with running sutures of 4/0 Prolene or Gore-tex. Closure, drainage and dressing are the same as for plaque excision and grafting (Figure 30.8d). Any further curvature at the most distal portion of the penis may require glanuloplasty through the use of plication of the glans penis dorsally onto the corporal shaft, as described by Ball.[2] This procedure, which is performed over the corpora cavernosa lateral to the dorsal and ventral structures, will eliminate distal penile curvature and the SST deformity.

## References


1. Balconi, G., Angeli, E., Nessi, R., de Flaviis, L. (1988) Ultrasonic evaluation of Peyronie's disease. *Urologic Radiology,* **10**, 85
2. Ball, T. P. (1980) Surgical repair of penile 'SST' deformity. *Urology,* **15**, 603
3. Bertram, R. A., Carson, C. C., Altaffer, L. F. (1988) Severe penile curvature after implantation of an inflatable penile prosthesis. *Journal of Urology,* **139**, 743
4. Billig, R., Baker, R., Immergut, M., Maxted, W. (1975) Peyronie's disease. *Urology,* **6**, 409
5. Bivins, C. H., Marecek, R. L., Feldman, J. M. (1973) Peyronie's disease – a presenting complaint of the carcinoid syndrome. *New England Journal of Medicine,* **289**, 844
6. Carson, C. C. (1981) François Gigot de la Peyronie. *Investigative Urology,* **19**, 62
7. Carson, C. C., Coughlin, P. W. F. (1985) Radiation therapy for Peyronie's disease: is there a place? *Journal of Urology,* **134**, 684
8. Carson, C. C., Hodge, G. B., Anderson, E. E. (1983) Penile prosthesis in Peyronie's disease. *British Journal of Urology,* **55**, 417
9. Chilton, C. P., Castle, W. M., Westwood, C. A., Pryor, J. P. (1982) Factors associated in the aetiology of Peyronie's disease. *British Journal of Urology,* **54**, 5748
10. Coughlin, P. W. F., Carson, C. C., Paulson, D. F. (1984) Surgical correction of Peyronie's disease: the Nesbitt procedure. *Journal of Urology,* **131**, 282
11. Desai, K. M., Gingell, J. C. (1988) Penile corporal fibrosis complicating papaverine self-injection therapy for erectile impotence. *European Urology,* **15**, 132
12. Devine, C. J. (1991) Peyronie's disease. In: Glenn, J. F. (ed) *Urologic Surgery*. L. B. Lippincott Company, Philadelphia, p. 864
13. Devine, C. J., Horton, C. E. (1974) Surgical treatment of Peyronie's disease with dermal graft. *Journal of Urology,* **111**, 44
14. Dini, G., Grappone, C., del Rosso, M. *et al.*, (1986) Intracellular collagen in fibroblasts of Peyronie's disease. *Journal of Submicroscopic Cytology,* **18**, 605
15. Eigner, E. B., Kabalin, J. N., Kessler, R. (1991) Penile implants in the treatment of Peyronie's disease. *Journal of Urology,* **145**, 69
16. Fallon, B. (1990) Cadaveric dura mater graft for correction of penile curvature in Peyronie's disease. *Urology,* **35**, 127
17. Fishman, I. J. (1989) Corporal reconstruction procedures for complicated penile implants. *Urologic Clinics of North America,* **16**, 73
18. Furlow, W. L., Swenson, H. E., Lee, R. E. (1975) Peyronie's disease: a study of its natural history and treatment with orthovoltage radiotherapy. *Journal of Urology,* **114**, 69
19. Gasior, B. L., Levine, F. J., Howannesian, A. *et al.*, (1990) Plaque-associated corporal veno-occlusive dysfunction in idiopathic Peyronie's disease: a pharmacocavernosometric and pharmacocavernosographic study. *World Journal of Urology,* **8**, 90
20. Gelbard, M. K. (1988) Dystrophic penile calcification in Peyronie's disease. *Journal of Urology,* **139**, 738
21. Gelbard, M. K., Dorey, F., James, K. (1990) The natural history of Peyronie's disease. *Journal of Urology,* **144**, 1376
22. Gelbard, M. K., Lindner, A., Kaufman, J. J. (1983) The use of collagenase in the treatment of Peyronie's disease. *Journal of Urology,* **134**, 280
23. Gauldieri, L., Valentini, G., Lupoli, S., Giordano, M. (1988) Peyronie's disease in systemic sclerosis: report of two cases. *Journal of Rheumatology,* **15**, 380
24. Hamilton, R. G., Mintx, G. R., Gelbard, M. K. (1986) Humoral immune responses in Peyronie's disease patients receiving clostridial collagenase therapy. *Journal of Urology,* **135**, 641
25. Hasche-Klunder, R. (1983) conservative treatment of Peyronie's disease with potassium para-amino benzoate. *Progress in Reproductive Biology and Medicine,* **9**, 57

26. Heslop, R. W., Oakland, D. J., Maddix, B. T. (1967) Ultrasonic therapy in Peyronie's disease. *British Journal of Urology,* **39**, 415
27. Kalami, A. (1977) Surgical treatment of Peyronie's disease using human dura. *European Urology,* **3**, 191
28. Leffell, M. S., Devine, C. J., Horton, C. E. *et al.*, (1982) Non-association of Peyronie's disease with HLA B7 cross-reactive antigens. *Journal of Urology,* **127**, 1223
29. Lowe, D. H., Hoe, P. C., Parsons, C. L. (1982) Surgical treatment of Peyronie's disease with dacron graft. *Urology,* **19**, 609
30. Mattson, R. H., Cramer, J. A., McCutchen, C. B. (1989) Barbiturate-related connective tissue disorder. *Archives of Internal Medicine,* **149**, 911
31. Melman, A., Holland, T. F. (1978) Evaluation of the dermal graft inlay technique for the surgical treatment of Peyronie's disease. *Journal of Urology,* **120**, 421
32. Mersdorf, A., Goldsmith, P. C., Diederichs, W. *et al.*, (1991) Ultrastructural changes in impotent penile tissue: comparison of sixty-five patients. *Journal of Urology,* **145**, 749
33. Metz, P., Ebbho, J. J., Uhrenholdt, A., Wagner, G. (1983) Peyronie's disease in erectile failure. *British Journal of Urology,* **130**, 1103
34. Miller, H. C., Ardizzone, J. (1983) Peyronie's disease treated with ultrasound and hydrocortisone. *Urology,* **21**, 584
35. Nesbitt, R. M. (1965) Congenital curvature of the phallus: report of three cases with description of corrective operation. *Journal of Urology,* **93**, 230
36. Nyberg, L. M., Bias, W. B., Hochberg, M. C., Walsh, P. C. (1982) Identification of an inherited form of Peyronie's disease with autosomal dominant inheritance and association with Dupuytren's contracture in histocompatibility B7 cross-reacting antigens. *Journal of Urology,* **128,** 48
37. Osborne, D. R. (1977) Propranolol and Peyronie's disease. Letter to the editor. *Lancet,* **1**, 1111
38. Palomar, J. M., Halikiopouloush, T. R. (1980) Evaluation of the surgical treatment of Peyronie's disease. *Journal of Urology,* **123**, 680
39. Peyronie, F. de la (1743) Sur quelques obstacles qui s'opposent a l'ejaculation naturelle de la semance. *Mem Acad R Chir,* **425**, 1743
40. Pryor, J. P. (1988) Peyronie's disease in impotence. *Acta Urologica Belgica,* **56**, 317
41. Pryor, J. P., Fitzpatrick, J. M. (1979) A new approach to the correction of penile deformity in Peyronie's disease. *Journal of Urology,* **122**, 622
42. Rossman, B., Mieza, M., Melman, A. (1990) Penile vein ligation for corporal incompetence in evaluation of short-term, and long-term results. *Journal of Urology,* **144,** 679
43. Scardino, P. L., Scott, W. W. (1949) The use of tocopherols in the treatment of Peyronie's disease. *Annals of the New York Academy of Sciences,* **52**, 390
44. Schiffman, Z. J., Gursel, E. O., Laor, R. (1985) Use of dacron patch in Peyronie's disease. *Urology*, **25**, 38
45. Smith, B. H. (1966) Peyronie's disease. *American Journal of Clinical Pathology,* **45**, 670
46. Somers, K. D., Sismour, E. N., Wright, G. L. *et al.*, (1989) Isolation and characterization of collagen in Peyronie's disease. *Journal of Urology,* **141**, 629
47. Somers, K. D., Winters, P. A., Dawson, D. M. *et al.*, (1987) Chromosome abnormalities in Peyronie's disease. *Journal of Urology,* **137**, 672
48. Stranchan, J. R., Pryor, J. P. (1988) Prostacyclin in the treatment of painful Peyronie's disease. *British Journal of Urology,* **61**, 516
49. Van de Berg, J. S., Devine, C. J., Horton, C. E. *et al.*, (1982) Mechanisms of calcification in Peyronie's disease. *Journal of Urology,* **127**, 52
50. Wild, R. M., Devine, C. J., Horton, C. E. (1979) Dermal repair of Peyronie's disease: survey of fifty patients. *Journal of Urology,* **121**, 47
51. Willscher, M. K., Cwazka, W. F., Novicki, D. E. (1979) The association of histocompatibility antigens of the B7 cross-reacting group with Peyronie's disease. *Journal of Urology,* **122**, 34
52. Winter, C. C., Khanna, R. (1975) Peyronie's disease: results with dermo-jet injection of dexamethasone. *Journal of Urology,* **111**, 898
53. Yudkin, J. S. (1977) Peyronie's disease in association with metoprolol. Letter to the Editor. *Lancet,* **2**, 1355
54. Zarafonetis, C. J. D., Horrax, T. M. (1959) Treatment of Peyronie's disease with potassium para-amino benzoate (Potaba). *Journal of Urology,* **81**, 770

# Index

# HOLY MOTHER!

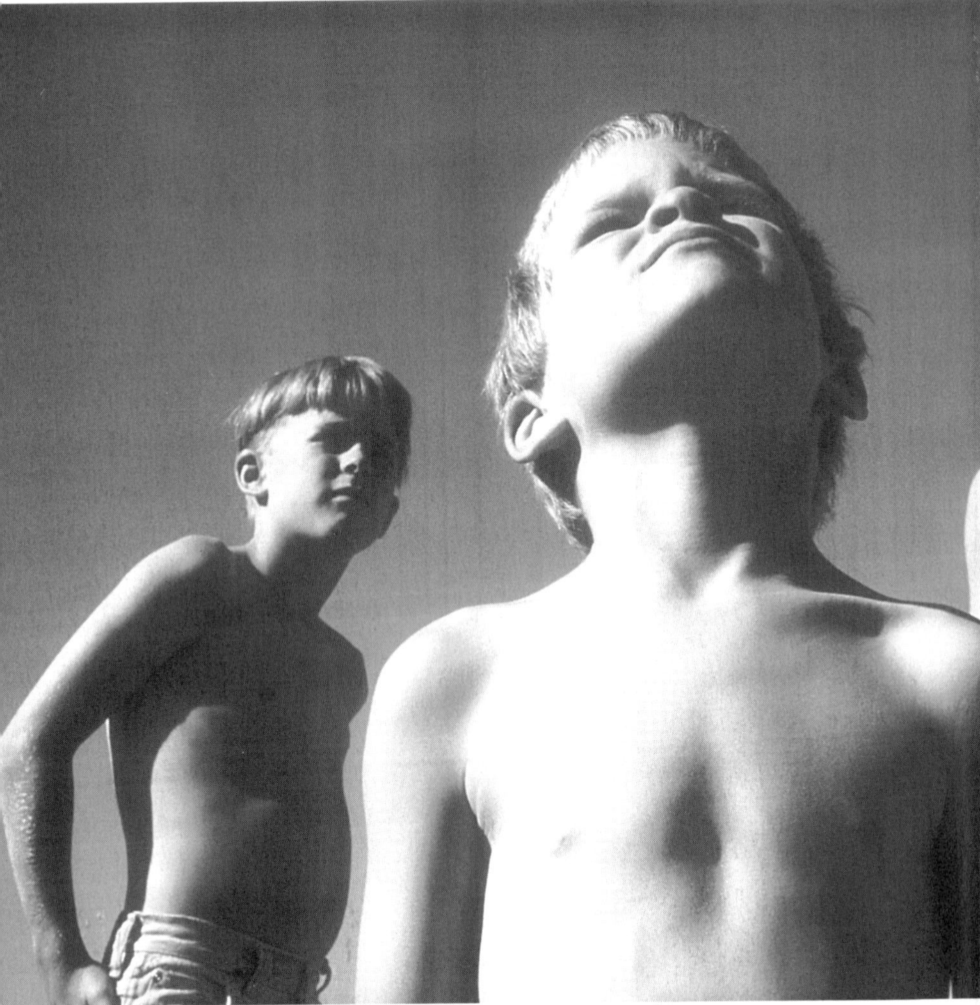

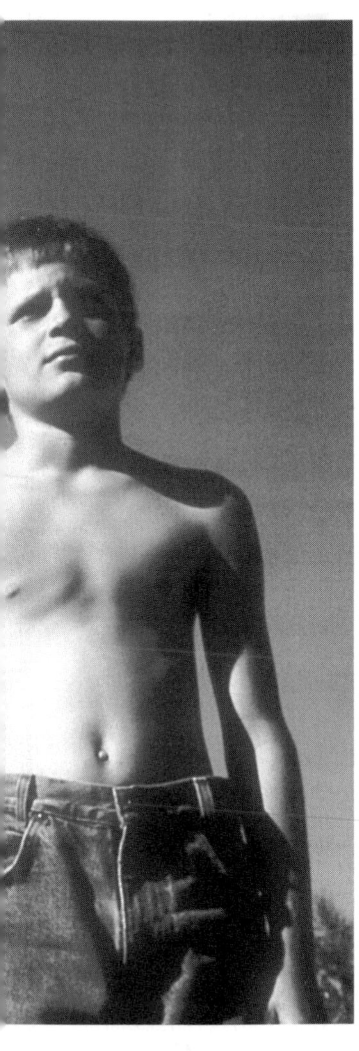

# HOLY MOTHER!

## *Seriously Weird* SIGHTINGS OF THE VIRGIN MARY

DANNY PICCOLO

AND STACEY HOOD

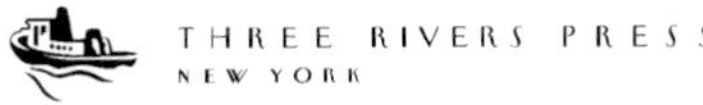

THREE RIVERS PRESS
NEW YORK

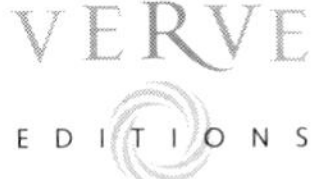

Published by Three Rivers Press, New York, New York.
Member of the Crown Publishing Group, a division of Random House, Inc.

www.randomhouse.com

THREE RIVERS PRESS is a registered trademark
and the Three Rivers Press colophon is a trademark of Random House, Inc.

Printed in the United States of America

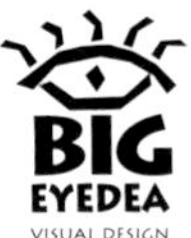


Design and images by Stacey Hood,
Big Eyedea Visual Design, Waitsfield, Vermont

Library of Congress Cataloging-in-Publication Data is available upon request
ISBN 0-609-80916-4
10 9 8 7 6 5 4 3 2 1

**Photography Credits:** AP Photo/Chris O'Meara, cover; Image Bank/Vicky Kasala pp.2-3; Image Bank p. 10; Archive Photos/Reuters/Carol Cleere p. 12; Archive Photos p. 14; Stacey Hood p. 16; Image Bank/Marvin E. Newman p. 18; Image Bank p. 20; Archive Photos/Hebert p. 22; Image Bank/Grant V. Faint p. 28; Image Bank/Kaz Mori p. 30; Image Bank/Stephen Wilkes p. 32; Image Bank/Pete Turner p. 34; Image Bank/Alfred Gescheidt p. 36; Geoffrey Moss p. 39; Archive Newsphotos/Tina Paul p. 40; Archive Photos/Express Newspapers p. 42; Archive Photos p. 44; Image Bank/A. Boccaccio p. 46; Image Bank/Marvin E. Newman p. 48; Image Bank/Alain Chambon p. 50; Archive Photos p. 54; Archive Photos & Image Bank/Joao Paulo p. 56; Image Bank p. 60; Archive Photos p. 62; Magnum Photos/Leonard Freed p. 64; Archive Photos p. 66; Image Bank/Chuck Fishman p. 68; Magnum Photos/Abbas p. 70; Archive Photos/Reuters/Lou Dematteis p. 72; Imapress/S. Viegas p. 74; Magnum Photos/Bob Adelman p. 78; The Washington Times/Mary F. Calvert p. 82; Corbis/Bettmann-UPI p. 84; Archive Photos p. 86; Archive Photos p. 88; The Post-Standard/Li-Hua Lan p. 90; AP Photo/Diane Bondareff p. 92; Archive Photos p. 94; Image Bank/Tim Bieber p. 94.

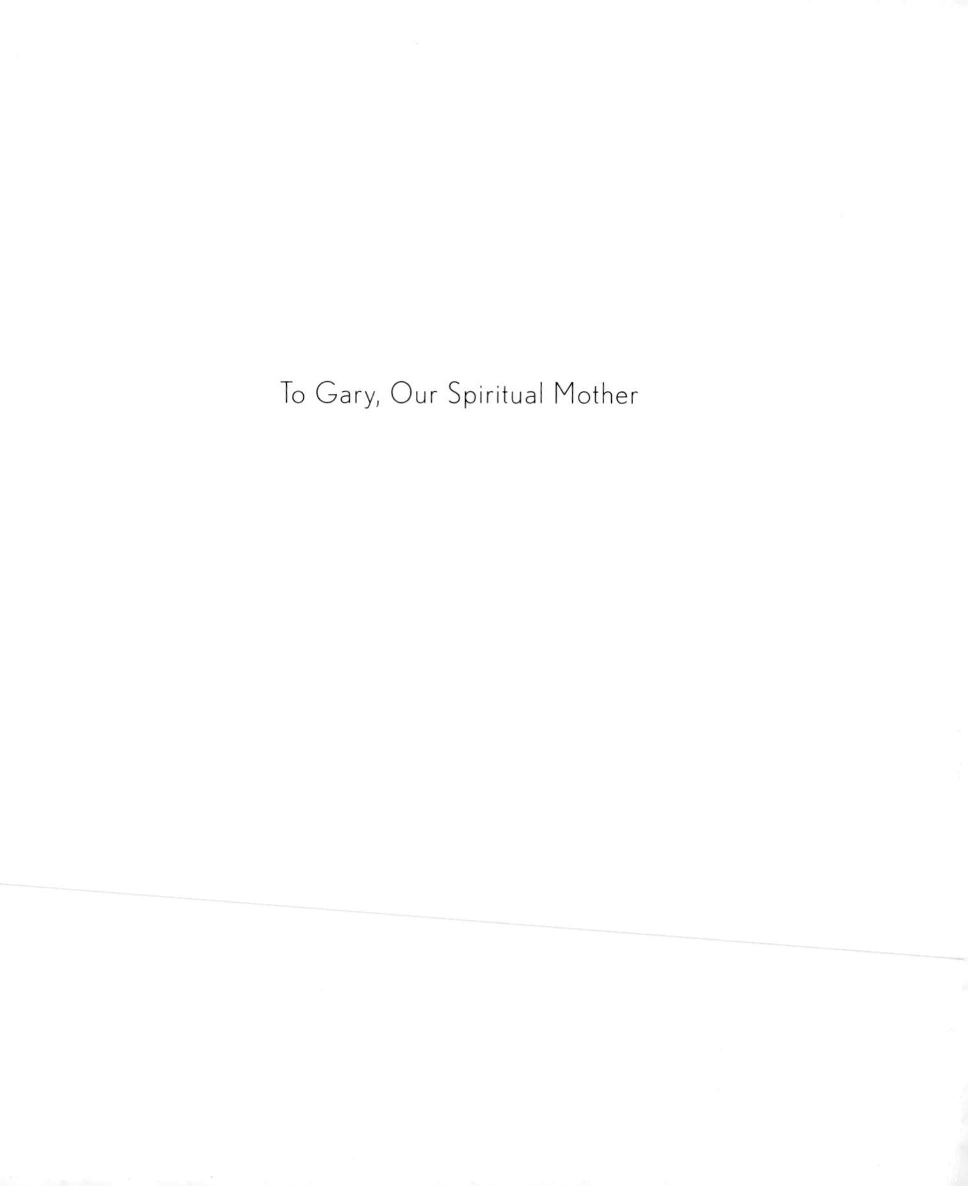

To Gary, Our Spiritual Mother

# Acknowledgments

We would like to thank Sister Mary Elizabeth, Sister Mary Louise, Sister Mary Frances, Sister Mary Joanne, and Sister Mary Gwendolyn. Our knuckles still remember you, but what the heck, where would we be without you?

Not a day goes by without the Virgin Mary making a miraculous and mysterious appearance. A short-order cook cuts open a danish in Tallahassee, and there she is, nestled in a cinnamon swirl. A spinster in Milwaukee stares out a rain-streaked window, and there she is, illuminated in the window pane. A sick child in Milan prays at her bedside, and there she is again!

# Introduction

In fact, in 1999 alone, the Virgin was sighted 117 more times than Elvis! (The Elvis sightings are entirely phony, of course–hallucinatory products of mass hysteria).

We at the Institute of Seriously Weird Virgin Mary Sightings (ISWVMS) have been cataloging these sightings for almost two thousand years now (with a brief hiatus during The Plague). Our archival library in Rome takes up several catacombs. Our files brim with on-site sketches (one, by Leonardo da Vinci, shows The Virgin Mother interceding for a lion at the Colosseum) and photographs. Our field workers have traveled as far as the South Pacific (Our Lady of Bali Hai), the North Pole (Our Lady of the Dog Sleds), and New Jersey (Our Lady of the Dumpster) to document seriously weird appearances of the Mother of God.

And in our state-of-the art laboratory, experts in spiritual forensics pour over hundreds of photographs each day, eliminating photographic trickery and Mary impersonators from the masses of submissions we receive.

It is exacting, painstaking work, but the rewards are supremely gratifying: authenticated sightings of the Magical Madonna.

Yet it is only in the past fifteen years that our job at ISWVMS has been made immensely easier by the close cooperation of the VM herself, who telephones us about seriously weird appearances ahead of time so that we can record them on film. What is more, The Eternal Mother has submitted to the occasional post-photo-op background interview, filling us in on the whys and wherefores of the mountainous schedule of daily miracles. (For example, why an appearance in Newark and not Jersey City?)

Our mission is strictly scientific. We are not polemicists; we do not wish to rub anybody's nose in elephant dung. We are simply truth seekers.

Here then, for the first time in book form, are the best, most provocative, and inspiring Seriously Weird Virgin Mary Sightings. It's a miracle, *nu*?

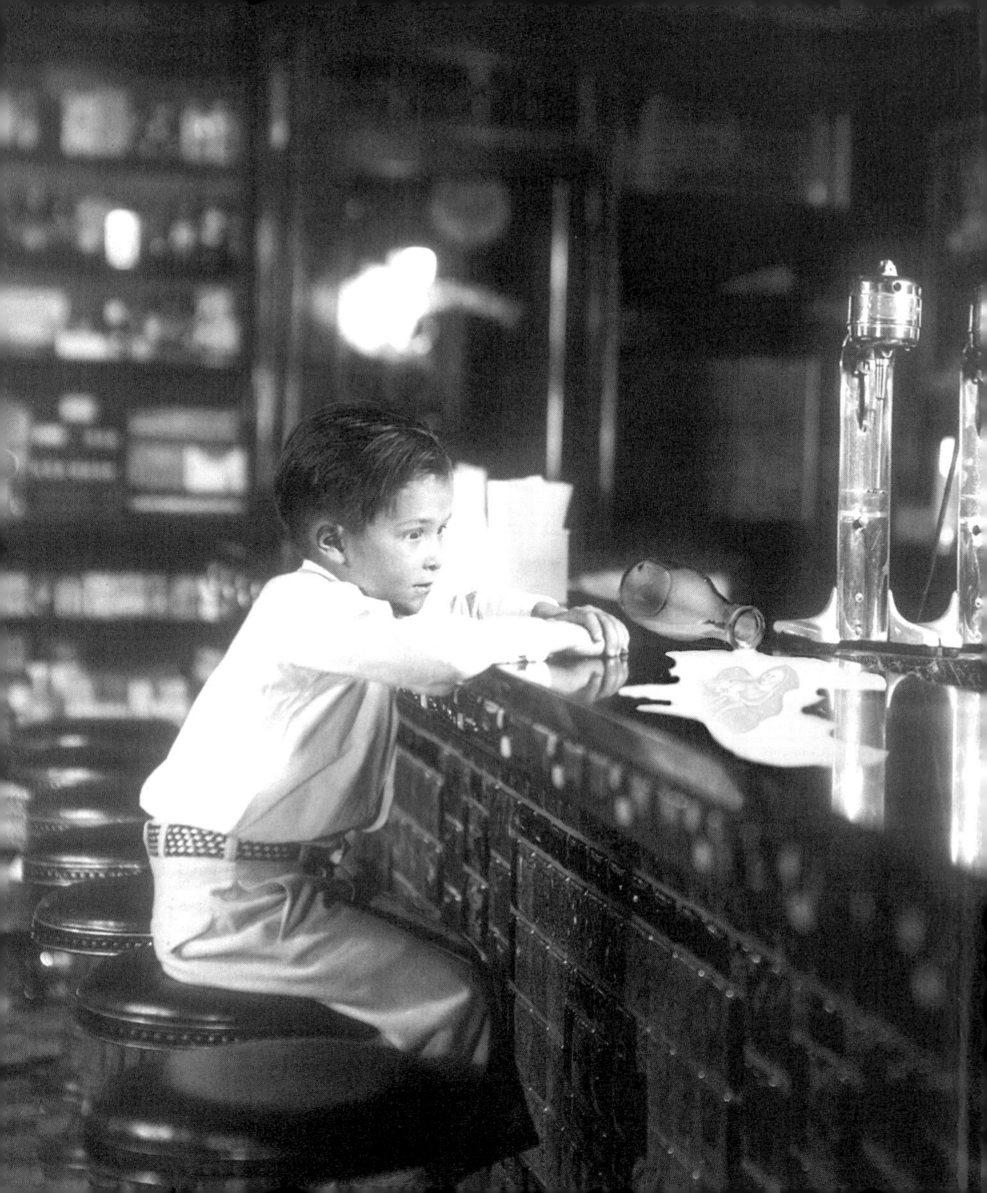

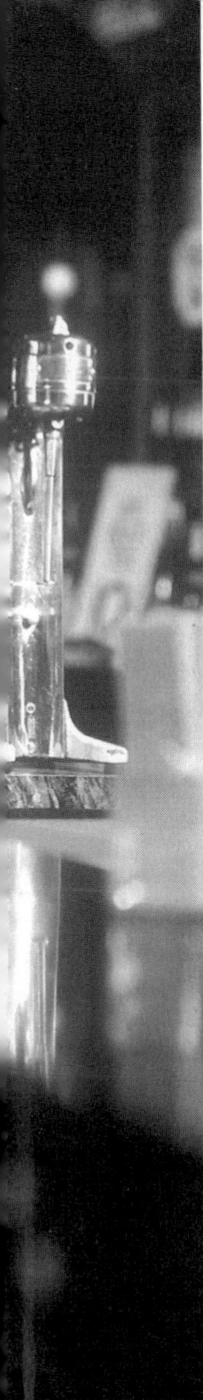

When Teddy "Buster" Malloy knocked over the milk bottle at Farnsworth's Drugs in Terre Haute in 1948, Mary made one of her miraculous "ooze" appearances. "Don't cry," the Virgin Mother whispered from the puddle.

# Miracle of The Malted

To this day, the Malted Mary Shrine still stands in Farnsworth's, where dairy farmers from every state in the union make an annual pilgrimage.

"Buster" Malloy, now 60, swears that he hasn't cried since '48.

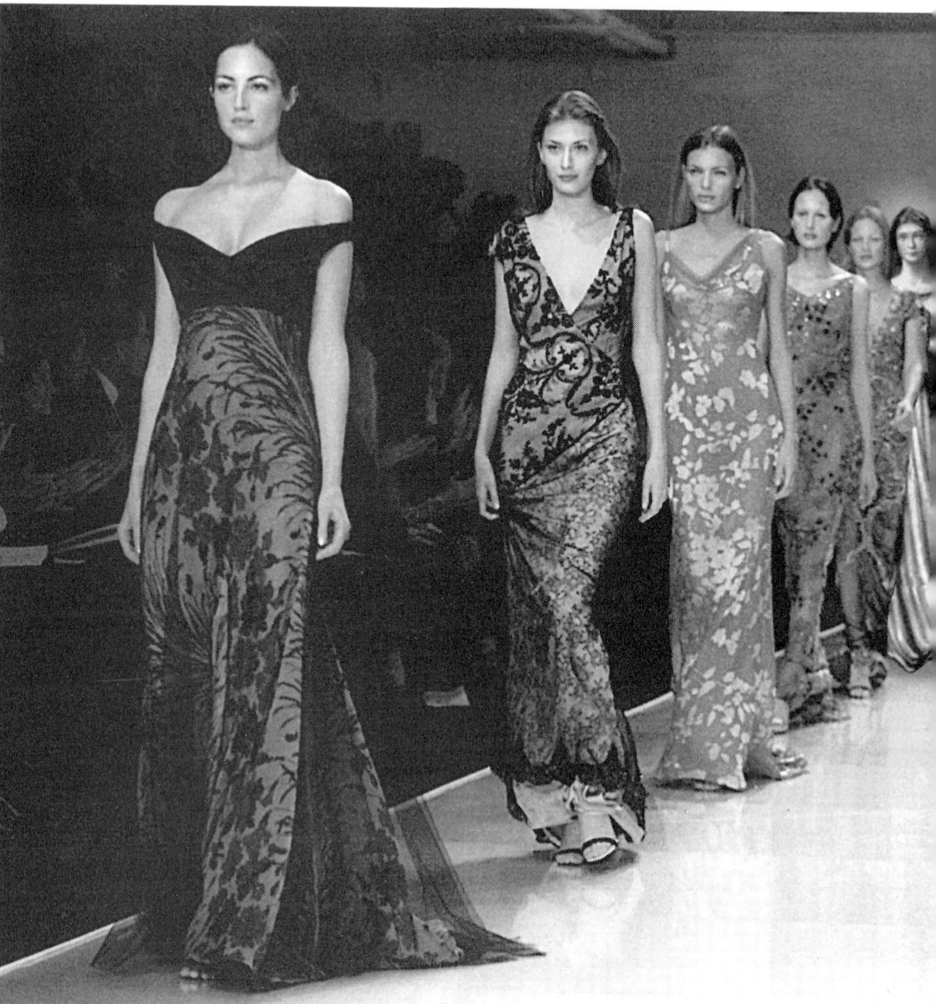

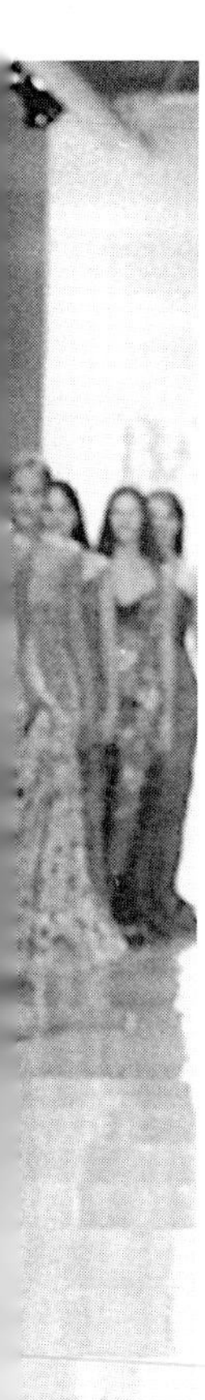

# Sister Mary Chic

With church attendance among yuppies at record lows, the Mother of God has initiated an outreach program just blocks away from St. Patrick's Cathedral in Manhattan.

"They come to see the dresses," Mary says, "but I drop Mass Cards into their Givenchy bags."

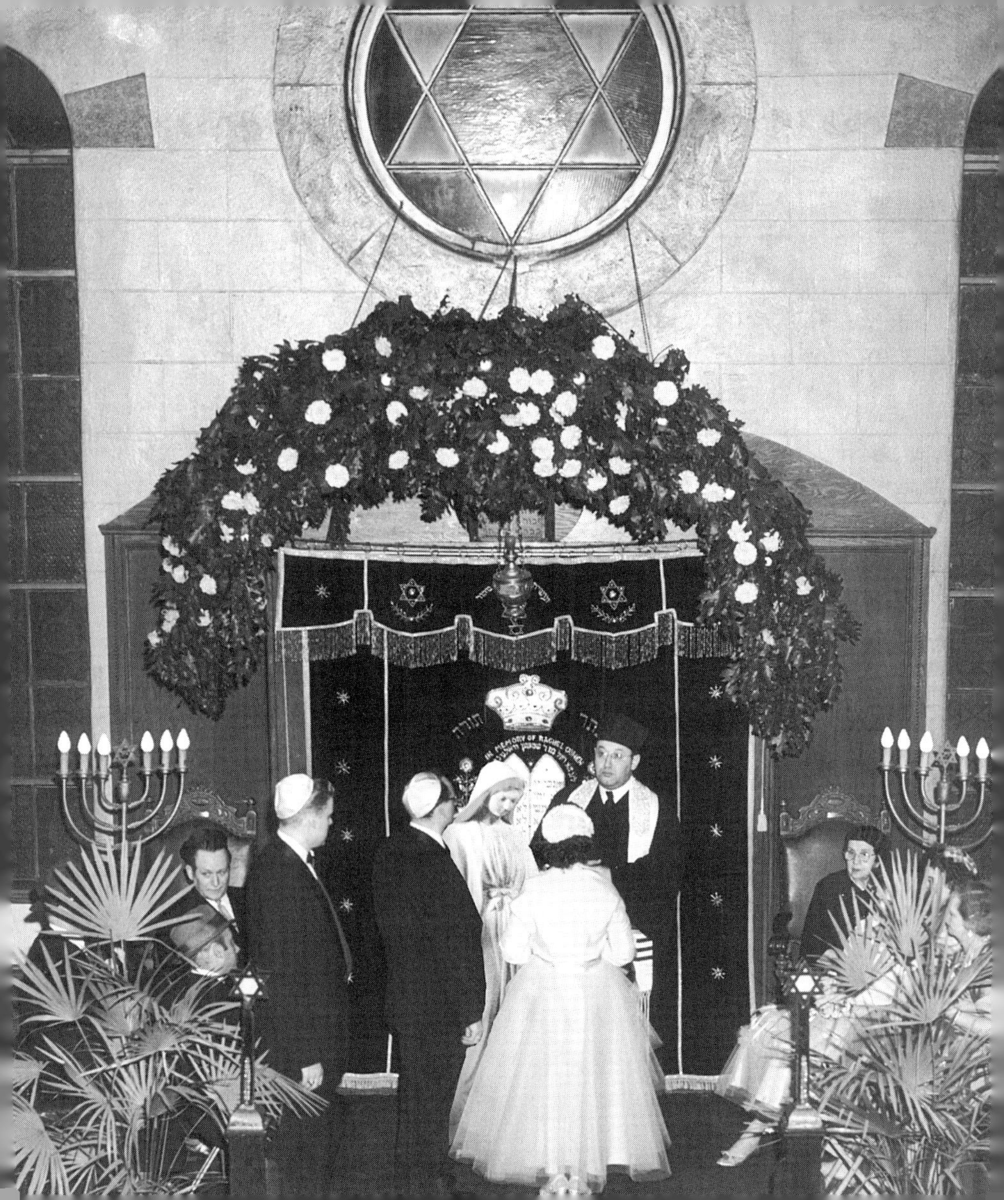
תורה
IN MEMORY OF RACHEL

"My boy, he never married," says the Virgin Mother ruefully. "I know, he didn't have a steady job, but still he was a real catch. Sometimes I wonder, could something have been wrong with Him?"

# Once A Jewish Mother

As a balm against this hole in her life, Mary attends as many weddings as she can squeeze into her busy schedule.

"Sure, it's a big thrill being the Mother of God," she says, "but think of it–no grandchildren!"

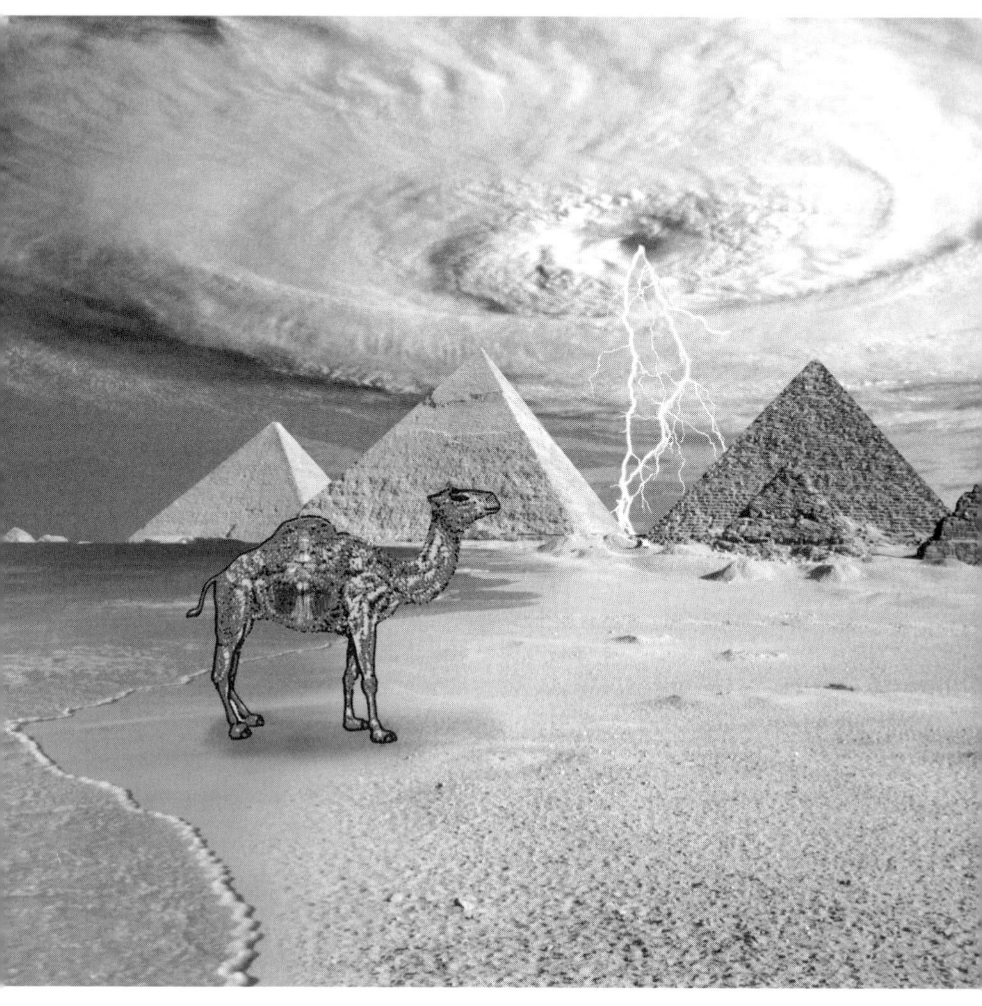

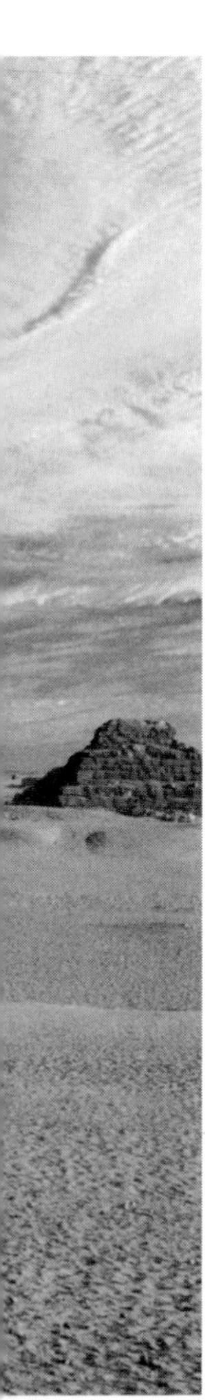

Now, in her early 2000s, the Virgin Mother has occasional mental lapses, as this photograph illustrates. Recalling her Son's famous words, "It is easier for a camel to pass through

# The Hump Conundrum

the eye of a needle than for a rich man to pass into the Kingdom of God," Mary was moved to perform a miracle. But in her confusion, she tried to pass through the camel.

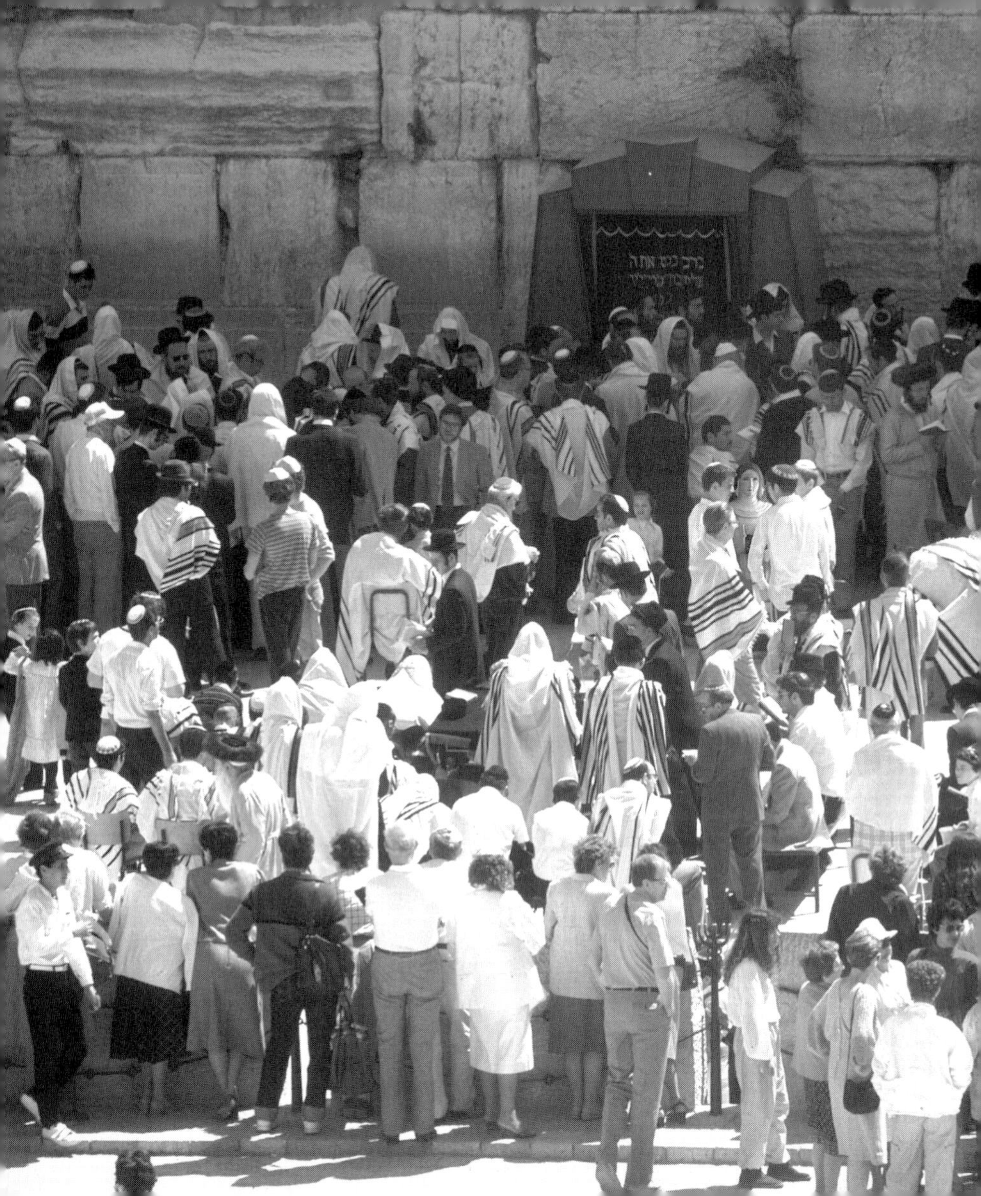

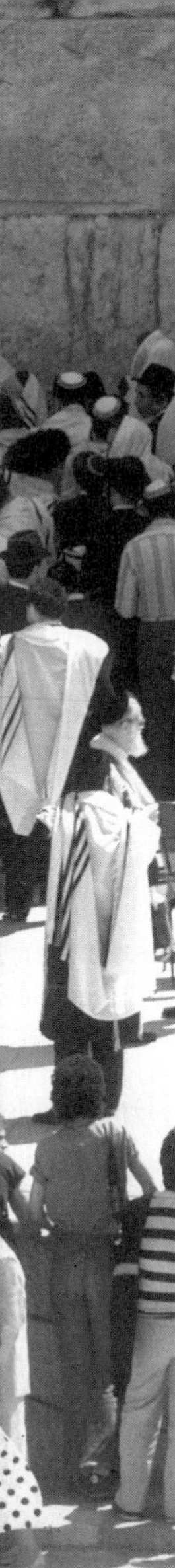

# Cry Me A River

"Old habits die hard," says the Mother of the First Christian, seen here praying at the Wailing Wall in Jerusalem. "Anyway, it's near home, and let's face it, it's a good place to meet men my age."

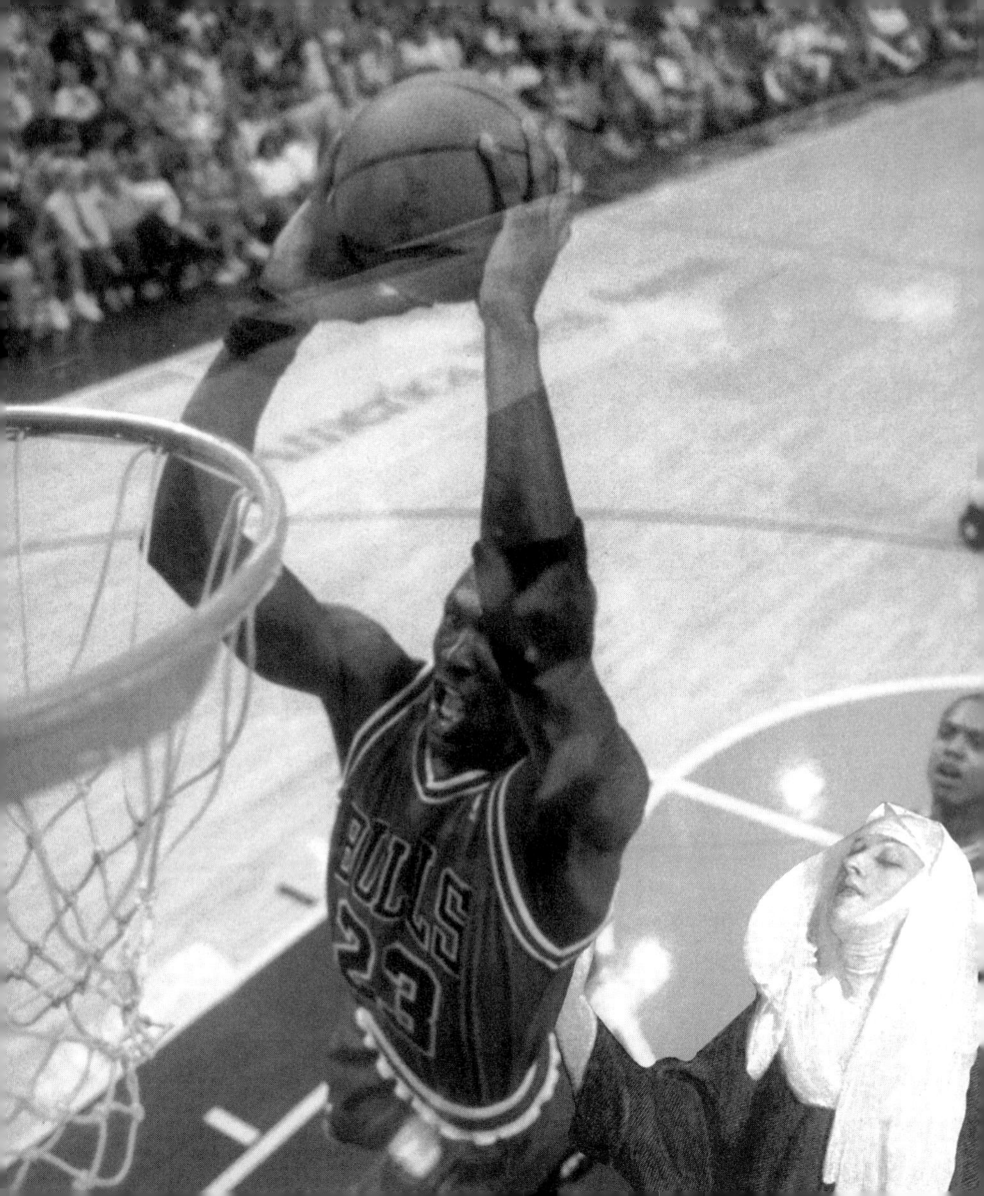
BULLS
23

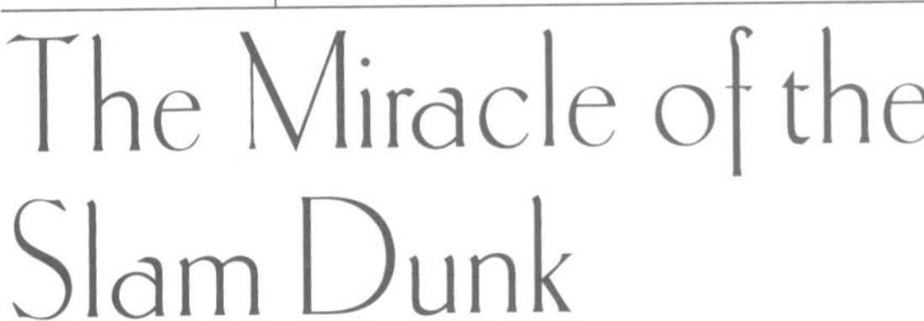

# The Miracle of the Slam Dunk

"They call him 'Air Jordan,'" says Sister Mary, "but let's be real, gravity is gravity. So I give a little helping hand."

When asked if she thought this was giving Jordan an unfair advantage, the Virgin replied, "Hey, who said miracles were fair?"

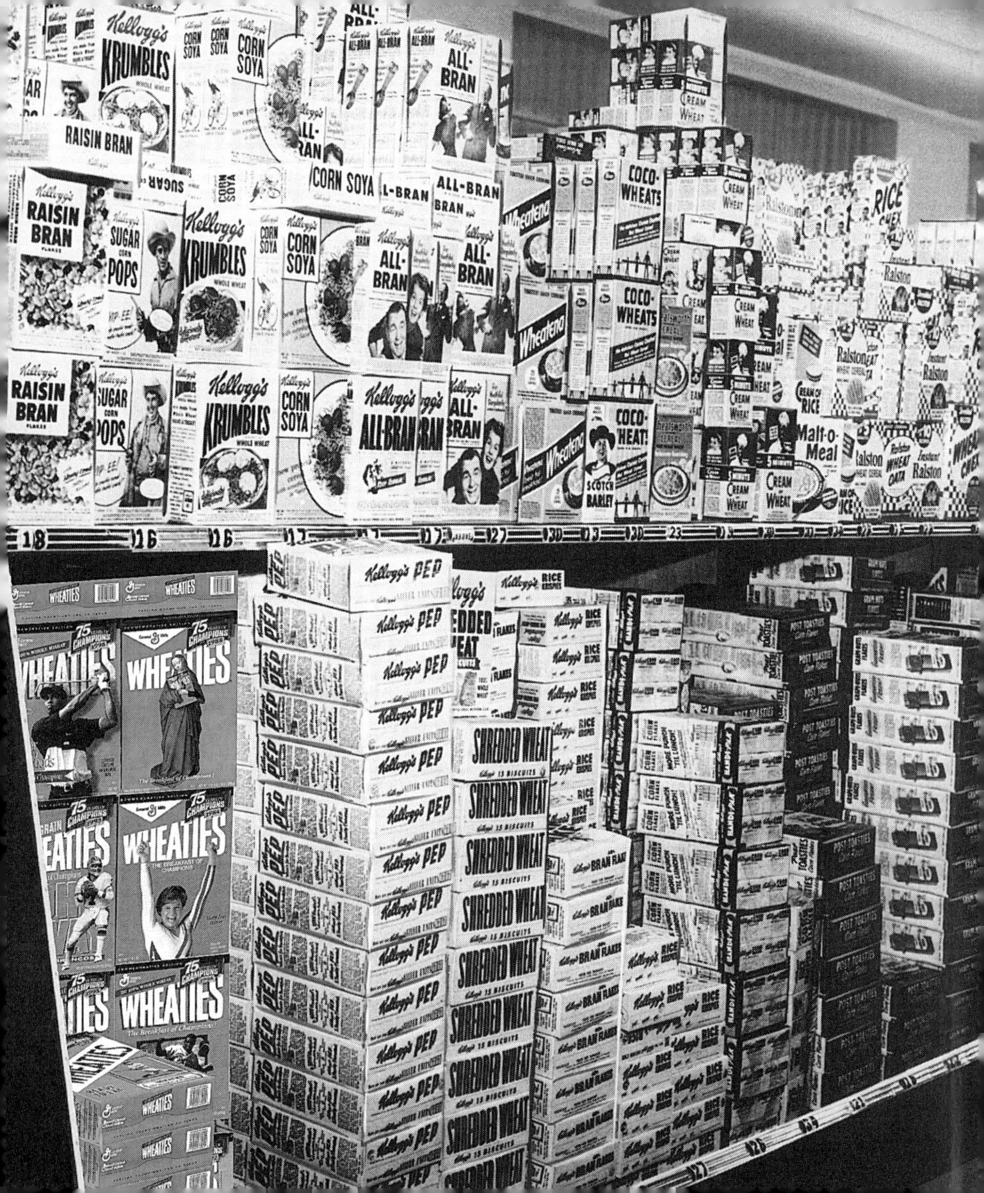

Kellogg's KRUMBLES WHOLE WHEAT
CORN SOYA
ALL-BRAN
RAISIN BRAN
Kellogg's RAISIN BRAN FLAKES
SUGAR CORN POPS
Wheatena
COCO-WHEATS
CREAM OF WHEAT
Ralston
RICE CHEX
Malt-o-Meal
CREAM OF RICE
Instant Ralston
WHEAT CHEX
SCOTCH BARLEY
WHEATIES
75 YEARS OF CHAMPIONS
The Breakfast of Champions
Kellogg's PEP
Kellogg's RICE KRISPIES
SHREDDED WHEAT
Kellogg's BRAN FLAKES
POST TOASTIES

A recent survey by the World Health Organization (WHO) revealed that Irish Catholics were more likely to skip breakfast than any other group.

"That's an awful way to start the day," says the Virgin Mother. "And

# Our Lady of the Flakes

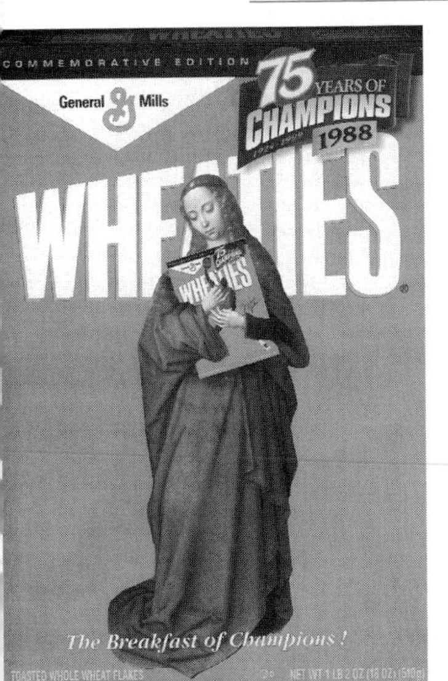


everyone knows that it's bad to drink on an empty stomach."

And that is why Sister Mary agreed to appear on the box of this popular General Mills product.

"We're currently in the talking stage about breakfast wafers," Mary confided to us.

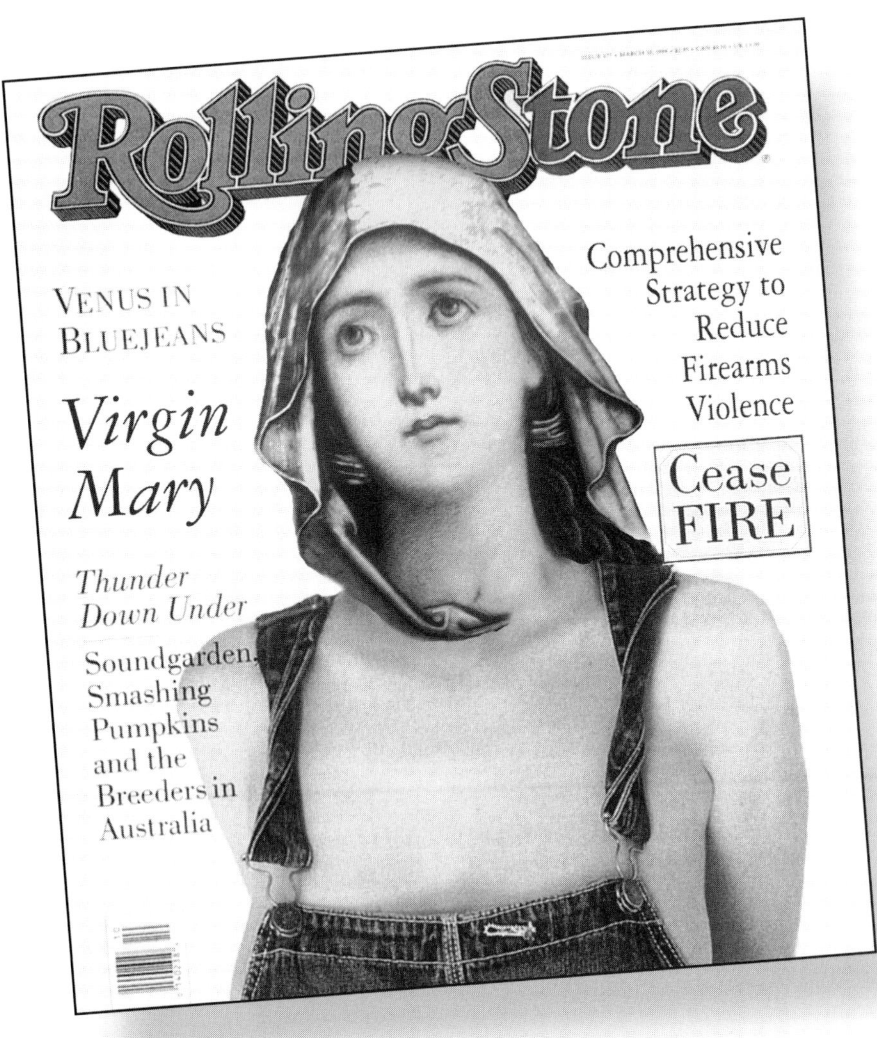

RollingStone
Comprehensive
Strategy to
Reduce
Firearms
Violence
VENUS IN
BLUEJEANS
Virgin
Mary
Cease
FIRE
Thunder
Down Under
Soundgarden,
Smashing
Pumpkins
and the
Breeders in
Australia

# Our Lady Who Gathers No Moss

In her current "Outreach To Slackers" campaign, Mary "Like A Virgin" Mother of God agreed to appear on the cover of *Rolling Stone*.

"The photo shoot went on and on," Mary complained. "'Look this way, look that way. Show me more feeling.' I'm telling you, Michelangelo took less time."

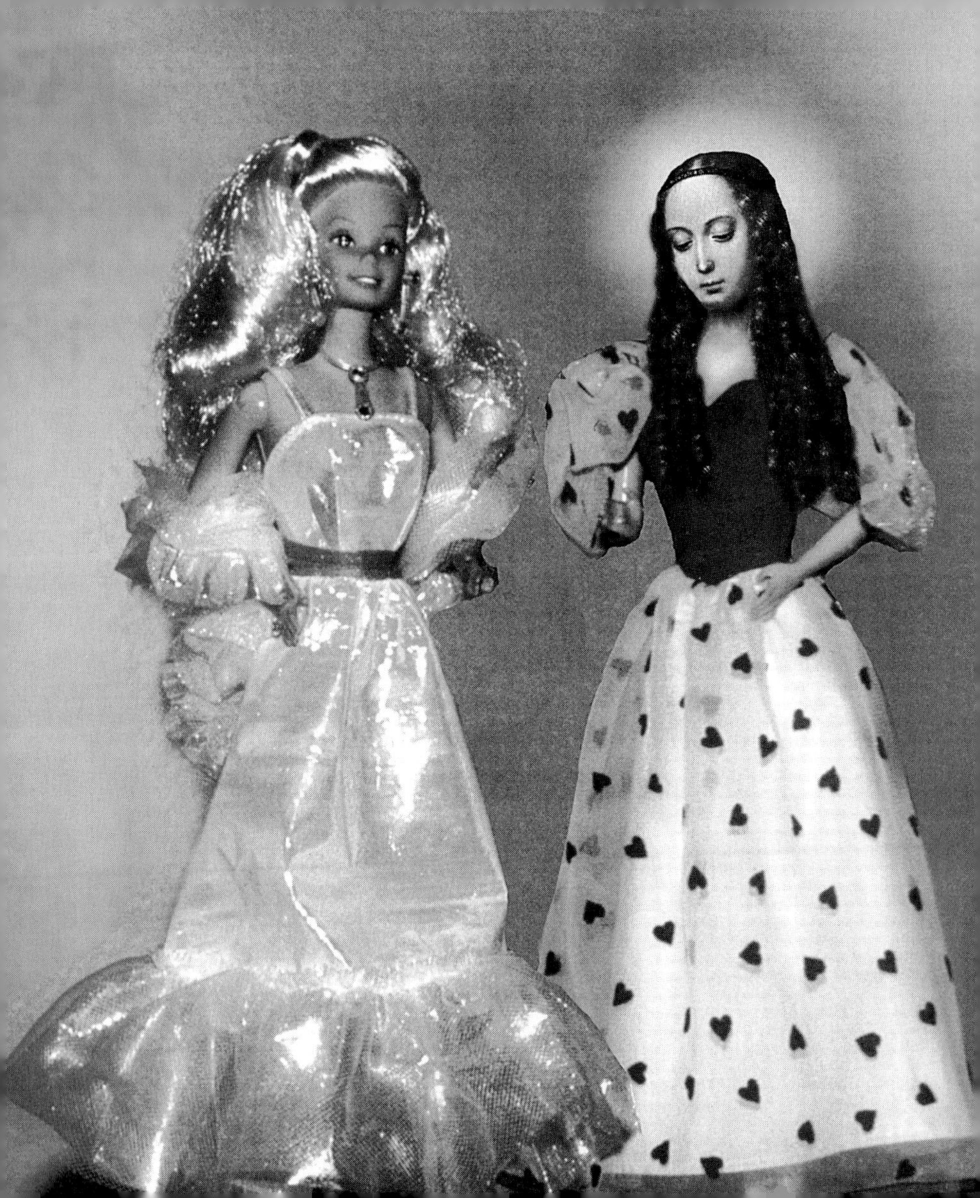

Lydia Westfall, 7, of Tom's River, New Jersey, took this photograph of her Barbie collection just seconds after Mary suddenly appeared as "Valentine Barbie."

# The Miracle of the Virgin Barbie

"I sure am glad I took this picture because the next minute she was gone, and my mother never would have believed me," the little girl said. "Like Mom woulda thought I was sniffing glue or something."

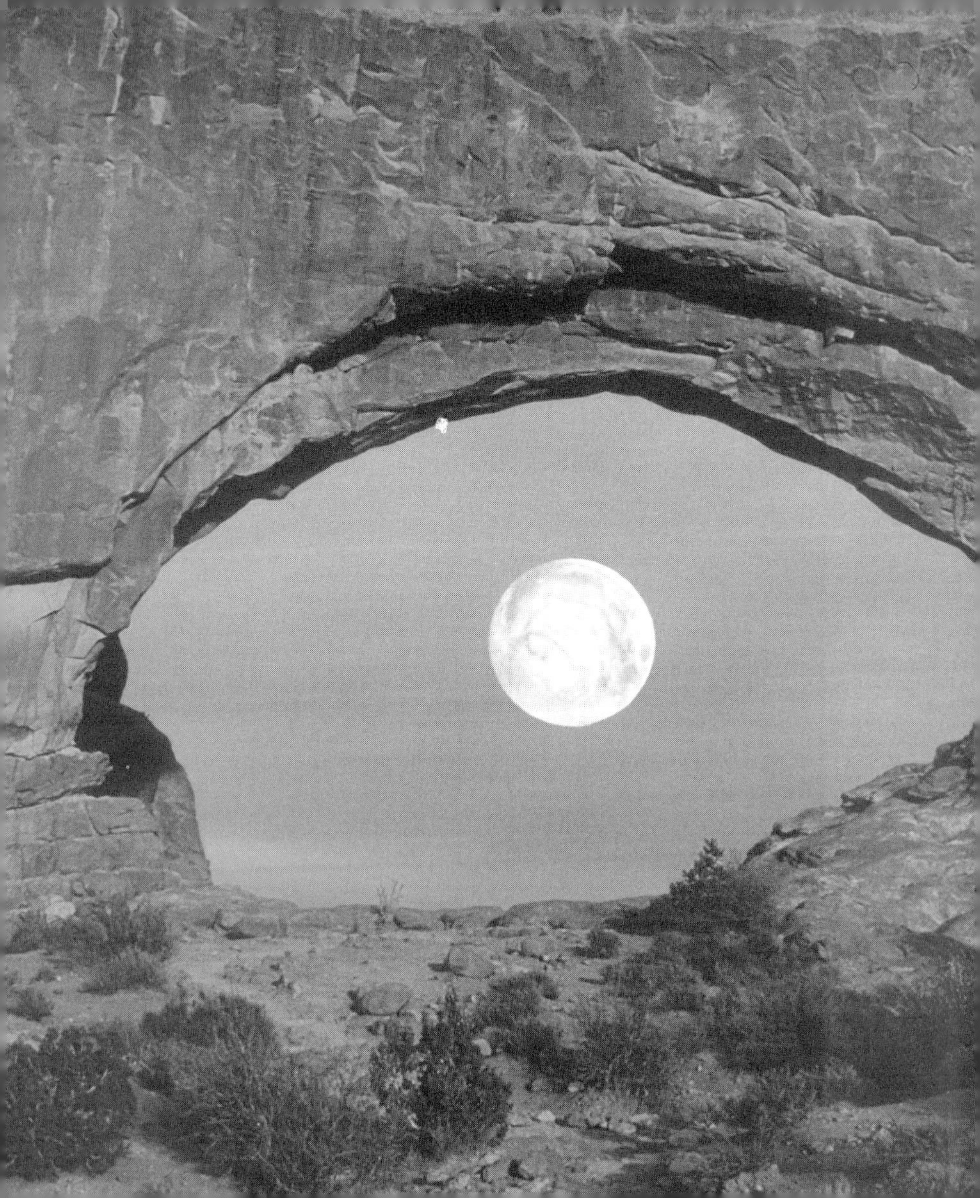

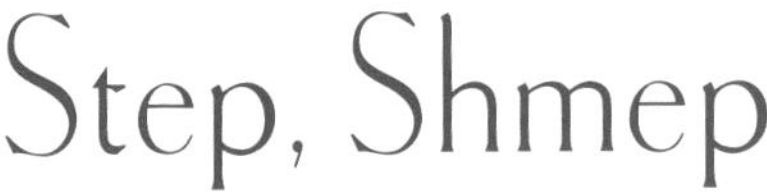

# Step, Shmep

"For Neil, it was 'One step for mankind' and all that hullabaloo," Mary says bemusedly. "But for me, it's just part of my daily rounds."

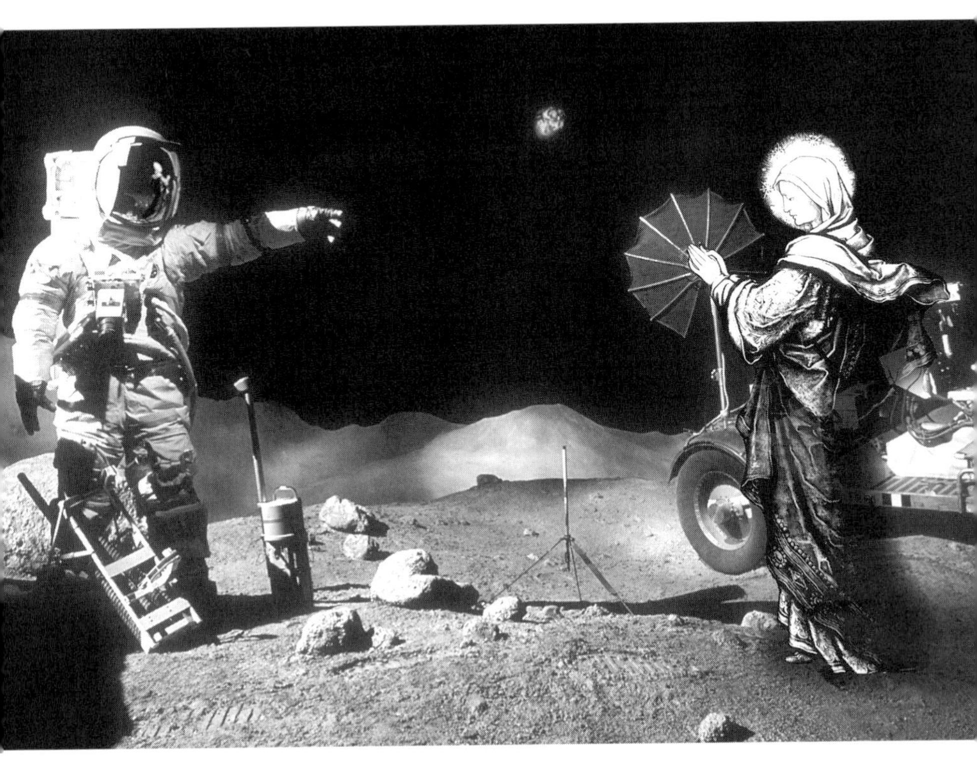

# The Miracle of NASA

On a tip, we discovered this photo in NASA's archives via the Freedom of Information Act.

"Okay, so it wasn't all booster rockets that got Armstrong up there," the Mother of God confessed to us. "But I just couldn't stand the idea of the Russians beating us."

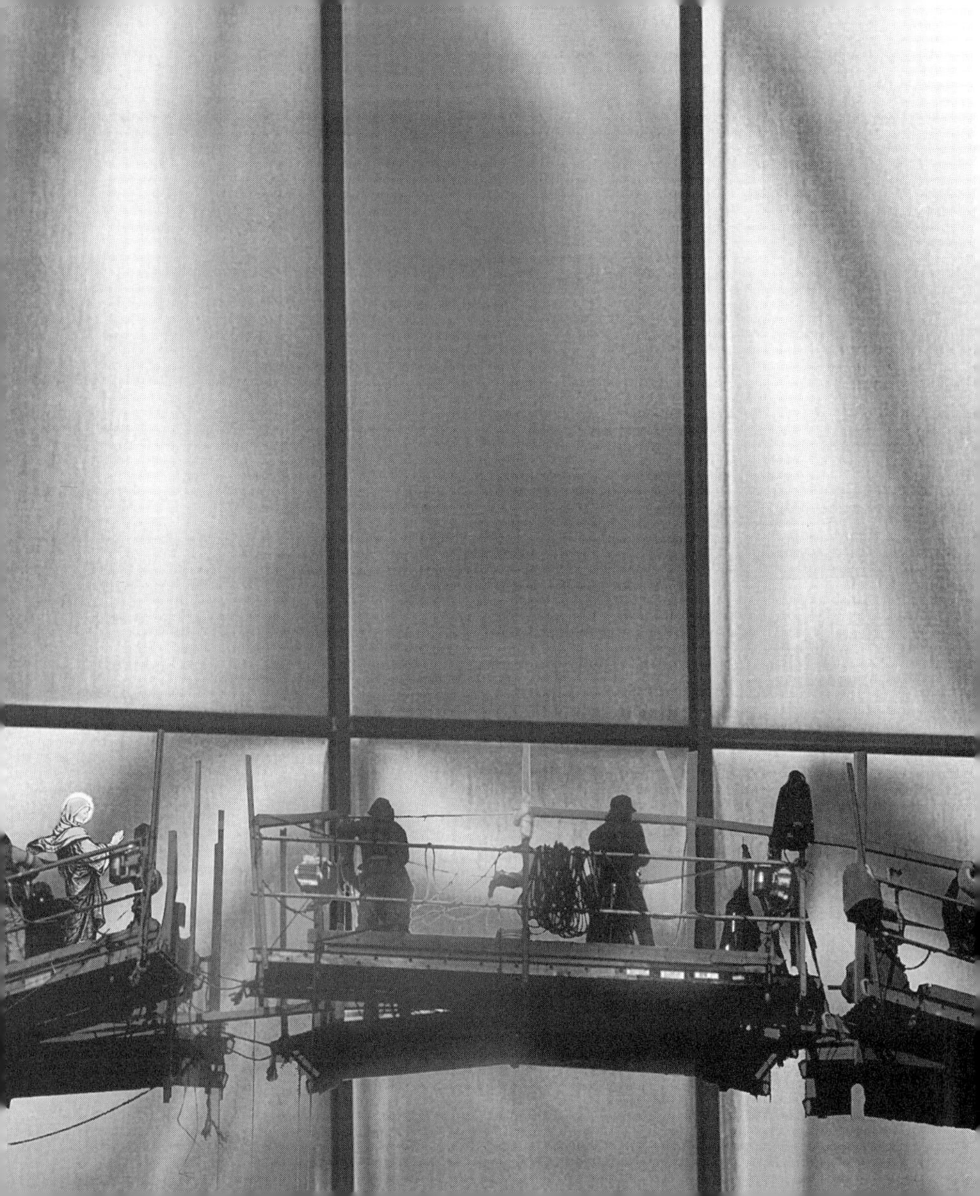

# "You Call This a Miracle?"

Responding to the all the excitement caused by the "Miracle of Mary in the Window" on the office building in Florida, the Mother of God came to town to check it out.

"It's a disgrace," she announced after viewing it. "Shoddy workmanship. Why I've seen better 'miracles' in Disneyland!"

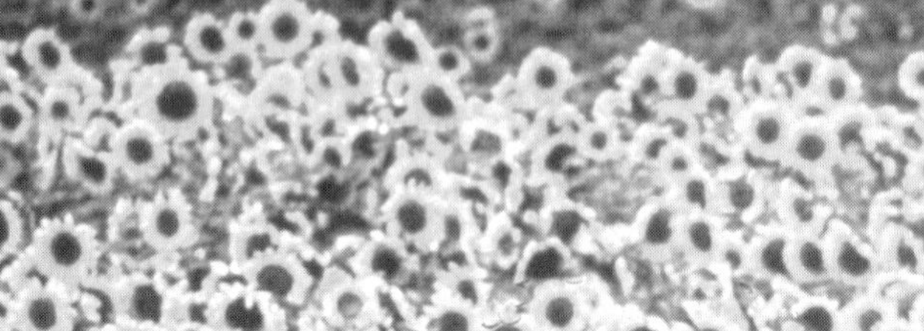

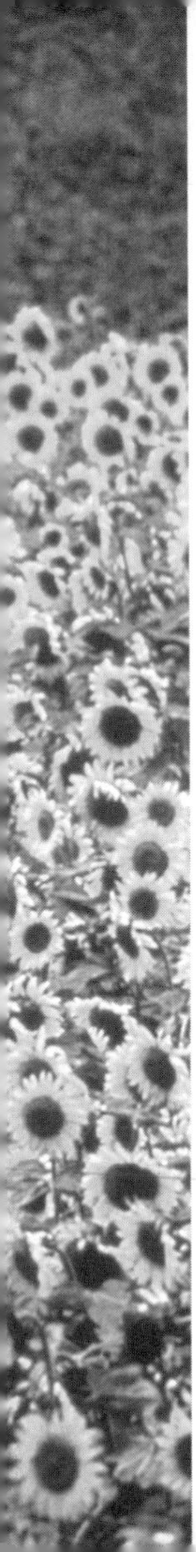

# Our Lady of the Sunflowers

It took our research department months to detect Mary's image in this photograph. When we questioned Sister Mary about its significance, she replied, "Actually, I was just fooling around. It was kind of a slow day for charitable works."

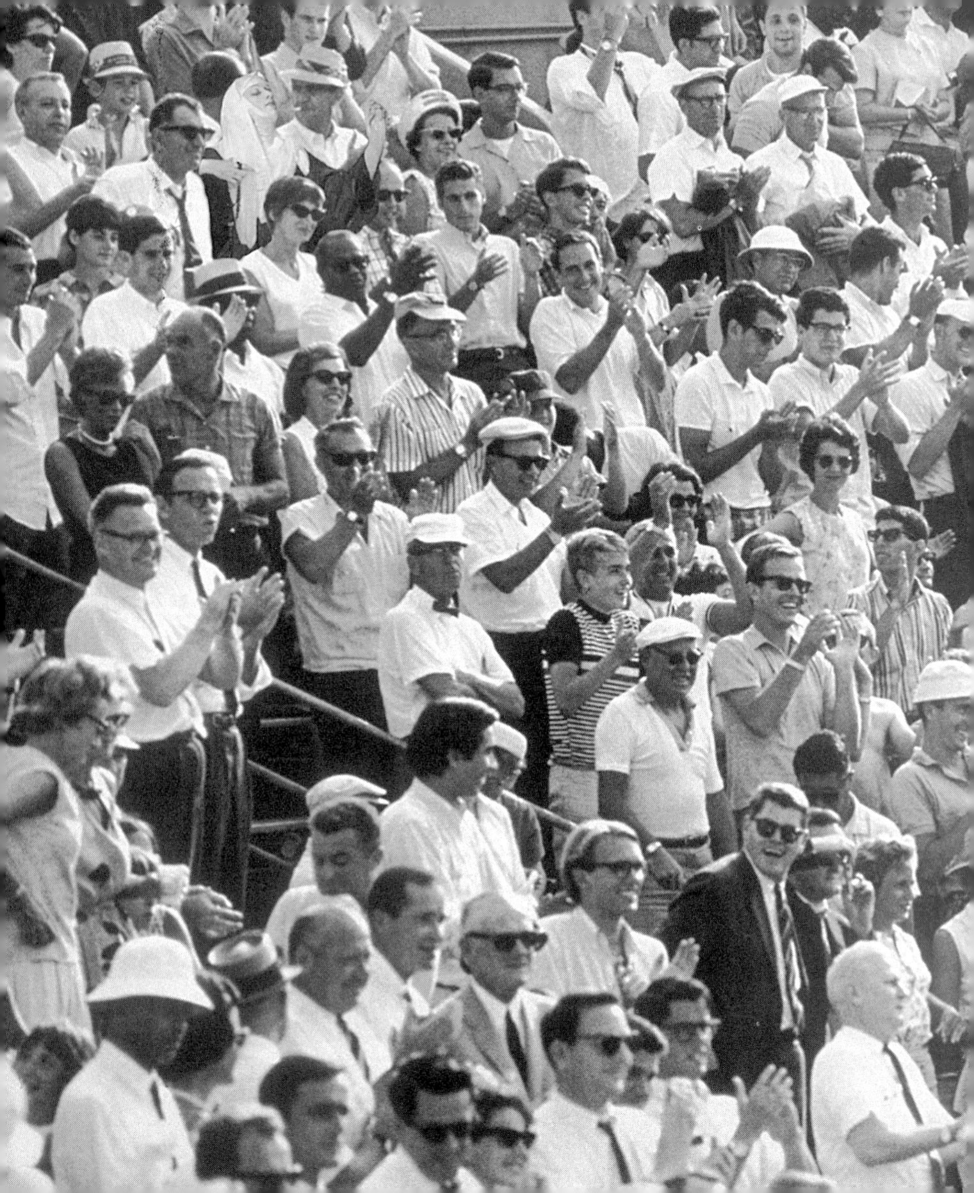

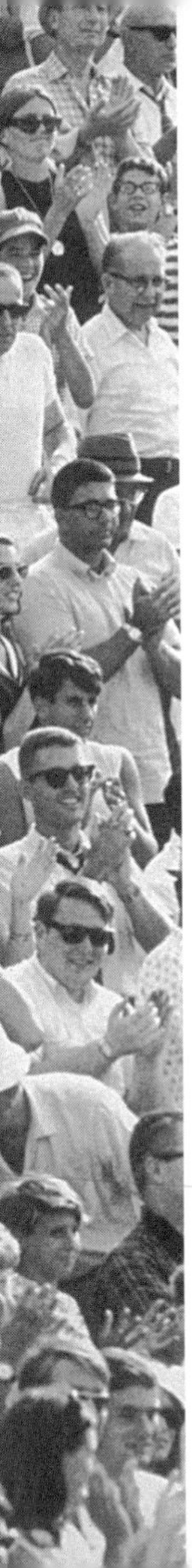

# Love/Thirty

Seen here at the U.S. Open, the Virgin Mother has a passion for tennis that goes back to 17th-century England, where she was a fan of court tennis.

"Not many people know this, but I'm the one who changed the 'zero' to 'love' in score-keeping," she informed us. "I think it sounds so much more Christian, don't you?"

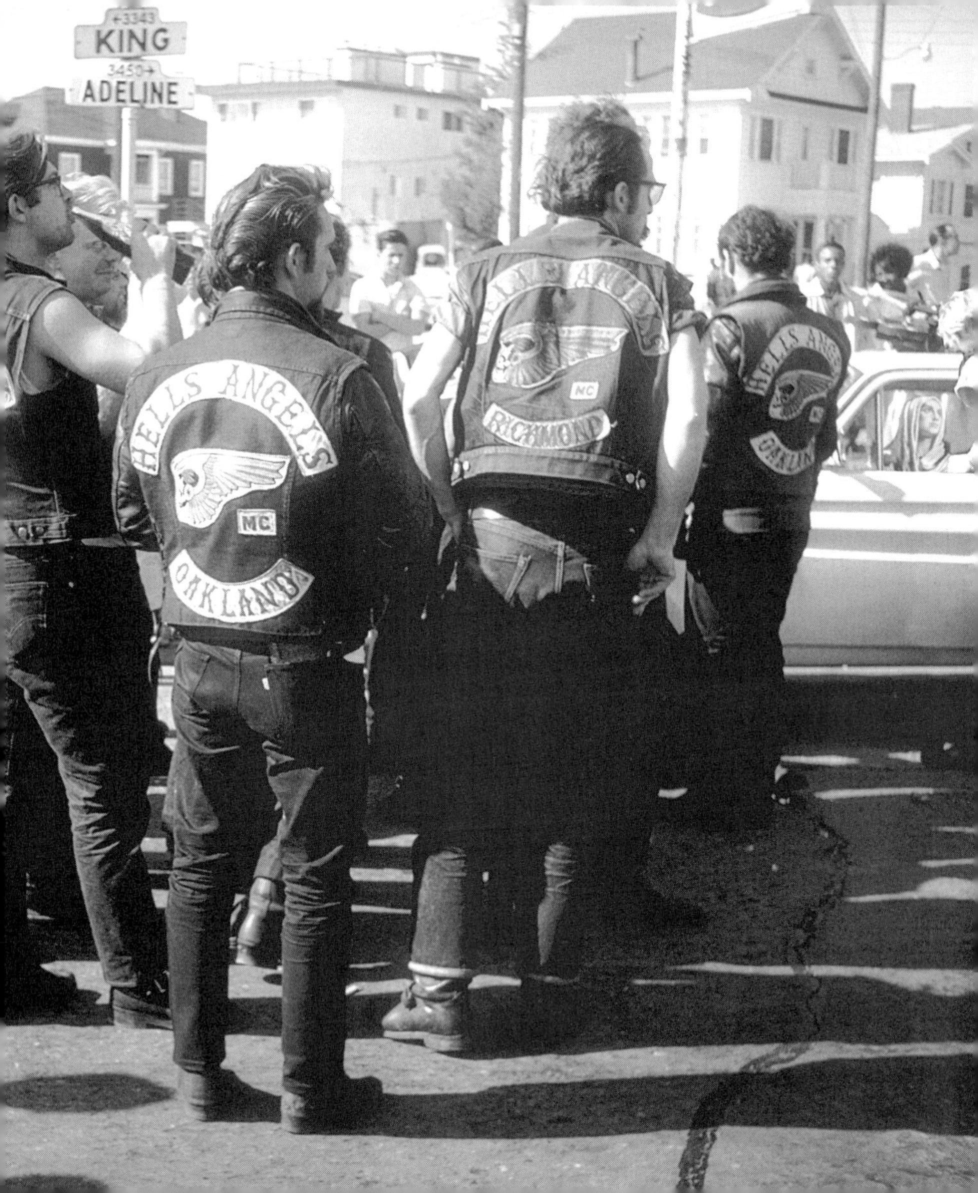
3343
KING
3450
ADELINE
HELLS ANGELS
MC
OAKLAND
MC
RICHMOND

# Our Lady of the Choppers

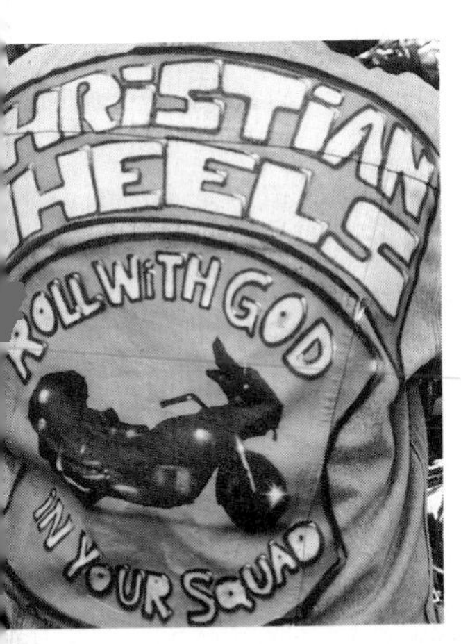


One of the Mother of God's longstanding crusades is to get the Hell's Angels to change their name, but negotiations keep breaking down.

"'Mary's Angels' would be nice. Or 'Mommy's Little Angels,'" Mary told us. "But they weren't buying."

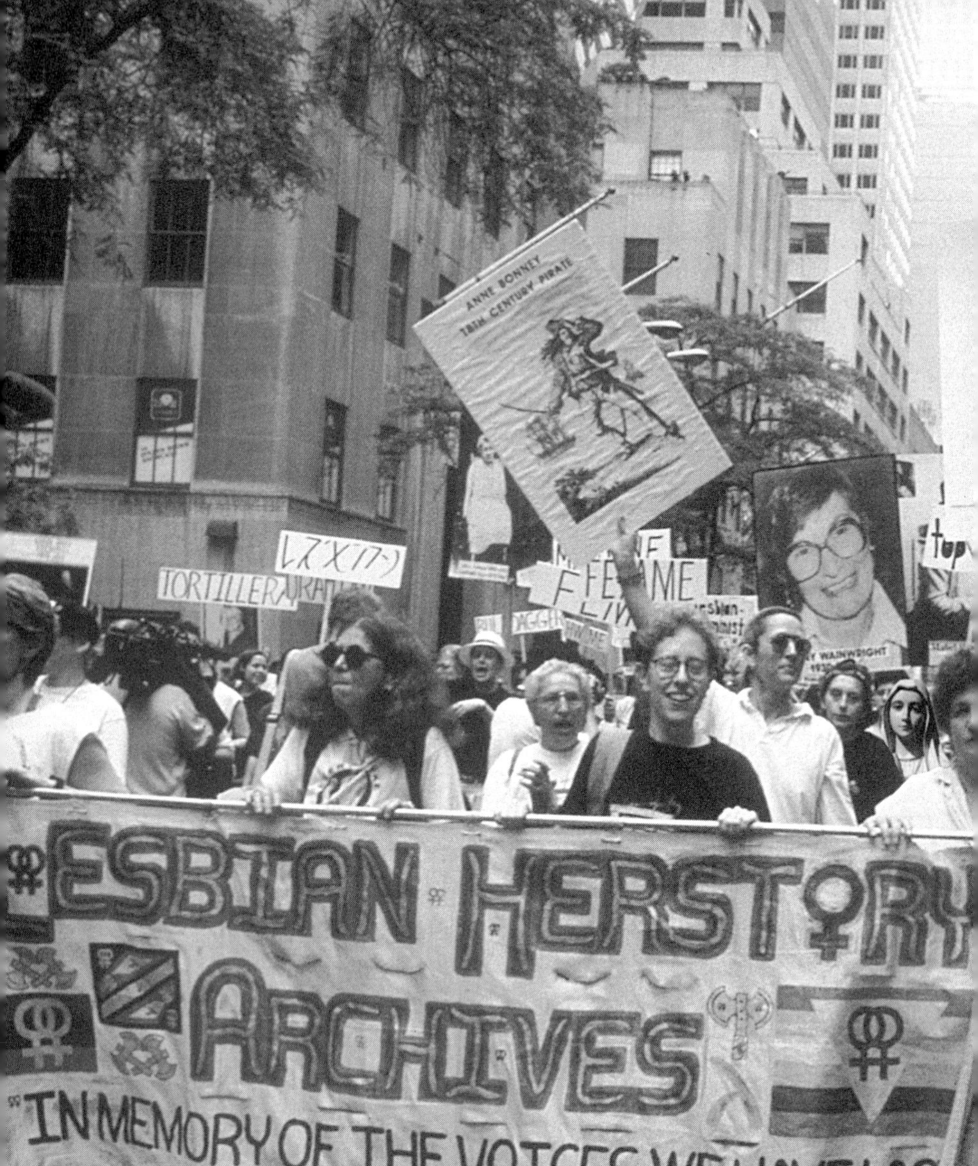
ANNE BONNEY
18TH CENTURY PIRATE
FEMME
ESBIAN HERSTORY
ARCHIVES
IN MEMORY OF THE VOICES WE HAVE LOS

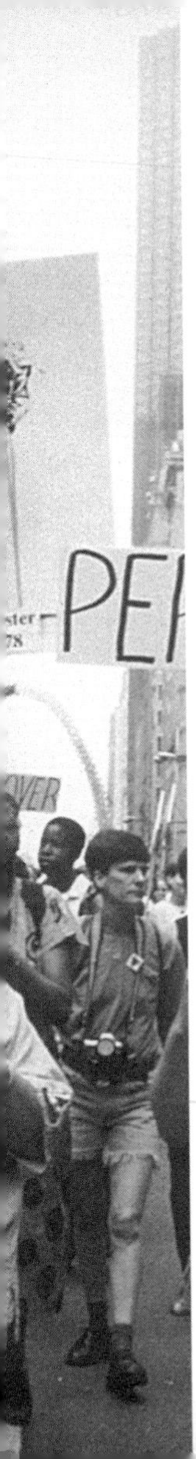

# Sisters of No Mercy

"One of my son's friends said that we should try to be all things to all people," Sister Mary told us, referring to one of the Gospels. "Well, God knows I'm trying, but these so-called 'sisters' feel more like brothers, if you know what I mean."

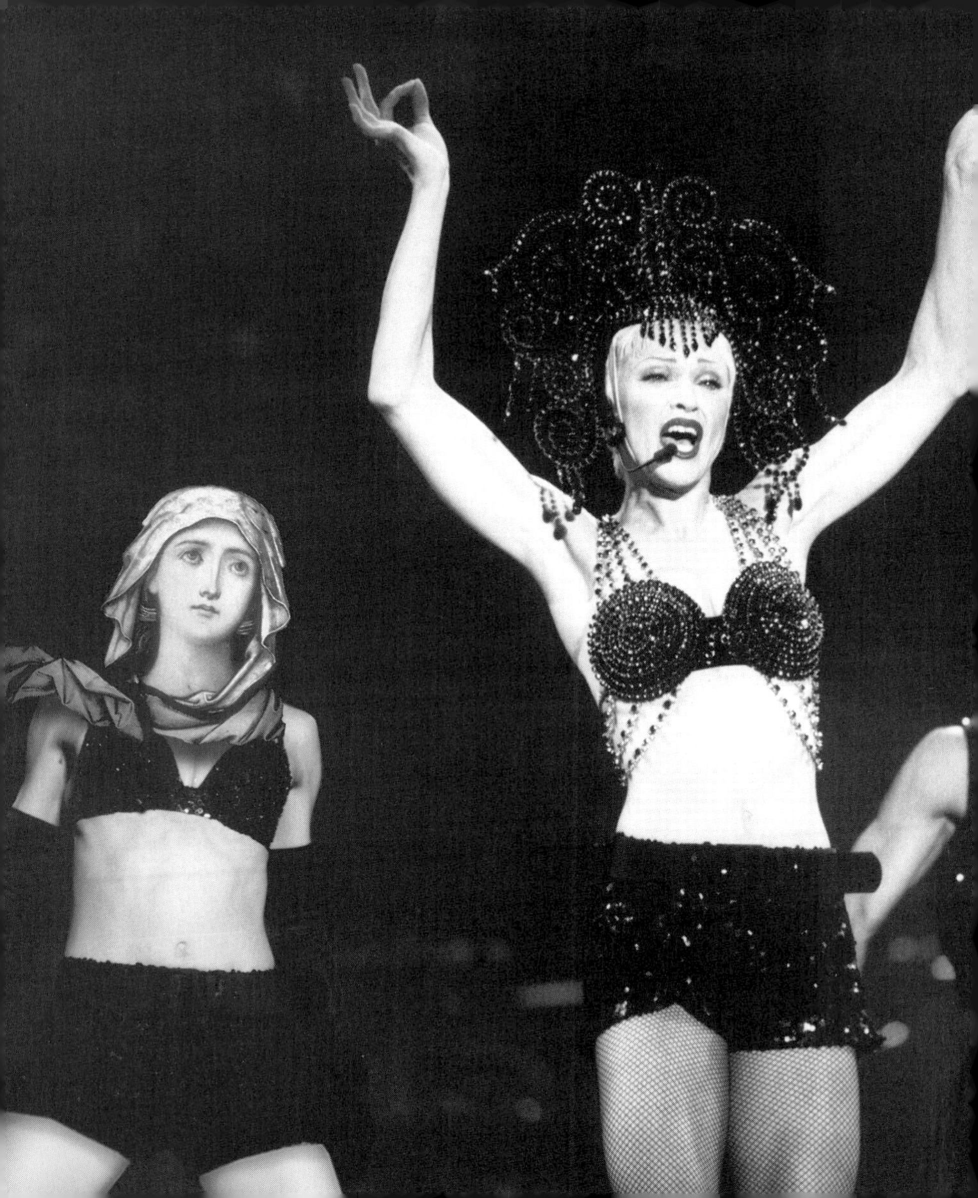

The Holy Madonna performs miracles of grace and charity at a rate of two to three thousand per day, so once in a while she performs one just for herself.

# Exactly Like a Virgin

"I always wondered what it would feel like to be a knockout," she says, photographed here performing in a music video with her namesake and heroine. "Joseph, may he rest in peace, always complained that I was too dowdy."

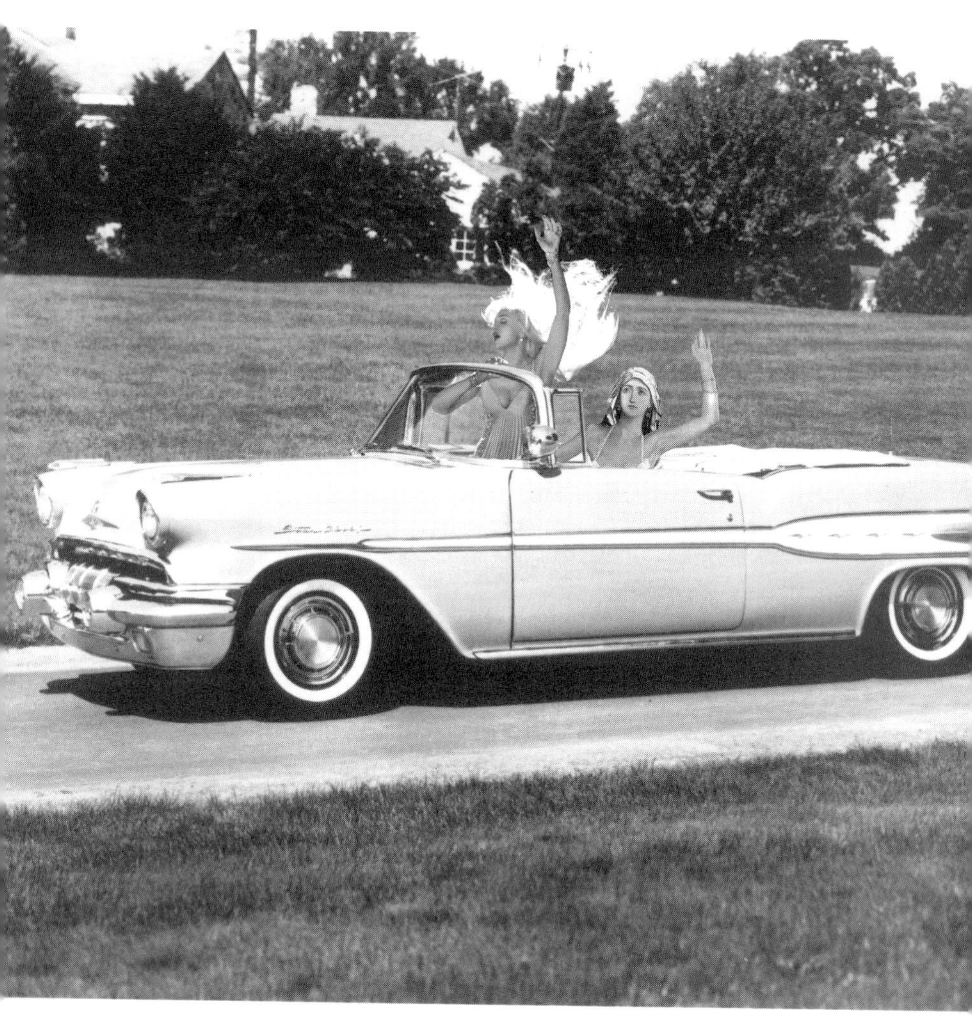

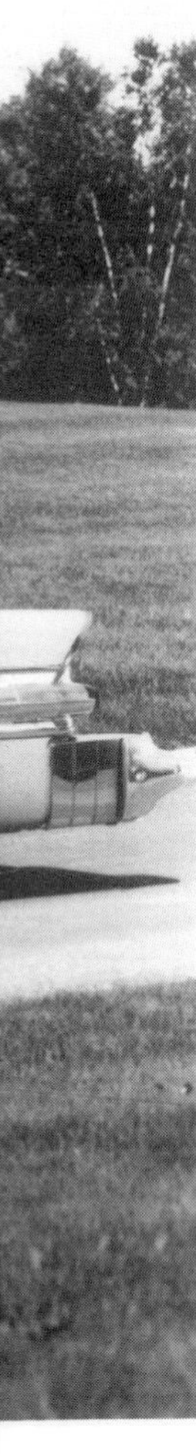

# Open-Air Virgin

In this recently unearthed 1957 photograph, the Virgin Mother is captured riding through the countryside with her friend, Veronica.

"It started out as a kind of crusade-on-wheels thing," she told us recently. "But in a matter of days it was all 'Thelma and Louise.'"

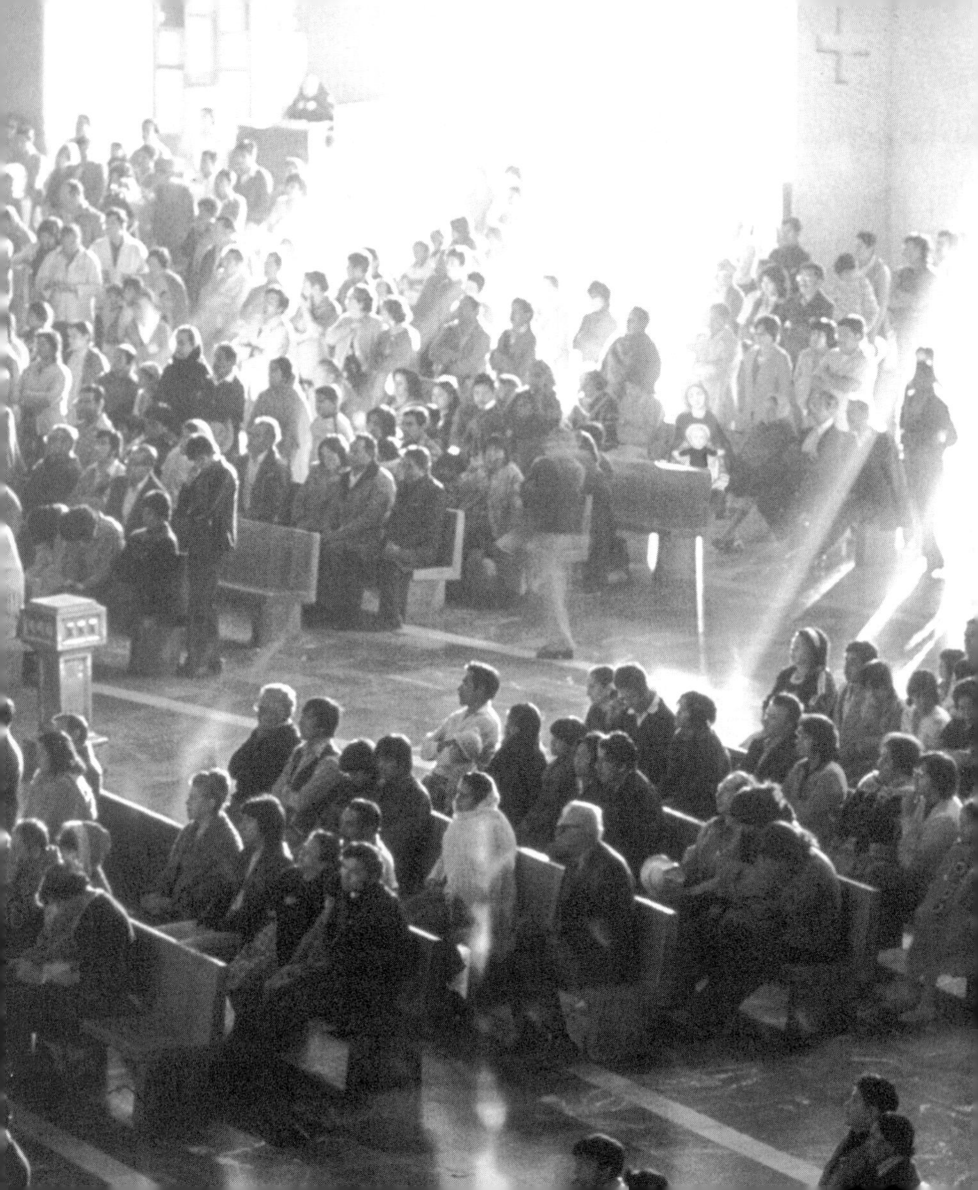

# Enough Already

Making miraculous appearances in churches is part of her job, but nonetheless, it sometimes makes Mary uncomfortable.

"It's the Hail Marys," she says, shrugging. "Such a fuss. You know?"

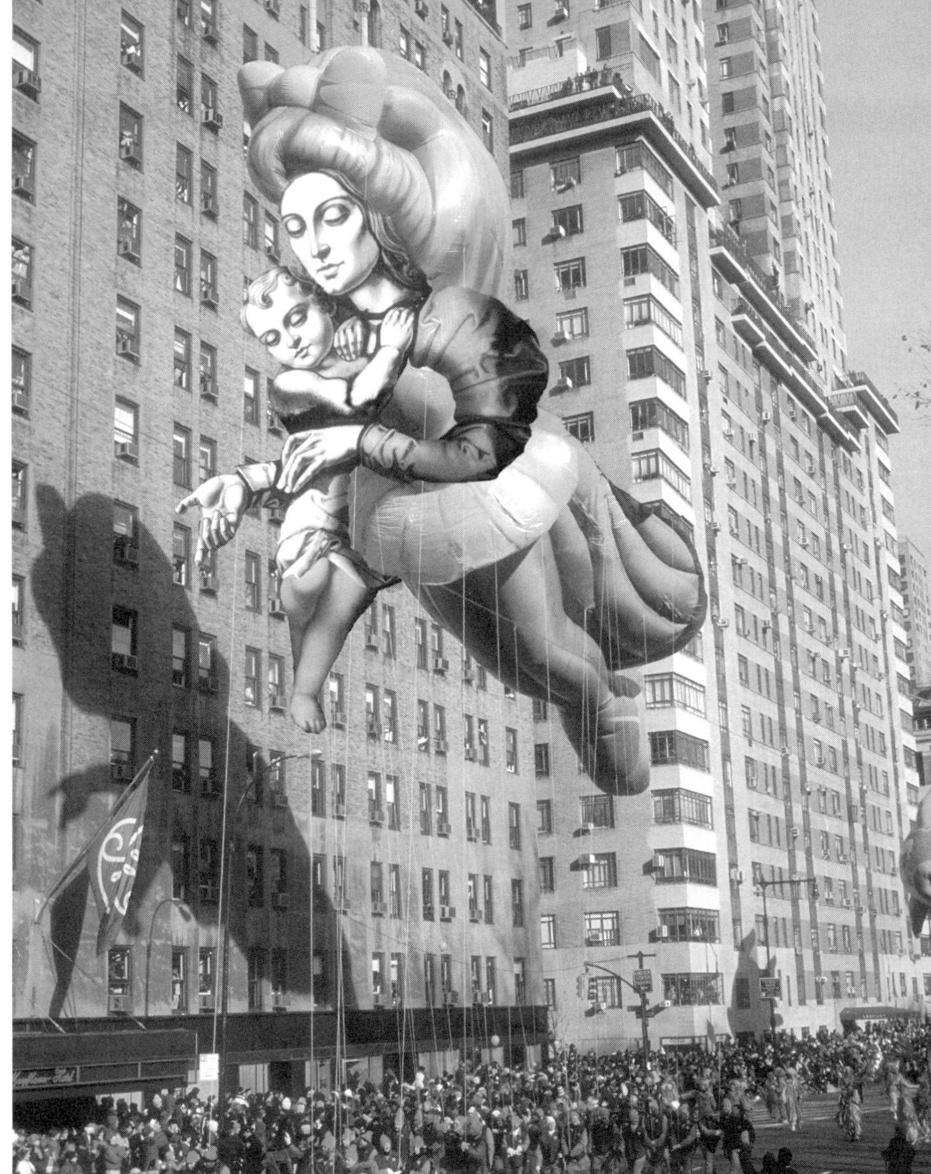

# Never Again

"Talk about gas!" Mary moaned. "I've never felt so bloated in my life. This is one gig I'll never do again—I don't care how many penitents it brings into St. Pat's."

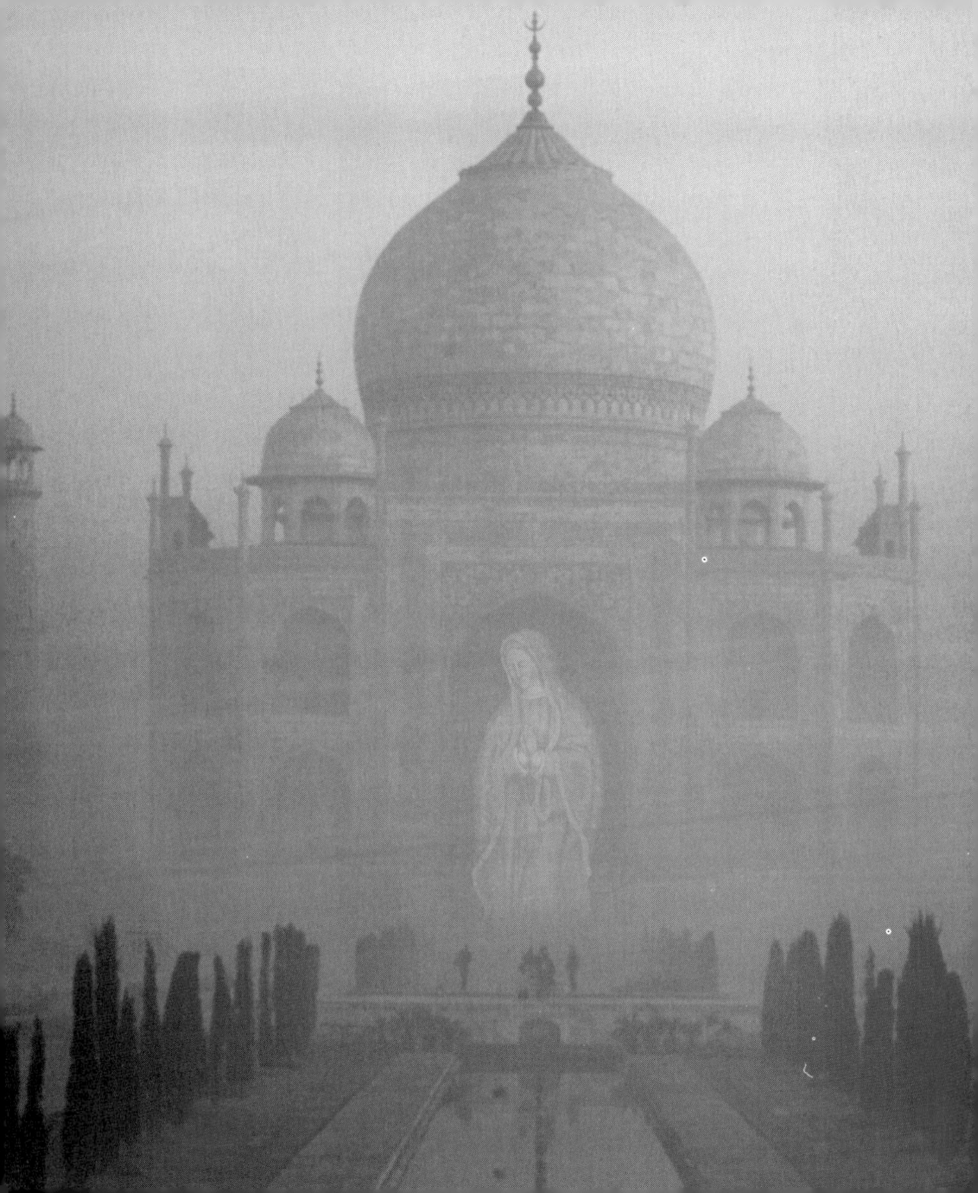

# Looking Good

Here is Mary in one of her favorite miraculous incarnations—as Our Lady of the Mist. "I happen to look good in droplets," she says.

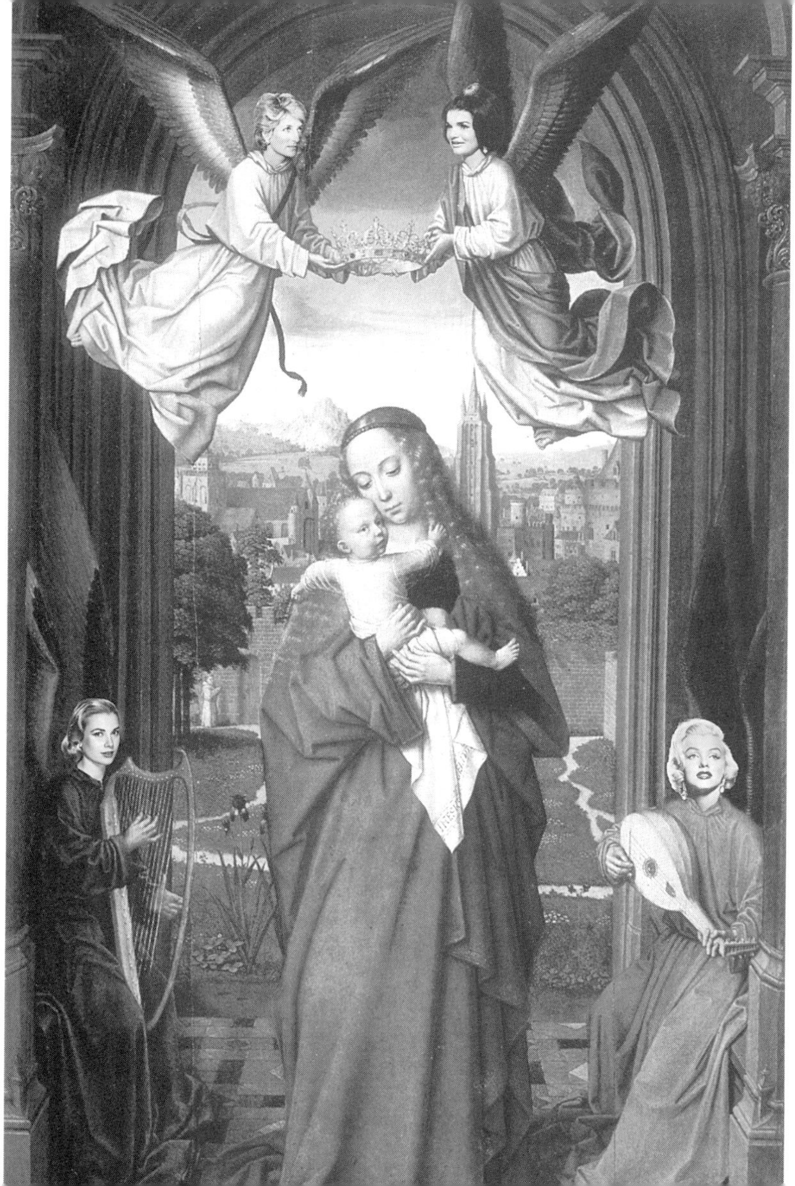

There are times when making miraculous appearances starts to get old for Mary. "It's all so me, me, me," she says. So for a change of pace, she let some other *grandes dames* make a miraculous appearance in this

# Enough About Me

painting, *Virgin and Child with Four Angels*, by Gerard David.

"But it was a waste," she said. "With the crowds at the Met, nobody noticed."

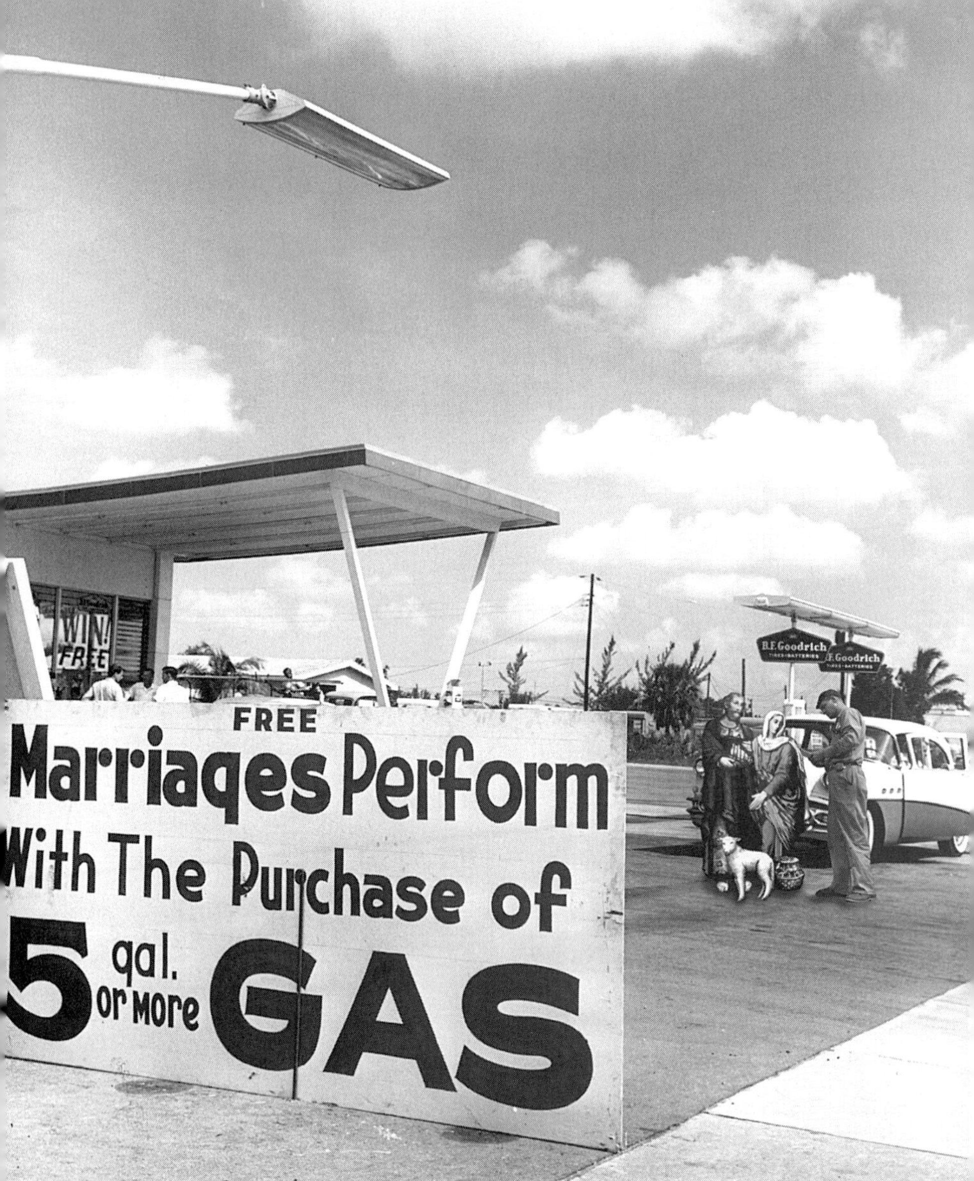
FREE
Marriages Perform
With The Purchase of
5 gal. or more GAS
WIN FREE
B.F.Goodrich
B.F.Goodrich

"Okay, I admit it—we never got married before," the Virgin Mother confided to us. "But then again, it wasn't Joe's baby anyhow."

# Better Late Than Never

Nonetheless, Mary could not pass up a deal like the one being offered at this highway gas station.

"I brought Joseph back from the dead for the occasion," she said. "Of course, he'd been out of the loop so long, he thought a tank of gas was some kind of ersatz Egyptian beer."

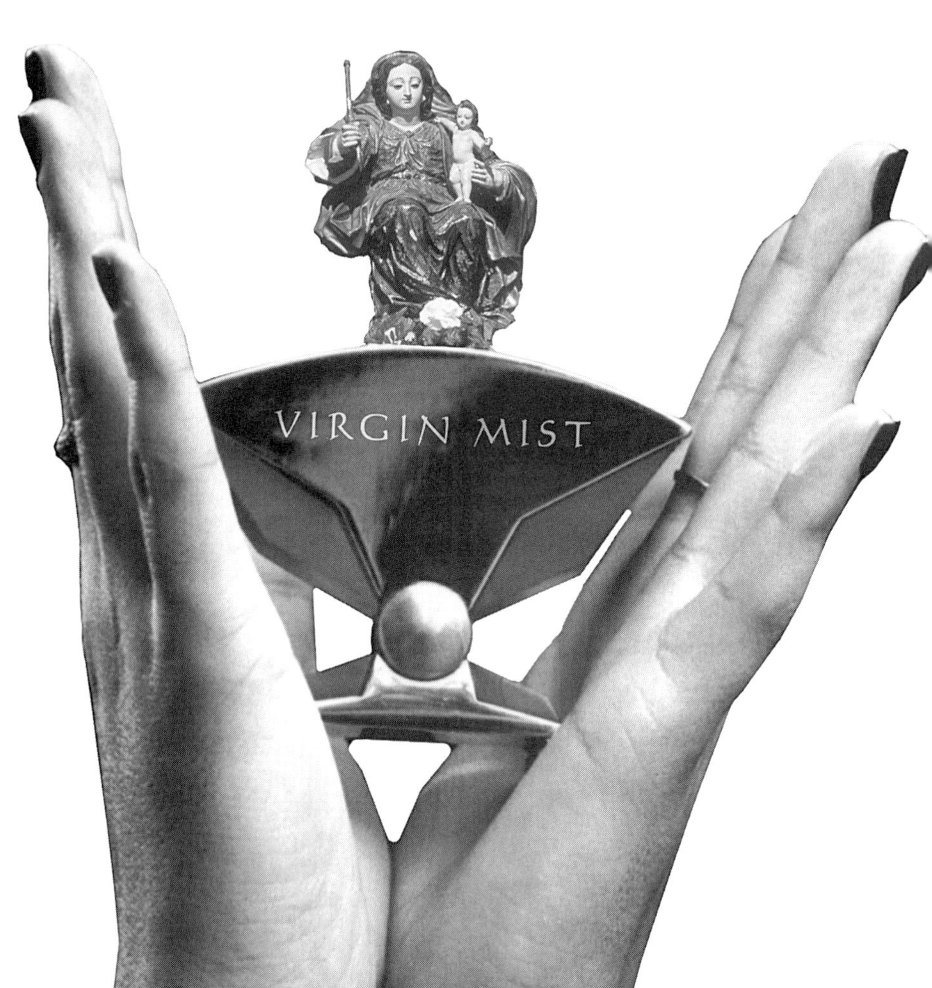
VIRGIN MIST

Like everything else these days, performing miracles has become more expensive. "It's the middle-men," Mary says, "they're now taking 30% off the top."

So the Virgin Mother has gone into personal marketing on the Home

# Niche Marketing

Shopping Network with her signature perfume, "Virgin Mist."

"We're positioning it as an alternative to all the erotic perfumes," she says. "It's a fragrance that says, 'sex doesn't interest me in the least.'

"We're doing very well in the Bible Belt."

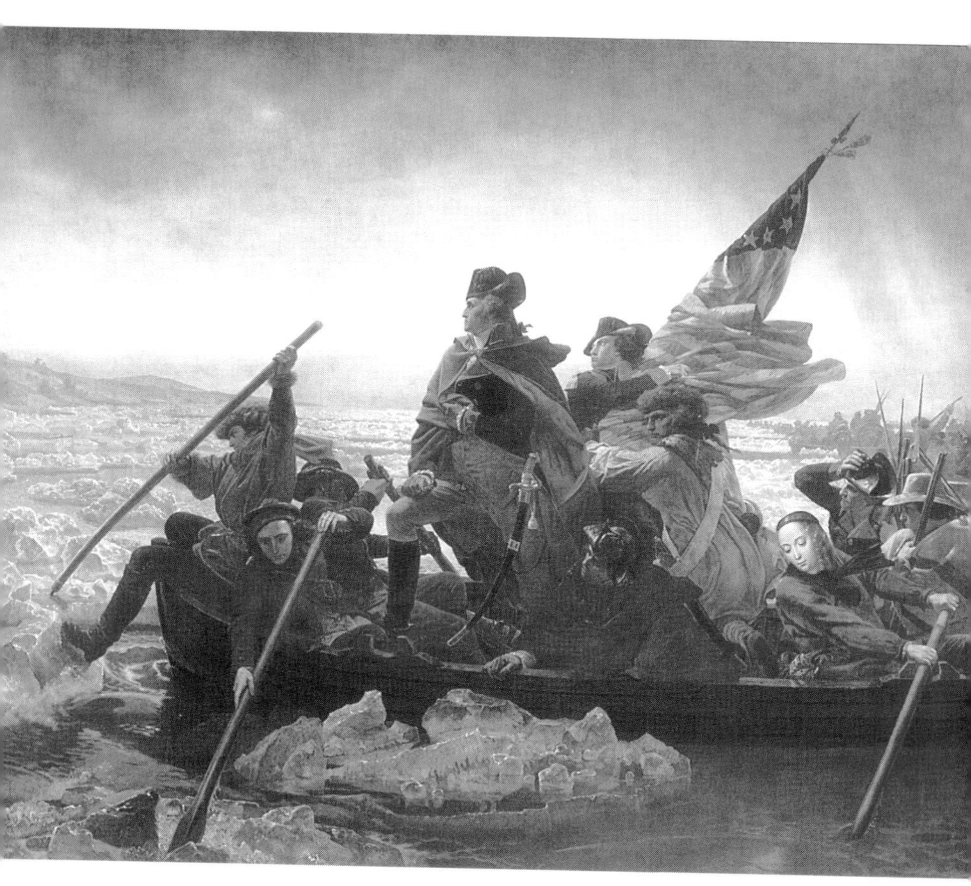

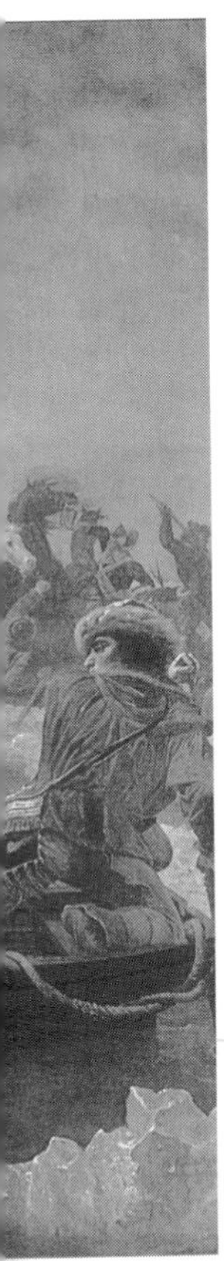

After art historians at the National Gallery in Washington, D.C., identified Sister Mary in this painting, we contacted the Virgin for background.

# Our Lady of the Oars

"It was a real b---h, pardon my French. Chunks of ice everywhere," she informed us. "And while we were breaking our backs, General George 'Capture-My-Profile' Washington was doing zip."

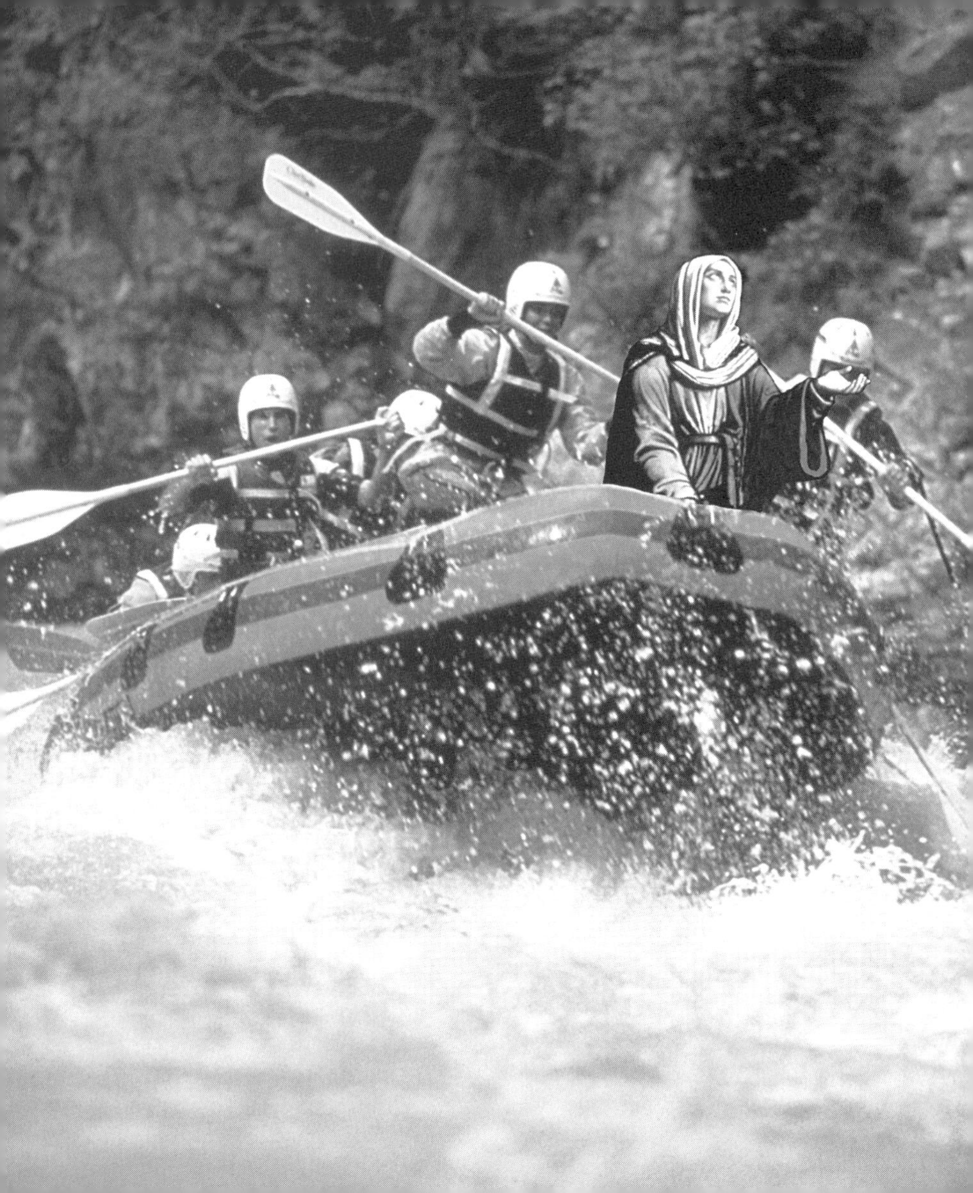

# Anchors Oy Vay

"Maybe I was too hard on George," Mary confessed. "After one day of white water rafting on the Colorado, I realize that all you can do is stare off at the horizon and try to keep your cookies down."

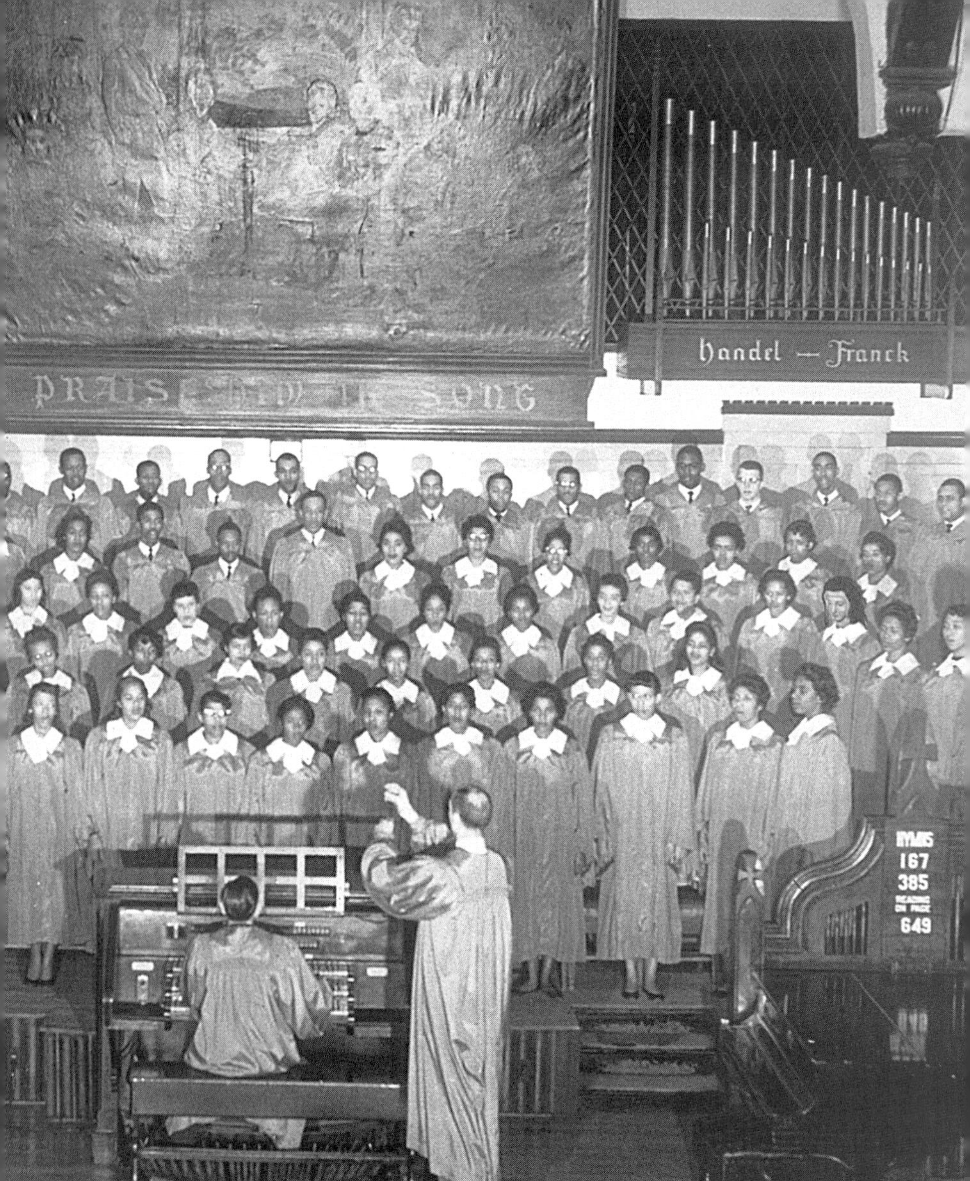
Handel — Franck
HYMNS
167
385
READING ON PAGE
649

Few people know that the Mother of God founded the original gospel choir, The Mangerettes, back in 3 A.D.

"We had a crossover hit with 'Frankincense and Myrrh,'" Mary told us.

# Gimme That Old-Time Religion

"But then Herod dropped out and started his own group, and it was all downhill from there."

These days, she is getting back into it with a church choir in Newark.

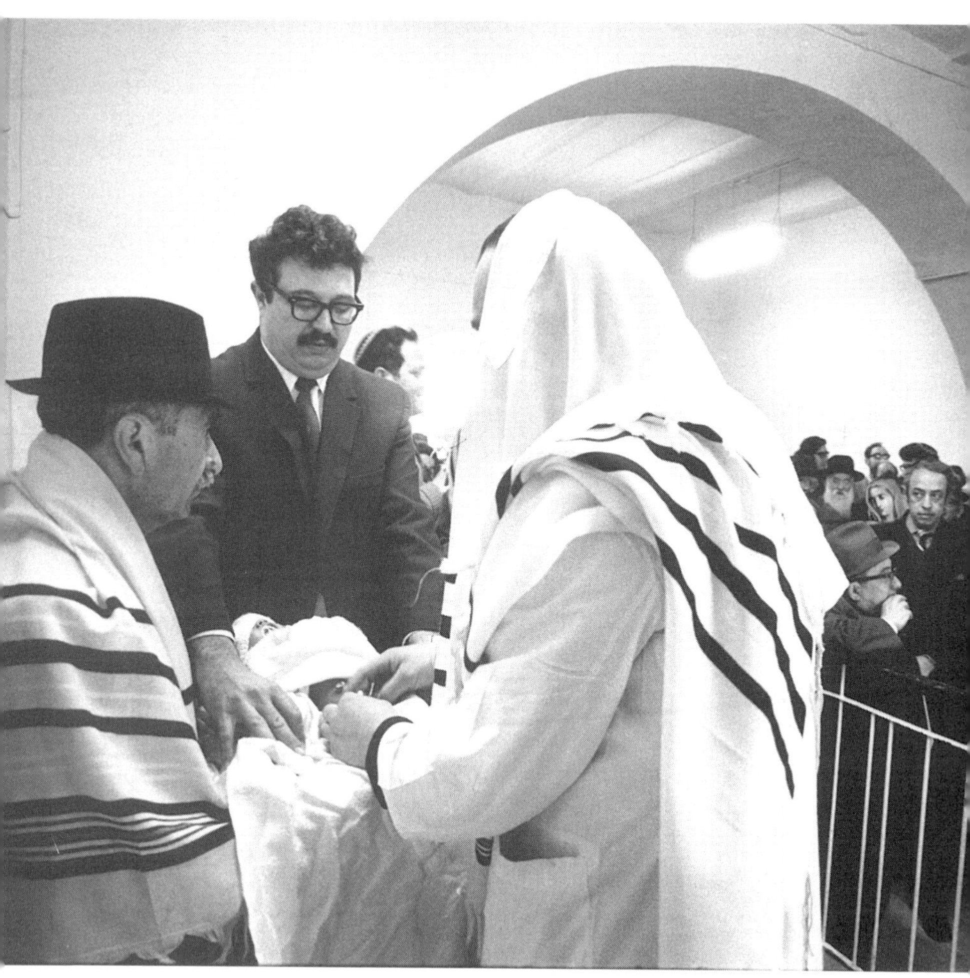

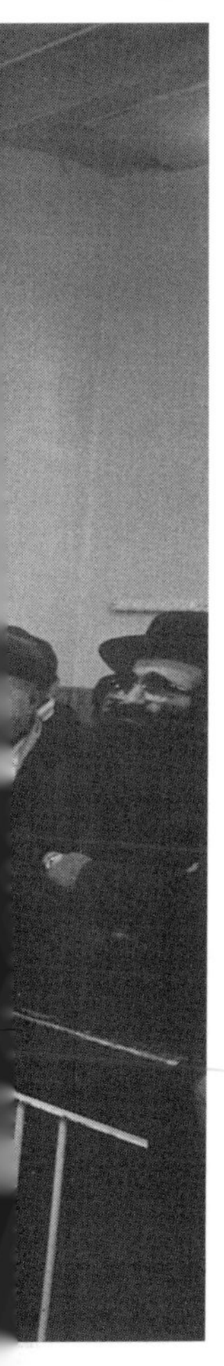

"One of the happiest days of my life was JC's bris. He didn't even cry. The Three Wise Men performed it right in the manger. Such a smell! Good thing they brought along some frankincense and myrrh."

# Tips

Anyway, all's well that ends well. (Or as one of the Wise Men said, "A stitch in time saves nine.")

"So that's why I try to take in a bris whenever I can."

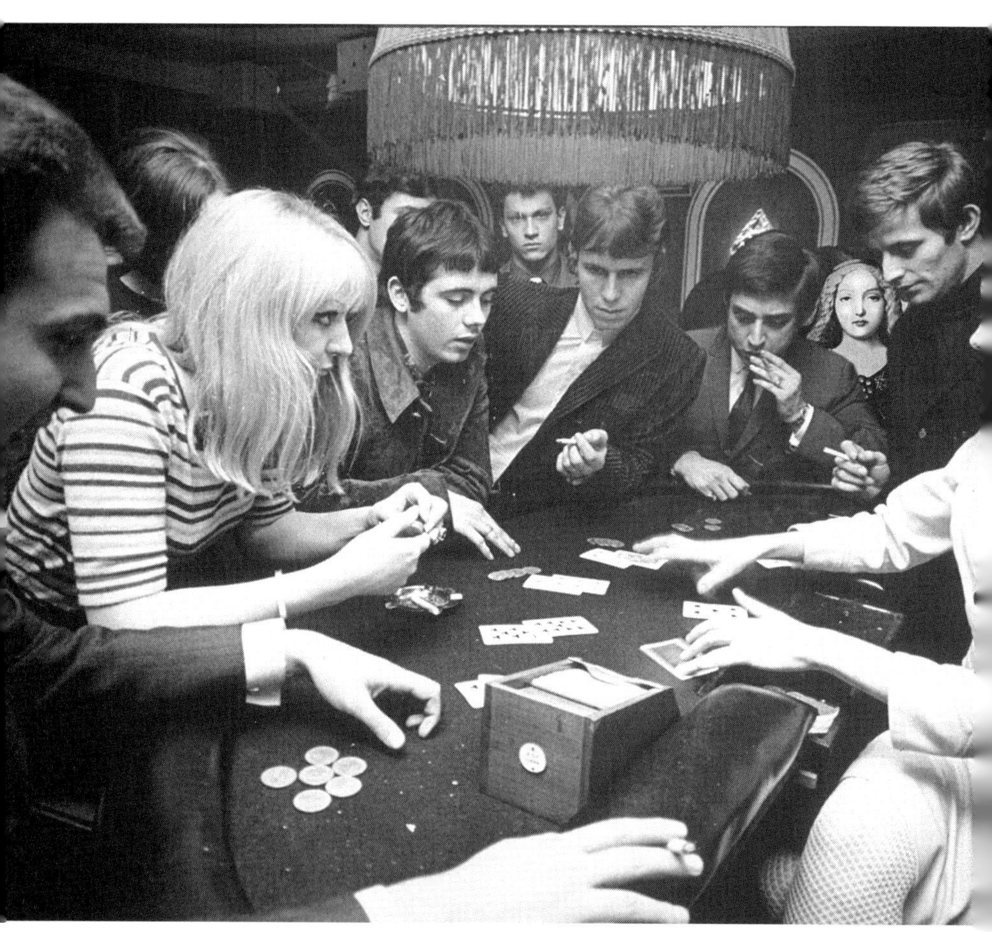

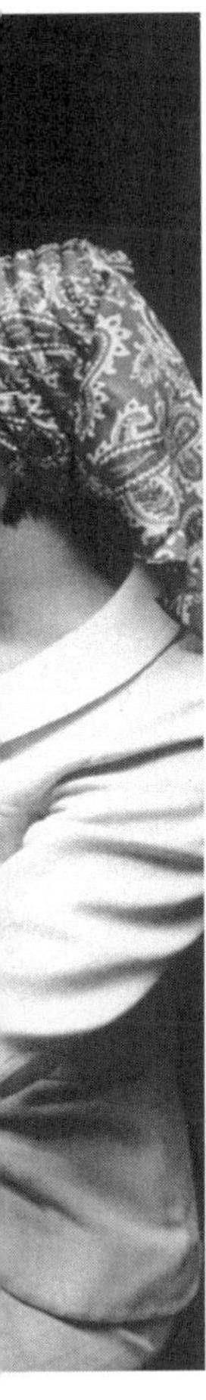

# Our Lady of Perpetual 21

"They say that gambling is addictive," Mary commented. "But that's only if you don't have total control over the cards. Actually, when you always win, blackjack gets old fast."

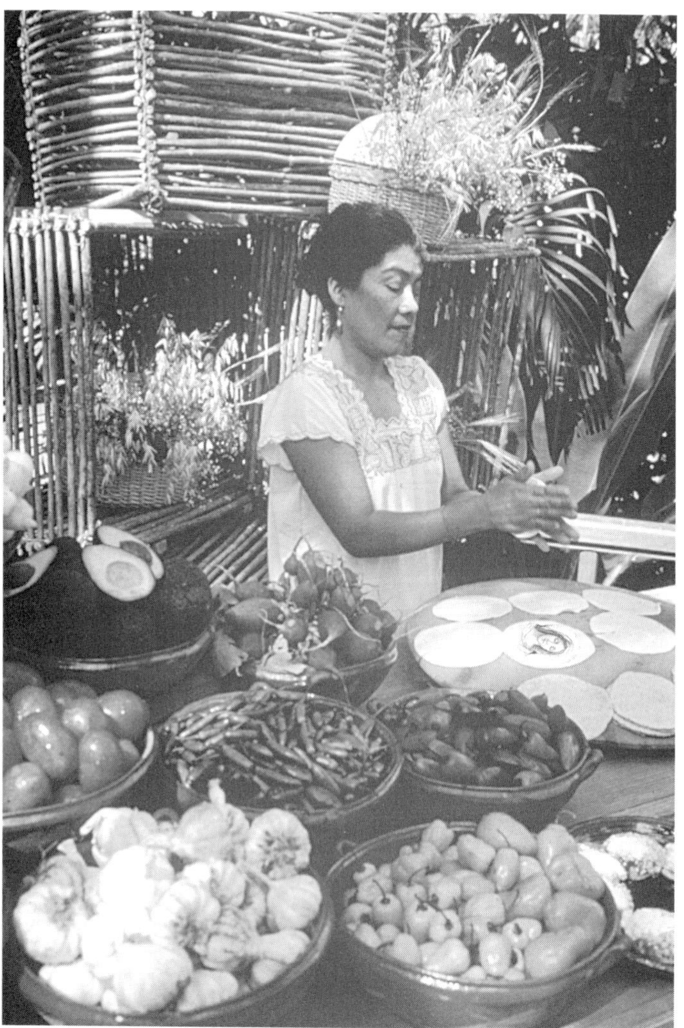

In this famous 1967 photograph, the Virgin Mother is recorded making a miraculous appearance at the tortilla stand of Señorita Nina Perez in Juarez.

"I had just started making the tortillas when I saw her," says Señorita Perez. "Of

# Our Lady of Masa Harina

course, I stopped immediately and prayed to the virgin."

Today, Perez has a chain of "Our Lady of Masa Harina" stands all over Mexico. Pilgrims come daily to the original stand, where, for a small fee, they can view the blessed tortilla. Perez now has a Swiss bank account.

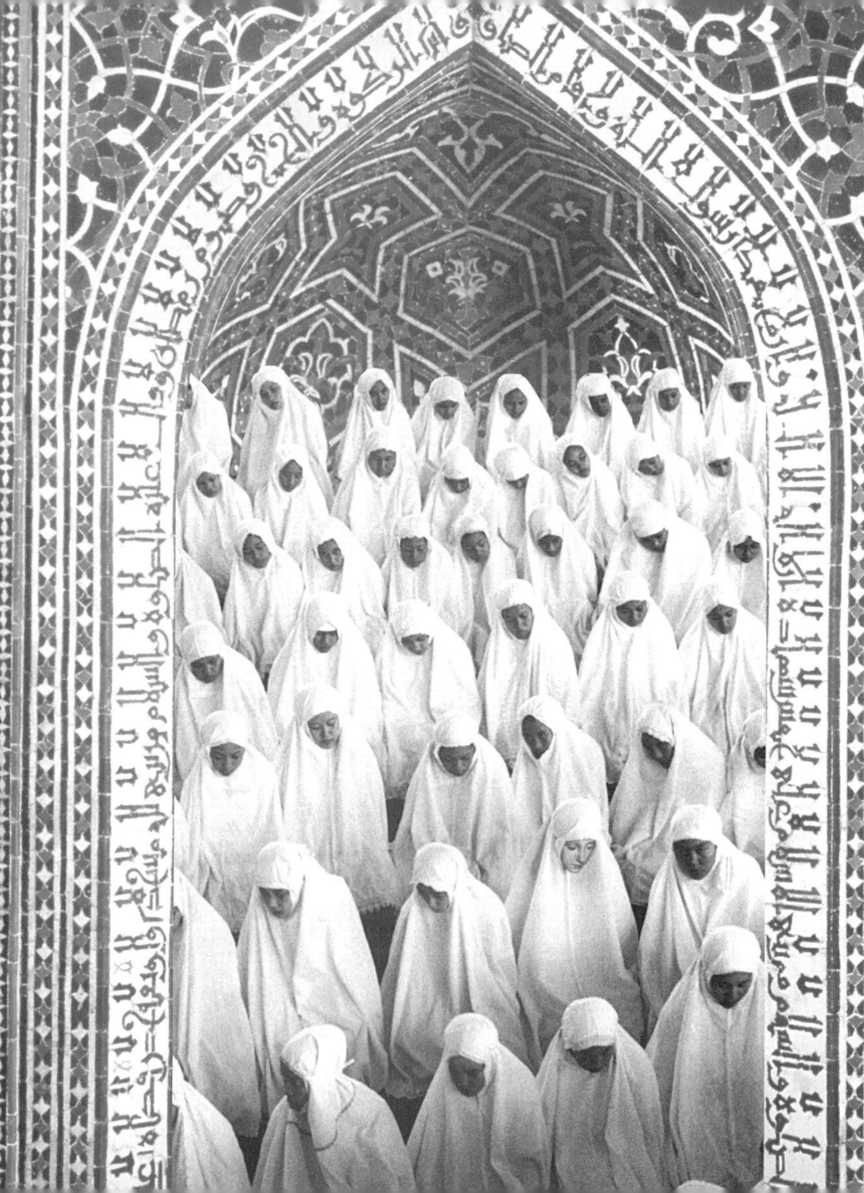

# Allah In The Family

In her lifelong commitment to ecumenicalism, Mary spends some time each week with her Muslim sisters.

"Hey, they gave me a walk-on in the Koran," she says. "So it's the least I can do."

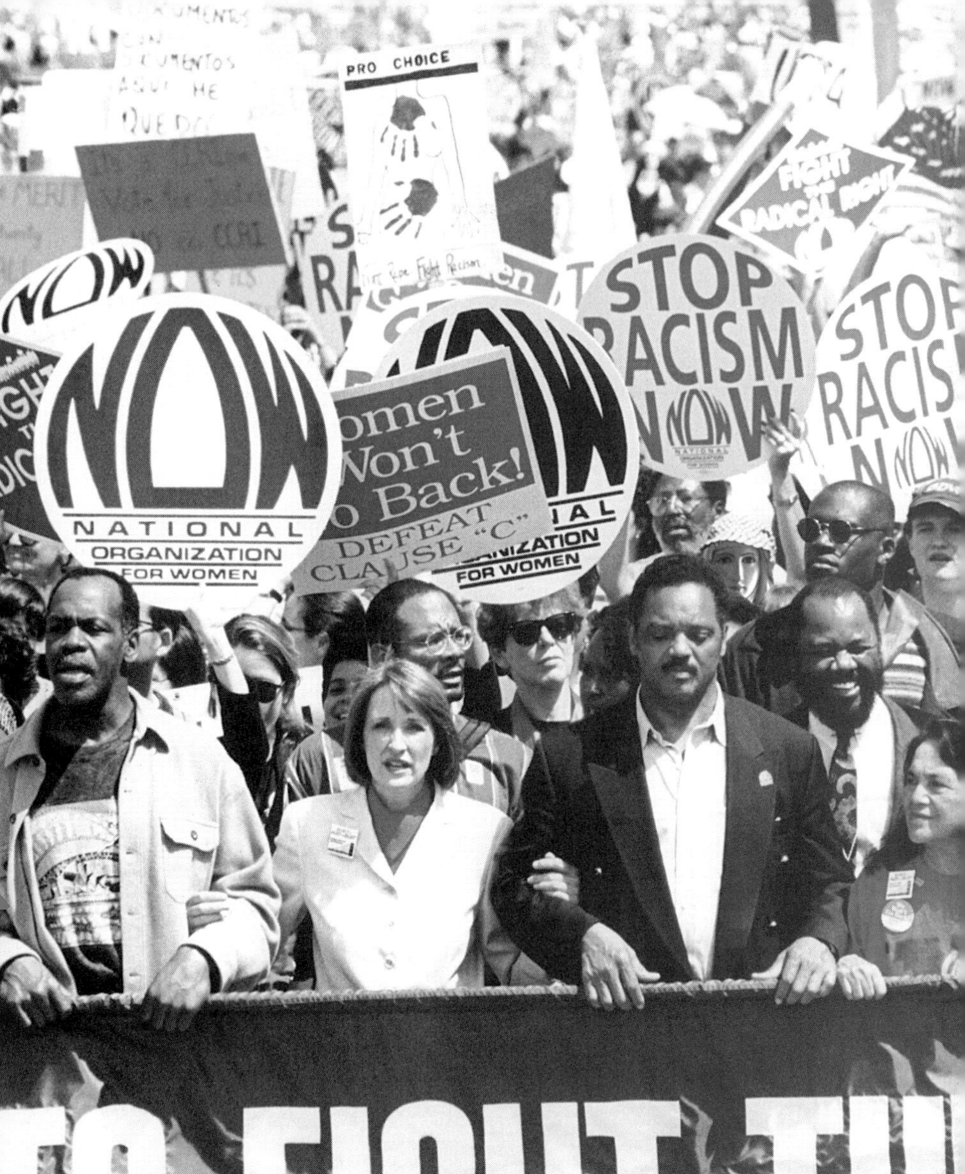

PRO CHOICE
NOW
NOW NATIONAL ORGANIZATION FOR WOMEN
omen Won't o Back! DEFEAT CLAUSE "C"
STOP RACISM NOW
NATIONAL ORGANIZATION FOR WOMEN
FIGHT RADICAL RIGHT
STOP RACIS N

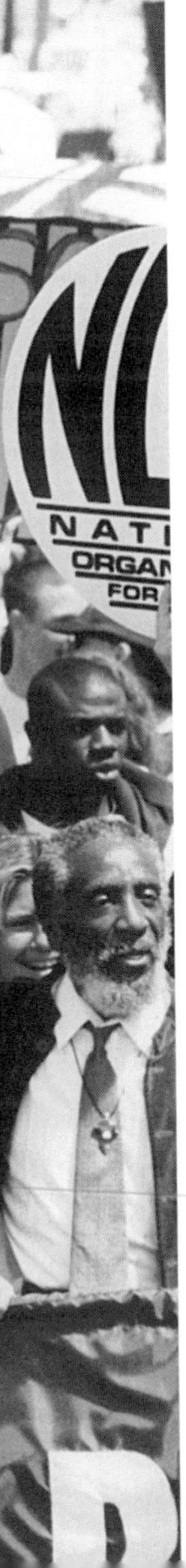


# Rally and Truly

Mary loves rallies of all kinds and attends as many as her schedule permits.

"You always meet such a nice people," she says. "I still remember my first rally. It was for animal rights outside the Colosseum."

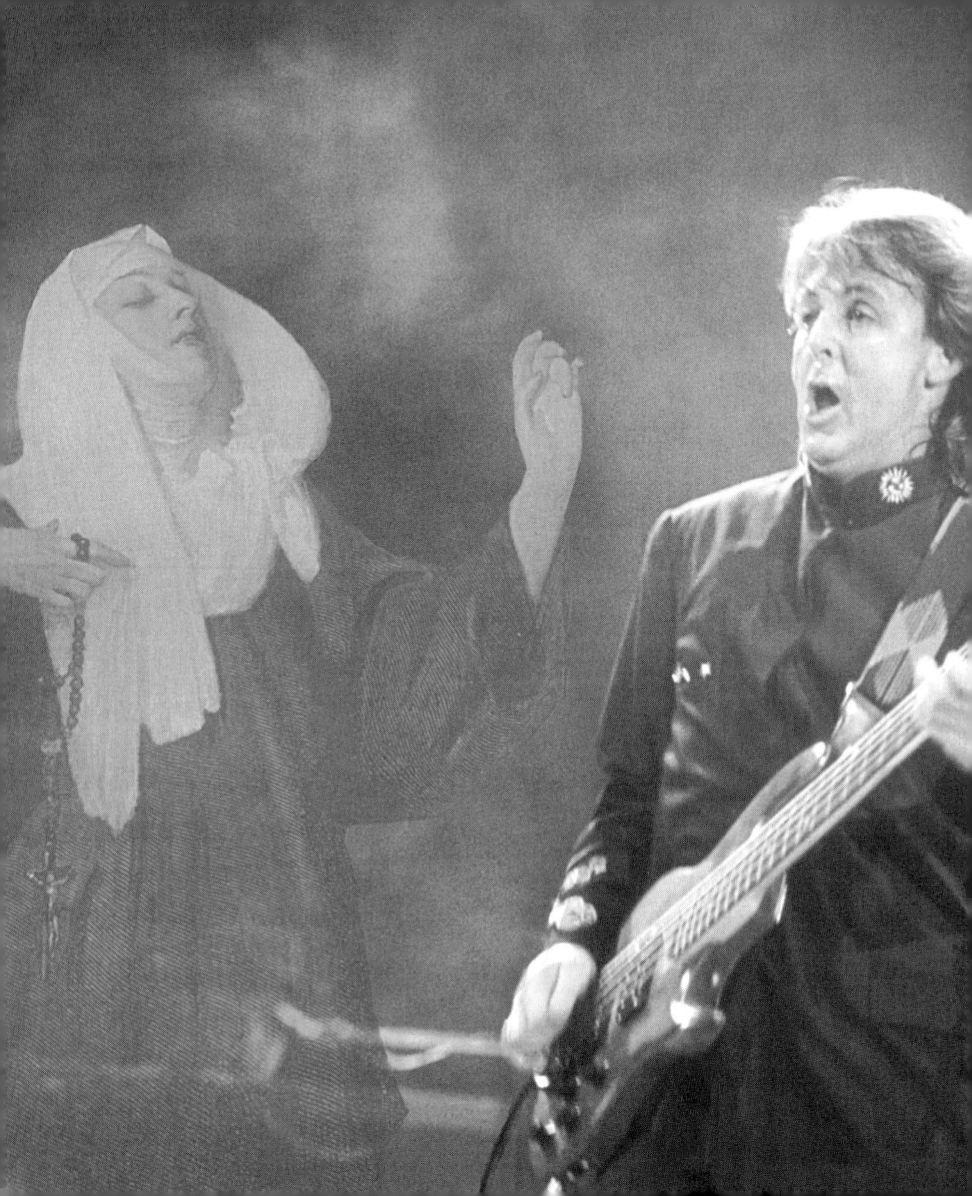

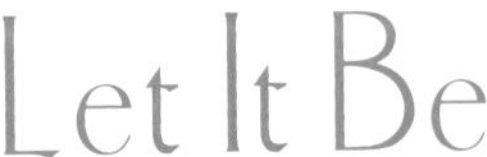

# Let It Be

Whenever Paul McCartney is performing "Let It Be" and comes to the line "Mother Mary comes to me...," the Mother of God makes a quick guest appearance, her schedule permitting.

"What can I say?" she says. "It's a gig."

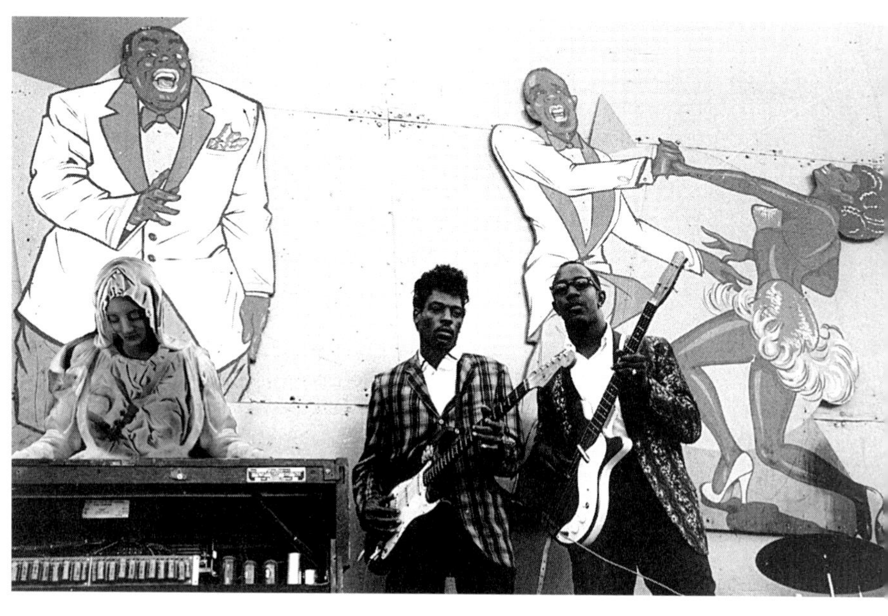

Whenever she's in her Black Madonna incarnation, the Mother of God likes to really get down with the blues.

"I've got enough heartache to fill a whole blues festival," she says.

# Sometimes I Feel Like A Childless Mother

Here she is doing her signature number, "I Got The Nobody-Believes-Me-When-I-Tell-Them-I'm-a-Virgin Blues."

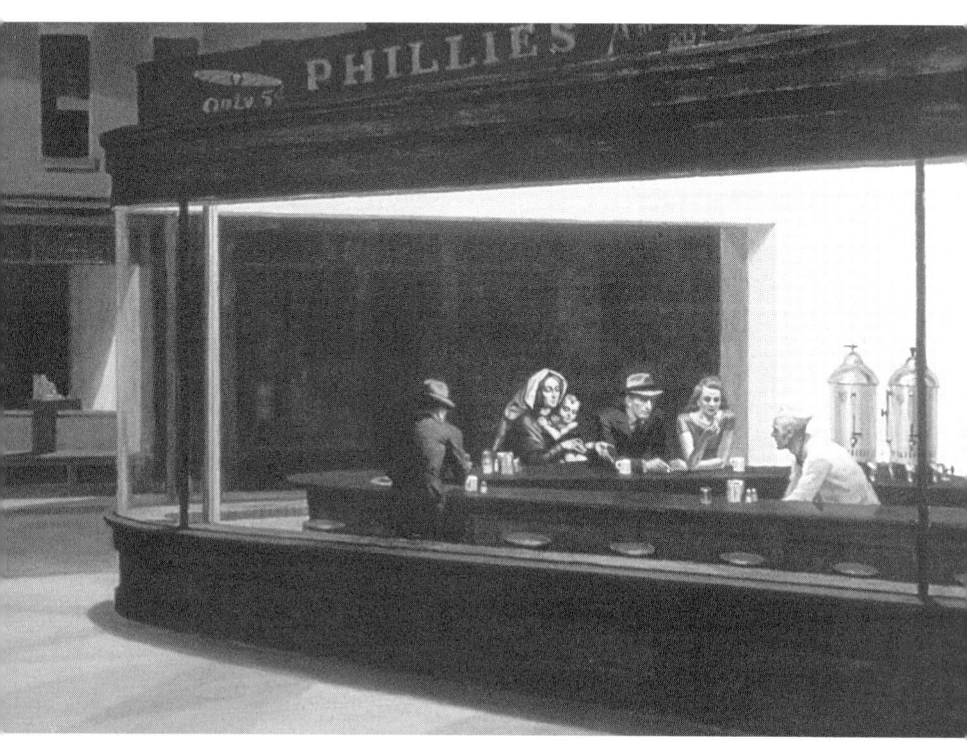
PHILLIES

After another long day of performing miracles and making mysterious appearances ("I make more guest appearances than Prince Charles and Hillary combined"), Mary

# Our Lady of Loneliness

often calls it a night with a last cup of java at Becky's Hash House.

In this oft-neglected authenticated sighting, the noted American painter, Edward Hopper, captures the Virgin Mother at her last lonely stop for the day.

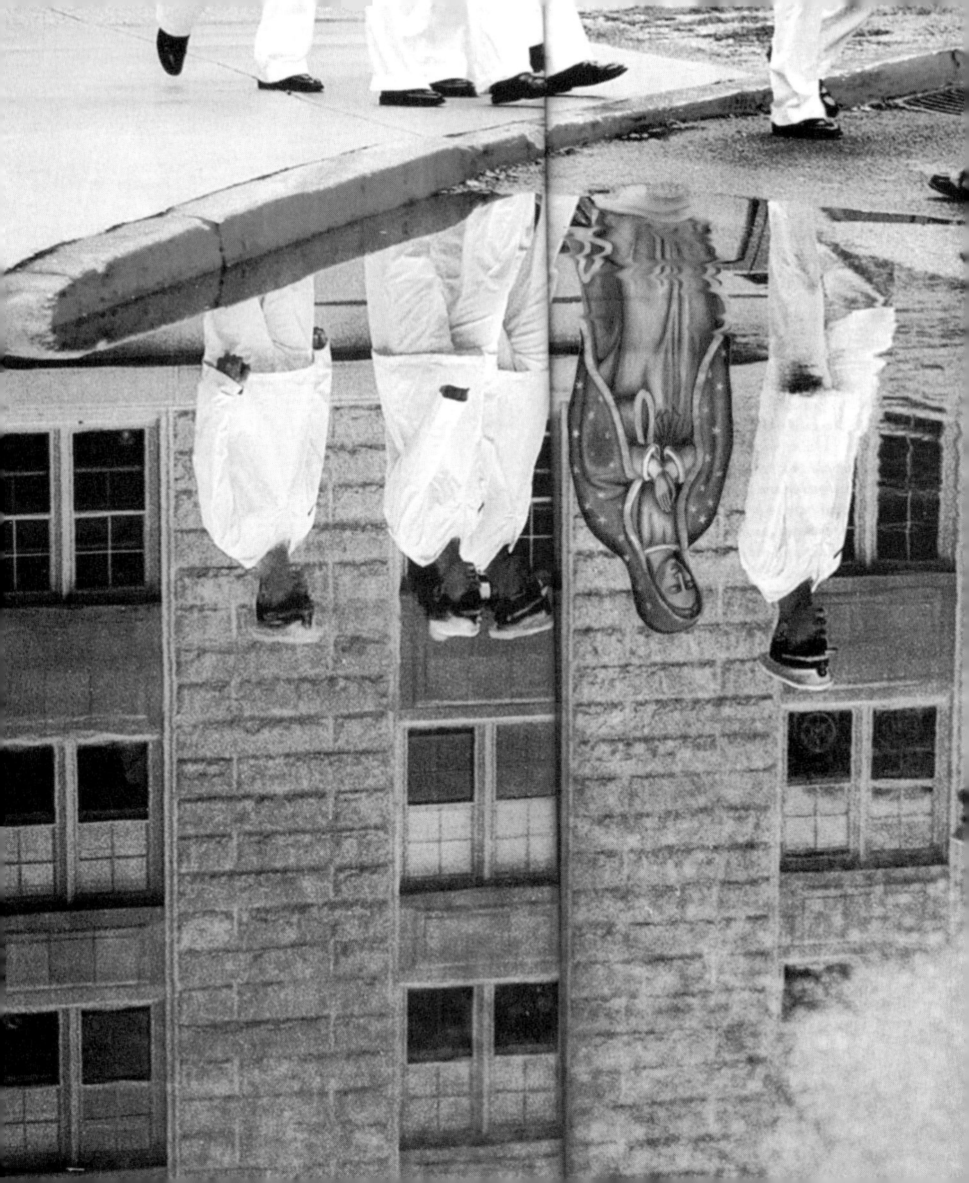

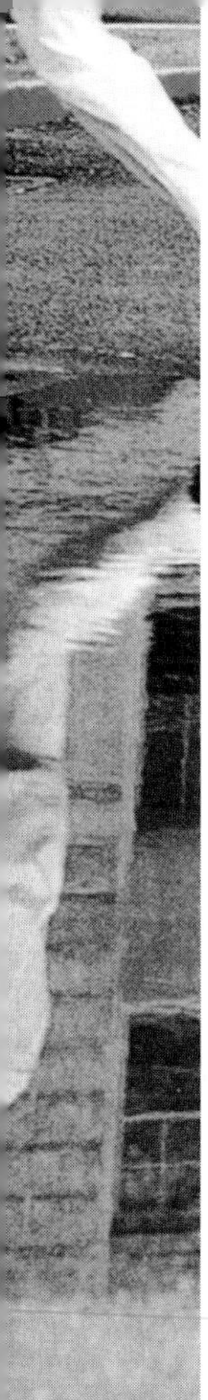

# No Reflection On Me

Occasionally, "just for a goof," Mary does a little trick she picked up from a vampire friend.

"But these guys are so stiff, they didn't even notice," she says.

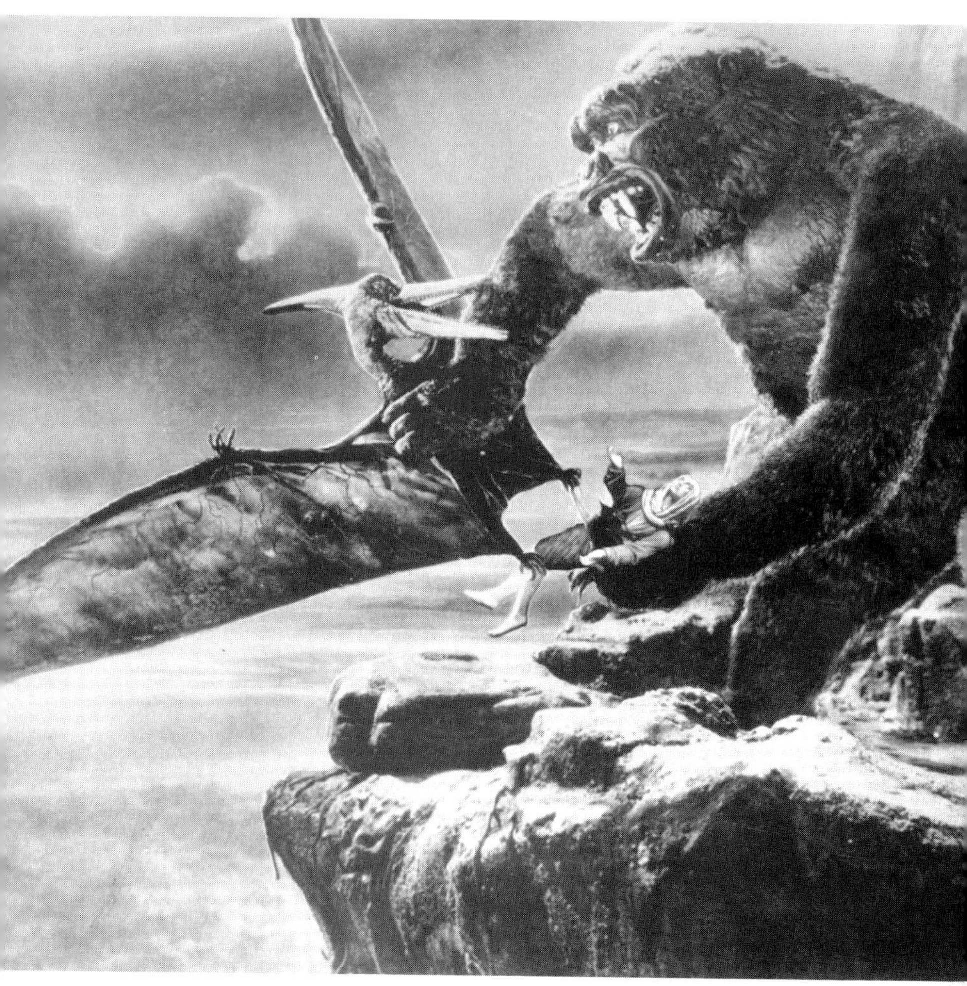

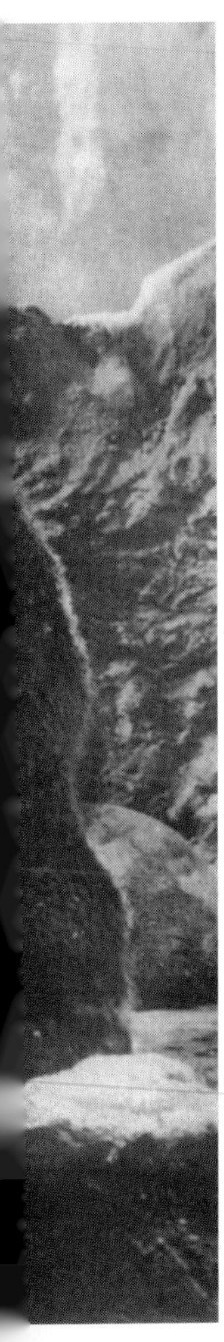

# A Stretch

Like others before her, Mary has had to contend with typecasting in Hollywood.

"It's always the same Fatima thing," she complains. "So when this part was offered to me, I jumped at it. Sure, it was a stretch for me, but I almost won an Oscar."

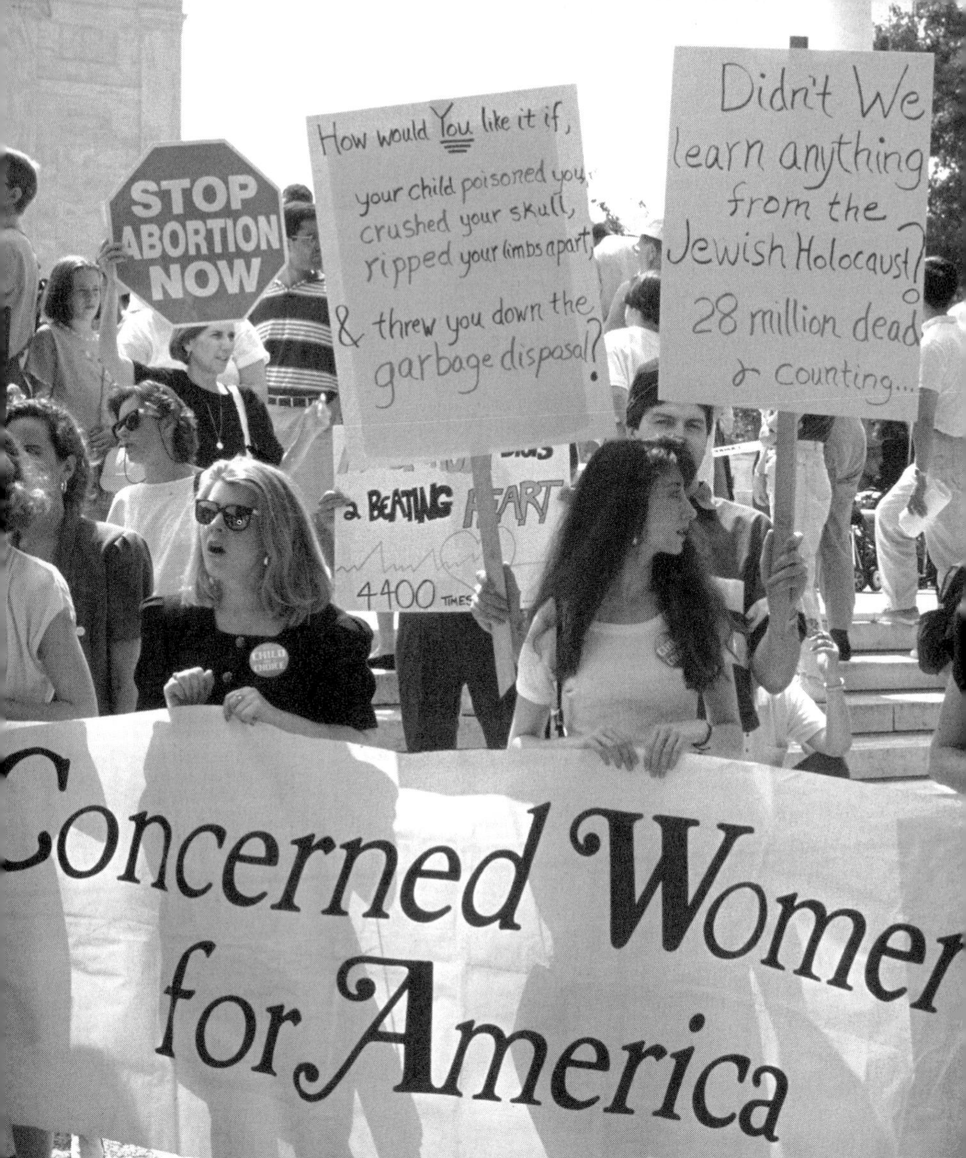
STOP ABORTION NOW
How would You like it if,
your child poisoned you,
crushed your skull,
ripped your limbs apart,
& threw you down the garbage disposal?
Didn't We learn anything from the Jewish Holocaust?
28 million dead & counting...
a BEATING
4400 TIMES
Concerned Wome
for America

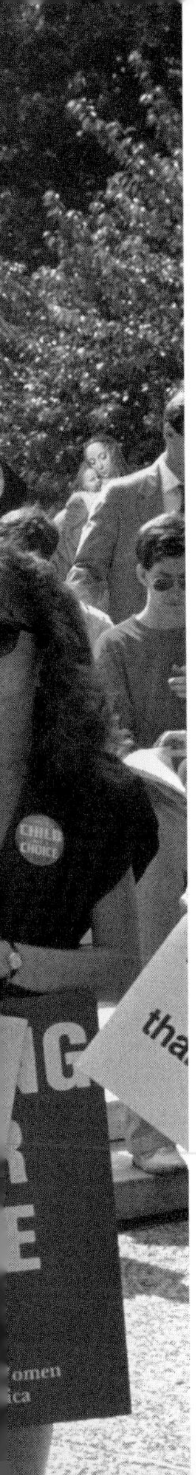

# Think About It

There is one issue that the Mother of God is adamant about, and that is her Pro-Life stance.

"I was a single pregnant woman," she says. "And you'd better believe there were people who thought I should 'take care of it.' But think about it—where would we all be today if I had listened to them?"

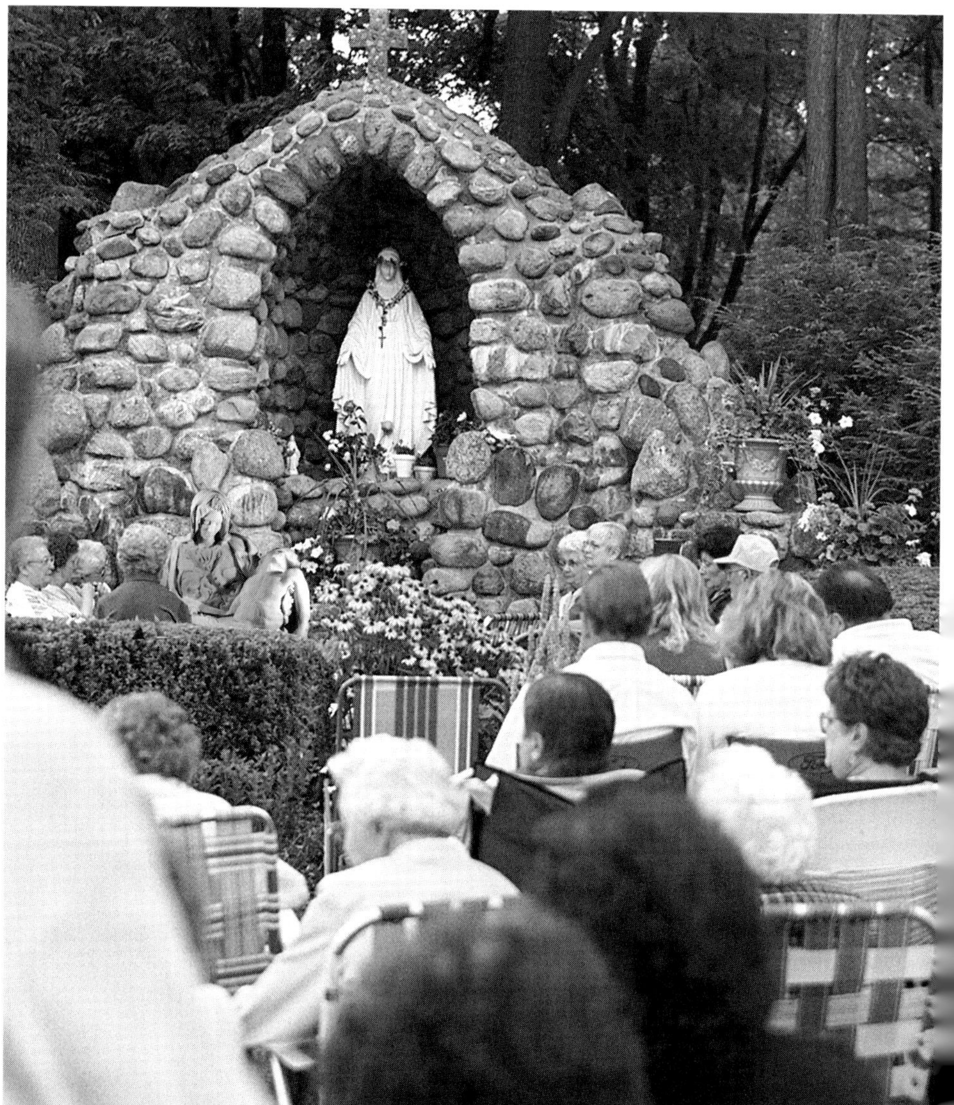

# Mary Statue in Grotto

"Little old ladies with blue hair never believe it's really me unless I'm covered with plaster," says Our Lady of the Backyard Grotto, making an appearance at a barbecue. "The worst part is when I get an itch."

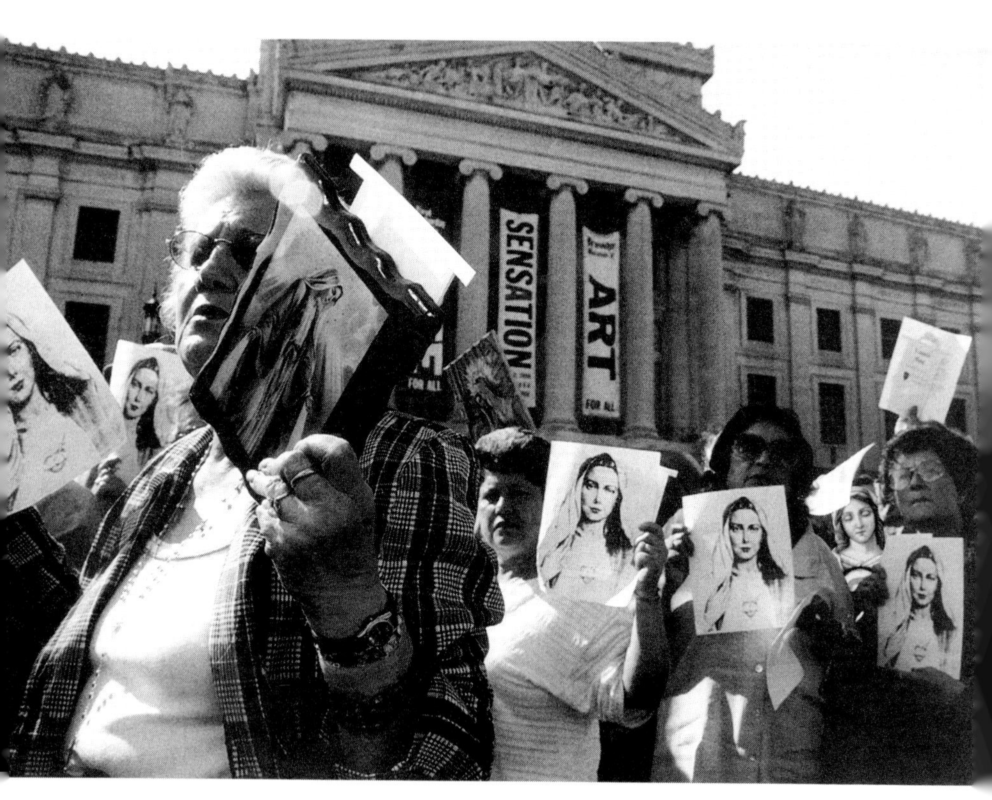
SENSATION
FOR ALL
ART
FOR ALL

# Sensation, Shmensation

"So I said to Rudy, 'Look, do you think I liked the way Michelangelo did me? All skin and bones with a butter-wouldn't-melt-in-my-mouth smile and no sex appeal at all?' But you know men—especially Italian men—they always want you to look like a Virgin."

# Authors

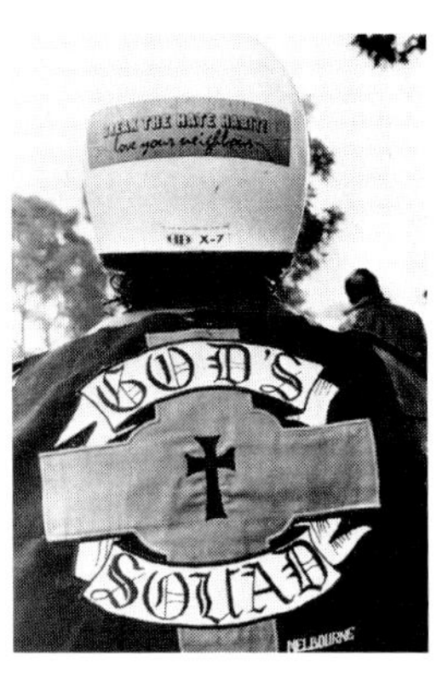


**Danny Piccolo** is the *nom de goof* of a product of the parochial-school system of Brooklyn, N.Y. Under another name, Danny is the author of numerous humor books. He has chosen anonymity to protect his relationship with his real mother.

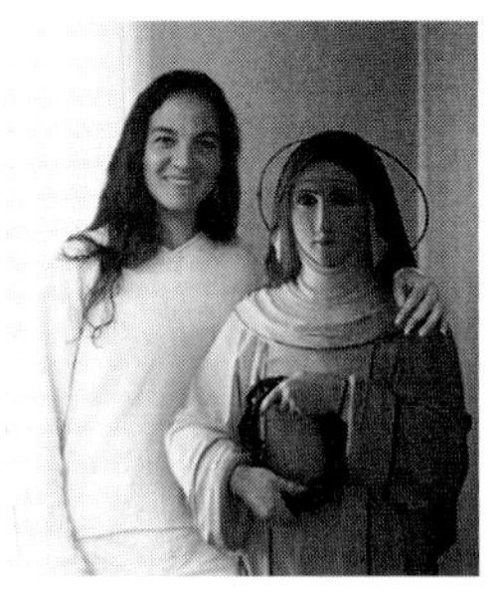

**Stacey Hood** is the name her mother gave her, God bless her. Stacey is the C.E.O. of Big Eyedea Visual Design. She has at least one thing in common with the Virgin Mother.

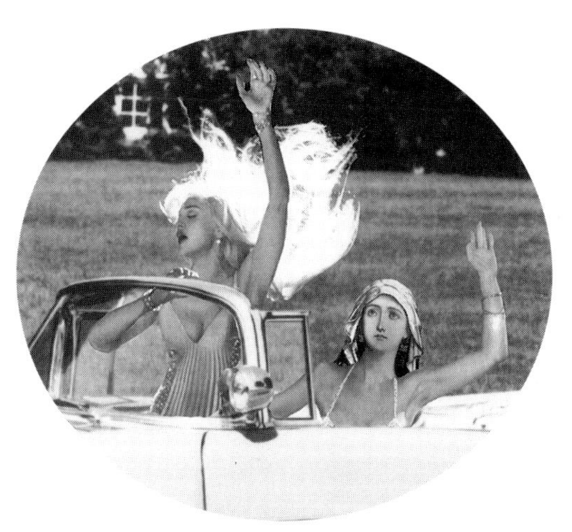

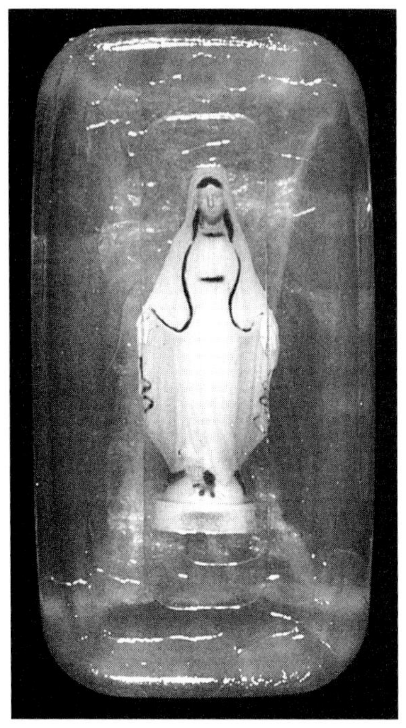

Here is the Virgin Mother in one of her frequent soap bar apearances as a reminder that "Mens sana in corpore sano"– which, loosely translated from the Latin, means: "You can get closer to God if you don't have B.O."